Clinical Textbook of Mood Disorders

Mood disorders affect around 1 in 5 people, but the diagnosis and management of these conditions can be challenging. This practical handbook presents a comprehensive overview of these disorders, as well as detailed guidelines for their treatment.

The handbook takes a transdisciplinary approach to mood disorders, focusing not only on the biological aspects but also on psychosocial features of importance for optimal diagnosis and management. Content covers nosological considerations, historical aspects, peculiarities along the lifespan, and the associations between mood disorders and other conditions, with a focus on their implications for the optimal management of patients. Practical and evidence-based information is discussed on the role of guidelines related to treatment in selected population groups, including youth, the elderly, and women.

With a practical, reader-friendly approach, this book will be invaluable for mental health professionals involved in the treatment of patients with mood disorders, including trainees from different mental health areas.

Professor Allan Young is the Chair of Mood Disorders and Director of the Centre for Affective Disorders in the Department of Psychological Medicine in the Institute of Psychiatry, Psychology and Neuroscience at King's College London.

Marsal Sanches is Associate Professor of Psychiatry at Baylor College of Medicine in Houston, Texas. He is also the Director of Research Education at The Menninger Clinic and an Associate Editor of the journal *Debates in Psychiatry*.

Jair C. Soares is Professor and Chair of Psychiatry and Behavioral Sciences at McGovern Medical School at UTHealth Houston, Texas. He is a past president of the International Society on Affective Disorders, and the American Association for Chairs of Departments of Psychiatry.

Mario Juruena is Professor (Reader) in Translational Psychiatry at the Institute of Psychiatry, Psychology and Neuroscience, Centre for Affective Disorders, in the Department of Psychological Medicine at King's College London. He is also an Associate Editor for the *British Journal of Psychiatry Open* and the *Journal of Affective Disorders*.

Clinical Textbook of Mood Disorders

Edited by

Allan Young
Chair of Mood Disorders, Institute of Psychiatry at King's College London

Marsal Sanches
Baylor College of Medicine, Texas

Jair C. Soares
Director, Center of Excellence on Mood Disorders, McGovern Medical School, The University of Texas

Mario Juruena
King's College London

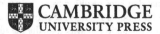
CAMBRIDGE
UNIVERSITY PRESS

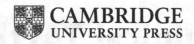
CAMBRIDGE
UNIVERSITY PRESS

Shaftesbury Road, Cambridge CB2 8EA, United Kingdom

One Liberty Plaza, 20th Floor, New York, NY 10006, USA

477 Williamstown Road, Port Melbourne, VIC 3207, Australia

314–321, 3rd Floor, Plot 3, Splendor Forum, Jasola District
Centre, New Delhi – 110025, India

103 Penang Road, #05–06/07, Visioncrest Commercial,
Singapore 238467

Cambridge University Press is part of Cambridge University
Press & Assessment, a department of the University of
Cambridge.

We share the University's mission to contribute to society
through the pursuit of education, learning and research at the
highest international levels of excellence.

www.cambridge.org
Information on this title: www.cambridge.org/9781108978279

DOI: 10.1017/9781108973922

First published 2024

*A catalogue record for this publication is available from the
British Library*

*A Cataloging-in-Publication data record for this book is available
from the Library of Congress*

ISBN 978-1-108-97827-9 Paperback

Cambridge University Press & Assessment has no responsibility
for the persistence or accuracy of URLs for external or third-party
internet websites referred to in this publication and does not
guarantee that any content on such websites is, or will remain,
accurate or appropriate.

....

Every effort has been made in preparing this book to provide
accurate and up-to-date information that is in accord with
accepted standards and practice at the time of publication.
Although case histories are drawn from actual cases, every effort
has been made to disguise the identities of the individuals involved.
Nevertheless, the authors, editors, and publishers can make no
warranties that the information contained herein is totally free
from error, not least because clinical standards are constantly
changing through research and regulation. The authors, editors,
and publishers therefore disclaim all liability for direct or
consequential damages resulting from the use of material
contained in this book. Readers are strongly advised to pay careful
attention to information provided by the manufacturer of any
drugs or equipment that they plan to use.

Contents

Contents

Contributors

Danilo Arnone
United Arab Emirates University,
United Arab Emirates

Gabriel Barg
Neuroscience & Learning Department,
Catholic University of Uruguay, Montevideo, Uruguay

Christopher Busby
Louis A. Faillace, MD, Department of Psychiatry and
Behavioral Sciences, McGovern Medical School
The University of Texas Health Science Center at
Houston, Houston, TX, USA

Amanda K. Ceniti
Centre for Depression & Suicide Studies, St. Michael's
Hospital, Toronto, Canada, and
Institute of Medical Science, University of Toronto,
Canada

Anthony J. Cleare
Centre for Affective Disorders,
Institute of Psychiatry, Psychology & Neuroscience
(IoPPN),
King's College London, UK

Dominic Cottrell
South London and Maudsley NHS Trust, UK

David Cousins
Translational and Clinical Research Institute,
Newcastle University, Newcastle upon
Tyne, UK, and
Cumbria, Northumberland, Tyne
and Wear NHS Foundation Trust,
Newcastle upon Tyne, UK

Ioanna Douka
Section of Clinical and Computational
Neuroscience, National Institute of Mental
Health, National Institutes of Health,
Bethesda, MD, USA

Rina Dutta
NIHR Maudsley Biomedical Research Centre (BRC),
UK,
King's Clinical Academic Training Office (KCATO),
Department of Psychological Medicine, Division of
Academic Psychiatry,
King's College London, UK, and
Carol Bell | Health Care Professionals' Affective
Disorders Service | The Maudsley Hospital, UK

Louis A. Faillace
Louis A. Faillace, MD, Department of Psychiatry and
Behavioral Sciences, McGovern Medical School
The University of Texas Health Science Center at
Houston, Houston, TX, USA

Gabriel Rodrigo Fries
Louis A. Faillace, MD, Department of Psychiatry and
Behavioral Sciences, McGovern Medical School
The University of Texas Health Science Center at
Houston, Houston, TX, USA

Romayne Gadelrab
Centre for Affective Disorders,
Institute of Psychiatry, Psychology & Neuroscience,
(IoPPN),
King's College London, UK

Peter Gallagher
Translational & Clinical Research Institute,
Faculty of Medical Sciences,
Newcastle University, Newcastle upon Tyne,
UK

Fiona Gaughran
National Psychosis Service,
South London and Maudsley NHS Foundation Trust,
UK, and
Institute of Psychiatry, Psychology & Neuroscience
(IoPPN),
King's College London, UK

Elizabeth Graves
Research Department, Clinical Trials Facility, Moorgreen Hospital, Southern Health NHS Foundation Trust, Southampton, UK

Anna I. Guerdjikova
Research Institute, Lindner Center of HOPE, Mason, OH, and
Department of Psychiatry and Behavioral Neuroscience, University of Cincinnati College of Medicine, Cincinnati, OH, USA

Angela M. Heads
Louis A. Faillace, MD, Department of Psychiatry and Behavioral Sciences, McGovern Medical School
The University of Texas Health Science Center at Houston, Houston, TX, USA

Danielle Hett
Birmingham and Solihull Mental Health Foundation Trust and Institute of Mental Health, University of Birmingham, UK

Joanna Hook
National Affective Disorders Service and OPTIMA Mood Disorders Service,
South London and Maudsley NHS Foundation Trust, London, UK

Robin B. Jarrett
Department of Psychiatry,
The University of Texas Southwestern Medical Center, Dallas, TX, USA

Sameer Jauhar
Department of Psychological Medicine, Institute of Psychiatry, Psychology & Neuroscience, (IoPPN),
King's College London, UK, and
COAST Early Intervention in Psychosis Team, South London and Maudsley NHS Foundation Trust, London, UK

Mario Juruena
Centre for Affective Disorders,
Institute of Psychiatry, Psychology & Neuroscience (IoPPN),
King's College London, UK

Sidney H. Kennedy
Centre for Depression & Suicide Studies, St. Michael's Hospital, Toronto, Canada, and

Department of Psychiatry, University of Toronto, Canada

Yunna Kwan
Section on Developmental Genetic Epidemiology, Genetic Epidemiology Branch,
National Institute of Mental Health, Bethesda, MD, USA

Jon A. Levenson
Department of Psychiatry, Columbia University, New York, NY, USA

Claudia Lex
Institute of Psychology, Alpen-Adria-University, Klagenfurt, Austria, and
Department of Psychiatry, General Hospital Villach, Austria

Julia N. Lukacs
Department of Psychology, Simon Fraser University, Burnaby, Canada

Karine Macritchie
South London and Maudsley NHS Foundation Trust, London, UK

Steven Marwaha
Birmingham and Solihull Mental Health Foundation Trust and Institute of Mental Health, University of Birmingham, UK

Paul McCrone
Institute for Lifecourse Development, University of Greenwich, London, UK

Susan L. McElroy
Research Institute, Lindner Center of HOPE, Mason, OH,
and Department of Psychiatry and Behavioral Neuroscience,
University of Cincinnati College of Medicine, Cincinnati, OH, USA

Kathleen R. Merikangas
Section on Developmental Genetic Epidemiology, Genetic Epidemiology Branch,
National Institute of Mental Health, Bethesda, MD, USA

Thomas D. Meyer
Louis A. Faillace, MD, Department of Psychiatry and Behavioral Sciences, McGovern Medical School

The University of Texas Health Science Center at Houston, Houston, TX, USA

Eilidh Miller
Translational and Clinical Research Institute, Newcastle University, Newcastle upon Tyne, UK

Camila Nayane de Carvalho Lima
Translational Psychiatry Program,
Louis A. Faillace, MD, Department of Psychiatry and Behavioral Sciences, McGovern Medical School
The University of Texas Health Science Center at Houston, Houston, TX, USA

Alexandre Paim Diaz
Center of Excellence on Mood Disorders & Translational Psychiatry Program,
Louis A. Faillace, MD, Department of Psychiatry and Behavioral Sciences, McGovern Medical School
The University of Texas Health Science Center at Houston, Houston, TX, USA

Luis Pereira
Department of Psychiatry, Columbia University, New York, NY, USA

Guillermo Perez Algorta
Division of Health Research,
Faculty of Health and Medicine,
Lancaster University, Lancaster, UK

Peter Phiri
School of Psychology,
University of Southampton, UK

Joao Quevedo
Center of Excellence on Mood Disorders & Translational Psychiatry Program,
Louis A. Faillace, MD, Department of Psychiatry and Behavioral Sciences, McGovern Medical School
The University of Texas Health Science Center at Houston, Houston, TX, USA

Mutahira M. Qureshi
South London and Maudsley NHS Foundation Trust, London, UK

Shanaya Rathod
Research Department, Clinical Trials Facility, Moorgreen Hospital, Southern Health
NHS Foundation Trust, Southampton, UK

Francisco Romo-Nava
Research Institute, Lindner Center of HOPE, Mason, OH, and
Department of Psychiatry and Behavioral Neuroscience, University of Cincinnati College of Medicine, Cincinnati, OH, USA

Susan Rotzinger
Centre for Depression & Suicide Studies, St. Michael's Hospital, Toronto, Canada, and
Department of Psychiatry, University of Toronto, Canada

Marsal Sanches
UT Health Center of Excellence on Mood Disorders, Louis A. Faillace, MD, Department of Psychiatry and Behavioral Sciences, McGovern Medical School
The University of Texas Health Science Center at Houston, Houston, TX, USA

Jan Scott
Institute of Neuroscience, Newcastle University, Newcastle, UK

Sudhakar Selvaraj
Depression Research Program,
Louis A. Faillace, MD, Department of Psychiatry and Behavioral Sciences, McGovern Medical School
The University of Texas Health Science Center at Houston, Houston, TX, USA

Lokesh Shahani
Louis A. Faillace, MD, Department of Psychiatry and Behavioral Sciences, McGovern Medical School
The University of Texas Health Science Center at Houston, Houston, TX, USA

Peter A. Shapiro
Department of Psychiatry, Columbia University, New York, NY, USA

Jair C. Soares
UT Health Center of Excellence on Mood Disorders, Louis A. Faillace, MD, Department of Psychiatry and Behavioral Sciences, McGovern Medical School
The University of Texas Health Science Center at Houston, Houston, TX, USA

Rebecca Strawbridge
Centre for Affective Disorders,
Institute of Psychiatry, Psychology & Neuroscience (IoPPN),
King's College London, UK

Argyris Stringaris
Section of Clinical and Computational
Neuroscience, National Institute of Mental
Health, National Institutes of Health,
Bethesda, MD, USA

Vaishali Tirumalaraju
Louis A. Faillace, MD, Department of Psychiatry and
Behavioral Sciences, McGovern Medical School
The University of Texas Health Science Center at
Houston, Houston, TX, USA

Sophie R. Vaccarino
Centre for Depression & Suicide Studies, St. Michael's
Hospital, Toronto, Canada, and
Institute of Medical Science, University of Toronto,
Canada

Roos van Westrhenen
Parnassia Psychiatric Institute/PsyQ,
Amsterdam, The Netherlands,
Department of Psychiatry & Neuropsychology,
Faculty of Health, Medicine and Life Sciences,
Maastricht University, Maastricht,
The Netherlands, and
Institute of Psychiatry, Psychology & Neuroscience
(IoPPN),
King's College London, UK

Jeffrey R. Vittengl
Department of Psychology,
Truman State University,
Kirksville, MO, USA

Michael Weaver
Center for Neurobehavioral Research on Addiction,
Louis A. Faillace, MD, Department of Psychiatry and
Behavioral Sciences, McGovern Medical School

The University of Texas Health Science Center at
Houston, Houston, TX,
USA

Victoria C. Wing
Translational and Clinical Research Institute,
Newcastle University, Newcastle upon Tyne,
UK, and
Cumbria, Northumberland, Tyne and Wear NHS
Foundation Trust, Newcastle upon Tyne, UK

Sui Liem Alexandre Wong
Institute of Psychiatry, Psychology & Neuroscience,
(IoPPN),
Kings College London, UK, and
COAST Early Intervention in Psychosis Team,
South London and Maudsley NHS Foundation Trust,
London, UK

Chineze Worthington
Behavioral Health Center, St. Vincent's Hospital,
White Plains, NY, USA

Allan Young
Centre for Affective Disorders,
Institute of Psychiatry, Psychology & Neuroscience
(IoPPN),
King's College London,
UK

Roland Zahn
National Service for Affective Disorders, South
London & Maudsley NHS Trust, London, UK, and
Centre for Affective Disorders,
Institute of Psychiatry, Psychology & Neuroscience
(IoPPN),
King's College London,
UK

Foreword

It is a pleasure to pen this Foreword to the latest textbook on mood disorders to arise from the collaborative team of Allan Young, Jair Soares, Marsal Sanches, and Mario Juruena. This book serves the purpose of providing an excellent summary to inform, clarify, and explain a subject at the same time as provoking its readers in pursuit of the same.

This excellent book demonstrates clearly what a textbook can provide that the latest journal articles rarely do. Chapters clarify the reasoning inherent in research and treatment and they re-frame an earlier consensus view in one area, preparing the reader for what will be available in the next wave of published work from leading investigators. At their best, a chapter or a review may propose a new synthesis or use a new or unexpected set of comparisons to provoke responses from their readers.

In particular, I would cite the chapters on the treatment of depression in children and adolescents and on the value and limits of pharmacogenetic tests as valuable to me. Last but by no means least, I give a high mark to the lead editor, Allan Young, and Mutahira M. Quershi for educating and provoking me with their chapter "Classification of Mood Disorders and the Unipolar/Bipolar Dichotomy". I confidently agree with their thesis, that despite a century of effort we have no satisfactory classification for disorders of mood. I enjoyed the erudite tour of the historical, philosophical approaches to classification. Among the ancients the authors cited Aristotle, ibn-sina [Avicenna] and Linnaeus I also appreciated their short review of current workers in the field especially Gin Mahli's take on classification. When reading part of their account on the unipolar/bipolar perspective, you may get a temporary dizzy feeling when traversing from Gödel's incompleteness theorem to the wave and particle nature of light. A few checks into PubMed and Google will get you back to equilibrium and at least for me better informed by a short but arduous intellectual trip.

J. Raymond DePaulo, MD
University Distinguished Service Professor
Co-Director, Johns Hopkins Mood Disorders Center
Department of Psychiatry & Behavioral Sciences
Johns Hopkins University School of Medicine

Mood Disorders in the Twenty-First Century

Allan Young, Marsal Sanches, Jair C. Soares, and Mario Juruena

Introduction

Mood disorders are among the most prevalent and potentially severe psychiatric disorders. In the case of major depressive disorder (MDD), despite great geographical variations, data from the World Health Organization point to approximately a 6% 12-month prevalence and a 20% lifetime prevalence [1]. With regard to bipolar disorders (BD), epidemiological findings indicate a lifetime prevalence of 0.6% for bipolar type I and 0.4% for bipolar type II, with a 2.4% prevalence when all bipolar spectrum conditions are considered [2]. In addition to their significant impact on functional status and quality of life, mood disorders are associated with considerable psychological suffering and elevated rates of suicide [3]. Moreover, available evidence shows association between mood disorders and an increased risk for different medical conditions, including cardiovascular disease, diabetes, metabolic disorders, obesity, dyslipidemia, hypertension, and dementia [4,5].

Considering all these potential implications of mood disorders for individuals, families, and communities, their early diagnosis and effective management are essential. Researchers have strived to better understand the pathophysiology of these conditions and to identify predictive factors related to response to treatment and outcome [6]. Nevertheless, despite important advances in the management of mood disorders, studies estimate that the currently available antidepressant treatments may be ineffective in 30–50% of patients with MDD [7–9].

In light of these limitations, as well as the complexity of society in the twenty-first century, which can make the management of mental disorders particularly challenging, a personalized approach for the treatment of mood disorders is highly desirable [10]. Multidisciplinary collaborations, including the combination of pharmacotherapy with different psychosocial interventions, are strongly recommended.

Diagnostic Aspects

A fundamental limitation of the currently adopted diagnostic systems is related to the inexistence of established biological markers for the different psychiatric conditions. Consequently, the diagnosis of mood disorders is based mostly on the presence of certain criteria, usually comprised by certain core symptoms and specific history data. The *Diagnostic and Statistical Manual of Mental Disorders* (DSM), currently in its fifth edition (DSM-5), is the best example of such approach.

While these systems usually offer a good degree of diagnostic reliability, they may face problems in contemplating the considerable phenotypical overlap found across different types of mood disorders. Alternative diagnostic formulations, utilizing a dimensional approach in contrast to the standard categorical diagnostic systems, try to take these limitations into consideration. These approaches are based on the idea of a continuum across different mood disorders, being aware of not only clinical but also biological factors shared by different mood disorders.

It is expected that these diagnostic and nosological limitations will be overcome by the identification of validated biomarkers for mood disorders. Based on neurobiological and genetic findings, biomarkers will allow the integration of neuroscience into psychiatric diagnostic practice. By routinely incorporating data on biomarkers, future diagnostic systems should allow the integration of clinical, etiological, and pathophysiological factors, improving our diagnostic accuracy and having the potential to revolutionize the practice of psychiatry.

Depressive Disorders

The impact of depression on individuals' lives results from a combination of genetic vulnerability and environmental risk factors [11,12]. While the biological mechanisms behind depressive disorders are not yet completely understood, they seem to involve the hypothalamic–pituitary–adrenal (HPA) axis, genetic and neurodevelopmental factors, monoaminergic deficiencies, and other possible mechanisms [13], such as alteration of the intestinal microbiota [14,15].

The influence of stress on the pathophysiology of depression is well known [16,17]. Many depressive patients experience disturbances in the regulation of the HPA axis, and these dysfunctions are often reflected in changes in cortisol concentrations in blood and saliva [18,19].

Similarly, abnormalities involving the gut microbiota and the bidirectional communication of the intestine-brain axis [20] have been found to be involved in the pathophysiology of depression. Changes in the composition of the intestinal microbiota, due to factors such as age, diet, stress, use of antibiotics, prebiotics and probiotics, immune status, and intestinal transit [15,21] may result in intestinal dysbiosis, which shows important correlations with depression and other mental disorders [15,22]. Numerous authors recognize this bidirectional gut-brain communication via the autonomic nervous system (ANS), enteric nervous system (ENS), and neuroendocrine and immune systems [23,24].

Approximately 50% of individuals who receive treatment for a depressive episode will experience a second episode over their lifetime, usually within 5 years, with a lifetime average of four depressive episodes [25,26]. Moreover, it is estimated that 30 to 50% of depressed patients do not achieve full remission [9,27], and patients with depression may have persistent and severe psychosocial and occupational impairments, even after recovery from an acute episode [28].

Last, as previously mentioned, suicide rates are elevated among individuals with depression. In the National Comorbidity Survey Replication, the risk of suicide attempts in MDD was found to be fivefold higher than in the general population in the United States [29].

Bipolar Disorders

Despite numerous advances observed in the last several decades with regards to the understanding of bipolar disorder (BD), its underlying neurobiological mechanisms remain far from being fully elucidated [30]. This results in several limitations involving its

diagnosis and treatment, especially with regard to depressive symptoms or episodes.

That is complicated by the fact that approximately 35% of patients with bipolar disorder experience a delay of up to 10 years between symptom onset and the correct diagnosis. Even though BD is typically characterized by alternating periods of depression with symptoms of mania or hypomania, depression is usually the main reason patients with BD seek treatment [31]. Thus, the misdiagnosis of BD as MDD is common, causing delays in the implementation of the most appropriate therapeutic measures [32].

Currently available treatment options for bipolar disorder are often insufficient to help patients achieve full remission and restore their premorbid functioning. However, in the past few years, we have witnessed a more wide-ranging understanding of the neural circuits and the various mechanisms of synaptic and neural plasticity, the molecular mechanisms of receptors, and the process by which genes code for specific functional proteins [33,34]. It is expected that these advances will help in the identification of novel therapeutic targets.

Moreover, while pharmacological treatment is considered essential for the management of this condition, a growing amount of evidence has emphasized the importance of nonpharmacological interventions, such as psychoeducation and different psychotherapy modalities, in improving patients' understanding of their illness and their treatment adherence, as well as helping with the identification of prodromal symptoms and early signs of relapse, providing family support, and offering psychosocial rehabilitation [35].

Mood Disorders, Neuroimaging, and Cognition

Cognitive deficits in patients with depression and BD have been the object of great interest, given their importance from a functional and psychopathological perspective [36]. Neuroimaging studies point to the involvement of dysfunctions in neural networks connecting the limbic system and cortical regions in the pathophysiology of mood symptoms and cognitive impairment [37,38]. Areas involved in the pathophysiology of cognitive dysfunction in depression include regions of the prefrontal cortex, cingulate cortex, hippocampus, striatum, amygdala, and thalamus [39].

For example, the neocortex and hippocampus collaborate by mediating cognitive aspects of depression, such as guilt, impaired working memory, feelings of worthlessness, and suicidal ideation. On the other hand, interactions between the amygdala and the hippocampus can mediate anhedonia, anxiety, and loss of motivation, in addition to mnemonic changes [40]. Naturally, these identified regions act in coordination with other parallel circuits, possibly forming a neural network underlying depression [39,41–43].

Within this perspective, cognitive impairments in depression may result from high levels of cortisol resulting from stressful situations or dysfunctions in the HPA axis. In response to the prolonged action of stress, the organism passes from a slower conscious control of the top-down type regulated by cognitive processes and memory to an emotional control of the bottom-up type, which is faster and reflexive and related to the amygdala and subcortical structures [44].

Depression has been linked to deficits in a wide variety of cognitive domains. During depressive episodes, the most well-known cognitive deficits are a decrease in performance in tasks involving a change of attention focus, memory impairment, and problems related to executive function [45,46]. In addition, studies have demonstrated the effects of mood disorders and stress on global cognitive performance [47,48], executive functioning [49,50], and memory [51–54], in addition to reward processing, processing of social and affective stimuli, and emotional regulation [55].

Studies investigating cognitive deficits in depressive patients have reported results similar to those with participants who suffered early stress, either in global cognitive performance [45], in executive functions [56–57], and memory [58]. Thus, the cognitive impairments that result from depression may overlap with deficits related to early stress. Therefore, authors must be aware of depression as a factor to be included in the analysis of the effects of early stress on cognition [59].

Biomarkers and Pathophysiology

The search for biological markers in psychiatry has proved arduous and somewhat thankless. According to the FDA-NIH Biomarker Working Group, a biological marker is "a defining characteristic that is measured as an indicator of normal biological processes, pathogenic processes or responses to an exposure or intervention" [60]; however, in clinical practice, a good biomarker must have high reproducibility, that

is, be present in the vast majority of patients with the same disease, and ideally be dynamically and reliably modified as the clinical picture progresses [61]. Unfortunately, these definitions determine biological markers for psychiatric diseases to be almost unobtainable, given the high rates of comorbidity between different conditions and the fact that dysfunctions in the same neural circuits seem to be involved in the pathophysiology of different mental disorders. Moreover, when discussing biomarkers, it is necessary to consider the importance of genetic polymorphisms and the fact that gene expression can be influenced by different factors and regulatory processes. Therefore, not only gene–gene but also gene–stress interactions are likely to play a cumulative role in the predisposition to mood disorders.

For example, evidence suggests that changes in the hormonal system from stress can induce distortions of thinking and memory and worsen depressive symptoms and bipolar disorder [62]. These abnormalities appear to be related to changes in the ability of circulating glucocorticoids to exert their negative feedback on the secretion of HPA axis hormones by binding to mineralocorticoid (MR) and glucocorticoid (GR) receptors in HPA tissues [63]. MR receptors in the brain are involved in regulating stress hormone secretion and complex behaviors such as emotion, memory, and sleep. In humans, the role of MR and GR receptors in the pathophysiology of stress-related psychiatric disorders has not yet been sufficiently characterized. However, studies indicate possibilities for new pharmacotherapies via modulation of the function of these receptors [64].

Furthermore, a growing body of evidence suggests that chronic inflammation and oxidative stress are involved in both the pathogenesis and progression of mood disorders, especially bipolar disorders [65], bringing about cellular dysfunction and, eventually, neuronal death. Changes in glutamatergic neurotransmission might represent the downstream effects of these processes, given the prominent role of glutamate in excitotoxicity – overstimulation of neurons via increased intracellular calcium, resulting in cell death [66].

Last, changes in brain maturation follow a trajectory of development throughout life [67]. Any environmental events generating inappropriate stimulation could alter neurotransmitters, neuroendocrine hormones, and neurotrophic factors crucial for normal brain development and precipitate affective conditions such as depression and bipolar disorder [68,69]. Early stress may impact the development of brain structures [70]. Among the neural systems most frequently implicated in the relationship between early stress and depression, those whose development is completed during childhood and adolescence, such as the amygdala, prefrontal cortex, and hippocampus, are of particular relevance [71].

In summary, pathophysiological research in mood disorders has moved from the classic monoaminergic theory of depression to more dynamic pathophysiological models emphasizing different levels of disruptions (genetic, neurodevelopmental, physiological, neuroanatomical/neurofunctional, and biochemical). Nonetheless, despite the strong evidence supporting the role of neurobiological abnormalities in the pathophysiology of mood disorders, a unified understanding of how these different abnormalities lead to the development of clinical mood symptoms is still missing.

Treatment

Given the complexity of mood disorders, the variability of characteristics of their clinical forms, and their course among patients, no single treatment or combination of treatments is ideal for all patients. However, appropriate treatment can drastically reduce the functional disability and high mortality associated with the disorder [35].

Diverse therapeutic approaches have been used to treat mood disorders, including medications, neurostimulation treatments, and different psychotherapy modalities [72]. While the selection of suitable pharmacological treatment is decisive for reaching a therapeutic response [73,74], the effectiveness of psychopharmacology is also considered modest in parts due to the low adherence rate (30%) to psychopharmacological agents [72]. Although contemporary pharmacological agents have revolutionized the treatment of mood disorders, long-term outcomes for many patients remain modest [9,75–77]. Therefore, exploring new therapeutic targets for mood disorders is a priority for translational research, with an urgent need for the identification of more effective treatments and the better characterization of treatment guidelines for the management of MDD and BD.

In the case of depression, although the concept of difficult-to-treat depression (DTD) helps to reframe binary definitions of treatment-resistant depression (TRD) and assess response to other treatment modalities [78], therapeutic options remain limited for individuals who do not respond to conventional biopsychosocial interventions. Traditionally, neurostimulation has been considered an effective strategy for those with DTD. The estimated response rate to electroconvulsive therapy (ECT) in DTD surpasses 50%, making it one of the most effective treatments in psychiatry [79,80]. Nevertheless, there is a trend toward decreasing the use of this effective treatment. That may be explained by the public stigma around ECT, given its historical misuse and concerns about cognitive complications [81]. Although better accepted, other neurostimulation options, such as transcranial magnetic stimulation (TMS), lack the comparative efficacy and require more prolonged treatment courses [82].

Furthermore, over the past 20 years, a large body of evidence has demonstrated the effects of ketamine as a rapid-acting and effective antidepressant, even in those who have failed to respond to previous treatments [83]. Despite being a novel treatment within psychiatry, ketamine has long been used in medical settings as an anesthetic due to its ability to provide conscious sedation with lower risks of hypotension and respiratory depression compared to other induction agents [84]. Sharp declines in suicidal ideation have been reported in association with quick improvements in mood among acutely depressed patients receiving ketamine, corroborating its potential as a valuable acute psychiatric treatment [85]. As the clinical response from ketamine continues to be clarified, research exploring its underlying neurobiological mechanisms has provided new perspectives on the pathophysiology of depression. Ketamine's antidepressant functions are largely explained through its actions as a noncompetitive antagonist of N-methyl-D-aspartate (NMDA) receptors. NMDA receptors have multiple neuronal loci, and thus, many mutually inclusive molecular pathways have been implicated [86–88].

Considering the variable response to available treatments, a more personalized approach to the management of mood disorders is of great interest. Thus, pharmacogenetics represents a promising tool for the individualization of pharmacological treatment [89]. Therapeutic response, tolerability, and recurrence are some of the outcomes that can be affected by genetic differences between individuals [74,90,91]. Genetic variants account for 42% of individual differences in antidepressant response [92]. The incorporation of pharmacogenetic tests in clinical practice might increase remission rates and response in TRD patients [93,94], in addition to decreasing healthcare costs and polypharmacy [94,95]. In the UK, the promising results obtained in several studies are compiled by the Clinical Pharmacogenetics Implementation Consortium (CPIC) and Pharmacogenomics Knowledge Base (PharmGKB), which resulted in the development of pharmacogenetic-informed antidepressant guidelines [96–98].

Conclusion

The beginning of the twenty-first century seems to be an era likely to see an essential integration of concepts and knowledge. The full understanding of the pathophysiological pathways involved in the development of mood disorders is of pivotal importance for the development of more precise, biomarker-based diagnostic systems and more effective biological treatments. The concept of neuroprogression in mood disorders supports the need for neuroprotection with biological properties. On the other hand, psychosocial interventions for the treatment of mood disorders are of great importance and a better characterization of their therapeutic role, alone and in combination with biological treatments, is essential. By better understanding, these interactions and their relevance to mood disorders, better treatments and, ultimately, better outcomes for individuals with depression and bipolar affective disorder will be achieved.

References

1. E. Bromet, L. H. Andrade, I. Hwang, et al. Cross-national epidemiology of DSM-IV major depressive episode. *BMC Med.* 2011;**9**:90. https://doi.org/10.1186/1741-7015-9-90.

2. K. R. Merikangas, R. Jin, J.-P. He, et al. Prevalence and correlates of bipolar spectrum disorder in the World Mental Health Survey Initiative. *Arch Gen Psychiatry.* 2011;**68**:241. https://doi.org/10.1001/archgenpsychiatry.2011.12.

3. B. Gaynes. Assessing the risk factors for difficult-to-treat depression and treatment-resistant depression. *J Clin Psychiatry.* 2016;**77**(Suppl 1):4–8. https://doi.org/10.4088/JCP.14077su1c.01.

4. K. B. Wells. The functioning and well-being of depressed patients. Results from the Medical Outcomes Study. *JAMA.* 1989;**262**:914–19. https://doi.org/10.1001/jama.262.7.914.

5. A. Danese, T. E. Moffitt, H. Harrington, et al. Adverse childhood experiences and adult risk factors for age-related disease: depression, inflammation, and clustering of metabolic risk markers. *Arch Pediatr Adolesc Med.* 2009;**163**: 1135–43. https://doi.org/10.1001/archpediatrics.2009.214.

6. A. Cleare, C. M. Pariante, A. H. Young, et al.; Members of the Consensus Meeting. Evidence-based guidelines for treating depressive disorders with antidepressants: a revision of the 2008 British Association for Psychopharmacology guidelines. *J Psychopharmacol.* 2015;**29**:459–525. https://doi.org/10.1177/0269881115581093.

7. M. Fava. Diagnosis and definition of treatment-resistant depression. *Biol Psychiatry.* 2003;**53**:649–59. https://doi.org/10.1016/s0006-3223(03)00231-2.

8. D. Souery, P. Oswald, I. Massat, et al.; Group for the Study of Resistant Depression. Clinical factors associated with treatment resistance in major depressive disorder: results from a European multicenter study. *J Psychiatry.* 2007;**68**:1062–70. https://doi.org/10.4088/jcp.v68n0713.

9. A. J. Rush, M. H. Trivedi, S. R. Wisniewski, et al. Acute and longer-term outcomes in depressed outpatients requiring one or several treatment steps: a STAR* D report. *Am J Psychiatry.* 2006;**163**:1905–17.

10. A. H. Young, M. F. Juruena. The neurobiology of bipolar disorder. *Curr Top Behav Neurosci.* 2021;**48**:1–20. https://doi.org/10.1007/7854_2020_179.

11. S. R. Dube, R. F. Anda, V. J. Felitti, et al. Childhood abuse, household dysfunction, and the risk of attempted suicide throughout the life span: findings from the Adverse Childhood Experiences Study. *JAMA.* 2001;**286**:3089–96. https://doi.org/10.1001/jama.286.24.3089.

12. K. S. Kendler, K. Sheth, C. O. Gardner, C. A. Prescott. Childhood parental loss and risk for first-onset of major depression and alcohol dependence: the time-decay of risk and sex differences. *Psychol Med.* 2002;**32**;1187–94. https://doi.org/10.1017/s0033291702006219.

13. R. H. Belmaker, G. Agam, Major depressive disorder. *N Engl J Med.* 2008;**358**:55–68. https://doi.org/10.1056/NEJMra073096.

14. H. Jiang, Z. Ling, Y. Zhang, et al. Altered fecal microbiota composition in patients with major depressive disorder. *Brain Behav Immun.* 2015;**48**:186–94. https://doi.org/10.1016/j.bbi.2015.03.016.

15. V. L. Nikolova, M. R. B. Smith, L. J. Hall, et al. Perturbations in gut microbiota composition in psychiatric disorders: a review and meta-analysis. *JAMA Psychiatry.* 2021;**78**:1343–54. https://doi.org/10.1001/jamapsychiatry.2021.2573.

16. F. Navarro-Mateu, M. J. Tormo, D. Salmerón, et al. Prevalence of mental disorders in the south-east of Spain, one of the European regions most affected by the economic crisis: the cross-sectional PEGASUS-Murcia Project. *PloS One*. 2015;**10**: e0137293. https://doi.org/10.1371/journal .pone.0137293.

17. R. M. Post. Transduction of psychosocial stress into the neurobiology of recurrent affective disorder. *Am J Psychiatry*. 1992;**149**:999–1010. https://doi.org/10.1 176/ajp.149.8.999.

18. P. W. Gold. The organization of the stress system and its dysregulation in depressive illness. *Mol Psychiatry*. 2015;**20**:32–47. https://doi.org/10.1038/mp.2014.163.

19. E. S. Brown, F. P. Varghese, B. S. McEwen. Association of depression with medical illness: does cortisol play a role? *Biol Psychiatry*. 2004;**55**:1–9. https://doi.org/10.1016/s0006-3223(03)00473-6.

20. J. F. Cryan, T. G. Dinan. Mind-altering microorganisms: the impact of the gut microbiota on brain and behaviour. *Nat Rev Neurosci*. 2012;**13**:701712. https://doi.org/10.1038/nrn3346.

21. T. Yatsunenko, F. E. Rey, M. J. Manary, et al. Human gut microbiome viewed across age and geography. *Nature*. 2012;**486**:222–7. https://doi.org/10.1038/ nature11053.

22. S. S. Yarandi, D. A. Peterson, G. J. Treisman, T. H. Moran, P. J. Pasricha. Modulatory effects of gut microbiota on the central nervous system: how gut could play a role in neuropsychiatric health and diseases. *J Neurogastroenterol Motil*. 2016;**22**:201–12. https://doi.org/10.5056/jnm15146.

23. G. Clarke, S. Grenham, P. Scully, et al. The microbiome-gut-brain axis during early life regulates the hippocampal serotonergic system in a sex-dependent manner. *Mol Psychiatry*. 2013;**18**:666–73. https://doi.org/10.1038/mp.2012.77.

24. K.-A. Neufeld, J. A. Foster. Effects of gut microbiota on the brain: implications for psychiatry. *J Psychiatry Neurosci*. 2009;**34**:230–1.

25. D. J. Kupfer. Long-term treatment of depression. *J Psychiatry*. 1991;**52**(Suppl):28–34.

26. G. A. Fava, S. K. Park, N. Sonino. Treatment of recurrent depression. *Expert Rev Neurother*. 2006;**6**:1735–40. https://doi.org/10.1586/ 14737175.6.11.1735.

27. S. Quraishi, S. Frangou. Neuropsychology of bipolar disorder: a review. *J Affect Disord*. 2002;**72**:209–26. https://doi.org/10.1016/s0165-0327(02)00091-5.

28. P. Ay-Woan, C. P. Sarah, C. Lyinn, C. Tsyr-Jang, H. Ping-Chuan. Quality of life in depression: predictive models. *Qual Life Res*. 2006;**15**:39–48. https://doi.org/10.1007/s11136-005-0381-x.

29. M. K. Nock, I. Hwang, N. A. Sampson, R. C. Kessler. Mental disorders, comorbidity and suicidal behavior: results from the National Comorbidity Survey Replication. *Mol Psychiatry*. 2010;**15**:868–76. https:// doi.org/10.1038/mp.2009.29.

30. M. F. Juruena, L. A. Jelen, A. H. Young, A. J. Cleare. New pharmacological interventions in bipolar disorder. *Curr Top Behav Neurosci*. 2021;**48**:303–24. https://doi.org/10.1007/7854_2020_181.

31. L. L. Judd, H. S. Akiskal. Depressive episodes and symptoms dominate the longitudinal course of bipolar disorder. *Curr Psychiatry Rep*. 2003;**5**:417–18. https://doi.org/10.1007/s11920-003-0077-2.

32. J. Angst, J.-M. Azorin, C. L. Bowden, et al.; BRIDGE Study Group. Prevalence and characteristics of undiagnosed bipolar disorders in patients with a major depressive episode: the BRIDGE study. *Arch Gen Psychiatry*. 2011;**68**:791–8. https://doi.org/10.10 01/archgenpsychiatry.2011.87.

33. R. M. Post. The Kindling/Sensitization Model and early life stress. *Curr Top Behav Neurosci*. 2021;**48**:255–75. https://doi.org/10.1007/7854_ 2020_172.

34. T. Barichello, V. V. Giridharan, G. Bhatti, et al. Inflammation as a mechanism of bipolar disorder neuroprogression. *Curr Top Behav Neurosci*. 2021;**48**:215–37. https://doi.org/10.1007/7854_2020_ 173.

35. K. N. Fountoulakis, E. Vieta. Treatment of bipolar disorder: a systematic review of available data and clinical perspectives. *Int J Neuropsychopharmacol*. 2008;**11**:999–1029. https://doi.org/10.1017/ S1461145708009231.

36. M. Sanches, I. E. Bauer, J. F. Galvez, G. B. Zunta-Soares, J. C. Soares. The management of cognitive impairment in bipolar disorder: current status and perspectives. *Am J Ther*. 2015;**22**:477–86. https://doi .org/10.1097/MJT.0000000000000120.

37. G. Rayner, G. Jackson, S. Wilson. Cognition-related brain networks underpin the symptoms of unipolar depression: evidence from a systematic review. *Neurosci Biobehav Rev*. 2016;**61**:53–65. https://doi .org/10.1016/j.neubiorev.2015.09.022.

38. J. Savitz, W. C. Drevets. Bipolar and major depressive disorder: neuroimaging the developmental-degenerative divide. *Neurosci Biobehav Rev*. 2009;**33**:699–771. https://doi.org/10 .1016/j.neubiorev.2009.01.004.

39. E. J. Nestler, M. Barrot, R. J. DiLeone, et al. Neurobiology of depression. *Neuron*. 2002;**34**:13–25. https://doi.org/10.1016/s0896-6273(02)00653-0.

40. M. P. Richardson, B. A. Strange, R. J. Dolan. Encoding of emotional memories depends on amygdala and

hippocampus and their interactions. *Nat Neurosci.* 2004;7:278–85. https://doi.org/10.1038/nn1190.

41. H. S. Mayberg. Limbic-cortical dysregulation: a proposed model of depression. *J Neuropsychiatry Clin Neurosci.* 1997;9:471–81. https://doi.org/10.1176/jnp.9.3.471.

42. H. S. Mayberg. Targeted electrode-based modulation of neural circuits for depression. *J Clin Invest.* 2009;119:717–25. https://doi.org/10.1172/JCI38454.

43. A. K. Afifi, R. A. Bergman. *Functional Neuroanatomy: Text and Atlas.* International ed. New York: McGraw-Hill, Health Professions Division, 1998.

44. S. Vogel, G. Fernández, M. Joëls, L. Schwabe. Cognitive adaptation under stress: a case for the mineralocorticoid receptor. *Trends Cogn Sci.* 2016;20:192–203. https://doi.org/10.1016/j.tics.2015.12.003.

45. T. Beblo, G. Sinnamon, B. T. Baune. Specifying the neuropsychology of affective disorders: clinical, demographic and neurobiological factors. *Neuropsychol Rev.* 2011;21:337–59. https://doi.org/10.1007/s11065-011-9171-0.

46. J. V. Taylor Tavares, W. C. Drevets, B. J. Sahakian. Cognition in mania and depression. *Psychol Med.* 2003;33:959–67. https://doi.org/10.1017/s0033291703008432.

47. M. M. Loman, K. L. Wiik, K. A. Frenn, S. D. Pollak, M. R. Gunnar. Postinstitutionalized children's development: growth, cognitive, and language outcomes. *J Dev Behav Pediatr.* 2009;30:426–34. https://doi.org/10.1097/DBP.0b013e3181b1fd08.

48. M. Rutter, T. G. O'Connor, English and Romanian Adoptees (ERA) Study Team. Are there biological programming effects for psychological development? Findings from a study of Romanian adoptees. *Dev Psychol.* 2004;40:81–94. https://doi.org/10.1037/0012-1649.40.1.81.

49. S. D. Pollak, C. A. Nelson, M. F. Schlaak, et al. Neurodevelopmental effects of early deprivation in postinstitutionalized children. *Child Dev.* 2010;81:224–36. https://doi.org/10.1111/j.1467-8624.2009.01391.x.

50. E. Colvert, M. Rutter, J. Kreppner, et al. Do theory of mind and executive function deficits underlie the adverse outcomes associated with profound early deprivation?: findings from the English and Romanian adoptees study. *J Abnorm Child Psychol.* 2008;36:1057–68. https://doi.org/10.1007/s10802-008-9232-x.

51. A. H. Young, P. Gallagher, S. Watson, et al. Improvements in neurocognitive function and mood following adjunctive treatment with mifepristone (RU-486) in bipolar disorder.

Neuropsychopharmacology. 2004;29:1538–45. https://doi.org/10.1038/sj.npp.1300471.

52. M. D. De Bellis, S. R. Hooper, D. P. Woolley, C. E. Shenk. Demographic, maltreatment, and neurobiological correlates of PTSD symptoms in children and adolescents. *J Pediatr Psychol.* 2010;35:570–7. https://doi.org/10.1093/jpepsy/jsp116.

53. R. F. Anda, V. J. Felitti, J. D. Bremner, et al. The enduring effects of abuse and related adverse experiences in childhood. A convergence of evidence from neurobiology and epidemiology. *Eur Arch Psychiatry Clin Neurosci.* 2006;256:174–86. https://doi.org/10.1007/s00406-005-0624-4.

54. C. P. Navalta, A. Polcari, D. M. Webster, A. Boghossian, M. H. Teicher. Effects of childhood sexual abuse on neuropsychological and cognitive function in college women. *J Neuropsychiatry Clin Neurosci.* 2006;18:45–53. https://doi.org/10.1176/jnp.18.1.45.

55. P. Pechtel, D. A. Pizzagalli. Effects of early life stress on cognitive and affective function: an integrated review of human literature. *Psychopharmacology.* 2011;214:55–70. https://doi.org/10.1007/s00213-010-2009-2.

56. S. U. Kaymak, B. Demir, S. Sentürk, et al. Hippocampus, glucocorticoids and neurocognitive functions in patients with first-episode major depressive disorders. *Eur Arch Psychiatry Clin Neurosci.* 2010;260:217–23. https://doi.org/10.1007/s00406-009-0045-x.

57. P. Neu, M. Bajbouj, A. Schilling, et al. Cognitive function over the treatment course of depression in middle-aged patients: correlation with brain MRI signal hyperintensities. *J Psychiatr Res.* 2005;39:129–35. https://doi.org/10.1016/j.jpsychires.2004.06.004.

58. S. Reppermund, M. Ising, S. Lucae, J. Zihl. Cognitive impairment in unipolar depression is persistent and non-specific: further evidence for the final common pathway disorder hypothesis. *Psychol Med.* 2009;39:603–14. https://doi.org/10.1017/S003329170800411X.

59. R. Grassi-Oliveira, C. F. de Azevedo Gomes, L. M. Stein. False recognition in women with a history of childhood emotional neglect and diagnose of recurrent major depression. *Conscious Cogn.* 2011;20:1127–34. https://doi.org/10.1016/j.concog.2011.03.005.

60. D. N. Cagney, J. Sul, R. Y. Huang, et al. The FDA NIH Biomarkers, EndpointS, and other Tools (BEST) resource in neuro-oncology. *Neuro Oncol.* 2018;20:1162–72. https://doi.org/10.1093/neuonc/nox242.

61. R. M. Califf. Biomarker definitions and their applications. *Exp Biol Med (Maywood).* 2018;243:213–21. https://doi.org/10.1177/1535370217750088.

62. S. Watson, P. Gallagher, J. C. Ritchie, I. N. Ferrier, A. H. Young. Hypothalamic-pituitary-adrenal axis function in patients with bipolar disorder. *Br J Psychiatry*. 2004;**184**:496–502. https://doi.org/10.1192/bjp.184.6.496.

63. M. F. Juruena, B. Agustini, A. J. Cleare, A. H. Young. A translational approach to clinical practice via stress-responsive glucocorticoid receptor signaling. *Stem Cell Investig*. 2017;**4**:13. https://doi.org/10.21037/sci.2017.02.01.

64. J. R. Geddes, D. J. Miklowitz. Treatment of bipolar disorder. *Lancet*. 2013;**381**:1672–82. https://doi.org/10.1016/S0140-6736(13)60857-0.

65. A. C. Andreazza, M. Kauer-Sant'anna, B. N. Frey, et al. Oxidative stress markers in bipolar disorder: a meta-analysis. *J Affect Disord*. 2008;**111**:135–44. https://doi.org/10.1016/j.jad.2008.04.013.

66. M. Berk, H. Plein, B. Belsham. The specificity of platelet glutamate receptor supersensitivity in psychotic disorders. *Life Sci*. 2000;**66**:2427–32. https://doi.org/10.1016/s0024-3205(00)80002-8.

67. A. Pascual-Leone, M. J. Taylor. A developmental framework of brain and cognition from infancy to old age. *Brain Topogr*. 2011;**24**:183–6. https://doi.org/10.1007/s10548-011-0197-7.

68. S. L. Andersen. Trajectories of brain development: point of vulnerability or window of opportunity? *Neurosci Biobehav Rev*. 2003;**27**:3–18. https://doi.org/10.1016/s0149-7634(03)00005-8.

69. M. Sanches, M. S. Keshavan, P. Brambilla, J. C. Soares. Neurodevelopmental basis of bipolar disorder: a critical appraisal. *Prog Neuropsychopharmacol Biol Psychiatry*. 2008;**32**:1617–27. https://doi.org/10.1016/j.pnpbp.2008.04.017.

70. M. H. Teicher, S. L. Andersen, A. Polcari, C. M. Anderson, C. P. Navalta. Developmental neurobiology of childhood stress and trauma. *Psychiatr Clin North Am*. 2002;**25**:397–426, vii–viii. https://doi.org/10.1016/s0193-953x(01)00003-x.

71. S. J. Lupien, B. S. McEwen, M. R. Gunnar, C. Heim. Effects of stress throughout the lifespan on the brain, behaviour and cognition. *Nat Rev Neurosci*. 2009;**10**:434–45. https://doi.org/10.1038/nrn2639.

72. S. Weich, I. Nazareth, L. Morgan, M. King. Treatment of depression in primary care. Socio-economic status, clinical need and receipt of treatment. *Br J Psychiatry*. 2007;**191**:164–9. https://doi.org/10.1192/bjp.bp.106.032219.

73. K. S. Al-Harbi. Treatment-resistant depression: therapeutic trends, challenges, and future directions. *Patient Prefer Adherence*. 2012;**6**:369–88. https://doi.org/10.2147/PPA.S29716.

74. R. van Westrhenen, K. J. Aitchison, M. Ingelman-Sundberg, M. M. Jukić. Pharmacogenomics of antidepressant and antipsychotic treatment: how far have we got and where are we going? *Front Psychiatry*. 2020;**11**:94. https://doi.org/10.3389/fpsyt.2020.00094.

75. M. J. Gitlin, J. Swendsen, T. L. Heller, C. Hammen. Relapse and impairment in bipolar disorder. *Am J Psychiatry*. 1995;**152**:1635–40. https://doi.org/10.1176/ajp.152.11.1635.

76. J. A. Lieberman, T. S. Stroup, J. P. McEvoy, et al.; Clinical Antipsychotic Trials of Intervention Effectiveness (CATIE) Investigators. Effectiveness of antipsychotic drugs in patients with chronic schizophrenia. *N Engl J Med*. 2005;**353**:1209–23. https://doi.org/10.1056/NEJMoa051688.

77. M. E. Thase. STEP-BD and bipolar depression: what have we learned? *Curr Psychiatry Rep*. 2007;**9**:497–503. https://doi.org/10.1007/s11920-007-0068-9.

78. R. H. McAllister-Williams, C. Arango, P. Blier, et al. The identification, assessment and management of difficult-to-treat depression: an international consensus statement. *J Affect Disord*. 2020;**267**:264–82. https://doi.org/10.1016/j.jad.2020.02.023.

79. N. Buley, E. Copland, S. Hodge, R. Chaplin. A further decrease in the rates of administration of electroconvulsive therapy in England. *J ECT*. 2017;**33**:198–202. https://doi.org/10.1097/YCT.0000000000000374.

80. A. U. Haq, A. F. Sitzmann, M. L. Goldman, D. F. Maixner, B. J. Mickey. Response of depression to electroconvulsive therapy: a meta-analysis of clinical predictors. *J Psychiatry*. 2015;**76**:1374–84. https://doi.org/10.4088/JCP.14r09528.

81. N. Ghaziuddin, G. Walter, editors. *Electroconvulsive Therapy in Children and Adolescents*. New York: Oxford University Press, 2014.

82. J.-J. Chen, L.-B. Zhao, Y.-Y. Liu, S.-H. Fan, P. Xie. Comparative efficacy and acceptability of electroconvulsive therapy versus repetitive transcranial magnetic stimulation for major depression: a systematic review and multiple-treatments meta-analysis. *Behav Brain Res*. 2017;**320**:30–6. https://doi.org/10.1016/j.bbr.2016.11.028.

83. R. S. McIntyre, J. D. Rosenblat, C. B. Nemeroff, et al. Synthesizing the evidence for ketamine and esketamine in treatment-resistant depression: an international expert opinion on the available evidence and implementation. *Am J Psychiatry*. 2021;**178**:383–99. https://doi.org/10.1176/appi.ajp.2020.20081251.

84. C. Morris, A. Perris, J. Klein, P. Mahoney. Anaesthesia in haemodynamically compromised emergency patients: does ketamine represent the best choice of induction agent? *Anaesthesia*.

2009;**64**:532–9. https://doi.org/10.1111/j.1365-2044.2008.05835.x.

85. S. T. Wilkinson, E. D. Ballard, M. H. Bloch, et al. The effect of a single dose of intravenous ketamine on suicidal ideation: a systematic review and individual participant data meta-analysis. *Am J Psychiatry*. 2018;**175**:150–8. https://doi.org/10.1176/appi.ajp.2017.17040472.

86. N. Diazgranados, L. Ibrahim, N. E. Brutsche, et al. A randomized add-on trial of an N-methyl-D-aspartate antagonist in treatment-resistant bipolar depression. *Arch Gen Psychiatry*. 2010;**67**:793–802. https://doi.org/10.1001/archgenpsychiatry.2010.90.

87. R. S. Duman, G. K. Aghajanian. Synaptic dysfunction in depression: potential therapeutic targets. *Science*. 2012;**338**:68–72. https://doi.org/10.1126/science.1222939.

88. B. Kadriu, L. Musazzi, I. D. Henter, et al. Glutamatergic neurotransmission: pathway to developing novel rapid-acting antidepressant treatments. *Int J Neuropsychopharmacol*. 2019;**22**:119–35. https://doi.org/10.1093/ijnp/pyy094.

89. T. L. Smith, C. B. Nemeroff. Pharmacogenomic testing and antidepressant response: problems and promises. *Braz J Psychiatry*. 2020;**42**:116–17. https://doi.org/10.1590/1516-4446-2019-0799.

90. A. Tornio, J. T. Backman. Cytochrome P450 in pharmacogenetics: an update. *Adv Pharmacol*. 2018;**833**:32. https://doi.org/10.1016/bs.apha.2018.04.007.

91. M. Veldic, A. T. Ahmed, C. J. Blacker, et al. Cytochrome P450 2C19 poor metabolizer phenotype in treatment resistant depression: treatment and diagnostic implications. *Front Pharmacol*. 2019;**10**:83. https://doi.org/10.3389/fphar.2019.00083.

92. C. Han, S.-M. Wang, W.-M. Bahk, et al. A pharmacogenomic-based antidepressant treatment for patients with major depressive disorder: results from an 8-week, randomized, single-blinded clinical trial. *Clin Psychopharmacol Neurosci*. 2018;**16**:469–80. https://doi.org/10.9758/cpn.2018.16.4.469.

93. F. Corponi, C. Fabbri, A. Serretti. Pharmacogenetics and depression: a critical perspective. *Psychiatry Investig*. 2019;**16**:645–53. https://doi.org/10.30773/pi.2019.06.16.

94. J. F. Greden, S. V. Parikh, A. J. Rothschild, et al. Impact of pharmacogenomics on clinical outcomes in major depressive disorder in the GUIDED trial: a large, patient- and rater-blinded, randomized, controlled study. *J Psychiatr Res*. 2019;**111**:59–67. https://doi.org/10.1016/j.jpsychires.2019.01.003.

95. J. G. Winner, J. M. Carhart, C. A. Altar, et al. Combinatorial pharmacogenomic guidance for psychiatric medications reduces overall pharmacy costs in a 1 year prospective evaluation. *Curr Med Res Opin*. 2015;**31**:1633–43. https://doi.org/10.1185/03007995.2015.1063483.

96. M. Hewett, D. E. Oliver, D. L. Rubin, et al. PharmGKB: the pharmacogenetics knowledge base. *Nucleic Acids Res*. 2002;**30**:163–5. https://doi.org/10.1093/nar/30.1.163.

97. M. V. Relling, T. E. Klein, R. S. Gammal, et al. The Clinical Pharmacogenetics Implementation Consortium: 10 years later. *Clin Pharmacol Ther*. 2020;**107**:171–5. https://doi.org/10.1002/cpt.1651.

98. C. F. Thorn, T. E. Klein, R. B. Altman. PharmGKB: the pharmacogenetics and pharmacogenomics knowledge base. *Methods Mol Biol*. 2005;**311**:179–91. https://doi.org/10.1385/1-59259-957-5:179.

Chapter 2

The Classification of Mood Disorders and the Unipolar/Bipolar Dichotomy

Mutahira M. Qureshi and Allan Young

Introduction

Mood classification in psychiatric nosology has been in a state of flux and faces an existential crisis [1–4]. The word "mood" tends to quickly be followed by "disorder(s)" [5] since it is perhaps the only psychiatric construct where pathology is not immediately apparent without the addition of "disorder" in the name. Since the beginning [6], concepts relating to the two extremes, namely mania and melancholy, have been instinctively understood. Hence it is surprising that the classification and diagnosis of mood disorders are replete with complexities, disagreements, and controversies. In current psychiatric practice, mood disorders are considered both under-diagnosed [7–9] and overdiagnosed [10] at the same time, while also being misdiagnosed in the process [11–13].

A long-standing debate in the field of mood disorders classification is the continuity or spectrum concept of mood disorders, which includes overlapping and dimensional disorders [14] against the categorical split. As we explore in this chapter, both these conceptualizations have been in and out of vogue in the extensive history of mood classification that can be traced back to the earliest formulations. The issue of mood classification reflects the crisis faced by psychiatric nosology, which is then merged with issues deeper still that have to do with the methodological muddles in research and other philosophical dilemmas faced by psychiatry as a specialty of medicine and science. In this chapter, we hope to examine these to grasp the nature of the problem that has engendered much debate and polarization of the psychiatric community. Mood may be like Light that behaves both as particles (or discrete quanta) and as a spectral waveform – an allegory that will be used throughout the chapter (alongside other leanings on physics and mathematics). In the evolution of modern physics there was

much back-and-forth on what the true nature of Light was (particulate or wave), but embracing both these properties has been the single most important paradigm shift that has led to a Kuhnian revolution [15] in the field of physics in the past two centuries. Something similar is needed within the field of affective disorders in psychiatry.

The Odyssey of Mood Classification: Plato's *Theia Mania*, Dürer's *Melancholia*, and Nietzsche's *Eternal Recurrence*

It is beyond the scope of this chapter to capture a full narrative of the history of mood classification from the beginning of recorded civilization to current times. However, in this section we aim to provide a brief overview of the rich and convoluted history steeped in metaphysics, divinity, and controversy, with recommendations for further reading indicated where relevant. While the history of mood classification is deeply interwoven with the history of psychiatric classification in general, we focus on the events that are pertinent only to the former. Histories of psychiatric nosology have been extensively studies by Berrios [16,17], Kendler [3,18–21], and Shorter [4,22] and should be referred to for in-depth knowledge on the subject.

The Distant Past

Our earliest known encounters with mood classification date back to the ancient world. The words "mania" and "melancholia" come from the Greeks and appear to be aetiopathological, conforming to the Greek understanding of neurohumoral mechanisms driving disease processes (e.g., *melancholia* meaning "black bile") [23]. This aetiopathological tradition of the Greeks has continued to dominate Western conceptualization of psychiatry to this day. The Eastern thinking, both in the ancient world of the Indian and the medieval world of the Islamic golden ages, informed by the classical Greek tradition has tended to classify psychiatric phenomena, especially mood, as symptom clusters [24]. In his *Canon,* still considered a seminal work in the field of medicine, Ibn-e-Sina divides mood states into "anxious-depressive cluster", "manic cluster", "psychotic cluster", "cognitive cluster", and "somatic cluster" [25], which then are used to dictate treatment pathways. In his *Kitab al-Adviyt-al-Qalbiye* [The Book on Drugs for Cardiac Diseases], a work less studied by psychiatric historians, Ibn-e-Sina devotes a chapter to depression-anxiety manifestations such as palpitations that are treated with cardiac medications [26]. This suggests that in the Arab medieval world all symptoms were considered transdiagnostic in essence, and Avicenna and his contemporaries would draw classificatory/diagnostic distinctions based on either treatment response or syndromatology [27–29]. Whether these ideas permeated to the West and were incorporated in the clinical practice of the time has been lost to what Angst and Marneros term "the long medieval night" [23]. The next wave in classification is seen in the post-Renaissance seventeenth and eighteenth centuries spurred largely by Linnaeus's taxonomical standards and the boom of botanical and medical taxonomies of the sixteenth and seventeenth centuries [18]. Linnaeus in *Genera Morborum* classifies affective illnesses, for example, as "amentia" (idiotic insanity), "mania" (chronic unsound mind in a furious manner), "daemonia" (partially unsound mind in a demonic, devilish, frightful, and terrible manner), "vesania" (chronic partial unsound manner in a sad and calm manner), and "melancholia" (chronic partially unsound mind in an earnestly sorrowful manner). At this point, the importance of prognostication seems to have appeared as one of the factors to classification, and we can see precursors to modern conceptualizations in this period.

The Recent Past

In the second half of the nineteenth century there was a spurt of interest in psychiatric classification that is beyond the scope of this chapter to discuss in the detail that it merits. Some key features of note, however, include the operationalization of key definitions as we know them today, determining the approaches to classification, and the differing schools of thought that were created as a result.

In the beginning of the nineteenth century the term "melancholia" did not mean depression, it meant any form of insanity [17,23] and "mania" meant any type of agitated excited state, including and often overlapping with general paresis of the insane and other organic syndromes [17,18,30]. Another important concept during this period is that of unitary psychosis, or *Einheitspsychose*, which included all affective and non-affective psychoses in one category that was largely supported by neurologists Neuman and Wernicke. However, towards the mid-nineteenth century with Esquirol's proposal of lypemania and monomania there seems to be a formal identification of the two mood states and their separation from other forms of psychoses [31]. This tradition was carried on by Esquirol's successors, in particular his trainee Falret, who proposed the concept of *la folie circulare* that later led to Kraepelin's unified mania-depressive illness (MDI). While Kraepelin's dichotomy (MDI and dementia praecox [DP]) is considered a key feature of this period; there are several other important concepts to consider. Firstly, this period marks an important point where society was moving away from alienist-led asylums and "scientists" needed to distance themselves as much as possible from the abstract phenomenology to discrete quantifiable and replicative classifications [32,33]. Hence, a psychiatric classification frenzy gripped Europe. This led to the creation of groups that rejected all forms of phenomenology in the interest of "lesional" thinking against those who called such an approach the myth of psychiatry (Jasper's critique of Wernicke) [34,35]. Jaspers purported the idea of embracing the "chaos of the phenomenon" during a formulation and staying away from hardlines of diagnoses. The split became more apparent with their later prodigies (Kraepelin–Schneider for Japers and Kleist–Leonhard for Wernicke). As this tale progresses, the differences between these two schools of thought would become the bedrock of psychiatric classification schemes. The third consideration during this time is the approach. In the classification of psychoses [36,37], Kahlbaum and Hecker postulated the notion of a close correspondence between aetiology, brain pathology, symptom patterns, and outcome as a criterion for assuming that seemingly distinct clinical states and syndromes belong together as a single disease entity. This initially led to the formation of two separate schools of thought:

the Kraepelinian–Bleueler group who proposed their dichotomous nosology of dementia praecox (DP) versus manic depressive psychosis (MDP) / manic depressive insanity (MDI) primarily on the basis that the former has an unfavourable long-term prognosis than the latter: DP was understood to be chronic, progressively deteriorating and MDP to be relapsing-remitting with near-full recovery in the intervening periods. The second group, led by Berze and Hoche (1912) [38], rejected diagnosis made on longitudinal course and instead proposed "cross-sectional" classification based on symptom clusters, which they defined as overlapping, thereby reflecting overlapping disease processes. However, it was the former group that prevailed and to this day we conceptualize psychiatric diagnosis and treatments in broadly Kraepelinian terms. Angst and Marneros dub him as the greatest "lumper" of diagnoses, but if anything, Kraepelin proposed the first proper split between the various endogenous psychoses previously lumped within the unitary class by creating two separate entities based on a lifetime of observational research on the longitudinal course: MDI/MDP (manic depressive insanity / manic depressive psychosis) and DP (dementia praecox). His six gradations of mixed states also fundamentally demonstrate his tendency to fine-tune rather than lump, and while longer term prognoses of favourable versus non-favourable course will remain contentious, especially between bipolar disorder as we understand it today and schizophrenia spectrum. Nevertheless, his observations on degenerative processes (or dementia) inherent to one and not the other remain intact to this day [39–42]. The fourth important development during this time is the idea of depression. Depression initially was split across several subtypes from "neurotic" (reactive, which Schneider did not consider "proper" to be termed true depressions if they emerged out of life changes) to involutional, climacteric, and so on. Depression too was unified as a single "unitary" entity during this period (excellent papers by Sir Martin Roth summarize this [43,44]) by the Mapother-Aubrey Lewis group in the UK, which at the time was opposed by Gillespie and Schneider [43]. Hence depression as we know it today with its extensive heterogeneity was conceptualized during this period. This period defines the boundaries of classification and sets the stage for the next wave of frenzy triggered by innovations in psychiatric pharmacology.

The Present Past

The 1950/60s saw the development of several key psychiatric drugs within a short succession, just as the West had come out of two wars that had shaped the consciousness of psychiatric practice with the forays of Nazis in eugenics and spurred the exodus of a great number of academics from all fields including psychiatry from Europe to the United States. This period is often described as the first wave of biological psychiatry, and the beginning of the US dominance (dubbed hegemony by some authors [45]) in psychiatry. In terms of mood classification, this period would start with the independent and simultaneous proposal by Jules Angst and Carlos Perris to break MDI into unipolar depression and bipolar affective illnesses (in a series of studies between 1911 and 1953 originally Kleist disagreed with Kraepelin's concept, differentiating between unipolar [*einpolig*] and bipolar [*zweipolig*] affective disorders). They also noted that Leonhard developed Kleist's approach in publications between 1934 and 1957, but they added that neither Kleist nor Leonhard considered monopolar mania to be a component of bipolar disorders in present-day terms, a tradition that was also built upon by Marneros, Winokur, and neo-Wernicke-Kleistians such as Neele and Leonhard. This period marks an exceptionally increased aversion to all forms of phenomenology and an equally overvalued idea of pinning down the hard biology of psychiatric phenomena: biomarkers, genes, and brain lesions. This plays out on a very complex backdrop of the rise of corporate pharmaceuticals, several key changes in legislature that enable these pharmaceuticals not only to embed as a stakeholder in healthcare but also to powerfully influence research and information handling within health systems.

In 1970s Dunner et al. added bipolar II (major depression and hypomania) to Angst-Perris's (mania and depression). During this time psychiatrists appear to have become increasingly aware of the heterogeneity of biological correlates, leading to Crow proposing a reunion of all psychoses back to the unitary status [46] of earlier, and Akiskal et al. proposing the concept of "soft bipolarity", thereby harkening back to Kraepelin's MDI [47–49]. Akiskal et al.'s concept of bipolar spectrum proposed at the turn of the millennium has gained traction [50], although the concept of bipolarity has more or less remained intact: the notion that depression can exist on its own in unipolar form, but mania cannot [51]. However, some recent contributions in this field, as will be discussed below, especially those by Ghaemi et al [52–56] and Benazzi et al. [14,57,58], are perhaps a move towards the unification of all moods on a single spectrum, as envisioned by Kraepelin.

The Anatomy of Classification

Classification involves the assignment of something to a class, which in turn is the collection of objects that share some property. In the broad sense this should involve the correct identification of the properties of the objects of study that set it apart from other seemingly similar objects [59] – an interesting conundrum for psychiatry. Moreover, since classification relies on identifying properties of the object being classified, perfect classification would require perfect knowledge of the object [59]. Otherwise, without both components the classification system produced would be consistent with Borges's fictitious taxonomy of a menagerie in his *The Analytical Language of John Wilkins* (which was intended as a critique of the named philosopher's treatise):

> It is written that animals are divided into: (a) those that belong to the Emperor, (b) embalmed ones, (c) those that are trained, (d) suckling pigs, (e) mermaids, (f) fabulous ones, (g) stray dogs, (h) those that are included in this classification, (i) those that tremble as if they were mad, (j) innumerable ones, (k) those drawn with a very fine camel's-hair brush, (l) others, (m) those that have just broken a flower vase, (n) those that resemble flies from a distance.

In medicine, classification ideally accompanies aetiopathological processes unifying cause, symptom cluster, treatment, and prognosis in a smooth and linear manner. There are medical specialties where this clean linearity is compromised such as in the field of oncology where aetiology remains multifactorial and largely unknown. Hence there, the reliance for classification in oncology is solely on histopathological findings or morphology of the tumour. However, the process of epistemological iteration holds true even then due to consistency in treatment response for patients with similar tumour morphology and so on. In psychiatry, epistemological iterative process while coveted [60] cannot be the sole summation of arriving at the goal, and as Kendler himself concedes, can only lead to "wobbly iterations". This is because the process of epistemological iteration relies on the principle that in order to have

one justified belief, one must have infinitely many justified beliefs of increasing complexity (and not all subjects can tolerate this extent of higher-order iteration). Berrios [16] argues the need for epistemological iterative models for *inexact* sciences such as psychology and psychiatry; however, other philosophers have argued that in science exactness is a myth and all absolute entities (temperature, distance, etc.) are relative to each other, with the universal absolute/constant unknown [61].

Conceptualizing classification as an epistemological iterative process, however, disregards the *a priori* principle that is inherent to most of psychiatry but especially mood. Unlike some other psychiatric entities like some forms of psychoses, we all inherently know what sorrow or joy, and their respective escalations, should feel like; and hence there are already boundary limitations in place of what mood can be or should be. This recalls Kantian transcendental idealism from which the classification exercise can try but never fully escape. Kant argues that transcendental ego (subject/perceiver) constructs knowledge out of sense impressions and from the universal concepts that it imposes upon them – a theory that has been existence since the ancient Greeks (Xenophanes) or medieval period (Algazel). As has already been demonstrated, this becomes important, since the earliest description of mania from the Classical period are those that were previously imbued in the metaphysical and have now been inherited almost intact in our current point in nosological history.

So why classify at all? Berrios [16] in his book on the history of descriptive psychopathology quotes the Sapir-Whorf hypothesis as laid out in Whorf's 1956 text *Language, Thought and Reality* to answer this. "We cut nature up, organize it into concepts, and ascribe significances as we do, largely because we are parties to an agreement that holds throughout our speech community and is codified in the patterns of our language ... we cannot talk at all except by subscribing to the organization and classification of data which the agreement decrees."

A similar thought is echoed by the physicist Heisenberg, who will ultimately give his name to the famous "uncertainty principle" in quantum physics, in his treatise *Physics and Philosophy*: "What we observe is not nature itself, but nature exposed to our method of questioning."

Thus, especially in case of psychiatry, where inexactness persists, it is important to start with the question of why a particular classification or diagnosis is being attempted in the first place, since the demands on a classification system vary from making treatment decisions to claiming reimbursement from insurance agencies [62]. Malhi et al. (2016) identify four distinct beneficiaries of a psychiatric classification system. These include patients and their families; clinicians; scientists/clinical researchers; and governmental agencies, insurance companies, and the legal profession [1] – all have differing needs, with different uses and requiring different applications from a diagnostic system. This is why it is imperative to be aware of the underlying "needs" of the classification process as well as the history of that shaped current concepts and perhaps gives rise to the notion that a single classification system will perhaps always be inadequate to satisfy these varying needs and society will shape the classification process with modification of anchors around which classification systems are built (the medieval people's need to ascribe the divine to mania and our own to ascribe a specific neurological pathway to it are a similar phenomenon at its core), and will evolve in the face of economic and political factors [62–64] in the cycle of Great Recurrence that Nietzsche believes all natural phenomenon undergo.

The Clash of Semantics and Other Tales of Physics, Poetics, and Philosophy

Semantics are the core of psychiatry because language is used to express its symptoms, diagnosis, and treatment (such as psychotherapy). In the case of mood classification there remain certain unresolved conflicts when it comes to terminologies.

In fact, to begin with, the very definition of "mood" has remained neglected. Is mood a feeling, emotion, thought, response of the body? Diagnostically it is all of these; and yet the concept remains embedded in colloquialism, literary romance, and philosophy. Within psychiatric terms, it is possible to be diagnosed with MDD without true deep melancholia, and mania without the classic "euphoria" [33]. Hence the *scientific* mood is different from the philosophical and instinctive understandings of the same concept – which perhaps are closer to singularities like "emotion" than the composite. The word "singularity" here is also not coincidental since it is apropos to the philosophical crisis of defining emotion, like mathematical singularities that are defined as points where a mathematical object is not

"well-behaved"; for example, it is either infinite or not differentiable. In philosophy, constitutive and causal evaluative theories for emotion emerge [65–68]. Constitutive theories state that emotions are cognitions or evaluations of particular kinds, whereas causal theories state that emotions are caused by cognitions or evaluations of particular kinds. Hence it is evident that despite an instinctual understanding of mood, we don't really have means to verbalize it without borrowing from domains of cognition and physical symptoms. (A similar observation is made by Buonomano [69] in relation to Time: despite being universally understood in our language, we only refer to time in terms of distance: looking *forward*, in *hindsight*, *long* day, etc., while the two are discrete concepts in physics).

When referring to any mood or psychiatric classifications, we naturally mean *Diagnostic and Statistical Manual / International Classification of Diseases* (DSM/ICD) systems; however, the former (and broadly both) are diagnostic systems per se. While little distinction is drawn between the two since they serve semantical quibbles on qualia, classification and diagnosis are subtly different processes; the former aims to find commonality between large patient groups and the latter to distil the ailment experienced by the individual patient into a single explanation. When disease aetiology is well defined such as in gout and Lyme disease, diagnostic and classification criteria may be very similar and used interchangeably [70]; however, in certain medical specialties like rheumatology and psychiatry, that is not always the case. Since the aim during the diagnostic process is to fit the morbidity of a patient inside one of the boxes in the available diagnostic classification, when performing a diagnosis, we also carry out a classification process [71]. For the purpose of this chapter, we will be treating them as the same.

Another semantic conflict in the current psychiatric literature is the simultaneous use of such words as "dimension", "syndromatology", "phenotype", "symptom-cluster", "continuum", "spectrum", and "domains" almost interchangeably to describe similar underlying concepts of the multifaceted nature of mood. Are they the same things and do clear operational definitions exist? In medicine, a syndrome is a validated symptom-complex (e.g., Horner's syndrome), whereas a disease (such as Berger's disease) is a validated phenotype, and the two are usually differentiated based on a defined cause. Symptom-clusters suggest the existence of categories, that is, entities of different essence. The same goes for dimensions and domains. Mathematically, dimensions are vectors or axes, whereas domains are areas of study that are bounded by coordinates in the axial space. In mood classification, "dimensional" approach is usually reserved when talking about personality overlaps, while "domains" are used to denote symptom clusters such as level of activity or cognition. However, both these terminologies can sometimes to be treated as synonymous within the literature (e.g., Henry et al.'s [72] "dimensional" approach to mood, which uses symptom cluster "domains" as diagnostic anchors).

Mathematically speaking; since math is the alleged language of all sciences, mood is complex because it can be conceptualized as the following:

1) a polynomial function in a multidimensional system to the nth dimension solved on the basis of Taylor approximations (which supports the transdiagnostic symptoms argument);

2) an ergodic measure-preserving dynamical system like that of Poincaré, which states that certain systems will, after a sufficiently long but finite time, return to a state very close to the initial state (which supports the spectrum/ continuum argument); and

3) as a Kolmogorov Complexity, which can be thought of as the minimal description of an arbitrary string that can include algorithms within Algorithmic Information Theory and is the basis of heuristics and compression solutions in machine learning. This latter is like the medieval concept of Occam's razor, which states that "entities" (or here mood symptom complexes with their many permutations) "should not be multiplied beyond necessity" (which supports the categorical classification argument) (Figure 2.1).

Eventually all classification is very much like the quantum phenomenon of the collapse of the Copenhagen waveform with the introduction of an observer. So, while the patient's experience of the mood symptoms in all its permutations can be varied and multiple outcomes possible, but diagnosis at a single point in time reduces those possibilities to singular entities, which supports the categorical approach to classification/diagnosis.

Other considerations in the mood classificatory process that are reliant on the research conducted within the area include methodological muddles [75–77] like randomized controlled trial (RCT) "supernatant effects" [78] selecting patients for response and the Silberzahn problem of "one data set and many analysts" [79,80] (examples from

history: two separate re-analyses of Aubrey Lewis's thesis come to different conclusions about the unitary nature of MDD) that have their own bearings in the empirical, data-driven, pure *a posteriori* aspiration towards classificatory schemes in mood.

Theoretical Modelling of Mood

The authors of this chapter, as per many in the field of mood classification today, subscribe to the view that the concept of mood on a continuum is not only plausible based on intuition and clinical observation but also natural. However, within this fluid spectrum are discrete mood phenomena that are diagnosable/ classifiable entities. The authors conceptualize the two ends of the spectrum to be bounded by pure activation/ excitement and pure depression, with transdiagnostic symptoms, such as sleep, cognition, that together form the composite that we understand as mood (see Figure 2.3). Hence it is possible, as in the tradition of oncological tumour–node–metastasis (TNM) staging, that mood would be expressed as a notation of its symptoms, for example, melancholia–sleep–volition– suicidality M5,S3,V4,Sd8, and so on. These individual mood states, when considered over time will in an individual patient form a definitive diagnosis. Hence each individual mood episode even in the same patient might not be alike but their crystallization overtime might generate a comparable commonality that could be termed as "classes" when they are seen within population groups (see Figure 2.2).

This is a highly idealized and theoretical approach (much like theoretical physics where any attempt to unravel the phenomenon of spacetime beyond a single particle brings down all known knowledge and tears the fabric of the known physical Universe apart); however, it is the hope of the authors that the reader takes away from this the ultimate point that without integration of both phenomenology in its infinite qualia with the neurobiology, classificatory systems will continue to fail psychiatry [35,82].

The Nature of Light: Arguments for Particle and Wave Theory

In current literature, there are several valid arguments made for both the discrete categorization of depression, mania, and schizophrenia/schizoaffective spectrum and the various "continuum" arguments with differing poles. In the continuum camp there are two

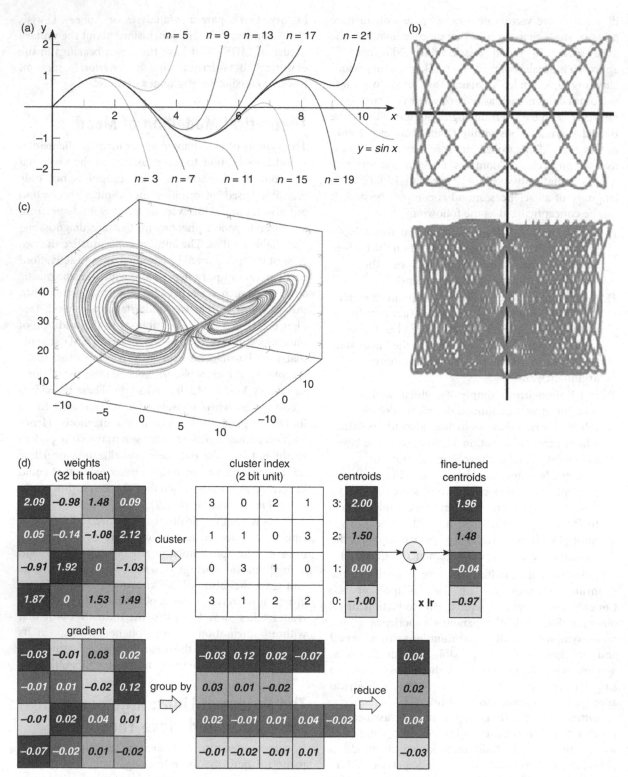

Figure 2.1 (a) Mood conceptualized as a Taylor series of a function, which is an infinite sum of terms that are expressed in terms of the function's derivatives at a single point (the episode where a mood diagnosis/ classification is considered), where n (the Taylor polynomial) can be understood both as the extent of core symptoms at presentation and number of episodes – that is, evidence accrued

schools of thought: one is of unifying all affective disorders along a continuum, and the second is unifying all chronic enduring affective psychotic disorders along a continuum (in the original unitary psychosis line of thinking). There is also a third, less adhered-to variant, which considers bipolarity and schizoaffective-schizophrenia as a single spectrum. The current DSM 5, while not fully conforming to it, does place bipolar disorder in between schizophrenia and depression "in recognition of their place as a bridge between the two diagnostic classes in terms of symptomatology, family history and genetics" [83], thereby demoting them as transitional states rather than an autonomous disorder complex of their own. In Table 2.1 we summarize the current argument for both [84–132]. The categorization camp draws most of its arguments in phenomenology and quality of depressive/affective states (described as pleomorphic [133]) experienced in all three diagnostic categories: schizophrenia/schizoaffective, bipolar disorder, and unipolar depression. The dimensional/continuum camp, however, draws its arguments from the fact that despite the introduction of the split in the 1960–1980s era, which was to aid with pinning down the biological tenets, there remains a great degree of heterogeneity and overlap in genetics, receptor and neurotransmitter profile, and neural circuitry [134].

The Four Questions of the Mood Classification

As Benazzi et al. [123] state, "in the extreme states, mood is very well delineated and categorical". Mania is perhaps the most conserved and valid clinical syndrome within psychiatry [6]. However, it is in "midway" disorders (BD2 and MDD plus bipolar signs) where a continuity/spectrum concept seems supported. In this section we discuss four mood concepts that throw current classification systems in a state of constant crisis.

Unipolar Mania

There is growing evidence from epidemiological, clinical and genetic studies that unipolar mania is a distinct disorder [135–138]. A recent analysis of data from seven epidemiological studies of adults found BD1 (mania with major depressive disorder) in 323 subjects and pure mania in 109, a relatively rare but separate diagnosis [139]. However, in current classification systems unipolar mania is not recognized as a standalone diagnosis, and its presence inevitably leads to a diagnosis of BD1. ICD/DSM recognize that a hypomanic episode should be carefully distinguished from euthymia during a period of recovery from a depressive episode [139]; however, a similar consideration is not extended to recovery from mania [140]. If unipolar mania is recognized as a diagnosis, then it will stand to reason that all mood states are bound between two "extremes" of mania and MDD and on a single spectrum, harkening back to Kraepelin's original manic-depressive illness.

Atypical Depression or Mixed Depressive States? The MDD Spectrum

Atypical depression is understood to have core features of depression accompanied by severe anxiety or by atypical vegetative symptoms, that is, increased appetite, weight, sleep, or libido in the early classifications, in particular Davidson et al. [141]. Many of the

---

Caption for Figure 2.1 (cont.)

across both cross-sectional and longitudinal morphology. Despite iterative attempts, an exact solution that overlies the graph of the function completely within the polynomial approximations is impossible. Another curious thing of note is that the accurate approximations are provided within a range, so too less information to start with ($n = 3$) and too many possible infinite sums of symptoms and presentations ($n = 21$) can both cause gross divergence away from the function – hence the considerations around fixing thresholds (knowing where to start – that is, where departure from normality has taken place and where to stop – that is, enough evidence has been accrued to satisfy classification) in the diagnostic process is of great import. **(b)** and **(c)** conceptualize mood as an ergodicity. **(b)** is a graphical two-dimensional system proposed by Boltzmann where for each value of x an infinity of values for y in any interval in its range are possible, and all points in the system are eventually crossed [73] (which supports the spectrum/continuum hypothesis and soft bipolarity). However, this is refuted under the Wernicke–Kleist–Leonhard (WKL) system where certain combinations of mood symptoms are simply not possible and hence would not conform to ergodic transformation. **(c)** is a case of the Lorenz system, where trajectories settle onto a "strange attractor", which is defined as an attractor that exhibits sensitive dependence on initial conditions, which is to say that two trajectories starting arbitrarily close together on the attractor rapidly diverge from each other [74], which supports the dimensional-domain approach where once domains are fixed as "anchors" all states within that domain are possible. **(d)** is an example of the deep learning mechanism in machine learning called "quantization", where the number of bits needed to store each weight in the Neural Network are reduced through weight sharing. This supports the categorical view that eventually key symptoms will conglomerate to form a diagnosis since it is not possible to factor all possible permutations within the classification/diagnostic systems.

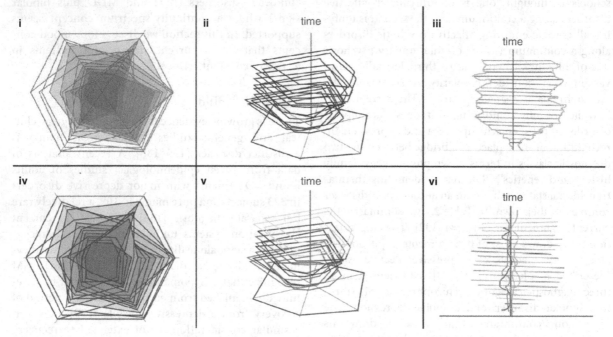

Figure 2.2 Hypothetical representation of the concept using a temporal radar plot [81] of individual mood episodes. (i–iii) show episodes over time in one single patient, and (iv–vi) show mood states for multiple patients. The symptoms plotted against severity and time, here limited to six, however, can, in theory, be extended further not just to incorporate symptom clusters but also quantifiable response to treatment trials, relevant biomarkers, polygenic risk scores, and so on. As evident, no two episodes in one patient or episodes in different patients are identical; however, they give rise to a manifold, that is, a topological space, that locally resembles Euclidean space near each point.

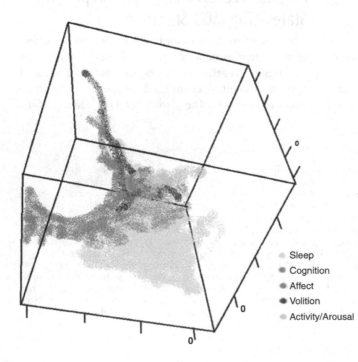

Figure 2.3 Multidimensional scaling with the 5D representations of mood notational staging of a single patient as a hyperbolic manifold in Euclidean space bounded, in Jasper and McHugh's tradition, within a patient's temperament, personality, life events, socio-cultural localization, level of functionality, comorbidities, and so on. It is here that the framework traverses from experimental to theoretical because while these changes can be clinically understood and stochastically factored in individual formulations, it would be impossible to quantify and code them within a predictive algorithm. Hence, while there will continue to be a drive towards numeric reduction of symptoms and matching them to both biological and genetic markers and treatments, a full diagnosis would only be possible within a combined neurobiological–phenomenological framework. So, *classification* at *population* levels, proviso clearly delineated zones of rarity emerge within symptom clusters is possible without inclusion of phenomenology; however, *diagnosis* at an *individual* patient level cannot escape from it – as theorized by Jaspers in his aptly worded view on grouping psychiatric presentations that one must instead embrace the "chaos of the phenomenon" [34].

Table 2.1 Categories versus continua

Categorization defence	Continuum of mood (BD+MDD) only	Continuum of psychoses (BD and SCZ/SAf spectrum)	The affective–psychotic continuum (MDD+BD+SCZ/SAf)
- Age of onset (MDD variable, BD/SCZ late adolescent) - Gender (MDD female preponderance, SCZ slight male, BD 1:1) - Onset (MDD: insidious vs. BD-mania abrupt, SCZ: variable) - Family History: BD more common in families of BD probands than in families of MDD probands - Varied duration of both depressions: BD depressions more prolonged and do not respond to traditional first line antidepressants - Higher suicidal ideation in bipolar depression, while unipolar depression has more anxiety features - MDD presents with more agitation which bipolar depression as retardation - Sleep: insomnia prevalent in MDD as opposed to hypersomnia in bipolar depression	- GWAS overlap between MDD and BD, with MDD being the most common mood disorder in BD families - Diagnostic conversion overtime from MDD to BD - Cyclicality and recurrence - Symptom profile: less frequent paranoid delusions / hallucinations and negative symptoms when compared to SCZ/SAf - The lithium test: therapeutic specificity of lithium to affective presentations - Similar psychosocial and cognitive impairments - No bimodality of lifetime manic and hypomanic symptoms in BD and MDD, and of cross-sectional hypomanic symptoms between bipolar depression and MDD - Frequent lifetime manic/hypo manic symptoms in MDD. Depression most prevalent mood state in all types of BD MDD spectrum: proof in response to antidepressants - Categorical classification of mood relies on the recognition of hypomanic episodes that often are not recognized by the patient and require extensive collateral history taking	- Psychotic episodes more prevalent in bipolar vs. unipolar depression - Higher prevalence of positive symptomatology in BD-SAf-SCZ spectrum - Risk of psychosis in first-degree relatives of probands - Similar treatment profiles both in acuity and maintenance phase of the illness as compared to MDD	- Similar shared polygenic component and lack of discriminative accuracy between them as discrete entities in severity. - Treatment parallels and overlaps with very little discrimination in treatment profiles as severity increases for all these disorders. - Grossly, all conform to the rule of thirds in their longitudinal course with at least a third of patients who have a chronic non-remitting and enduring illness profile. - Lack of the "zone of rarity" in clinical and biological features, which refers to the hiatus between the features of a biological disorder with a clear diagnosis and other conditions that do not carry this diagnosis.

Abbreviations: BD: bipolar disorder, GWAS: genome-wide association studies; MDD: major depressive disorder/unipolar depression, SAf: schizoaffective, SCZ: schizophrenia.

features associated with atypical depression are linked to an early onset of affective illness, including trait-like interpersonal sensitivity, comorbid social anxiety and agoraphobia, a history of childhood physical or sexual trauma, and indicators of the "soft" side of the bipolar spectrum. Neurophysiological studies also suggest that chronic, early-onset atypical depressions differ from both melancholia and normality [142]. Atypical depression came into being because of pharmacological specificity [143–145] to monoamine oxidase inhibitors (MAOIs) versus tricyclic anti-depressants (TCAs) (findings that were later dis-proved as more data accrued) and reinforces the categorical "typicality" (and thus atypicality) para-digm. Atypical features specifiers for MDD show weak internal consistency; the mandatory criterion of mood reactivity does not show specificity in rela-tion to any of the four accessory symptoms [146]. Within the class of bipolar disorders atypical depres-sion would be understood as depression with contra-polar symptoms, and hence a mixed episode or mixed feature specifier would be a more readily assumed diagnosis. Atypical depression shares features with BD2 or soft bipolar spectrum disorder, and studies have shown that a significantly higher frequency of atypical depressive symptoms such as hypersomnia and hyperphagia are found in bipolar than unipolar group. This has led to the proponents of mood spec-trum concept such as Benazzi and Akiskal to question whether atypical depression is a variant of BD2 or a bridge between MDD and BD2.

In recent years, the concepts of depressive mixed states and MDD spectrum have gained traction [147–154]. This is based on the increasing identification of hypomanic symptoms (using the Hypomania Checklist (HCL), etc.) in unipolar depression patients [107], often in more severe, chronic, and recurring forms of MDD. In one study, intuitive omitting of mood stem questions on Mini International Psychiatric Interview (MINI) in patients with MDD reveal a high prevalence of other hypomanic/manic symptoms. This also gives rise to the question of whether MDD with mixed features, atypical depres-sion, and bipolar depression are nuances of essentially the same concept that Ghaemi, Benazzi, and even Angst [155] recognize to be a feature of the entirety of mood spectrum, and whether cyclic and recurrent forms of unipolar depression should be included in a bipolar spectrum [141,156].

Ghaemi and Dalley [112] visualize depression as a spectrum from neurotic, vascular, pure, mixed, and melancholic in increasing severity and decreasing order of recurrence. This is supported by the argu-ment that the sobering conclusions from the NIMH-sponsored STEP-BD and STAR*D projects can in part be explained by failure to distinguish depressive con-ditions, particularly bipolar features, that are inher-ently less responsive to antidepressants [110].

Subsyndromal or "Soft Bipolarity" and the Bipolar Spectrum

The concept of soft bipolarity owes its rediscovery (since Kraepelin) to the efforts of Akiskal [106,157,158], who noticed persistence of subthreshold bipolarity clinically that would often converge on BD NOS type diagnoses. The concept was then further developed by Goodwin and Ghaemi, who proposed their definition/classifica-tion of the "bipolar spectrum" [159]. This included:

A. At least one major depressive episode

B. No spontaneous hypomanic or manic episodes

C. Either of the following, plus at least 2 items from criterion D, or both of the following plus 1 item from criterion D:

1. A family history of bipolar disorder in a first-degree relative

2. Antidepressant-induced mania or hypomania

D. If no items from criterion C are present, 6 of the following 9 criteria are needed:

1. Hyperthymic personality (at baseline, non-depressed state)

2. Recurrent major depressive episodes (> 3)

3. Brief major depressive episodes (on average, < 3 months)

4. Atypical depressive symptoms (DSM-IV criteria)

5. Psychotic major depressive episodes

6. Early age of onset of major depressive episode (< age 25)

7. Postpartum depression

8. Antidepressant "wear-off" (acute but not prophylactic response)

9. Lack of response to 3 antidepressant treatment trials

Clinical studies show that most mood episodes are not purely depressive or manic, but mixed, and hence it is difficult to create a stable and valid nosology on what is "uncommon" or distinct that sets apart one mood state from another [125,130]. This is further validated by weakening of the distinction between different "depressions" (bipolar vs. unipolar) in terms of treatment specificity, symptomatology, and family history, since treatment specificity was considered a diagnostic confirmation in the early years of psychopharmacology. This is reminiscent of Kraepelin's manic depressive psychosis category (and the reason for its enduring appeal) where all morphologies of mood are included under a single umbrella, including temperament, personality nuances, inter-episodic mood fluctuations, and mood fluctuations without formal or clearly delineated episodes that would not reach "caseness". He termed all of these "affective tendencies" that lie in between the two clearly demarcated and identifiable poles of unipolar mania and unipolar depression. Even in his own lifetime he attempted to refine these gradations further by classifying mixed states in six different subtypes, although these are states above the threshold of caseness and presenting with a mixture of symptoms from both poles.

The importance of understanding subsyndromal states and their natural course is of utmost import in furthering our understanding of true remission and relapse. How much of persistent symptomatology after an acute episode is too much and hence should be a relapse and how much of it is to be expected as part of the natural fluctuation on the normal spectrum?

While some of the original strict categorical proponents, especially Jules Angst and Goodwin have been won over to the spectrum approach, Ghaemi considers the classification to be antithetical to spectrum approach [112]. Some of the key critics of the bipolar spectrum today include Malhi et al. and Baldessarini based on typically "preserved" symptomatology and diagnostic validity of bipolar disorders [6], and David Healy, who cautions against the "epidemic" of diagnosis if the existing defined boundaries of bipolar syndromes are removed completely. Figure 2.4 [160] presents mood as a composite score, while Figure 2.5 represents mood as a spectrum using a quaternary phase diagram.

Affective Temperaments and Personalities: Kraepelin's View of "Affective Tendencies"

Affective temperaments are defined as relatively stable, trait-like expressions of affect that convey risk for mood psychopathology [161,162] and are

operationalized in four types: dysthymic, cyclothymic, irritable, and hyperthymic based on Kraepelin's classification. Affective temperaments have features that are common with "normal" dimensions of personality such as the Five-Factor Model (FFM) [163] and account for unique variance in measures of psychopathology, impairment, and daily-life experiences. Specifically, cyclothymic/irritable temperament is shown to predict bipolar disorders, impairment, borderline personality traits, urgency, and anger in daily life. Hyperthymic temperament, on the other hand, has been shown to predict hypomanic episodes, grandiosity, sensation seeking, and increased activity in daily life [163]. Psychiatric classification has oscillated between the placement of dysthymia and cyclothymia as mood disorders (state disorders) or as personality disorders (trait disorders) [140]. For emotionally unstable/borderline types and their relationship with the affective disorders there is a great difference of opinion. Ghaemi et al. perceive it to be markedly different: one is an illness / disease process, in the tradition of Kraepelin, and the other is a clinical picture but not a "disease" and dubs any symptom similarity between them to be purely superficial [112]. Akiskal [49,105,128,164–167] and Marneros and Angst [23] view personality disorders as a chronic type of mood disorder. Studies have shown that patients with hyperthymic temperaments belong to the bipolar spectrum and certain subtypes of personality disorders (histrionic, borderline, narcissistic) may also belong to cyclothymic temperaments. Angst and Marneros (2001) view temperaments-personalities to be both precursors to chronic mood disorder and a product of enduring mood changes [23].

Some studies, however, argue that the notion of personality disorders as stable and enduring as opposed to periodic-episodic mood have persisted despite evidence that mood can also run a chronic course, and personality disorders are not necessarily persistent over time [168,169]. The Collaborative Longitudinal Personality Disorder study, for example [170], demonstrated that 33–55% of personality disorder patients experienced a remission on a blind retest at 6 months, and at 2 years' follow-up 50–60% were below threshold for personality disorder diagnosis. When conceptualizing personality disorders, a chronic debilitating course is often assumed, whereas mood is largely conceptualized as relapsing–remitting with inter-episode gain of

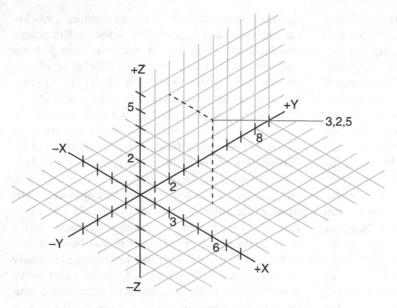

Figure 2.4 Mood as a composite of symptom type (–X = depression, X0 = euthymia, +X = mania), time (–Y = pre-index episode, Y0 = index episode, +Y = post-index episode), severity (–Z = subsyndromal, Z0 = threshold for "caseness", +Z = increasing severity). A hypothetical point X,Y,Z (3,2,5) corresponds to predominant severe manic symptoms that reach a threshold for a formal episode, and appears to be the third formal mood episode. Likely this conforms to a clinical diagnosis of BD1.

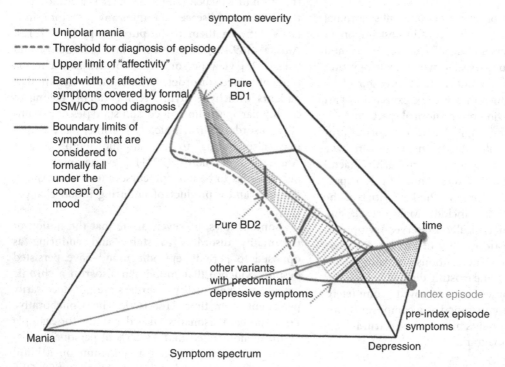

Figure 2.5 Mood represented as a quaternary phase diagram, bounded between symptoms, time, and symptom severity. As can be seen, current inclusion of affective symptoms is very strict from a diagnostic point of view. Affective symptoms prior to first formal mood episode are either understood as subsyndromal or prodromal or within the context of personality. The upper limit of affectivity is the threshold of symptom severity that usually leads to diagnostic revisions from a mood disorder to a psychotic disorder (usually schizoaffective) since current clinical understanding grasps mood to be less severe and intractable than schizoaffective and higher order psychotic illnesses. The empty space of the prism represents a gamut of affective symptoms in various combinations of symptom type, severity, and time that do not have a place within the categorical concept of mood.

functionality; however, this can often present interchangeably, such that mood can have a chronic course with loss of function and personality disorders can maintain functionality in between acute episodes.

Furthermore, in terms of family history, Skodol et al. [170] report that prevalence of mood disorder in borderline personality disorder ranges from 6 to 50% in various studies compared to age-adjusted morbidity risk of borderline PD in borderline PD, which is reported variously in literature as 1–25%. There are also considerations of overlap between BD2 that has many features suggestive of a chronic trait disorder (such as dysthymic mood) rather than an episodic state disorder. Hence, the exact placement of and relationship between temperament–personality– mood will be the subject of ongoing nosological and ontological [112] debate. The split is also further emphasized in DSM-5 and ICD-11, discussed in the next section.

As current evidence stands, each of these four concepts perhaps "bleeds into" the other, with atypical depression overlapping with the bipolar spectrum / soft bipolarity, which in turn overlaps with the cyclothymic / hyperthymic temperaments which then have an overlap with personality types such as borderline. This is diagrammatically represented in Figure 2.6, adapted from Kupier et al. [171].

Current State of the Art: Summary of Mood Classification in DSM-5 and ICD-11

Published online in 2018, ICD-11 is projected to replace the ICD-10 in clinical use by 2022. The ICD review process has taken over ten years, partly overlapping with the fifth revision of the DSM of the American Psychiatric Association (APA), the DSM-5, which was completed in 2013 [172]. Here we review the key features of both these diagnostic criteria for mood disorders and areas where they converge and diverge.

In terms of structure and organization, in DSM-5 bipolar disorders have been separated in their own chapter and placed between Schizophrenia and Depression, whereas in ICD-11 mood disorders are a superordinate grouping of Bipolar and Depressive Disorders. The DSM repositioning has been viewed by some authors to be an "intermediate position" of bipolar disorders, and their conceptualization as a transitional state is critical to the debate of unipolarity versus bipolarity of mood versus unitary psychoses. As far as depression is concerned, both DSM and ICD have remained consistent in the unitary approach to depression, as the composite major depressive disorder (MDD), and mania in both does not have a unipolar status. The ICD also followed the

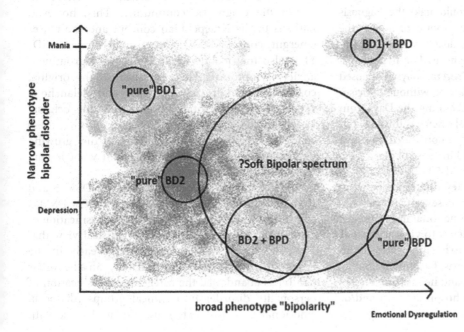

Figure 2.6 Adapted from Kuiper et al. [171] showing the overlap between classic manic-depressive illness, also referred by them as "narrow-phenotype BD", and subsyndromal mood instability, referred to as "broad phenotype BD" lying in between bipolar disorder (or pure affective spectrum) and borderline personality disorder (or affective personality constructs). BD1: bipolar disorder type 1, BD2: bipolar disorder type 2, and BPD: borderline personality disorder

DSM in introducing "qualifiers" (corresponding to DSM-5 "specifiers") to the diagnoses of mood disorders, based on specific aspects of symptomatology or course. While both DSM and ICD remain strictly categorical classificatory systems, DSM-5 with its recognition of "Depression with mixed features" and its new positioning of the chapters is perhaps a move towards recognizing one aspect of the "spectrum", while ICD's clinician-led distinction between chronic bipolar II disorder and personality disorder [140], including key modifications in the duration criteria for personality disorders, is a move towards recognition of another aspect of the spectrum of mood illness. In both DSM-5 and ICD-11, severity of the illness is not measured in terms of the number of symptoms but rather in the intensity of the individual symptom and the functional impairment as a result.

The gate question for mania/hypomania in both DSM and ICD has been modified to include not just euphoria, irritability, or expansiveness, but also increased activity or subjective experience of increased energy (criterion A). In addition, in ICD-11 "several" or three or more in DSM-5 of the seven symptoms (distractibility, flight of ideas, etc.) present for seven days or more are required for the diagnosis of mania. In case of criterion A this is viewed as both redundant [140] and restrictive [7], and perhaps derives from the semantic considerations and definitions of "mood", because it is possible to have depression without any melancholic mood or mania without any euphoric mood [33]. However, others argue that it would make the diagnosis more specific [173]. Another key point of note is the elimination of antidepressant-induced mania or hypomania as an exclusion for diagnosis. For hypomania, ICD-11 defines the duration as "several" days as opposed to 4 days in DSM-5, which is not without criticism (Malhi et al.'s 2019 editorial "Counting the Days from Bipolar II to Bipolar True!" [174] discusses this in excellent detail). This is also further demonstrated by Angst et al., who report almost twofold increase of diagnosing hypomania in ICD-11 versus DSM-5 [172].

Apart from duration, the key difference between mania and hypomania is based on severity (a composite of symptom intensity and functional impairment). While clinically there is a tendency to view severity as either a manic episode leading to hospitalization or an episode with features of psychosis, functional impairment requires clinical scrutiny and needs to be understood beyond the confines of hospitalization and/or severe risk incidents.

The DSM-5 also introduces the concept that BD2 is not a "milder" form of BD1, despite the fact that, according to clinical descriptions, the primary difference is the presence of hypomania rather mania [140]. Both DSM and ICD are identical in their criteria for BD2: one major depressive episode (lasting at least 2 weeks) and a hypomanic episode (lasting at least 4 days / several days).

For depression, both DSM and ICD stand unified in the stem criteria, which includes depressed mood or diminished interest or pleasure occurring most of the day for 2 weeks along with at least five other depressive symptoms causing significant impairment. The ICD-11 requires at least 5 out of a list of 10 (instead of 9 in the DSM-5). The additional symptom is "hopelessness", which has been found to outperform more than half of DSM symptoms in differentiating depressed from non-depressed people [175]. Another difference is the exclusion of bereavement in DSM-5, whereas ICD-11 includes bereavement in the diagnosis of MDD; however, it requires a longer period of symptom duration. Two important differences that further split the two classifications include DSM-5 acknowledging the diagnostic relevance of manic symptoms in persons who do not have bipolar disorder, that is, MDD with mixed features specifier, which is defined as the presence of non-overlapping mood symptoms from the opposite mood states, can be applied to either manic, hypomanic, or depressive episodes, and has received polarizing reactions from within the diagnostic community. This, however, harkens to the Kraepelinian concept and the newer emerging concept of MDD-spectrum. Unique to ICD-11 is also the qualifier depression "with prominent anxiety symptoms". This also suggests the original conflict between unitary depression and melancholic versus reactive/neurotic depression in the original Kraepelinian–Schneiderian scheme. Both these changes, however, are testament to the growing understanding of the heterogeneity of what is currently described as a unitary MDD.

One of the key divergences between DSM-5 and ICD-11 is the classification of personality. The DSM-5 continues to adhere to the categorical classification of distinct personality types and the classical view that these are trait disorders that emerge early in the developmental period. The ICD-11, on the other hand, has abandoned the categorical classification of personality disorder into clinical groups (dissocial, emotionally unstable, etc.) and replaced these with dimensional classes that can be mild, moderate, or severe. Furthermore, the clinical criteria for personality disorder no longer require that the symptoms begin in early adulthood if they have been present for 2 years. This has a key impact on the diagnosis of BD2 within ICD-11 since hypomanic features such as irritability, impulsivity, disinhibition, reckless behaviour, and excitement are also those of "poorly regulated emotional expression and behaviour", consistent with personality disorders. Hence, ICD 11 relies on the clinician's interpretation of the overall patterns of "emotional experience, emotional expression, and behaviour that are maladaptive" in order to differentiate between chronic BD2 and personality disorder [140]. This is also interesting because this challenges the classical view of the evolution of personality disorders and raises the alternative view that affective personality types are chronic, enduring mood states and their adaptive sequelae. It would be interesting to follow up several decades from now how this change has impacted the understanding, diagnosis, and diagnostic interchangeability of the pure affective–pure personality threshold.

While these diagnostic revisions have had some crucial changes, they are both considered flawed for the purposes of furthering understanding of psychiatric nosology and future research that can have meaningful therapeutic impact. Since the current "classes" within this system are a constellation of transdiagnostic, highly heterogeneous symptoms, with no emergent "zone of rarity", and embedded in the *a priori* conceptualizations of the earlier nineteenth century, it stands to reason that only a proportion of patients respond to current medications (the rule of one-thirds). As is argued, it is not because the medications do not work, but rather the heterogeneity of the diagnosis masks the embedded targets that respond to a particular treatment [33]. Hence, there is a clear need to come up with a classificatory approach that satisfies this need, and some that have been proposed in lieu are discussed in the section below.

Future Perspectives

The common theme that emerges in this examination is that consensus statements like the DSM and ICD fail to capture the cadence of the symptoms that together form the mood composite [176]. These symptoms cluster uniquely in various permutations to form a mood state that is both categorical/unitary in that moment in time but dynamic across the longitudinal course. In this section, we discuss some of the models that have been proposed to better classify and understand mood (in lieu of or in combination with the DSM/ICD frameworks) – all of them incorporate some part of the theoretical model proposed earlier. The common theme that emerges in all of them is that mood is not an aggregate but rather a variable arrangement of individual symptoms where temporal progression of these symptoms and their interactions over time should drive both classification and diagnosis.

Malhi et al.'s ACE model [177]

Malhi et al. in their paper propose unification of all moods in a single continuum and divide affective symptomatology into three domains: Activity, Cognition, and Emotion. These domains, and the symptoms they contain, are conceptualized as dimensional constructs rather than categories. This model considers the temporal strengthening of associations between each domain and factors the level of disability incurred across time in each of these symptom domains.

Cuthbert-Insel's Research Domain Criteria (RDoC) [178]

In 2010, the RDoC was launched by Bruce Cuthbert and Thomas Insel because of frustration with the DSM classification systems [179–184]. The objective of the RDoC was to develop end points for psychiatric research based on the biological substrate involved in the shaping of mental activity and/or altered in abnormal mental activity, much in line with Wernicke's original thinking [185].

To achieve this objective, "fundamental domains" of "behavioural functioning" are related to their underlying neurobiology by the identification of the "sites of dysregulation" (Wernicke's lesional approach) that become manifest and are postulated to crystalize on discrete "neurobiological circuit maps". Thus, in the RDoC, there are five "domains" of "neurobiological circuits," labelled as "negative affect", "positive affect", "cognition", "social processes", and "arousal/regulatory system" within which human behaviour and functioning are investigated across multiple units of analysis (e.g., genetic, molecular, clinical metrics, and circuitry) [186]. While studies have been undertaken to map mood phenotypes on RDoC, there is lack of replication between the studies of the phenotypes' treatment prediction value [186], which limits generalizability and widespread use of the criteria at this stage [63,187].

Foucher et al.'s appeals for a Wernicke–Kleist–Leonhard (WKL) phenotypic revival [188]

In their recent paper, neo-WKLians Foucher et al. [188] propose a phenotypic classification of mood where descriptions do not focus on what phenotypes have in common, but rather in what aspects they differ from one another. They argue that certain symptoms might occur in many phenotypes and hence are not helpful per se (e.g., nonspecific medical signs such as pyrexia) and meaningful symptom clusters can only be created with recognizing wherein they differ, or where there is "deficit" (in line with Wernicke's pure neurological thinking of lesions that create deficits that create symptoms, that, once localized, would result in diagnosis). However, the clinical implementations, including replicated cross-cultural validity, remain unknown.

Läge–Möller Multidimensional Scaling Based on Association for Methodology and Documentation in Psychiatry (AMDP) Symptom Profiles [189]

This concept has been recently introduced as an attempt to unify dimensional and categorical approaches by creating diagnostic maps. In this study, a manic, a depressive, and a non-affective cluster clearly emerged. At the same time, the mania dimension ($r = 0.82$), the depression dimension ($r = 0.68$), and the apathy dimension ($r = 0.74$) showed high multiple regression values in the map. The authors proposed that a multidimensional diagnostic map of this nature could serve as an automated diagnostic tool based on psychopathological symptom profiles; however, further studies in this are awaited.

Phillips and Kupfer's Classes of Illness [190]

Philips and Kupfer [190], endorsed by Jules Angst [7], propose an integrated biological systems approach to the affective disorders continuum. They propose new neurobiologically defined classes of affective disorders based on biosignatures of dimensions of pathology expressed at genetic, molecular, neural circuitry, and behavioural levels. They propose that overlaps in these dimensions will create "classes" of affective disorders that will be consistent in both diagnostic investigations and treatment response.

Henry and Etain's Dimensionality Anchors [72]

These authors propose the most simplified yet immediately implementable diagnostic system. The authors identify six dimensions based on those that are either being discussed or implemented within the DSM-5, may orientate towards the choice of specific treatments, or represent more homogeneous and thus more appropriate subgroups for research purposes. These include 1) predominant polarity, 2) psychotic symptoms, 3) inhibition/activation behavioural level, 4) emotional reactivity, 5) impulsivity/suicidality/substance misuse, and 6) cognitive impairment. The authors propose that each mood episode must be defined within these dimensions in order to covey the flavour of the episode more succinctly and guide targeted treatment decisions.

Kendler's Mechanistic Property Cluster (MPC) Model [191]

In 2011, Kendler et al. proposed the "mechanistic property cluster" (MPC) model of mental disorders. In this view, mental disorders are mechanistically mediated clusters of multilevel (bio-psycho-social) properties. The MPC-model is a non-reductionist form of realism born out of extensive research on the history of psychiatry in the context of the philosophy of psychiatry. This model tries to account for mental disorders in terms of the causal structure of the natural world, and because it views mental disorders as clusters of multilevel properties it is also non-reductionist [192].

One of the most obvious recommendations for future research would be to subject these models to the statistical rigour that is mostly just reserved for therapeutic trials in modern psychiatry since almost all of them are either purely theoretical or have not been replicated repeatedly and importantly cross culturally. The authors also recommend a shift of perspective in classification. Perhaps psychiatry needs to forgo the dream of emulating watertight specialties where the [193–195] cause to treatment course runs in a smooth and linear manner like cardiology and neurology and turn to specialties like rheumatology and oncology where there is a more chaotic (often unknown or multifactorial) relationship between aetiology, pathology, and management for classification templates.

Based on the choice of "classification parameters" [193] (aetiopathological, syndromic, treatment response, laboratory/neuroimaging evidence, etc.), varying classifications may be produced, with their own unique abstraction (nosology, syndromatology). The classes arising out of these different systems are the result of an idealizing abstraction (on the principles of Kant) and selection process [193] and hence cannot correspond to actual existing entities. The actual phenomenon of mood can never be known and will also not remain the same as the human evolution continues. The societal and cultural norms within which Kraepelin and contemporaries proposed the concepts of mood are phenomenally different from the "Exponential Age" of technology today.

It is also important to remain mindful of the stakeholders/beneficiaries of the diagnosis/classification system; including the potential conscious and unconscious gains of those who make the diagnosis, those who receive it, and those who stand in as audience (industry, society) while this exchange is enacted.

There is also an argument to bring phenomenology back into the fold of psychiatry [196,197], as nearly a century of dedicated research and concerted efforts to make psychiatry purely "biological" have not yielded sharp results like a single gene or a specific treatment. Exceptions include dementias and obsessive-compulsive disorder (OCD) where specific localized neurological mechanisms have allowed for diagnostic and treatment specificity. Hence, it stands to reason that if such defined mechanisms existed for the rest of psychiatry, in particular mood disorders, then some pattern would by now have probably started to emerge. Hence, there is also a need to re-examine the checklist culture of making diagnoses and reducing the phenomenon of diagnosis (that according to Jaspers must be the last thing that should be attempted in psychiatry) to an app/algorithm checklist administered by people with varying backgrounds in training, and coded for various financial/administrative reasons, sometimes at the very first interaction with the patient. This argument then feeds into and comes a full circle to the original debate of categorical versus dimensional. If mood was purely categorical, then a simple checklist, administered by any professional, should always yield the same results. However, this is not the case, and the "quality" of the assessment and the intuitions behind scoring have a tangible bearing on the results. It seems that currently a categorical approach will be continued and combined with a dimensional subtype/subdifferentiation [193,194]. It will be interesting to see how this continuum concept evolves, and what its extreme poles are eventually demarcated to be: whether we will arrive back at unitary psychoses or re-embrace the Kraepelinian MDI.

Gödel's Incompleteness Theorem and Some Key Conclusions

The authors of this chapter subscribe to the view that mood is conceptualized as a continuum bounded by unipolar mania and unipolar depression (instead of other proposed continuums discussed in this chapter), so our conclusions should be interpreted in that context. We also view mood, in the semblance of the Light analogy, to be made of discrete categories or symptom clusters that will remain relevant as nosographical reference points for diagnosis and prognosis purposes. The conceptualization of mood will also continue to evolve, and in this perhaps we are no different from our ancient and medieval ancestors who ascribed mania or psychotic phenomena with the divine or the hard vacuum of biology to which it was relegated in the 1960s because it was embedded within the societal understandings of time. Hence, the full conceptualization of mood would always be incomplete, as Gödel's incompleteness theorem to explain complexities of spacetime, and would always rely on a degree of heuristic compressions and approximations. Semantic harmonization is perhaps the first step before any classification is even attempted, especially in psychiatry, which operates primarily within the realm of communication and observation. Mood, in particular, will likely remain a diagnostic challenge because it is one of the few concepts in psychiatry where thresholds between normality and disorder are as important as gradations of the disorder. Based on the current clinical knowledge, as argued by Möller et al. [195], there is insufficient evidence to completely break up current categorical classifications that have, as noted by Baldessrini [6] and Soares and Gershon [198], remained a clinically stable and identifiable syndrome for over a century. There is also enough evidence to consider the transdiagnostic symptom clustering / symptom domain criteria and test them further; however, there is insufficient evidence to start using them clinically. While not without criticism, some key changes in DSM and ICD harken to a slow but tangible shift in view of how mood will be conceptualized in future. However, whether mood disorders take the eventual quantum leap of faith, embracing Heisenberg's uncertainty and Gödel's incompleteness [199], and render similar treatment to mood as physics has to Light (where Light is now a trinity of particle, energy, and electromagnetic waveform that spans across all bands of visible/"classical" light and the rest of the EM spectrum) remains to be seen.

References

1. Gitlin M, Malhi GS. The existential crisis of bipolar II disorder. *Int J Bipolar Disord* [Internet]. 2020;8(1):5. Available from: https://doi.org/10.1186/s40345-019-0175-7

2. Joober R, Tabbane K. From the neo-Kraepelinian framework to the new mechanical philosophy of psychiatry: regaining common sense. *J Psychiatry Neurosci* [Internet]. 2019 Jan 1;44(1):3–7. Available from: https://pubmed.ncbi.nlm.nih.gov/30565447

3. Kendler KS. The transformation of American psychiatric nosology at the dawn of the twentieth century. *Mol Psychiatry* [Internet]. 2016;21(2):152–8. Available from: https://doi.org/10.1038/mp.2015.188

4. Shorter E. The history of nosology and the rise of the Diagnostic and Statistical Manual of Mental Disorders. *Dialogues Clin Neurosci* [Internet]. 2015 Mar;17(1):59–67. Available from: https://pubmed.ncbi.nlm.nih.gov/25987864

5. Nettle D, Bateson M. The evolutionary origins of mood and its disorders. *Curr Biol* [Internet]. 2012;22(17):R712–21. Available from: www.sciencedirect.com/science/article/pii/S09609822212006653

6. Baldessarini RJ. A plea for integrity of the bipolar disorder concept. *Bipolar Disord*. 2000;2(1):3–7.

7. Angst J. Bipolar disorders in DSM-5: strengths, problems and perspectives. *Int J Bipolar Disord* [Internet]. 2013;1(1):12. Available from: https://doi.org/10.1186/2194-7511-1-12

8. Pelletier L, O'Donnell S, Dykxhoorn J, McRae L, Patten SB. Under-diagnosis of mood disorders in Canada. *Epidemiol Psychiatr Sci* [Internet]. 2017;26(4):414–23. Available from: www.cambridge.org/core/article/underdiagnosis-of-mood-disorders-in-canada/68581D51E09F9955DABEE8E0450DC0E2

9. Smith DJ, Ghaemi N. Is underdiagnosis the main pitfall when diagnosing bipolar disorder? Yes. *BMJ* [Internet]. 2010 Feb 22;340:c854. Available from: www.bmj.com/content/340/bmj.c854.abstract

10. Zimmerman M. Is underdiagnosis the main pitfall in diagnosing bipolar disorder? *BMJ* [Internet]. 2010 Feb 22;340:c855. Available from: www.bmj.com/content/340/bmj.c855.abstract

11. de Leon J. Paradoxes of US psychopharmacology practice in 2013: undertreatment of severe mental illness and overtreatment of minor psychiatric problems. *J Clin Psychopharmacol*. 2014;34(5):545–8.

12. Glick ID. Undiagnosed bipolar disorder: new syndromes and new treatments. *Prim Care Companion J Clin Psychiatry* [Internet]. 2004;6(1):27–33. Available from: https://pubmed.ncbi.nlm.nih.gov/15486598

13. Singh T, Rajput M. Misdiagnosis of bipolar disorder. *Psychiatry (Edgmont)* [Internet]. 2006 Oct;3(10):57–63. Available from: https://pubmed.ncbi.nlm.nih.gov/20877548

14. Benazzi F. Borderline personality–bipolar spectrum relationship. Prog *Neuropsychopharmacol Biol Psychiatry* [Internet]. 2006;30(1):68–74. Available from: www.sciencedirect.com/science/article/pii/S0278584605002058

15. Kuhn TS. *The Structure of Scientific Revolutions*. Vol. 111. Chicago: University of Chicago Press, 1970.

16. Berrios GE. *The History of Mental Symptoms: Descriptive Psychopathology since the Nineteenth Century*. Cambridge: Cambridge University Press, 1996.

17. Berrios GE. Melancholia and depression during the 19th century: a conceptual history. *Br J Psychiatry* [Internet]. 2018/01/02. 1988;153(3):298–304. Available from: www.cambridge.org/core/article/melancholia-and-depression-during-the-19th-century-a-conceptual-history/5257E8A5BA6C993A023F32462378CC92

18. Kendler KS. An historical framework for psychiatric nosology. *Psychol Med* [Internet]. 2009 Dec;39(12):1935–41. Available from: https://pubmed.ncbi.nlm.nih.gov/19368761

19. Kendler KS, Parnas J, eds. *Philosophical Issues in Psychiatry*. Vol. II: *Nosology*. Oxford: Oxford University Press, 2013. Available from: https://oxfordmedicine.com/view/10.1093/med/9780199642205.001.0001/med-9780199642205-chapter-015001

20. Kendell RE. *The Classification of Depressive Illnesses*. Vol. 18. Oxford: Oxford University Press, 1968.

21. Kendler KS. The transformation of American psychiatric nosology at the dawn of the twentieth century. *Mol Psychiatry* [Internet]. 2016;21(2):152–8. Available from: https://doi.org/10.1038/mp.2015.188

22. Shorter E. History of psychiatry. *Curr Opin Psychiatry*. 2008;21(6):593.

23. Angst J, Marneros A. Bipolarity from ancient to modern times: conception, birth and rebirth. *J Affect Disord* [Internet]. 2001;67(1):3–19. Available from: www.sciencedirect.com/science/article/pii/S0165032701004293

24. Charney AW, Mullins N, Park YJ, Xu J. On the diagnostic and neurobiological origins of bipolar disorder. *Transl Psychiatry* [Internet]. 2020;**10**(1):118. Available from: https://doi.org/10.1038/s41398-020-0796-8

25. Pies R. The historical roots of the "bipolar spectrum": Did Aristotle anticipate Kraepelin's broad concept of manic-depression? *J Affect Disord* [Internet]. 2007;**100**(1):7–11. Available from: www.sciencedirect.com/science/article/pii/S0165032706004940

26. Chamsi-Pasha MAR, Chamsi-Pasha H. Avicenna's contribution to cardiology. *Avicenna J Med* [Internet]. 2014 Jan;**4**(1):9–12. Available from: https://pubmed.ncbi.nlm.nih.gov/24678465

27. Omrani A, Holtzman NS, Akiskal HS, Ghaemi SN. Ibn Imran's 10th century treatise on melancholy. *J Affect Disord.* 2012;**141**(2–3):116–19.

28. Amar Z, Lev E, Serri Y. On Ibn Juljul and the meaning and importance of the list of medicinal substances not mentioned by Dioscorides. *J R Asiat Soc.* 2014;**24**(4):529–55.

29. Leonti M, Casu L. Ethnopharmacology of love. *Front Pharmacol* [Internet]. 2018;**9**. Available from: www.frontiersin.org/article/10.3389/fphar.2018.00567

30. Goldney RD. The utility of the DSM nosology of mood disorders. *Can J Psychiatry.* 2006;**51**(14):874–8.

31. Goldstein JE. *Console and Classify: The French Psychiatric Profession in the Nineteenth Century.* Chicago: University of Chicago Press, 2001.

32. Decker HS. How Kraepelinian was Kraepelin? How Kraepelinian are the neo-Kraepelinians? – from Emil Kraepelin to DSM-III. *Hist Psychiatry* [Internet]. 2007 Sep 1;**18**(3):337–60. Available from: https://doi.org/10.1177/0957154X07078976

33. Geddes JR, Andreasen NC, Goodwin GM, et al. *New Oxford Textbook of Psychiatry.* Oxford: Oxford University Press, 2020. Available from: https://oxfordmedicine.com/view/10.1093/med/9780198713005.001.0001/med-9780198713005-chapter-7

34. Stanghellini G, Fuchs T. *One Century of Karl Jaspers' General Psychopathology.* Oxford: Oxford University Press, 2013.

35. de Leon J. DSM-5 and the research domain criteria: 100 years after Jaspers' General Psychopathology. *Am J Psychiatry* [Internet]. 2014 May 1;**171**(5):492–4. Available from: https://doi.org/10.1176/appi.ajp.2013.13091218

36. Kendler KS, Engstrom EJ. Kahlbaum, Hecker, and Kraepelin and the transition from psychiatric symptom complexes to empirical disease forms. *Am J Psychiatry.* 2017;**174**(2):102–9.

37. Kraam A. On the Origin of the Clinical Standpoint in Psychiatry: by Dr Ewald Hecker in Görlitz. *Hist Psychiatry* [Internet]. 2004 Sep 1;**15**(3):345–60. Available from: https://doi.org/10.1177/0957154X04044598

38. Schioldann J, Berrios G. "The meaning of the symptom in psychiatry. An overview", by Hans W. Gruhle (1913). *Hist Psychiatry.* 2015 Jun 1;**26**:214–32.

39. Kendler KS. The development of Kraepelin's concept of dementia praecox: a close reading of relevant texts. *JAMA Psychiatry* [Internet]. 2020 Nov 1;**77**(11):1181–7. Available from: https://doi.org/10.1001/jamapsychiatry.2020.1266

40. Kendler KS. The genealogy of the clinical syndrome of mania: signs and symptoms described in psychiatric texts from 1880 to 1900. *Psychol Med* [Internet]. 2017/10/11. 2018;**48**(10):1573–91. Available from: www.cambridge.org/core/article/genealogy-of-the-clinical-syndrome-of-mania-signs-and-symptoms-described-in-psychiatric-texts-from-1880-to-1900/91DA305CB1DB842D9F97C9A74C27B8D2

41. Klerman GL, Barrett JE. The affective disorders: clinical and epidemiological aspects. In S Gershon, B Shopsin, editors. *Lithium: Its Role in Psychiatric Research and Treatment* [Internet]. Boston, MA: Springer US, 1973; 201–36. Available from: https://doi.org/10.1007/978-1-4684-2022-7_12

42. Jablensky A, Hugler H, von Cranach M, Kalinov K. Kraepelin revisited: a reassessment and statistical analysis of dementia praecox and manic-depressive insanity in 1908. *Psychol Med* [Internet]. 2009/07/09. 1993;**23**(4):843–58. Available from: www.cambridge.org/core/article/kraepelin-revisited-a-reassessment-and-statistical-analysis-of-dementia-praecox-and-manicdepressive-insanity-in-1908/2AEB1AA7AB6E80EC2BE7B9C382DD8891

43. Roth SM. Unitary or binary nature of classification of depressive illness and its implications for the scope of manic depressive disorder. *J Affect Disord* [Internet]. 2001;**64**(1):1–18. Available from: www.sciencedirect.com/science/article/pii/S0165032700002378

44. Roth M. Problems in the classification of affective disorders. *Acta Psychiatr Scand* [Internet]. 1981 Apr 1;**63**(s290):42–51. Available from: https://doi.org/10.1111/j.1600-0447.1981.tb00706.x

45. Wallace ER IV, Gach J. *History of Psychiatry and Medical Psychology: With an Epilogue on Psychiatry and the Mind-Body Relation.* New York: Springer, 2008.

46. Crow TJ. The continuum of psychosis and its implication for the structure of the gene.

Br J Psychiatry [Internet]. 2018/01/29. 1986;**149** (4):419–29. Available from: www.cambridge.org/cor e/article/continuum-of-psychosis-and-its-implica tion-for-the-structure-of-the-gene/4ECDA141D36 A08E246 CAA84208C367F0

47. Akiskal HS. The bipolar spectrum – the shaping of a new paradigm in psychiatry. *Curr Psychiatry Rep*. 2002;**4**(1):1–3.

48. AKISKAL HS. The prevalent clinical spectrum of bipolar disorders: beyond DSM-IV. *J Clin Psychopharmacol* [Internet]. 1996;**16**(2). Available from: https://journals.lww.com/psychopharma cology/Fulltext/1996/04001/The_Prevalent_Clinical_ Spectrum_of_Bipolar.2.aspx

49. Perugi G, Akiskal HS. The soft bipolar spectrum redefined: focus on the cyclothymic, anxious-sensitive, impulse-dyscontrol, and binge-eating connection in bipolar II and related conditions. *Psychiatr Clin North Am* [Internet]. 2002;**25**(4):713–37. Available from: www.sciencedir ect.com/science/article/pii/S0193953X02000230

50. Perugi G, Akiskal HS, Lattanzi L, et al. The high prevalence of "Soft" bipolar (II) features in atypical depression. *Comp Psychiatry* [Internet]. 1998;**39** (2):63–71. Available from: www.sciencedirect.com/ science/article/pii/S0010440X98900803

51. Angst J. Will mania survive DSM-5 and ICD-11? *Int J Bipolar Disord* [Internet]. 2015;**3**(1):24. Available from: https://doi.org/10.1186/s40345-015-0041-1

52. Ghaemi SN. Bipolar spectrum: a review of the concept and a vision for the future. *Psychiatry Investig* [Internet]. 2013/09/16. 2013 Sep;**10**(3):218–24. Available from: https://pubmed.ncbi.nlm.nih.gov/ 24302943

53. Ghaemi SN, Hippocratic psychopharmacology: a non-DSM approach to practice. In *Clinical Psychopharmacology Principles and Practice*. Oxford: Oxford University Press, 2019. Available from: https://oxfordmedicine.com/view/10.1093/med/9780 199995486.001.0001/med-9780199995486-chapter-16

54. Ghaemi SN, Selker HP. Maintenance efficacy designs in psychiatry: randomized discontinuation trials– enriched but not better. *J Clin Transl Sci*. 2017;**1** (3):198–204.

55. Goodwin FK, Ghaemi SN. Prospects for a scientific psychiatry. *Acta Neuropsychiatr* [Internet]. 1997;**9** (2):49–51. Available from: www.cambridge.org/ core/article/prospects-for-a-scientific-psychiatry/ 630867EDFFC8E69C053ACB565E58B2CB

56. Goodwin FK, Whitham EA, Ghaemi SN. Maintenance treatment study designs in bipolar disorder. *CNS Drugs*. 2011;**25**(10):819–27.

57. Benazzi F. Mixed depression: a clinical marker of bipolar-II disorder. *Prog Neurosychopharmacol BiolPsychiatry*. 2005;**29**(2):267–74.

58. Benazzi F. Mood patterns and classification in bipolar disorder. *Curr Opin Psychiatry*. 2006;**19**(1):1–8.

59. Sperberg-McQueen CM. Classification and its structures. In S Shreibman, R Siemens, J Unsworth, editors. *A Companion to Digital Humanities*. Oxford: Blackwell, 2004: chap. 14.

60. Kendler KS. Psychiatric nosology, epistemic iteration, and pluralism. In KS Kendler, J Parnas, editors. *Philosophical Issues in Psychiatry*. Vol. IV: *Classification of Psychiatric Illness*. Oxford: Oxford University Press, 2017; 246.

61. Helmer O, Rescher N. On the epistemology of the inexact sciences. *Manage Sci* [Internet]. 1959;**6** (1):25–52. Available from: www.jstor.org/stable/ 2627474

62. Blackwell B. Corporate corruption in the psychopharmaceutical industry (revised). International Network for the History of Neuropsychopharmacology. March; 2017.

63. Ban TA. Academic psychiatry and the pharmaceutical industry. *Prog Neuropsychopharmacol Biol Psychiatry*. 2006;**30**(3):429–41.

64. Ban TA. Development of the language of psychiatry. In TA Ban, et al., editors. *International Network for the History of Neuropsychopharmacology*. INHN 2013 (INHN Historical Record). 2020: chap. 17.

65. Farrell DM. Recent work on the emotions. *Analyse Kritik*. 1988;**10**(1):71–102.

66. Marks J. A theory of emotion. *Philos Stud*. 1982;**42** (2):227–42.

67. Bedford E. Emotions. *Proceed Aristotelian Soc*. 1956;**57**:281–304.

68. Marks J. A theory of emotion. *Philos Stud*. 1982;**42** (2):227–42.

69. Buonomano D. *Your Brain Is a Time Machine: The Neuroscience and Physics of Time*. New York: WW Norton, 2017.

70. Aggarwal R, Ringold S, Khanna D, et al. Distinctions between diagnostic and classification criteria? *Arthritis Care Res (Hoboken)* [Internet]. 2015 Jul;**67** (7):891–7. Available from: https://pubmed.ncbi.nlm .nih.gov/25776731

71. Belmonte-Serrano MA. The myth of the distinction between classification and diagnostic criteria. *Reumatol Clin*. 2015;**11**(3):188–9.

72. Henry C, Etain B. New ways to classify bipolar disorders: going from categorical groups to symptom clusters or dimensions. *Curr Psychiatry Rep*

[Internet]. 2010 Dec;**12**(6):505–11. Available from: https://pubmed.ncbi.nlm.nih.gov/20878275

73. Baran L. Dynamical systems and a brief introduction to ergodic theory. Self-published paper. 2014;

74. Uffink J. Compendium of the foundations of classical statistical physics. In J Butterfield, J Earman, editors. *Philosophy of Physics*. North Holland, 2006; 923–1074.

75. Elliott KC. Epistemic and methodological iteration in scientific research. *Stud Hist Philos Sci Pt A* [Internet]. 2012;**43**(2):376–82. Available from: www.sciencedir ect.com/science/article/pii/S0039368112000039

76. Möller HJ. Methodological issues in psychiatry: psychiatry as an empirical science. *World J Biol Psychiatry* [Internet]. 2001 Jan 1;**2**(1):38–47. Available from: https://doi.org/10.3109/15622970109039983

77. Cassano GB, Dell'Osso L, Frank E, et al. The bipolar spectrum: a clinical reality in search of diagnostic criteria and an assessment methodology. *J Affect Disord* [Internet]. 1999;**54**(3):319–28. Available from: www.sciencedirect.com/science/article/pii/S016503279800158X

78. Gillman K. Stepped trials: magnifying methodological muddles – the supernatant effect. *PsychoTropical Res.* 2019.

79. Silberzahn R, Uhlmann EL, Martin DP, et al. Many analysts, one data set: making transparent how variations in analytic choices affect results. *Adv Methods Pract Psychol Sci* [Internet]. 2018 Aug 23;**1**(3):337–56. Available from: https://doi.org/10.1177/2515245917747646

80. Uhlmann EL, Ebersole CR, Chartier CR, et al. Scientific Utopia III: crowdsourcing science. *Perspect Psychol Sci* [Internet]. 2019 Jul 1;**14**(5):711–33. Available from: https://doi.org/10.1177/1745691619850561

81. Peters S. Dynamics of spatially extended phenomena – visual analytical approach to movements of lightning clusters. Ph.D. thesis, University of South Australia. 2014.

82. De Leon J. Is psychiatry scientific? A letter to a 21st century psychiatry resident. *Psychiatry Investig* [Internet]. 2013/09/16. 2013 Sep;**10**(3):205–17. Available from: https://pubmed.ncbi.nlm.nih.gov/24302942

83. American Psychiatric Association. *Diagnostic and Statistical Manual of Mental Disorders: DSM-5.* 5th ed. Washington, DC: American Psychiatric Association, 2013.

84. Wille L, McMahon FJ. Coherence through incongruence – can genetic markers inform nosology after all? *JAMA Psychiatry* [Internet]. 2018 Jan 1;**75**(1):7–8. Available from: https://doi.org/10.1001/jamapsychiatry.2017.3484

85. Angst J, Azorin JM, Bowden CL, et al. Prevalence and characteristics of undiagnosed bipolar disorders in patients with a major depressive episode: the BRIDGE study. *Arch Gen Psychiatry.* 2011;**68**(8):791–9.

86. Möller HJ, Jäger M, Riedel M, et al. The Munich 15-year follow-up study (MUFUSSAD) on first-hospitalized patients with schizophrenic or affective disorders: comparison of psychopathological and psychosocial course and outcome and prediction of chronicity. *Eur Arch Psychiatry Clin Neurosci* [Internet]. 2010;**260**(5):367–84. Available from: https://doi.org/10.1007/s00406-010-0117-y

87. Mullins N, Forstner AJ, O'Connell KS, et al. Genome-wide association study of more than 40,000 bipolar disorder cases provides new insights into the underlying biology. *Nat Genet* [Internet]. 2021;**53**(6):817–29. Available from: https://doi.org/10.1038/s41588-021-00857-4

88. Witt SH, Streit F, Jungkunz M, et al. Genome-wide association study of borderline personality disorder reveals genetic overlap with bipolar disorder, major depression and schizophrenia. *Transl Psychiatry* [Internet]. 2017 Jun 20;**7**(6): e1155–e1155. Available from: https://pubmed.ncbi.nlm.nih.gov/28632202

89. Léger M, Wolff V, Kabuth B, Albuisson E, Ligier F. The mood disorder spectrum vs. schizophrenia decision tree: EDIPHAS research into the childhood and adolescence of 205 patients. *BMC Psychiatry* [Internet]. 2022 Mar 18;**22**(1):194. Available from: https://pubmed.ncbi.nlm.nih.gov/35300648

90. Amare AT, Vaez A, Hsu YH, et al. Bivariate genome-wide association analyses of the broad depression phenotype combined with major depressive disorder, bipolar disorder or schizophrenia reveal eight novel genetic loci for depression. *Mol Psychiatry* [Internet]. 2020;**25**(7):1420–9. Available from: https://doi.org/10.1038/s41380-018-0336-6

91. Schulze TG, Akula N, Breuer R, et al. Molecular genetic overlap in bipolar disorder, schizophrenia, and major depressive disorder. *World J Biol Psychiatry* [Internet]. 2012/03/09. 2014 Apr;**15**(3):200–8. Available from: https://pubmed.ncbi.nlm.nih.gov/22404658

92. Alarcón RD. Culture, cultural factors and psychiatric diagnosis: review and projections. *World Psychiatry* [Internet]. 2009 Oct;**8**(3):131–9. Available from: https://pubmed.ncbi.nlm.nih.gov/19812742

93. Dudek D, Siwek M, Zielińska D, Jaeschke R, Rybakowski J. Diagnostic conversions from major

depressive disorder into bipolar disorder in an outpatient setting: results of a retrospective chart review. *J Affect Disord*. 2013;**144**(1–2):112–5.

94. Wendt FR, Pathak GA, Tylee DS, Goswami A, Polimanti R. Heterogeneity and polygenicity in psychiatric disorders: a genome-wide perspective. *Chronic Stress (Thousand Oaks)* [Internet]. 2020 Jan 1;4:2470547020924844. Available from: https://doi.org/10.1177/2470547020924844

95. Malhi GS, Geddes JR. Carving bipolarity using a lithium sword. *Br J Psychiatry* [Internet]. 2014;**205**(5):337–9. Available from: www.cambridge.org/core/article/carving-bipolarity-using-a-lithium-sword/A81A879C5C80B070F3C7641F00EB7EB9

96. Kontos N, Freudenreich O, Querques J. Out-patient institutionalisation. *Br J Psychiatry* [Internet]. 2014;**205**(5):339–339. Available from: www.cambridge.org/core/article/outpatient-institutionalisation/F74D3B70CB9771635CB6272426E57942

97. Taylor MA, Abrams R. Reassessing the bipolar-unipolar dichotomy. *J Affect Disord* [Internet]. 1980;**2**(3):195–217. Available from: www.sciencedirect.com/science/article/pii/0165032780900051

98. Parker G, Hall W, Boyce P, et al. Depression sub-typing: unitary, binary or arbitrary? *Aust N Z J Psychiatry* [Internet]. 1991 Mar 1;**25**(1):63–76. Available from: https://doi.org/10.3109/00048679109077720

99. Ghaemi SN, Ko JY, Goodwin FK. "Cade's disease" and beyond: misdiagnosis, antidepressant use, and a proposed definition for bipolar spectrum disorder. *Can J Psychiatry*. 2002;**47**(2):125–34.

100. Angst J. The bipolar spectrum. *Br J Psychiatry* [Internet]. 2007;**190**(3):189–91. Available from: www.cambridge.org/core/article/bipolar-spectrum/418765D7EB2BDB1EB16B1EFA407BF724

101. Akiskal HS, Maser JD, Zeller PJ, et al. Switching from "unipolar" to bipolar II: an 11-year prospective study of clinical and temperamental predictors in 559 patients. *Arch Gen Psychiatry*. 1995;**52**(2):114–23.

102. Akiskal HS, Walker P, Puzantian VR, et al. Bipolar outcome in the course of depressive illness: phenomenologic, familial, and pharmacologic predictors. *J Affect Disord*. 1983;**5**(2):115–28.

103. Ghaemi SN, Stoll AL, Pope Jr HG. Lack of insight in bipolar disorder. The acute manic episode. *J Nerv Ment Dis*. 1995;**183**(7):464–7.

104. Klerman GL. The spectrum of mania. *Comp Psychiatry*. 1981;**22**(1):11–20.

105. Akiskal HS, Djenderedjian AH, Rosenthal RH, Khani MK. Cyclothymic disorder: validating criteria for inclusion in the bipolar affective group. *Am J Psychiatry*. 1977;**134**(11):1227–33.

106. Akiskal HS, Pinto O. The evolving bipolar spectrum: prototypes I, II, III, and IV. *Psychiatr Clin North Am*. 1999;**22**(3):517–34.

107. Smith DJ, Forty L, Russell E, et al. Sub-threshold manic symptoms in recurrent major depressive disorder are a marker for poor outcome. *Acta Psychiatr Scand* [Internet]. 2009 Apr 1;**119**(4):325–9. Available from: https://doi.org/10.1111/j.1600-0447.2008.01324.x

108. Liu X, Jiang K. Should major depressive disorder with mixed features be classified as a bipolar disorder? *Shanghai Arch Psychiatry* [Internet]. 2014 Oct;**26**(5):294–6. Available from: https://pubmed.ncbi.nlm.nih.gov/25477723

109. Savitz J, Drevets WC. Bipolar and major depressive disorder: neuroimaging the developmental-degenerative divide. *NeurosciBiobehav Rev* [Internet]. 2009;**33**(5):699–771. Available from: www.sciencedirect.com/science/article/pii/S0149763409000062

110. Nassir Ghaemi S. Why antidepressants are not antidepressants: STEP-BD, STAR*D, and the return of neurotic depression. *Bipolar Disord* [Internet]. 2008 Dec 1;**10**(8):957–68. Available from: https://doi.org/10.1111/j.1399-5618.2008.00639.x

111. Akiskal HS, Grinspoon L. *Psychiatry Update: The American Psychiatric Association Annual Review*. Vol 2. Washington, DC, 1983; 271.

112. Ghaemi SN, Dalley S. The bipolar spectrum: conceptions and misconceptions. *Aust N Z J Psychiatry* [Internet]. 2014 Mar 7;**48**(4):314–24. Available from: https://doi.org/10.1177/0004867413504830

113. Akiskal HS, Pinto O. The evolving bipolar spectrum: prototypes I, II, III, and IV. *Psychiatr Clin North Am*. 1999;**22**(3):517–34.

114. Akiskal HS, Akiskal KK, Lancrenon S, et al. Validating the bipolar spectrum in the French National EPIDEP Study: overview of the phenomenology and relative prevalence of its clinical prototypes. *J Affect Disord*. 2006;**96**(3):197–205.

115. Angst J. The etiology and nosology of endogenous depressive psychoses. *Foreign Psychiatry*. 1973;**2**:1–108.

116. Angst J. The emerging epidemiology of hypomania and bipolar II disorder. *J Affect Disord*. 1998;**50**(2–3):143–51.

117. Benazzi F. Depressive mixed states: unipolar and bipolar II. *Eur Arch Psychiatry Clin Neurosci*. 2000;**250**(5):249–53.

118. Angst J, Azorin JM, Bowden CL, et al. Prevalence and characteristics of undiagnosed bipolar disorders in patients with a major depressive episode: the BRIDGE study. *Arch Gen Psychiatry*. 2011;**68**(8):791–9.

119. Benazzi F. Depressive mixed state: testing different definitions. *Psychiatry ClinNeurosci*. 2001;**55**(6):647–52.

120. Benazzi F. Depressive mixed state frequency: age/gender effects. *Psychiatry Clin Neurosci*. 2002;**56**(5):537–43.

121. Benazzi F. Mixed depression: a clinical marker of bipolar-II disorder. *Prog Neuropsychopharmacol BiolPsychiatry*. 2005;**29**(2):267–74.

122. Benazzi F, Akiskal HS. Delineating bipolar II mixed states in the Ravenna–San Diego collaborative study: the relative prevalence and diagnostic significance of hypomanic features during major depressive episodes. *J Affect Disord*. 2001;**67**(1–3):115–22.

123. Benazzi F. Mixed depression and the dimensional view of mood disorders. *Psychopathology*. 2007;**40**(6):431–9.

124. Akiskal HS. The dark side of bipolarity: detecting bipolar depression in its pleomorphic expressions. *J Affect Disord* [Internet]. 2005;**84**(2):107–15. Available from: www.sciencedirect.com/science/article/pii/S0165032704001843

125. Koukopoulos A, Faedda G, Proietti R, et al. Mixed depressive syndrome. *L'encephale*. 1992;**18**:19–21.

126. Ghaemi SN. *On Depression: Drugs, Diagnosis, and Despair in the Modern World*. JHU Press, 2013.

127. Benazzi F. Mood patterns and classification in bipolar disorder. *CurrOpin Psychiatry* [Internet]. 2006;**19**(1). Available from: https://journals.lww.com/co-psychiatry/Fulltext/2006/01000/Mood_patterns_and_classification_in_bipolar.2.aspx

128. Akiskal HS, Bourgeois ML, Angst J, et al. Re-evaluating the prevalence of and diagnostic composition within the broad clinical spectrum of bipolar disorders. *J Affect Disord* [Internet]. 2000;**59**:S5–30. Available from: www.sciencedirect.com/science/article/pii/S0165032700002032

129. Gama Marques J, Ouakinin S. Schizophrenia-schizoaffective–bipolar spectra: an epistemological perspective. *CNS Spectrums* [Internet]. 2021;**26**(3):197–201. Available from: www.cambridge.org/core/article/schizophreniaschizoaffectivebipolar-spectra-an-epistemological-perspective/BCD44BC80E44989D8F7AAD8F71582E9F

130. Koukopoulos A, Sani G, Koukopoulos AE, et al. Endogenous and exogenous cyclicity and temperament in bipolar disorder: review, new data and hypotheses. *J Affect Disord* [Internet]. 2006;**96**(3):165–75. Available from: www.sciencedirect.com/science/article/pii/S0165032706003661

131. Haslam N. Categorical versus dimensional models of mental disorder: the taxometric evidence. *Aust N Z J Psychiatry* [Internet]. 2003 Dec 1;37(6):696–704. Available from: https://doi.org/10.1080/j.1440-1614.2003.01258.x

132. Grisanzio KA, Goldstein-Piekarski AN, Wang MY, et al. Transdiagnostic symptom clusters and associations with brain, behavior, and daily function in mood, anxiety, and trauma disorders. *JAMA Psychiatry* [Internet]. 2018 Feb 1;**75**(2):201–9. Available from: https://pubmed.ncbi.nlm.nih.gov/29197929

133. Akiskal HS. The dark side of bipolarity: detecting bipolar depression in its pleomorphic expressions. *J Affect Disord* [Internet]. 2005;**84**(2):107–15. Available from: www.sciencedirect.com/science/article/pii/S0165032704001843

134. Cassano GB, Rucci P, Frank E, et al. The mood spectrum in unipolar and bipolar disorder: arguments for a unitary approach. *Am J Psychiatry* [Internet]. 2004;**161**(7):1264–9. Available from: https://doi.org/10.1176/appi.ajp.161.7.1264

135. Perugi G, Passino MCS, Toni C, Maremmani I, Angst J. Is unipolar mania a distinct subtype? *Comp Psychiatry* [Internet]. 2007;**48**(3):213–7. Available from: www.sciencedirect.com/science/article/pii/S0010440X07000120

136. Angst J, Grobler C. Unipolar mania: a necessary diagnostic concept. *Eur Arch Psychiatry Clin Neurosci* [Internet]. 2015;**265**(4):273–80. Available from: https://doi.org/10.1007/s00406-015-0577-1

137. Merikangas KR, Cui L, Heaton L, et al. Independence of familial transmission of mania and depression: results of the NIMH family study of affective spectrum disorders. *Mol Psychiatry*. 2014;**19**(2):214–9.

138. Baek JH, Eisner LR, Nierenberg AA. Epidemiology and course of unipolar mania: results from the national epidemiologic survey on alcohol and related conditions (NESARC). *Depress Anxiety*. 2014;**31**(9):746–55.

139. Angst J, Rössler W, Ajdacic-Gross V, et al. Differences between unipolar mania and bipolar-I disorder: evidence from nine epidemiological studies. *Bipolar Disord*. 2019;**21**(5):437–48.

140. Luty J. Bordering on the bipolar: a review of criteria for ICD-11 and DSM-5 persistent mood disorders. *BJPsych Advances* [Internet]. 2020;**26**(1):50–7. Available from: www.cambridge.org/core/article/bordering-on-the-bipolar-a-review-of-criteria-for-

icd11-and-dsm5-persistent-mood-disorders/
D73A8F4F22A635353B17DFF36AB9301B

141. Davidson JRT, Miller RD, Turnbull CD, Sullivan JL. Atypical depression. *Arch Gen Psychiatry* [Internet]. 1982 May 1;**39**(5):527–34. Available from: https://doi.org/10.1001/archpsyc.1982.04290050015005

142. Thase ME. Atypical depression: useful concept, but it's time to revise the DSM-IV criteria. *Neuropsychopharmacology* [Internet]. 2009;**34**(13):2633–41. Available from: https://doi.org/10.1038/npp.2009.100

143. Sargant W. The treatment of anxiety states and atypical depression by the MAOI drugs. *J Neuropsychiatry*. 1962;**3**(1):96–103.

144. Liebowitz MR, Quitkin FM, Stewart JW, et al. Antidepressant specificity in atypical depression. *Arch Gen Psychiatry*. 1988;**45**(2):129–37.

145. Quitkin FM, Stewart JW, McGrath PJ, et al. Phenelzine versus imipramine in the treatment of probable atypical depression: defining syndrome boundaries of selective MAOI responders. *Am J Psychiatry*. 1988;**145**(3):306–11.

146. Parker G, Roy K, Mitchell P, Wilhelm K, Malhi G, Hadzi-Pavlovic D. Atypical depression: a reappraisal. *Am J Psychiatry* [Internet]. 2002 Sep 1;**159**(9):1470–9. Available from: https://doi.org/10.1176/appi.ajp.159.9.1470

147. Sani G, Vöhringer PA, Barroilhet SA, Koukopoulos AE, Ghaemi SN. The Koukopoulos Mixed Depression Rating Scale (KMDRS): an International Mood Network (IMN) validation study of a new mixed mood rating scale. *J Affect Disord*. 2018;**232**:9–16.

148. Sato T, Bottlender R, Sievers M, Möller HJ. Evidence of depressive mixed states. *Am J Psychiatry*. 2005;**162**(1):193-a.

149. Koukopoulos A, Albert MJ, Sani G, Koukopoulos AE, Girardi P. Mixed depressive states: nosologic and therapeutic issues. *Int Rev Psychiatry*. 2005;**17**(1):21–37.

150. Benazzi F, Akiskal H. Irritable-hostile depression: further validation as a bipolar depressive mixed state. *J Affect Disord*. 2005;**84**(2–3):197–207.

151. Akiskal HS, Benazzi F. Atypical depression: a variant of bipolar II or a bridge between unipolar and bipolar II? *J Affect Disord*. 2005;**84**(2–3):209–17.

152. Benazzi F. The continuum/spectrum concept of mood disorders: is mixed depression the basic link? *Eur Arch Psychiatry Clin Neurosci*. 2006;**256**(8):512–15.

153. Akiskal HS, Benazzi F, Perugi G, Rihmer Z. Agitated "unipolar" depression re-conceptualized as a depressive mixed state: implications for the antidepressant-suicide controversy. *J Affect Disord*. 2005;**85**(3):245–58.

154. Akiskal HS, Benazzi F. The DSM-IV and ICD-10 categories of recurrent [major] depressive and bipolar II disorders: evidence that they lie on a dimensional spectrum. *J Affect Disord*. 2006;**92**(1):45–54.

155. Angst J, Gamma A. Diagnosis and course of affective psychoses: was Kraepelin right? *Eur Arch Psychiatry Clin Neurosci* [Internet]. 2008;**258**(2):107. Available from: https://doi.org/10.1007/s00406-008-2013-2

156. Saggese JM, Lieberman DZ, Goodwin FK. The role of recurrence and cyclicity in differentiating mood disorder diagnoses. *Primary Psychiatry*. 2006;**13**(11):43–8.

157. Akiskal HS, Djenderedjian AM, Rosenthal RH, Khani MK. Cyclothymic disorder: validating criteria for inclusion in the bipolar affective group. *Am J Psychiatry*. 1977;**134**(11):1227–33.

158. Akiskal HS, Akiskal K. Reassessing the prevalence of bipolar disorders: clinical significance and artistic creativity. *Psychiatry Psychobiol*. 1988;**3**(S1):29s–36s.

159. Ghaemi SN, Ko JY, Goodwin FK. The bipolar spectrum and the antidepressant view of the world. *J Psychiatr Pract*. 2001;**7**(5):287–97.

160. Healy D. *Mania: A Short History of Bipolar Disorder*. JHU Press, 2008.

161. Akiskal HS, Akiskal KK. TEMPS: Temperament Evaluation of Memphis, Pisa, Paris and San Diego. *J Affect Disord*. 2005;**85**(1–2):1–2.

162. Rihmer Z, Akiskal KK, Rihmer A, Akiskal HS. Current research on affective temperaments. *Curr Opin Psychiatry* [Internet]. 2010;**23**(1). Available from: https://journals.lww.com/co-psychiatry/Fulltext/2010/01000/Current_research_on_affective_temperaments.4.aspx

163. Kwapil TR, DeGeorge D, Walsh MA, et al. Affective temperaments: Unique constructs or dimensions of normal personality by another name? *J Affect Disord* [Internet]. 2013;**151**(3):882–90. Available from: www.sciencedirect.com/science/article/pii/S0165032713005995

164. Akiskal HS, Placidi GF, Maremmani I, et al. TEMPS-I: delineating the most discriminant traits of the cyclothymic, depressive, hyperthymic and irritable temperaments in a nonpatient population. *J Affect Disord*. 1998;**51**(1):7–19.

165. Akiskal HS, Akiskal KK, Lancrenon S, et al. Validating the bipolar spectrum in the French National EPIDEP Study: overview of the phenomenology and relative prevalence of its

clinical prototypes. *J Affect Disord*. 2006;**96** (3):197–205.

166. Scandinavica AP, Akiskal HS. Demystifying borderline personality: critique of the concept and unorthodox reflections on its natural kinship with the bipolar spectrum. *Acta Psychiatr Scand*. 2004;**110**:401–7.

167. Akiskal HS, Akiskal KK, Haykal RF, Manning JS, Connor PD. TEMPS-A: progress towards validation of a self-rated clinical version of the Temperament Evaluation of the Memphis, Pisa, Paris, and San Diego Autoquestionnaire. *J Affect Disor*d. 2005;**85**(1–2):3–16.

168. Paris J. Borderline or bipolar? Distinguishing borderline personality disorder from bipolar spectrum disorders. *Harv Rev Psychiatry*. 2004;**12**(3):140–5.

169. Zimmerman M. Diagnosing personality disorders: a review of issues and research methods. *Arch Gen Psychiatry*. 1994;**51**(3):225–45.

170. Skodol AE, Shea MT, Yen S, White CN, Gunderson JG. Personality disorders and mood disorders: perspectives on diagnosis and classification from studies of longitudinal course and familial associations. *J Pers Disord* [Internet]. 2010 Feb 1;**24**(1):83–108. Available from: https://doi.org/ 10.1521/pedi.2010.24.1.83

171. Kuiper S, Curran G, Malhi GS. Why is soft bipolar disorder so hard to define? *Aus N Z J Psychiatry* [Internet]. 2012 Oct 26;**46**(11):1019–25. Available from: https://doi.org/10.1177/0004867412464063

172. Angst J, Ajdacic-Gross V, Rössler W. Bipolar disorders in ICD-11: current status and strengths. *Int J Bipolar Disord* [Internet]. 2020 Jan 20;**8**(1):3. Available from: https://pubmed.ncbi.nlm.nih.gov/31956923

173. Tandon R. Bipolar and depressive disorders in Diagnostic and Statistical Manual of Mental Disorders-5: clinical implications of revisions from Diagnostic and Statistical Manual of Mental Disorders-IV. *Indian J Psychol Med* [Internet]. 2015;**37**(1):1–4. Available from: https://pubmed.ncbi.nlm.nih.gov/25722503

174. Malhi GS, Irwin L, Outhred T. Counting the days from bipolar II to bipolar true! *Acta Psychiatr Scand*. 2019;**139**(3):211–13.

175. di Cerbo A. convergences and divergences in the ICD-11 vs. DSM-5 classification of mood disorders. *Turk Psikiyatri Dergisi*. 2021;**32**(4):293.

176. Westen D, Malone JC, DeFife JA. An empirically derived approach to the classification and diagnosis of mood disorders. *World Psychiatry* [Internet]. 2012 Oct;**11**(3):172–80. Available from: https://pubmed.ncbi.nlm.nih.gov/23024677

177. Malhi GS, Bell E, Boyce P, Mulder R, Porter RJ. Unifying the diagnosis of mood disorders. *Aust N Z J Psychiatry* [Internet]. 2020 Jun 1;**54**(6):561–5. Available from: https://doi.org/10.1177/ 0004867420926241

178. Insel TR. Disruptive insights in psychiatry: transforming a clinical discipline. *J Clin Invest* [Internet]. 2009/04/01. 2009 Apr;**119**(4):700–5. Available from: https://pubmed.ncbi.nlm.nih.gov/ 19339761

179. Insel T, Cuthbert B, Garvey MK, et al. Research domain criteria (RDoC): toward a new classification framework for research on mental disorders. *Am J Psychiatry*. 2010;**167**:748–51.

180. Cuthbert B, Insel T. The data of diagnosis: new approaches to psychiatric classification. *Psychiatry*. 2010;**73**(4):311–4.

181. Insel TR, Cuthbert BN. Brain disorders? precisely. *Science (1979)*. 2015;**348**(6234):499–500.

182. Cuthbert BN, Insel TR. Toward new approaches to psychotic disorders: the NIMH Research Domain Criteria project. *Schizophr Bull*. 2010;**36**(6):1061–2.

183. Cuthbert BN, Insel TR. Toward the future of psychiatric diagnosis: the seven pillars of RDoC. *BMC Med*. 2013;**11**(1):1–8.

184. Cuthbert BN, Insel TR. Toward precision medicine in psychiatry: the NIMH research domain criteria project. In DS Charney, JD Buxbaum, P Sklar, EJ Nestler, editors. *Neurobiology of Mental Illness*. Oxford: Oxford University Press, 2013:1076–88.

185. Clark LA, Cuthbert B, Lewis-Fernández R, Narrow WE, Reed GM. three approaches to understanding and classifying mental disorder: ICD-11, DSM-5, and the National Institute of Mental Health's Research Domain Criteria (RDoC). *Psychol Sci Public Interest* [Internet]. 2017 Nov 1;**18** (2):72–145. Available from: https://doi.org/10.1177/ 1529100617727266

186. Ahmed AT, Frye MA, Rush AJ, et al. Mapping depression rating scale phenotypes onto research domain criteria (RDoC) to inform biological research in mood disorders. *J Affect Disord* [Internet]. 2018 Oct 1;**238**:1–7. Available from: https://pubmed.ncbi.nlm.nih.gov/29807322

187. Ban TA. Thomas A. Ban: RDoC In Historical Perspective: Redefining Mental Illness by Tanya M. Luhrmann. Samuel Gershon's question. Collated Document Olaf Fjetland. 2017.

188. Foucher JR, Gawlik M, Roth JN, et al. Wernicke-Kleist-Leonhard phenotypes of endogenous psychoses: a review of their validity. *Dialogues Clin Neurosci* [Internet]. 2020 Mar;**22**(1):37–49. Available from: https://pubmed.ncbi.nlm.nih.gov/ 32699504

189. Läge D, Egli S, Riedel M, Strauss A, Möller HJ. Combining the categorical and the dimensional perspective in a diagnostic map of psychotic disorders. *Eur Arch Psychiatry Clin Neurosci* [Internet]. 2011;**261**(1):3–10. Available from: https://doi.org/10.1007/s00406-010-0125-y

190. Phillips ML, Kupfer DJ. Bipolar disorder diagnosis: challenges and future directions. *Lancet* [Internet]. 2013;**381**(9878):1663–71. Available from: www.sciencedirect.com/science/article/pii/S0140673613609897

191. Kendler KS, Zachar P, Craver C. What kinds of things are psychiatric disorders? *Psychol Med*. 2011;**41**(6):1143–50.

192. Ghaemi SN. Taking disease seriously: beyond "pragmatic" nosology. In KS Kendler, J Parnas, editors, *Philosophical Issues in Psychiatry*. Vol. II: *Nosology*. Oxford: Oxford University Press, 2012; 42–53.

193. Möller H. Development of DSM-V and ICD-11: tendencies and potential of new classifications in psychiatry at the current state of knowledge. *Psychiatry Clin Neurosci*. 2009;**63**(5):595–612.

194. Möller HJ. Systematic of psychiatric disorders between categorical and dimensional approaches. *Eur Arch Psychiatry Clin Neurosci* [Internet]. 2008;**258**(2):48–73. Available from: https://doi.org/10.1007/s00406-008-2004-3

195. Möller HJ, Bandelow B, Bauer M, et al. DSM-5 reviewed from different angles: goal attainment, rationality, use of evidence, consequences – part 2: bipolar disorders, schizophrenia spectrum disorders, anxiety disorders, obsessive–compulsive disorders, trauma- and stressor-related disorders, personality disorders, substance-related and addictive disorders, neurocognitive disorders. *Eur Arch Psychiatry Clin Neurosci* [Internet]. 2015;**265**(2):87–106. Available from: https://doi.org/10.1007/s00406-014-0521-9

196. Fernandez AV. Reconsidering the affective dimension of depression and mania: towards a phenomenological dissolution of the paradox of mixed states. *J Psychopathol*. 2014;**20**(4).

197. Joober R, Karama S. Randomness and nondeterminism: from genes to free will with implications for psychiatry. *J Psychiatry Neurosci* [Internet]. 2021 Aug 20;**46**(4):E500–5. Available from: https://pubmed.ncbi.nlm.nih.gov/34415691

198. Soares JC, Gershon S. The diagnostic boundaries of bipolar disorder. *Bipolar Disord* [Internet]. 2000 Mar 1;**2**(1):1–2. Available from: https://doi.org/10.1034/j.1399-5618.2000.020101.x

199. Berto F. *There's Something about Gödel: The Complete Guide to the Incompleteness Theorem*. New York: John Wiley & Sons, 2011.

Chapter 3

Epidemiology of Mood Disorders across the Life Span

Kathleen R. Merikangas and Yunna Kwan

Background: Epidemiology

There has been a major transformation in the field of psychiatric epidemiology across the past decade. Whereas previous generations of epidemiology developed the tools and methods to estimate prevalence of mental disorders in the general population, there has been a shift to characterize samples from health registries and biobanks, and to define the impact of mental disorders in terms of disability and impact across the life span.

The expansion of epidemiological research from North America, Europe, and developed pan-Pacific countries to less economically advantaged countries across the world has documented the tremendous burden of mental disorders and the glaring gap in access to treatment. There has also been an increasing focus on mental–medical comorbidity and estimation of their impact on impairment and mortality. Finally, increased awareness of diversity of gender, age, ethnicity, and class is leading to increased efforts to address differences in risk profiles in population strata.

This chapter provides a summary of (i) prevalence rates and correlates of mood disorder subtypes in adults and youth; (ii) patterns of comorbidity of mood disorders; (iii) treatment patterns in community and registry samples; and (iv) impact of mood disorders in population-based samples.

Prevalence of Mood Disorders

The prevalence of both major subtypes of mood disorders has now been well documented through international studies that have employed structured diagnostic interviews to ascertain DSM-IV criteria.

Bipolar Disorder

The largest series of international studies that provide prevalence rates of DSM-IV mood disorders is the World Health Organization (WHO) World Mental Health (WMH) surveys. Data on Bipolar Disorder (BPD) was collected in a subset of eleven population-based surveys that were carried out in the Americas (Sao Paulo metropolitan area, Brazil; Colombia; Mexico; and the United States), Europe (Bulgaria and Romania), Asia (Shenzhen, People's Republic of China; Pondicherry region, India; and nine metropolitan areas in Japan), Lebanon, and New Zealand. Apart from Japan (unclustered two-stage probability sample), all surveys were based on stratified multistage clustered area probability samples. In the past few decades, the lifetime prevalence of Bipolar I (BPI) Disorder has generally been estimated at about 1.0%. Recent studies have begun to include estimates for Bipolar II (BPII) and Bipolar Spectrum (BPS) disorders as well as BPI. As would be expected, prevalence tends to increase with successively more inclusive disorder definitions. For example, in the WMH surveys, the cross-national lifetime prevalence of BPS disorders was 2.4%; of which 0.6% met criteria for BPI, 0.4% for BPII, and 1.4% for subthreshold Bipolar Disorder (sub-BPD) [1]. In many (but not all) studies assessing BPII, its prevalence is actually lower than that of BPI; this may indicate that the majority of people who experience hypomanic episodes also experience manic episodes, or may be explained by the Major Depressive Episode (MDE) requirement for diagnosis of BPII.

Lifetime prevalence estimates for BPD in the largest survey in the United States, the National Epidemiologic Survey on Alcohol and Related Conditions (NESARC), were 2.19% for BPI and 1.12% for BPII, with corresponding 12-month rates of 0.87% and 0.32%, respectively [2]. The only population-based study that produced prevalence rates for DSM-5-defined BPD was the NESARC-III sample. Lifetime prevalence of BPI was 2.1 (2.2 males; 2.0 females) and 12-month prevalence was 1.5 (1.6 male; 1.5 female) [3]. A more recent summary of population-based studies that aggregated across nine community samples in five countries including

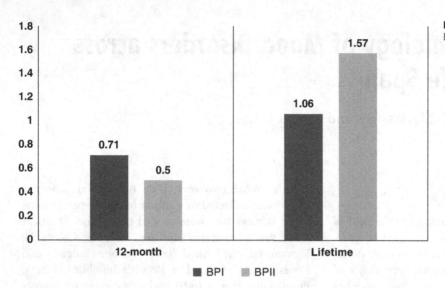

Figure 3.1 Pooled prevalence of Bipolar Disorder.

Switzerland, the Netherlands, Brazil, the United States, and Germany reported a range of prevalence rates from of BPI that ranged from 0.19% to 5.13% [4]. Variability in prevalence rates was most strongly attributable to the diagnostic interview employed and the diagnostic criteria. The pooled prevalence of BPD is presented in Figure 3.1.

An increasing number of studies have estimated the occurrence of BPD in youth. A nationally representative survey of youth aged 13–18 in the United States yielded prevalence rates of 2.1% (12-month) for BPD [5]. More recently, a meta-analysis of 19 studies published between 1985 and 2019 was conducted to estimate the prevalence of BPS in pediatric samples aged 5–19 years [6]. The weighted average prevalence of BPS was 3.9% across the full age span of youth, and increased to 8.3% when the analysis was limited to studies conducted on adolescents aged 12–19 years. Among the 11 studies that examined lifetime prevalence, the weighted average prevalence of BPS was 6.4%. Significant heterogeneity was reported among the research findings depending on the diagnostic criteria and assessment tools utilized, even in relatively recent studies. While clinical studies have found evidence of BPS in children even before adolescence, nationally representative community studies on this are lacking.

Major Depression

The WMH surveys also provided the largest aggregate data on the prevalence of Major Depressive Disorder (MDD). Lifetime and 12-month prevalence rates were estimated in 18 countries, divided according to high- and low-middle income. The lifetime prevalence estimates average 11.1 (range 8.0–18.4) in low-income and 14.6 (range 6.6–21.0) in high-income countries, whereas the 12-month prevalence rates average 5.5 in high-income (range 2.2–8.3) and 5.9 (range 3.8–10.4) in low-income countries [7]. The most recent analysis including 17 surveys from 15 countries participating in the WMH surveys reported a 12-month prevalence of MDD based on DSM-IV diagnostic criteria as 4.8% [8]. Recent prevalence estimates from the NESARC study were 13.2 for lifetime and 5.3 for 12-month MDD [9]. Although there is a wide range of estimates, the average rates of both lifetime and 12-month depression are consistent across studies that employ comparable methodology.

Several cross-sectional and prospective studies have also reported rates of MDD in youth. A recent meta-analysis of 41 studies conducted in 27 countries worldwide yielded a 12-month estimate of any depressive disorder at 2.6% (95% confidence interval [CI]: 1.7–3.9). The prevalence of MDD increases significantly across adolescence, more marked among females than males. The prevalence of MDD by age group in the United States is presented in Figure 3.2. Most cases of MDD are associated with psychiatric comorbidity and severe role impairment, and a substantial minority reported suicidality.

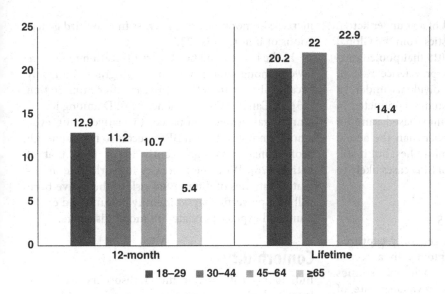

Figure 3.2 Major Depressive Disorder prevalence by age group in the United States.

Electronic Health Records

There has also been an increasing effort to estimate the prevalence of mood disorders in data from health claims, registries, and electronic health record (EHR) databases. Analyses from these studies only identify people who have sought professional treatment for their conditions. The prevalence rates derived from the Kaiser Permanente Northwest (KPNW) cohort study, which encompasses EHR data from clinics in nine states of the United States, were 1.2% for BPD and 7.8% for nonpsychotic MDD [10]. Lifetime prevalence rates From the UK biobank were 6.4% for single MDE, 12.2% for recurrent MDD (moderate), 7.2% for recurrent MDD (severe), and 1.3% for BPD [11]. In contrast, nationwide patient registry data from the Scandinavian countries indicated treatment rates of 3.1% for MDD in Sweden, 3.2% in Denmark, and 4.4% in Norway [12], and 0.58% for BPD in both Sweden and Norway [13, 14]. The 12-month prevalence rates for mood disorders at 0.35% for MDD and 0.16% for BPD were reported in the National Health Insurance database from Taiwan [15].

Correlates of Mood Disorders

Sex/Gender

The most consistent finding across all the studies on the prevalence and incidence of MDD is that it is approximately twofold more common among women than men (odds ratio [OR] = 1.4~2.8) [16]. This gender difference begins in early adulthood, is most pronounced in people between the ages of 30 and 45, and persists in the elderly. There is a more pronounced gender disparity in the prevalence of MDE among women in countries with higher adherence to traditional gender roles, indicating the contribution of psychosocial factors [17]. In contrast to MDD, the gender ratio in BPD (all subtypes combined) is approximately 1:1. However, women have higher rates of BPII and the gender disparity increases as the prominence of depression symptoms is included in the diagnostic nomenclature.

Age of Onset

The onset of BPD generally occurs in the late teens and early twenties and is substantially lower than that of unipolar depression. Men with BPD appear to have 4–5 years of earlier onset than women. In more than half of the cases, onset is before the age of 20, frequently in late adolescence. In contrast, onset of mania rarely occurs after midlife. The ages of onset of BPI and BPII are similar, but there is a slight tendency for a later age of onset in BPII patients (the mean age of onset for BPI is 18.4, BPII is 20.0, and sub-BPD is 21.9 based on the WMH survey) [1]. Despite the consistent evidence provided by clinical studies regarding early onset BPD occurring prior to adolescence, there is a lack of community-based studies on pediatric and adolescent BPD [6], exhibiting an inability to exclude the likelihood of a younger actual average age of onset. In fact, statistics from the Global Health Data Exchange (GHDx) 2019 that pooled estimate prevalence rates suggest a prevalence rate of approximately 1% for BPD in individuals under 15 years of age, incorporating both studies conducted in clinical populations and community-based samples [18]. This estimation may be higher than the actual rate due to the inclusion of clinical studies, but it still indicates a considerable number of BPD cases likely to manifest before adolescence.

Postpartum Mood Disorders

Postpartum mood disorders are generally captured in the form of depressive symptoms. In a recent large-scale meta-analysis that included studies conducted in 80 countries, the prevalence rate of postpartum depression was found to be 17.22% (95% CI: 16.00–18.51) when only considering postpartum females without MDD or other psychiatric conditions [19]. This study identified significant variations in the prevalence rates depending on the developmental level of countries and regions. A meta-analysis showed that women with BPD are particularly susceptible to postpartum depression, with more than one-third experiencing a postpartum mood episode and two-thirds of women who are not taking medication [20]. There is still a general lack of awareness regarding the existence of bipolar postpartum depression, leading to misdiagnosis as unipolar depression, and postpartum hypomania often goes unrecognized [21].

Race and Ethnicity

It is well known that cultural differences may influence the clinical presentation of depression and mania, leading to unreliable figures in prevalence studies performed under standard methodology. However, there is now consistent evidence that rates of mood disorders are lower in Blacks and Hispanic than in Whites in the United States [22]. Because of their increased exposure to psychosocial stress and other risk factors for mood disorders, the lower rates in these ethnic subgroups are paradoxical. However, there has been growing interest in mood disorders in immigrants because of the recent influx of people from several countries into North American and Europe. Previous work has shown that there is an increase in mood disorders across first to third generations of immigrants [23,24].

In the UK, overall healthcare utilization rates were lower among first-generation immigrants and only became similar to natives 10 years after immigration [25]. In Canada, the prevalence of BPD among immigrants was lower compared to natives, but even among immigrants with BPD, access to mental health professionals was significantly lower than that of natives [26]. With the increases in worldwide immigration, studies of differential risk to the native-born will be a powerful way to identify cultural and environmental exposures related to mood disorders.

Comorbidity

Individuals with major mood disorders are at an increased risk of having one or more additional comorbid DSM-IV Axis-I disorders. The most frequent disorders are alcohol use disorder and anxiety disorders [1,16]. Conversely, individuals with substance use disorders (SUDs) and anxiety disorders also have an elevated risk of comorbid mood disorders [27]. In both MDD and BPD, men more frequently present with SUDs, whereas women more frequently present with anxiety and eating disorders. In general, BPD patients more frequently show comorbidity of SUDs and anxiety disorders than do patients with MDD [28], with the highest rate in the BPII subgroup in both clinical and epidemiological studies. Because comorbid SUDs and anxiety disorders worsen the prognosis of the illness and markedly increase the risk of suicide among those with mood disorders, the data presented above are consistent with previous findings showing that those with BPD (particularly BPII) are at the highest risk of suicide [28]. These findings also indicate that Axis-I comorbidity might be among the most important contributing factor to that risk. However, there is a substantial overlap between mood and SUDs [29]. Data from the NESARC study revealed that 41% of those with alcohol use disorders met criteria for primary depression, 17% for concurrent depression, and 42% for secondary depression. This finding supports and extends the results of previous studies conducted among alcoholics in treatment and has strong diagnostic and treatment implications.

There is growing interest in studies of comorbidity of mood disorders with medical conditions.

Systematic collection of data on chronic conditions in the WMH surveys provided systematic evaluation of patterns of comorbidity of mental disorder subtypes with the full range of common medical disorders, their impact on severity, and course [30]. Prospective studies have continued BPD. There is growing effort to identify biomarkers, particularly inflammatory/immunological factors related to the stress system, as potential explanations for comorbidity of mood disorders with cardiovascular disease, diabetes, and cancer. However, it has not been possible to distinguish whether there may be underlying common pathophysiological factors, or that the comorbidity was attributable to common risk factors, such as substance use, sedentary behavior, and other unhealthy behaviors that are elevated among people with mood disorders.

Service Patterns

Adults

Despite the great progress in the diagnosis and treatment of depressions in the past two decades, they remain underdiagnosed and undertreated. Globally, approximately half of those who develop mood disorders seek treatment for them, but only a small fraction (about one-third) of those receive appropriate treatment for a mood disorder [8,31,32]. Interestingly, people with manic episodes were less likely than those with MDE to seek disorder-specific treatment. An increasing rate of health service utilization is related to increasing severity of depression and to comorbid psychiatric and medical disorders.

Even though many patients with depressive disorders seek help in primary care, general practitioners still have difficulties recognizing and treating depression. Because severe major depression is much more common among those with comorbid chronic medical disorders, depression with significant somatic comorbidity remain unrecognized in primary care.

Youth

Despite the magnitude and serious consequences of depression in youth, less than half of those with mental disorders receive mental health services [33]. Factors associated with service utilization include ethnicity, high global impairment, comorbidity, prior history of depression, suicide attempt, and impact of the child's problem on the family. School services are the most common point of entry for children seeking services, although those who enter through the education sector are least likely to transition to specialty mental health services. The actual diagnostic process and services provided differ dramatically by the context of entry to service. There has been accumulating controlled research on the effects of antidepressants in youth, but few studies of either the comparative efficacy of various agents that are commonly used in clinical practice or of individual and family therapies either in conjunction with or independent from pharmacological treatments. There is now growing evidence for a stepped care approach with increasingly intensive interventions moving from psychosocial to pharmacological interventions, as well as their combinations.

Impact of Mood Disorders

The importance of role disability has become increasingly recognized as a major source of indirect costs of illness because of its high economic impact on ill workers, their employers, and society. MDD is the primary cause of disability, ranking among the top 10 sources of disease burden for individuals aged 10 to 49 [34]. In the most recent estimates of the impact of chronic diseases by the World Health Organization, 1.47% of the total proportion of Disability Adjusted Life Years (DALYs) was attributable to MDD, and 0.3% to BPD [34]. Among mental disorders, 37.4% was attributable to MDD and 6.8% to BPD [35]. Of particular concern is the impact of MDD in youth, with 17.64% of DALYs due to mental disorders in the 0–19 age group, while BPD accounted for 4.85% [36]. Comparative studies of role disability reveal that the effects of mood disorders outweigh those of most other mental and neurological disorders with a few exceptions. The dramatic impact of mood disorders on lifetime disability highlights the importance of epidemiology in surveillance, understanding, and control of the major mental disorders.

Mortality and Mood Disorders

There are now several prospective studies that have investigated mortality among those with a range of mental disorders. Data from large population registries in Sweden and Denmark have shown that BPD is associated with substantial elevation in risk of both mortality in general, particularly death by suicide. The mortality risk associated with mood disorders tends to decrease with age; that is, the high risk of death by suicide associated with affective disorders in the Danish Registry was much greater during the first 12 months following the initial admission compared to later years. No differences in excess mortality have been shown for different subgroups of mood disorders in either of these registries. A more recent prospective population-based study with direct examinations of both psychiatric and medical conditions, the CoLaus|PsyCoLaus study, found that current MDD was associated with a nearly threefold increase in mortality after adjustment for socio-demographic and lifestyle characteristics, comorbid anxiety disorders, antidepressant use, and cardiovascular risk factors and diseases [37].

Suicide Attempts

The most alarming consequences of mood disorders are suicide attempts and death by suicide. Untreated major mood disorders (and particularly BPD) carry extremely high risk of both completed and attempted suicide. In a recent meta-analysis, the risk of death by suicide was found to be 7.64 times higher in individuals with MDD and 6.05 times higher in individuals with BPD [38]. Regarding the prevalence, the WHO reported that 2–15% of individuals with MDD and 3–20% of those with BPD die by suicide [39]. A study that followed a nationally representative cohort in Denmark for up to 36 years reported the cumulative incidence rates of suicide to be 7.77% for BPD and 6.67% for MDD in males, as well as 4.78% for BPD and 3.77% for MDD in females, which are considered the most accurate current estimates. Consequently, the early recognition and appropriate acute and long-term treatment of mood disorders are crucial for suicide prevention [40]. The careful and systematic exploration of clinically detectable suicide risk factors helps clinicians to identify suicidal patients, but unfortunately, at the stage of our present knowledge we cannot predict and prevent all suicides.

Summary

There is now a large body of evidence from community-based samples that provides information on the magnitude of mood disorders across the world. These studies show that BPS is far more common than earlier estimates, with an aggregate estimate of 2.4% of the general population. Recent studies of BPS in youth indicate that the peak prevalence of BPS emerges in late adolescence and early adulthood. Comorbidity between both BPD and MDD with other mental disorders is pervasive, with the greatest co-occurrence being anxiety disorders and substance use disorders. Despite a large increase in the proportion of people with mood disorders who receive professional treatment, there is still a large gap between those with impairing mood disorders who remain untreated. There is still substantial under-recognition of bipolarity among those in treatment for depression. The global burden of MDD equals that of many other common chronic diseases, and there is tremendous impact of subtypes of mood disorders at both the individual and societal levels. Mood disorders are the major source of suicide attempts and deaths, and people with these conditions have increased morbidity from chronic diseases and mortality. The growing international efforts to build registries that can track people with mood disorders is providing important information on treatment outcomes and courses of these conditions that can inform efforts to prevent the devastating consequences of mood disorders. There is still a huge gap in information on prevalence, course, and treatment of mood disorders in developing and low-income countries, as well as information on the impact of recent global challenges such as COVID-19 and climate change. Efforts to obtain this information are critical to provide a broader scope of affective disorders in those with the greatest vulnerability.

Acknowledgments

This work was supported by the Intramural Research Program of the National Institute of Mental Health (grant ZIAMH002953). The views and opinions expressed in this chapter are those of the authors and should not be construed to represent the views of any of the sponsoring organizations, agencies, or the US government.

References

1. Merikangas KR, Jin R, He JP, et al. Prevalence and correlates of bipolar spectrum disorder in the world mental health survey initiative. *Arch Gen Psychiatry*. 2011;**68**(3):241–51.

2. Hoertel N, Le Strat Y, Angst J, Dubertret C. Subthreshold bipolar disorder in a US national representative sample: prevalence, correlates and perspectives for psychiatric nosography. *J Affect Disord*. 2013;**146**(3):338–47.

3. Blanco C, Compton WM, Saha TD, et al. Epidemiology of DSM-5 bipolar I disorder: results from the National Epidemiologic Survey on Alcohol and Related Conditions–III. *J Psychiatr Res*. 2017;**84**:310–17.

4. Angst J, Rossler W, Ajdacic-Gross V, et al. Differences between unipolar mania and bipolar-I disorder: evidence from nine epidemiological studies. *Bipolar Disord.* 2019;**21**(5):437–48.

5. Kessler RC, Avenevoli S, Costello EJ, et al. Prevalence, persistence, and sociodemographic correlates of DSM-IV disorders in the National Comorbidity Survey Replication Adolescent Supplement. *Arch Gen Psychiatry.* 2012;**69**(4):372–80.

6. Van Meter A, Moreira ALR, Youngstrom E. Updated meta-analysis of epidemiologic studies of pediatric bipolar disorder. *J Clin Psychiatry.* 2019;**80**(3):21938.

7. Bromet E, Andrade LH, Hwang I, et al. Cross-national epidemiology of DSM-IV major depressive episode. *BMC Med.* 2011;**9**:90.

8. Vigo D, Haro JM, Hwang I, et al. Toward measuring effective treatment coverage: critical bottlenecks in quality- and user-adjusted coverage for major depressive disorder. *Psychol Med.* 2022;**52** (10):1948–58.

9. Hasin DS, Grant BF. The National Epidemiologic Survey on Alcohol and Related Conditions (NESARC) Waves 1 and 2: review and summary of findings. *Soc Psychiatry Psychiatr Epidemiol.* 2015;**50**:1609–40.

10. Yarborough BJH, Perrin NA, Stumbo SP, Muench J, Green CA. Preventive service use among people with and without serious mental illnesses. *Am J Prev Med.* 2018;**54**(1):1–9.

11. Smith DJ, Nicholl BI, Cullen B, et al. Prevalence and characteristics of probable major depression and bipolar disorder within UK biobank: cross-sectional study of 172,751 participants. *PloS One.* 2013;**8**(11): e75362.

12. Pasman JA, Meijsen JJ, Haram M, et al. Epidemiological overview of major depressive disorder in Scandinavia using nationwide registers. *Lancet Reg Health Eur.* 2023;**29**:100621

13. Nesvåg R, Knudsen GP, Bakken IJ, et al. Substance use disorders in schizophrenia, bipolar disorder, and depressive illness: a registry-based study. *Soc Psychiatry Psychiatr Epidemiol.* 2015;**50**:1267–76.

14. Ekman M, Granström O, Omérov S, Jacob J, Landén M. The societal cost of bipolar disorder in Sweden. *Soc Psychiatry Psychiatr Epidemiol.* 2013;**48**:1601–10

15. Chien I-C, Chou Y-J, Lin C-H, Bih S-H, Chou P. Prevalence of psychiatric disorders among National Health Insurance enrollees in Taiwan. *Psychiatr Serv.* 2004;**55**(6):691–7.

16. Gutiérrez-Rojas L, Porras-Segovia A, Dunne H, Andrade-González N, Cervilla JA. Prevalence and correlates of major depressive disorder: a systematic review. *Braz J Psychiatry.* 2020;**42**:657–72.

17. Seedat S, Scott KM, Angermeyer MC, et al. Cross-national associations between gender and mental disorders in the World Health Organization World Mental Health Surveys. *Arch Gen Psychiatry.* 2009;**66** (7):785–95.

18. Network GBo DC. *Global Burden of Disease Study 2019 (GBD 2019) Results Seattle, United States*: Institute for Health Metrics and Evaluation (IHME); 2020.

19. Wang Z, Liu J, Shuai H, et al. Mapping global prevalence of depression among postpartum women. *Transl Psychiatry.* 2021;**11**(1):543.

20. Wesseloo R, Kamperman AM, Munk-Olsen T, et al. Risk of postpartum relapse in bipolar disorder and postpartum psychosis: a systematic review and meta-analysis. *Am J Psychiatry.* 2016;**173**(2):117–27.

21. Sharma V, Doobay M, Baczynski C. Bipolar postpartum depression: an update and recommendations. *J Affect Disord.* 2017;**219**:105–11.

22. Akinhanmi MO, Biernacka JM, Strakowski SM, et al. Racial disparities in bipolar disorder treatment and research: a call to action. *Bipolar Disord.* 2018;**20** (6):506–14.

23. Pignon B, Geoffroy PA, Thomas P, et al. Prevalence and clinical severity of mood disorders among first-, second- and third-generation migrants. *J Affect Disord.* 2017;**210**:174–80.

24. Osooli M, Ohlsson H, Sundquist J, Sundquist K. Major depressive disorders in young immigrants: a cohort study from primary healthcare settings in Sweden. *Scand J Public Health.* 2021:**51** (3):315–32.

25. Saunders CL, Steventon A, Janta B, et al. Healthcare utilization among migrants to the UK: cross-sectional analysis of two national surveys. *J Health Serv Res Policy.* 2021;**26**(1):54–61.

26. Schaffer A, Cairney J, Cheung A, et al. Differences in prevalence and treatment of bipolar disorder among immigrants: results from an epidemiologic survey. *Can J Psychiatry.* 2009;**54**(11):734–42.

27. Martin P. The epidemiology of anxiety disorders: a review. *Dialogues Clin Neurosci.* 2022;**5**(3):81–98.

28. Kessler RC, Merikangas KR, Wang PS. Prevalence, comorbidity, and service utilization for mood disorders in the United States at the beginning of the twenty-first century. *Annu Rev Clin Psychol.* 2007;**3**:137–58.

29. Hasin D, Kilcoyne B. Comorbidity of psychiatric and substance use disorders in the United States: current issues and findings from the NESARC. *Curr Opin Psychiatry.* 2012;**25**(3):165.

30. Scott KM, Von Korff M, Alonso J, et al. Mental–physical co-morbidity and its relationship with disability: results from the World Mental Health Surveys. *Psychol Med.* 2009;**39**(1):33–43.

31. Mekonen T, Chan GCK, Connor JP, Hides L, Leung J. Estimating the global treatment rates for depression: a systematic review and meta-analysis. *J Affect Disord.* 2021;**295**:1234–42.

32. Mackenzie CS, Reynolds K, Cairney J, Streiner DL, Sareen J. Disorder-specific mental health service use for mood and anxiety disorders: associations with age, sex, and psychiatric comorbidity. *Depress Anxiety.* 2012;**29**(3):234–42.

33. Merikangas KR, Nakamura EF, Kessler RC. Epidemiology of mental disorders in children and adolescents. *Dialogues Clin Neurosci.* 2022;**11**(1)7_20.

34. Vos T, Lim SS, Abbafati C, et al. Global burden of 369 diseases and injuries in 204 countries and territories, 1990–2019: a systematic analysis for the Global Burden of Disease Study 2019. *Lancet.* 2020;**396** (10258):1204–22.

35. Collaborators GMD. Global, regional, and national burden of 12 mental disorders in 204 countries and territories, 1990–2019: a systematic analysis for the Global Burden of Disease Study 2019. *Lancet Psychiatry.* 2022;**9**(2):137–50.

36. Piao J, Huang Y, Han C, et al. Alarming changes in the global burden of mental disorders in children and adolescents from 1990 to 2019: a systematic analysis for the Global Burden of Disease study. *Eur Child Adolesc Psychiatry.* 2022;**31**(11):1827–45.

37. Lasserre AM, Marti-Soler H, Strippoli M-PF, et al. Clinical and course characteristics of depression and all-cause mortality: a prospective population-based study. *J Affect Disord.* 2016;**189**:17–24.

38. Moitra M, Santomauro D, Degenhardt L, et al. Estimating the risk of suicide associated with mental disorders: a systematic review and meta-regression analysis. *J Psychiatr Res.* 2021;**137**:242–9.

39. World Health Organization. Preventing suicide: a global imperative. 2014.

40. Nordentoft M, Mortensen PB, Pedersen CB. Absolute risk of suicide after first hospital contact in mental disorder. *Arch Gen Psychiatry.* 2011;**68** (10):1058–64.

The Mood Spectrum Concept: Clinical Implications

Rebecca Strawbridge and Anthony J. Cleare

History

The concept of a bipolar spectrum has a long history, some of which has been covered in Chapter 2. Early conceptualisations of a continuum, for example by Kretschmer [1], have been elaborated as more modern concepts and data emerged [2]. The spectrum encompasses both polarity and severity, including subthreshold presentations.

Angst conceived of minor (d) and major (D) forms of depression, and minor (m) and major (M) forms of hypomania/mania, suggesting that this produced a spectrum from unipolar mania (M) or hypomania through to unipolar minor (d) or major (D) depression, with a large group of bipolar patients in between. The bipolar patients also existed on a spectrum, which included Mania and major Depression (MD), through Mania with minor depression (Md) and major Depression with hypomania (Dm) to cyclothymia (md) [3].

Perhaps the most detailed attempts to delineate the bipolar spectrum have come from Akiskal, who expanded the existing type 1 and type 2 subcategories of bipolar disorder (BD) as shown in Table 4.1. All of these have a clinical, suprathreshold severity of at least one of the poles of illness. However, for Bipolar 2½

onwards, the presentations are of depression with a variety of subthreshold forms of hypomanic symptoms, which fall short of the DSM/ICD definitions as discussed in the next section. It should be noted that patients do move between these presentations, and that individuals are usually categorised into their highest lifetime state; for example, patients with Bipolar 2 will often also experience antidepressant-induced states and may have periods of subthreshold mania [2].

Clinically, we could even take this spectrum further. One is often struck by the presentation of patients with highly recurrent and cycling depressive conditions, with predictable periodicity, often relatively brief durations, and with both onset and offset occurring rapidly. Very careful history-taking or clinical observation can sometimes (though by no means always) detect subtle changes – such as irritability, interest, energy, or sleep – in the days before onset or after offset that could be conceived as subthreshold hypomanic features. Similarly, seasonal depression with the characteristic Spring recovery with feelings of activation and invigoration may also fit as an extension of the spectrum [2].

We turn now to the current classification of bipolar spectrum disorders (BSDs).

Table 4.1 Akiskal soft bipolar spectrum

Bipolar ½	Schizomanic/schizobipolar disorder
Bipolar 1	Depression and mania
Bipolar 1½	Depression and protracted hypomania
Bipolar 2	Depression and hypomania
Bipolar 2½	Depression with cyclothymia
Bipolar 3	Depression with antidepressant-induced hypomania
Bipolar 3½	Depression with substance-induced hypomania
Bipolar 4	Depression with hyperthymic temperament

Current Classification/Diagnosis

The current DSM-5 classification of 'bipolar and related disorders' includes the main categories of BD type I (BD-I) and type II (BD-II), as well as cyclothymic disorder, BDs induced by substance use or medical condition, specified and unspecified BDs. Current criteria for those not qualifying for a BD-I or BD-II diagnosis permits one of four other diagnoses. For all, the symptoms must not be better explained by a psychotic disorder, or indeed another diagnosis, and cause clinically significant distress and/or functional impairment.

* *Cyclothymic Disorder:* Over a > 2-year period (or 1 year if age < 18), symptoms of hypomania and/or depression present for > 50% of time, without a symptom free period exceeding 2 months. Neither within this period, nor previously, can criteria have been met for a major depressive or hypomanic episode.

* *Substance/Medication-Induced BD and Related Disorder:* Here, hypomanic (with or without depressive) symptoms are evidenced as emerging during or soon after substance exposure, intoxication, or withdrawal, with said substance known to be capable of producing these symptoms. The symptoms must not be exclusive to delirious states. Commonly, these substances are antidepressants, stimulants, steroids, phencyclidine or recently cathinone derivatives ('bath salts') with timing of affective symptom onset and offset dependent on the substance.

* *Bipolar and Related Disorder Due to Another Medical Condition:* Here, the hypomanic symptoms are attributed with supporting evidence as being directly consequential to another medical condition. The symptoms must not be exclusive to delirious states. Commonly, these conditions are multiple sclerosis, Cushing's syndrome, stroke, and traumatic brain injuries, with timing of affective symptom onset and offset dependent on the condition (although often aligning with the development and/or remittance of the co-occurring illness).

* *Other Specified or Unspecified Bipolar and Related Disorder:* Specified if symptoms are impairing, and where a specific reason is given for not meeting full criteria of other bipolar diagnoses. This reason might be a short duration of hypomania and/or depression, or episodes with insufficient symptoms to meet criteria for a full episode. The DSM-5 also lists a substantive hypomanic episode without history of a major depressive episode in this category.

It is worth noting here that bipolar spectrum disorders (other than type I and type II) most typically comprise patients with cyclothymic disorder or the latter catch-all not otherwise specified (NOS) category, but it is considered that substance- or medical-condition induced bipolar disorders are often indicative of a latent bipolar diathesis and other bipolar spectrum conditions often emerge in such patients.

The DSM allows multiple other specifiers to delineate affective disorder, including not only the current or most recent episode type and severity, but also the presence of several specifiers, including anxious distress, mixed features, rapid cycling, melancholic features, atypical features, mood-congruent psychotic features, mood-incongruent psychotic features, catatonia, peripartum onset, and seasonal pattern.

Recent Updates

One of the main changes between DSM-IV and DSM-5 was the requirement for people to have experienced both increased mood *and* activity to meet criteria for (hypo)mania. Some have criticised this change, suggesting that it reduces the prevalence of (hypo)manic episodes and that this could 'distort' detection of those with BD [4], supported by a recent study reporting that half of participants with a BD diagnosis and elevated mood did not concurrently record increased activation [5]. Other research contradicts this, finding that the change in this criterion does not impact BD diagnosis rates [6] and many welcome the change as reflecting the evidence to date of (hypo)mania as a multidimensional affective state, rather than one reflective only of mood – particularly as elevated mood can range from elation to irritability [7]. All iterations of the DSM have been criticised for including unipolar mania as a bipolar disorder [8]. DSM-IV had been criticised for not being evidence-derived (e.g., incorporating activity) but also excluding many people with a bipolar disorder with clinically significant but brief manic episodes. This has not changed in the primary criteria for mania/hypomania in DSM-5, although the NOS category exists for the latter. DSM-5 criteria now specifically note, under NOS, hypomania of a short duration (2 to 3 days) or with insufficient (fewer) symptoms) and this has been met also with mixed views and evidence. One large study comparing various hypomania durations (1 day, 2 to 3 days, 4 to 6 days) with other external validators identified 4 days as the optimal duration threshold [9], while other evidence has suggested no differences between individuals with Bipolar II ($\geq$ 4 day hypomania duration) and others with depressive episodes and brief hypomania (< 4 days; not meeting the duration criterion) [10].

The loosening of BD-NOS DSM criteria has the strength of permitting a diagnosis for many individuals who would not previously have been eligible but who required treatment for mood disorders, but the NOS category is still considered to be non-specific and heterogeneous, and the 'activity' requirement for a (hypo)manic episode would also result in the re-diagnosis of some individuals to NOS instead of type I/II BD [8].

ICD-11

In previous iterations, the ICD was criticised for not including a BD-II classification, but ICD-11 now specifies this and also includes cyclothymic disorder. Many have praised a convergence of ICD-11 to DSM-5 (e.g., in terms of BD-II inclusion) and appreciate the scope for clinical judgement that ICD-11 offers. For example, there is not a precise number of symptoms or minimum duration for hypomania (the latter specifying 'at least several days'). ICD-11 permits a hypomanic episode within a diagnosis of cyclothymic disorder, where appropriate, while DSM only permits cyclothymic features as a specifier of BD-II [11]. Although both BD-II and cyclothymia can be diagnosed more frequently in ICD-11 [12], there continues to be some criticism for not including a formal category to recognise subthreshold bipolar disorders and resultantly classifying the full bipolar spectrum [13].

BD Timing and Risk

A further controversial issue is the retrospective diagnosis of people with bipolar disorders. For most patients, the first affective episode is major depressive as opposed to (hypo)manic. Although in an initial depressive episode, major depressive disorder (MDD) would be a valid diagnosis, receiving this diagnosis (and corresponding intervention) can have problematic consequences for people who later manifest bipolar disorder. The large BRIDGE study found that 47% of bipolar patients had at least for a time been

mistakenly diagnosed with unipolar depression [14]. This cannot be definitively avoided, but illustrates an argument for identifying those *at risk for* BD separately from a definite unipolar disorder. These at-risk features include a positive family history for BD, substance use (disorders), recurrent depressive episodes, anxiety disorders (particularly panic disorder, but also generalised anxiety disorder [GAD], social phobia, and potentially obsessive-compulsive disorder [OCD]), mixed or atypical depressive symptoms, early age of onset, other comorbidities such as personality disorders [15], or those with trait affective lability [16]. Treatment responsiveness to antidepressants is also relevant: in a large Taiwanese cohort, those who responded to their first antidepressant treatment had rates of manic switch of about 6–9%, whereas those who needed at least two treatment changes had switch rates of over 25% [17]. It is acknowledged that the DSM does note some of these as risk factors for BD in one section or other, but these are seldom used in clinical practice when considering treatment for an individual without a BD diagnosis who is experiencing a depressive episode. For a potential solution to this challenge, we may turn to the psychosis field where (following frequent use of a research-defined 'at-risk' prodromal state), much dialogue has debated the optimal solution for halting or mitigating the development of a first full psychotic episode. A popular solution would be adding criteria for a risk syndrome into DSM revisions [18] despite concerns over false-positive diagnoses, unnecessary medication treatment, and stigma [19].

Weighing the Benefits of Broadening Diagnostic Criteria

When considering what should, and shouldn't, be classified diagnostically (relevant for at-risk mental states and broader BSD) it is worth remembering the goals of diagnosis. Ultimately, the main objective is to treat impairing conditions appropriately to reduce or eliminate impairment. Since the most common alternative diagnoses for people with latent bipolar disorders largely recommend monoaminergic antidepressants (and that these when used monotherapeutically can worsen symptoms), there is an argument for increased classification. A secondary goal is to homogenise definitions used in research, which will advance our understanding and progress towards enhanced management of these illnesses.

Table 4.2 Selection of proposed BSD definitions

Author(s)	Definition description
Akiskal (1987)[23] Akiskal & Pinto (1999)[2]	[see Table 4.1] Subaffective disorders: bipolar II ½ (MDE + cyclothymic disorder), bipolar III (antidepressant-associated hypomania), bipolar III ½ (bipolarity masked/unmasked by substance use), and bipolar IV (MDE + hyperthymic temperament)
Ghaemi et al. (2002)[24]	'Bipolar spectrum disorder'; compromise between categorical and dimensional. Depression without (hypo)mania + either BD affected 1st-degree relative or antidepressant induced (hypo)mania, or 6/9 tertiary criteria (hyperthymic temperament, recurrent depression, brief depression, atypical depression, psychosis during depression, depression onset age <25, post-partum depression, unsustained antidepressant response or non-response to >3 antidepressants).
Muzina (2007)[25]	Modification of above BSD definition. Depression *or* single mania. If no mania, distinct hypomania (if antidepressant induced, plus three tertiary) or recurrent / brief depressive episodes (plus two tertiary). Tertiary: BD affected 1st-degree relative, hyperthymic temperament, atypical depression, psychotic depression, depression onset age <25, post-partum depression, non-response to >3 antidepressants or repeated tolerance to antidepressants.
Angst et al. (2003)[26]	+ minor bipolar disorder (dysthymia, minor depression or recurrent brief depression associated with hypomanic syndrome/symptoms) and pure hypomania.
Phelps et al. (2008)[27]	Three diagnostic groups: 1. Antidepressant-associated hypomania 2. 'Subthreshold' hypomania with depression 3. 'Soft bipolar': Non-hypomania bipolar features (e.g., recurrent MDE, family history, early onset, mixed features)

This is also something that has been lacking to date. These appear to be arguments in favour of increased classification but it has also been contended that, despite overall consensus on the implications of a current under-classification, there is not robust *enough* evidence of the harms of (possibly) mistreatment to warrant its expansion, and that such an expansion of the bipolar section could impede future research progress as well as potentially diminish the value of a B[S]D diagnosis [20].

One key debate here is whether temperament/personality factors should or should not be considered in BSD definitions. On one hand, BDs are associated with trait cyclothymic temperament and affective lability that precede BD diagnosis [16] (although, despite an ongoing presence in the literature, there is conflicting evidence surrounding hyperthymic temperament [21]). On the other hand, one of the differentiating factors between bipolar and borderline personality disorder is episodicity of affective instability [22]. Thus, many advise temperament constructs to be considered as important and relevant for bipolar spectrum disorders, but as a tertiary dimension with less priority than severity and diagnostic criteria [15].

Table 4.2 contains a non-exhaustive summary of BSD definitions that have been proposed.

Epidemiology

Regardless of exactly how the affective disorders are classified, a large number of people fall into the 'gap' between a clearcut unipolar depressive disorder and a definitive bipolar disorder (BD-I or BD-II) as defined in current classification systems. These subthreshold presentations can include:

Within episode: MDD with mixed symptoms; stand-alone subthreshold hypomania; stand-alone subthreshold mixed affective symptoms.

Longitudinal: MDD with a history of subthreshold hypomanic symptoms; MDD with a history of subthreshold mixed symptoms; history of subthreshold depressive and hypomanic symptoms, that is, cyclothymia.

While overdiagnosis has been raised as a concern of expanding BSD criteria [20], it is important to highlight that at present we observe underdiagnosis of all affective disorders, referring here to individuals that definitively meet existing criteria. It is widely documented that many people meeting criteria for bipolar disorders are undiagnosed [9,28], and even unipolar MDD is under-recognised in services [29]. The rates of BD-NOS/BSD/cyclothymia appear particularly low, and this specific under-diagnosis has been emphasised in landmark national survey data [30]. We posit, though, that misdiagnosis may extend to those with existing BD diagnoses, with individuals diagnosed as having BD-II actually meeting criteria for BD-type I in routine healthcare services.

Considering in slightly more depth the rates of BSD in samples of people ostensibly with MDD, this may approximate at 50%: several studies indicate a rate of around 15–20% for BD type I and type II combined [9,31–33] while estimates incorporating a variety of broader 'spectrum' definitions are around 40–55% [9,33–35]. One recent study of individuals referred to a UK primary care psychological therapies service (not considered suitable for people with bipolar disorders) reported a rate of approximately 70%, although it was estimated that around 5% may have had a BD diagnosis [28]. At a population level, and in contrast to diagnosis rates, the prevalence rates of subthreshold bipolar spectrum disorders appear higher (around 2.5% lifetime) than BD type I and II (around 1% each) [30].

In interpreting these aforementioned studies, it is important to emphasise that the prevalence estimates of these illnesses depend partially on definitions employed, with lower rates identified when stricter criteria are applied [33].

Clinical Assessment

Clinical assessment of patients with depression (perhaps particularly in those with antidepressant resistance) should always explore the potential presence of hypomanic symptoms, both cross sectionally and longitudinally. Diagnoses according to current criteria for BD type I and II demonstrate good agreement, although agreement is lower for unipolar MDD [36] (and, as implied above, each of these not be applied as reliably in many routine practice settings).

Evidently greater consensus is required on what constitutes a clinically relevant bipolar *spectrum* disorder and standardised clinical assessments pertaining to DSM criteria are lacking for NOS. A systematic review, seeking to determine accuracy of BSD diagnosis when assessed using validated assessments, focused on rating scales evaluating hypomania [37]. The review and meta-analysis of 14 such tools found a generally good discrimination between BD and non-BD although this was hindered by extensive unexplained heterogeneity between studies and measures. The greatest accuracy was observed overall with four measures noted below, which had an area under the curve (AUC) from receiver operating characteristic (ROC) analysis of 0.76 after adjusting for covariates; this was reported to be both

'clinically informative' and significantly better than non-standardised clinical judgement [37]. All four tools are patient rated: the Hypomanic Checklist (HCL) [38] was designed to screen for previous hypomanic symptoms; the Mood Disorder Questionnaire (MDQ) [39] and Bipolar Spectrum Diagnostic Scale (BSDS) [40] were specifically intended to detect BSDs, and finally the Internal State Scale (ISS) [41], which was actually developed as a measure of current symptomatology (24-hour period) for people with BD. Nevertheless, all of these measures have been criticised for being over-sensitive/over-inclusive for BDs [33,42] and there are concerning implications of both false-positive and false-negative BD diagnoses. Additionally, while this review suggested that the use of screening tools outperformed non-standardised clinical judgement, they were essentially comparing screening tools to standardised diagnostic interviews, but diagnostic assessments (e.g., MINI) are sometimes rapid and can also be over-inclusive [28].

Associated Characteristics

A number of clinical features are associated with the presence of a bipolar diathesis. These include a family history of bipolar and related disorders, increased substance use (disorders), comorbid anxiety-related disorders and other psychiatric conditions (e.g., personality disorders, attention deficit hyperactivity disorder [ADHD]), physical health conditions and body mass index (BMI), stressful life events (including early in childhood), and dysfunctional (self) assumptions. More centrally, experience of psychosis; occupational, functional, and cognitive difficulties; suicidality; and an early age of psychiatric illness onset are affective characteristics associated with bipolarity. Features of depressive illness indicative of BSD also include high recurrence, affective lability and atypical features/symptoms. As a rule, these characteristics are found not only in individuals with a BD-I or BD-II diagnosis, but also in people with a subthreshold/spectrum BSD [9,28]. In those at risk for BD, their presence can predict diagnostic conversion [16,43].

These characteristics, alongside the challenges in diagnosing BSDs, have led to the development of a bipolarity index. This is intended not only to bolster diagnostic confidence but also to highlight individuals at risk of diagnostic conversion (note, this does not pertain specifically to 'spectrum' disorders). To do so, the bipolarity index detects, alongside symptomatology/episodes, some of these associated characteristics (age of onset, illness course, family history, treatment response). Its ability to detect current bipolar disorders has a reported sensitivity of 0.91 and specificity of 0.90 (AUC 0.97) suggesting its superiority over self-reported screening tools [44]. Given recommendations that to improve detection and treatment, clinicians should screen for BSDs in patients who may be at risk, the Bipolarity Index could be used routinely by clinicians to assess risk for a BSD – for example, in people with antidepressant-resistant depression.

Treatment

The treatment of patients with clearcut bipolar disorder or clearcut unipolar disorder is outside of the scope of this chapter. We focus on the treatment of those cases with sub-threshold bipolarity. When doing so, one is soon struck by the paucity of evidence to guide treatment approaches. Much of the treatment approach is extrapolated from the bipolar or unipolar depression literature, with few studies specifically focussing on the various presentations discussed earlier. We discuss some specific categories here.

BD-NOS

A recent, broad review suggested an absence of an evidence base regarding treatment options for BD-NOS/BSD. Across 15 original studies (the majority being case reports/series), the treatments mentioned in multiple articles were valproate (three positive), quetiapine (two positive, one negative), and lithium and lamotrigine (one positive, two negative). Of the two randomised studies reviewed, neither reported efficacious results (one of lithium and quetiapine, mentioned above, and the other of ziprasidone). This review also included expert opinion and/or review papers, which largely suggested that antidepressant monotherapy is not helpful for people with BSD, most citing mood stabilisers / anticonvulsants as the optimal treatment options albeit with an insufficient evidence base (either monotherapuetically or adjunct to antidepressants), with some indications that people with BSD should be broadly treated in line with BD guidelines, although there does not appear to be consensus on that issue. It is worth noting that the studies included in this review assessed participants meeting various BSD criteria as well as various methodologies and treatments [45]. To our knowledge, non-pharmacological interventions have been rarely discussed for BSD.

Cyclothymia

Although there is a scant evidence base and no specific pharmacological treatments for cyclothymia approved by the US Food and Drug Administration (FDA), mood stabilisers are considered first line (one recent review recommended valproate for prominent anxiety, lamotrigine for anxious-depression prominence, lithium for affective lability) [46]. Atypical antipsychotics are also used, albeit with some caution around sensitivity to D2-antagonists inducing negative symptoms [47]. Antidepressants, particularly selective serotonin reuptake inhibitors (SSRIs), are not recommended [46], although tricyclics can be helpful in some cases [47]. Some have specifically recommended lithium, while others contradict this, although suggestions of poor treatment response for people with cyclothymic disorder are not specific to lithium [47].

Psychoeducation is considered important for this, as with other, BSDs. Cognitive behavioural therapy is also used [46].

Depression with Mixed Features

Although a major depressive episode with mixed features is not always considered a formal BSD, its presence is clearly indicative (depression with mixed features has a prevalence of around 46–73% in BD-diagnosed individuals, and 7–49% of notionally unipolar MDD). Despite these high rates of presentation, and the clear clinical challenge it brings, there is a limited evidence base for treating mixed depression. A recent systematic review identified 11 randomised controlled trials (RCTs) of pharmacological therapies (six unipolar, five bipolar). In unipolar MDD (i.e., subthreshold BSD), five of six were posthoc studies from one parent study of lurasidone, which showed promising effects. A second study using ziprasidone did not show benefits over placebo (for BSD; grouped with unipolar MDD due to consistency of illness criteria used between them). In those with a BD diagnosis, single studies of lurasidone and ziprasidone were positive, as was olanzapine and olanzapine-fluoxetine combination [48]. There is also recent evidence that cariprazine is effective across the bipolar spectrum, including for mixed states [49].

The Pragmatic Approach

Many clinicians take a pragmatic approach to treating patients with a bipolar spectrum presentation. It is likely to be the case that many patients, especially those with a predominant depressive presentation, will have been included within unipolar depression trials as they will not have met exclusionary criteria for a diagnosis of BD-I or BD-II. Thus, it is not unreasonable to extrapolate from trials in MDD and use antidepressants as initial treatment, unless specifically contraindicated (see above). However, clinicians should be aware of the heightened risk of exacerbating mixed symptoms or precipitating hypomanic switch, and there should be a low threshold for adding mood stabilisers to antidepressants in these patients. In that regard, one is then largely extrapolating from the bipolar literature.

Similarly, in patients who are not responding well to antidepressant monotherapy, the use of mood-stabilising medication as an early treatment step would be warranted. As with suprathreshold bipolarity, in some cases antidepressants simply do not work or worsen the presentation acutely or longitudinally, by destabilising mood or accelerating recurrences. In these cases, mood stabilisers in monotherapy or combination may be preferred to the use of antidepressants. The choice of mood stabiliser can be targeted to the type of presentation, with the knowledge that some are preferentially effective against depressive symptoms, such as lamotrigine and quetiapine, and may be preferred where depressive symptoms are the most prominent part of the presentation. On the other hand, in cases where there is historically more of a concern about hypomanic symptoms, mood stabilisers with actions against both poles, like lithium, may be preferred. Patient preference is of course very important, and it is a matter of regret that few good studies have looked at the influence of this on treatment. In a recent study comparing lithium and quetiapine, it was notable that patients' concerns about the use of lithium in advance of treatment, such as frequent blood testing, were less apparent once treatment had been initiated [50].

We have focussed on pharmacological treatment, but there is even less research on the use of non-pharmacological therapies in these patients. Given the propensity for recurrence, the use of psychological therapies to aid relapse prevention is of particular benefit (although some trials, e.g., of mindfulness-based cognitive therapy [51], have not supported their use in BSD).

The overriding message from this section is the urgent need for good RCTs that specifically recruit patients with a bipolar diathesis that falls short of current definitions. That these presentations are so common in clinical practice and yet still so understudied in the research literature is one of psychiatry's greatest mysteries.

Concluding Remarks

There is no perfect way to categorise mood disorders, but there is undoubtedly a large group of patients who experience recurrent mood illness that does not fit neatly into a unipolar or bipolar category as currently defined. For these individuals, the concept of a bipolar spectrum is helpful.

Nevertheless, the conceptualisation of BSD subsumes substantial heterogeneity in terms of clinical presentations. There is a need to fully standardise the definition of BSD, procedures for assessment and management, with there currently being no clear guidelines on how to treat individuals with impairing affective disorder that is not quite unipolar or substantively bipolar. Perhaps most importantly of all, well-designed studies that specifically recruit these individuals are urgently needed to provide a sufficient evidence base upon which to guide our treatments.

References

1. Kretschmer E. *Körperbau und Charakter. Untersuchungen zum Konstitutions-Problem und zur Lehre von den Temperamenten.* [Physique and character. Investigations on the constitution problem and on the doctrine of the temperaments]. Oxford: Springer, 1936: 243 p.

2. Akiskal HS, Pinto O. The evolving bipolar spectrum. Prototypes I, II, III, and IV. *Psychiatr Clin North Am.* 1999 Sep;**22**(3):517–34, vii.

3. Angst J. The course of affective disorders. II. Typology of bipolar manic-depressive illness. *Arch Psychiatr Nervenkr.* 1978 Oct 9;**226**(1):65–73.

4. Grunze A, Born C, Fredskild MU, Grunze H. How does adding the DSM-5 criterion increased energy/activity for mania change the bipolar landscape? *Front Psychiatry.* 2021;**12**:123.

5. Faurholt-Jepsen M, Christensen EM, Frost M, et al. Hypomania/Mania by DSM-5 definition based on daily smartphone-based patient-reported assessments. *J Affect Disord.* 2020 Mar 1;**264**:272–8.

6. Gordon-Smith K, Jones LA, Forty L, Craddock N, Jones I. Changes to the diagnostic criteria for bipolar disorder in DSM-5 make little difference to lifetime diagnosis: findings from the U.K. Bipolar Disorder

Research Network (BDRN) study. *Am J Psychiatry.* 2017 Aug 1;**174**(8):803.

7. Severus E, Bauer M. Diagnosing bipolar disorders in DSM-5. *Int J Bipolar Disord.* 2013 Aug 23;**1**(1):14.

8. Angst J. Bipolar disorders in DSM-5: strengths, problems and perspectives. *Int J Bipolar Disord.* 2013 Aug 23;**1**(1):12.

9. Angst J, Azorin JM, Bowden CL, et al. Prevalence and characteristics of undiagnosed bipolar disorders in patients with a major depressive episode: the BRIDGE study. *Arch Gen Psychiatry.* 2011 Aug;**68**(8):791–8.

10. Parker G, Graham R, Synnott H, Anderson J. Is the DSM-5 duration criterion valid for the definition of hypomania? *J Affect Disord.* 2014 Mar;**156**:87–91.

11. Severus E, Bauer M. Diagnosing bipolar disorders: ICD-11 and beyond. *Int J Bipolar Disord.* 2020 Jan 20;**8**(1):4.

12. Angst J, Ajdacic-Gross V, Rössler W. Bipolar disorders in ICD-11: current status and strengths. *Int J Bipolar Disord.* 2020 Jan 20;**8**(1):3.

13. Kaltenboeck A, Winkler D, Kasper S. Bipolar and related disorders in DSM-5 and ICD-10. *CNS Spectr.* 2016 Aug;**21**(4):318–23.

14. Angst J, Gamma A, Bowden CL, et al. Evidence-based definitions of bipolar-I and bipolar-II disorders among 5,635 patients with major depressive episodes in the Bridge Study: validity and comorbidity. *Eur Arch Psychiatry Clin Neurosci.* 2013 Dec;**263**(8): 663–73.

15. ANGST J. Problems in the current concepts and definitions of bipolar disorders. *World Psychiatry.* 2011 Oct;**10**(3):191–2.

16. Taylor RH, Ulrichsen A, Young AH, Strawbridge R. Affective lability as a prospective predictor of subsequent bipolar disorder diagnosis: a systematic review. *Int J Bipolar Disord.* 2021 Nov 1;**9**(1):33.

17. Li CT, Bai YM, Huang YL, et al. Association between antidepressant resistance in unipolar depression and subsequent bipolar disorder: cohort study. *Br J Psychiatry J Ment Sci.* 2012 Jan;**200**(1):45–51.

18. Carpenter WT. Anticipating DSM-V: should psychosis risk become a diagnostic class? *Schizophr Bull.* 2009 Sep 1;**35**(5):841–3.

19. Zachar P, First MB, Kendler KS. The DSM-5 proposal for attenuated psychosis syndrome: a history. *Psychol Med.* 2020 Apr;**50**(6):920–6.

20. Strakowski SM, Fleck DE, Maj M. Broadening the diagnosis of bipolar disorder: benefits vs. risks. *World Psychiatry.* 2011;**10**(3):181–6.

21. Vazquez GH, Kahn C, Schiavo CE, et al. Bipolar disorders and affective temperaments: a national family study testing the 'endophenotype' and 'subaffective' theses using the TEMPS-A Buenos Aires. *J Affect Disord.* 2008 May;**108**(1–2):25–32.

22. Paris J. Differential diagnosis of bipolar and borderline personality disorders. *Neuropsychiatry.* 2011 Jun;**1**(3):251–7.

23. Akiskal HS, Mallya G. Criteria for the 'soft' bipolar spectrum: treatment implications. *Psychopharmacol Bull.* 1987;**23**(1):68–73.

24. Ghaemi SN, Ko JY, Goodwin FK. 'Cade's disease' and beyond: misdiagnosis, antidepressant use, and a proposed definition for bipolar spectrum disorder. *Can J Psychiatry Rev Can Psychiatr.* 2002 Mar;**47** (2):125–34.

25. Muzina DJ. Bipolar spectrum disorder: differential diagnosis and treatment. *Prim Care Clin Off Pract.* 2007 Sep 1;**34**(3):521–50.

26. Angst J, Gamma A, Benazzi F, et al. Toward a re-definition of subthreshold bipolarity: epidemiology and proposed criteria for bipolar-II, minor bipolar disorders and hypomania. *J Affect Disord.* 2003 Jan;**73**(1–2):133–46.

27. Phelps J, Angst J, Katzow J, Sadler J. Validity and utility of bipolar spectrum models. *Bipolar Disord.* 2008 Feb;**10**(1 Pt 2):179–93.

28. Strawbridge R, Alexander L, Richardson T, Young A, Cleare A. Is there a 'bipolar iceberg' in UK primary care psychological therapy services? *Psycol Med.* 2023 Sep;**53**(12):5385–94.

29. Strawbridge R, McCrone P, Ulrichsen A, et al. Care pathways for people with major depressive disorder: a European Brain Council Value of Treatment study. *Eur Psychiatry.* 2022 Jun 15;**65** (1):1–21.

30. Merikangas KR, Akiskal HS, Angst J, et al. Lifetime and 12-month prevalence of bipolar spectrum disorder in the National Comorbidity Survey Replication. *Arch Gen Psychiatry.* 2007 May 1;**64** (5):543–52.

31. Hantouche EG, Akiskal HS, Lancrenon S, et al. Systematic clinical methodology for validating bipolar-II disorder: data in mid-stream from a French national multi-site study (EPIDEP). *J Affect Disord.* 1998 Sep;**50**(2–3):163–73.

32. Hirschfeld RMA, Cass AR, Holt DCL, Carlson CA. Screening for bipolar disorder in patients treated for depression in a family medicine clinic. *J Am Board Fam Pract.* 2005 Jul 1;**18**(4):233–9.

33. Smith DJ, Griffiths E, Kelly M, et al. Unrecognised bipolar disorder in primary care patients with depression. *Br J Psychiatry J Ment Sci.* 2011 Jul;**199** (1):49–56.

34. Zimmermann P, Brückl T, Nocon A, et al. Heterogeneity of DSM-IV major depressive disorder

as a consequence of subthreshold bipolarity. *Arch Gen Psychiatry*. 2009 Dec 1;**66**(12):1341–52.

35. Angst J, Cui L, Swendsen J, et al. Major depressive disorder with subthreshold bipolarity in the National Comorbidity Survey Replication. *Am J Psychiatry*. 2010 Oct 1;**167**(10):1194–201.

36. Freedman R, Lewis DA, Michels R, et al. The initial field trials of DSM-5: new blooms and old thorns. *Am J Psychiatry*. 2013 Jan 1;**170**(1):1–5.

37. Youngstrom EA, Egerton GA, Genzlinger J, et al. Improving the global identification of bipolar spectrum disorders: meta-analysis of the diagnostic accuracy of checklists. *Psychol Bull*. 2018 Mar;**144**(3):315–42.

38. Angst J, Adolfsson R, Benazzi F, et al. The HCL-32: towards a self-assessment tool for hypomanic symptoms in outpatients. *J Affect Disord*. 2005 Oct;**88**(2):217–33.

39. Hirschfeld RM, Williams JB, Spitzer RL, et al. Development and validation of a screening instrument for bipolar spectrum disorder: the Mood Disorder Questionnaire. *Am J Psychiatry*. 2000 Nov;**157**(11):1873–5.

40. Nassir Ghaemi S, Miller CJ, Berv DA, et al. Sensitivity and specificity of a new bipolar spectrum diagnostic scale. *J Affect Disord*. 2005 Feb;**84**(2–3):273–7.

41. Bauer MS, Crits-Christoph P, Ball WA, et al. Independent assessment of manic and depressive symptoms by self-rating: scale characteristics and implications for the study of mania. *Arch Gen Psychiatry*. 1991 Sep 1;**48**(9):807–12.

42. Wang YY, Xu DD, Liu R, et al. Comparison of the screening ability between the 32-item Hypomania Checklist (HCL-32) and the Mood Disorder Questionnaire (MDQ) for bipolar disorder: a meta-analysis and systematic review. *Psychiatry Res*. 2019 Mar;**273**:461–6.

43. Ratheesh A, Cotton SM, Betts JK, et al. Prospective progression from high-prevalence disorders to bipolar disorder: exploring characteristics of pre-illness stages. *J Affect Disord*. 2015 Sep 1;**183**:45–8.

44. Aiken CB, Weisler RH, Sachs GS. The Bipolarity Index: a clinician-rated measure of diagnostic confidence. *J Affect Disord*. 2015 May 15;**177**:59–64.

45. Hede V, Favre S, Aubry JM, Richard-Lepouriel H. Bipolar spectrum disorder: what evidence for pharmacological treatment? A systematic review. *Psychiatry Res*. 2019 Dec 1;**282**:112627.

46. Bielecki JE, Gupta V. Cyclothymic disorder. In *StatPearls* [Internet]. Treasure Island (FL): StatPearls Publishing; 2022 [cited 2022 May 31]. Available from: www.ncbi.nlm.nih.gov/books/NBK557877/

47. Perugi G, Hantouche E, Vannucchi G. Diagnosis and treatment of cyclothymia: the 'primacy' of temperament. *Curr Neuropharmacol*. 2017 Apr;**15**(3):372–9.

48. Shim IH, Bahk WM, Woo YS, Yoon BH. Pharmacological treatment of major depressive episodes with mixed features: a systematic review. *Clin Psychopharmacol Neurosci*. 2018 Nov;**16**(4):376–82.

49. Stahl SM, Laredo S, Morrissette DA. Cariprazine as a treatment across the bipolar I spectrum from depression to mania: mechanism of action and review of clinical data. *Ther Adv Psychopharmacol*. 2020 Jan 1;**10**:2045125320905752.

50. McKeown L, Taylor RW, Day E, et al. Patient perspectives of lithium and quetiapine augmentation treatment in treatment-resistant depression: a qualitative assessment. *J Psychopharmacol*. 2022 May;**36**(5):557–65.

51. Miklowitz DJ, Semple RJ, Hauser M, et al. Mindfulness-based cognitive therapy for perinatal women with depression or bipolar spectrum disorder. *Cogn Ther Res*. 2015 Oct;**39**(5):590–600.

Clinical Screening for Unipolar and Bipolar Disorders

Claudia Lex and Thomas D. Meyer

Introduction

Accurate diagnoses of affective disorders are essential for an effective treatment. While structured clinical interviews are the gold standard, they are time consuming and the interviewer needs training to administer them reliably [1]. However, most individuals with an affective index episode are seen by general practitioners or in non-specialty clinics that are unlikely to use such interviews, which increases the risk that a disorder might remain undetected [2,3]. Furthermore, at least for bipolar disorders (BD), it has been shown that diagnostically irrelevant information and heuristic biases of clinicians affect the likelihood of a diagnosis [4,5]. Such undetected unipolar depression (UD) and BD are problematic because they are associated with higher rates of recurrences, risk of chronicity, and treatment resistance [6,7].

An additional problem is the accurate diagnosis of BD in individuals who have already been diagnosed with (unipolar) depression. In about 50% of cases the onset of BD is a depressive episode [8]; thus, at first onset, UD should always be considered a temporary, working diagnosis. Especially in younger people, an early onset of UD is related to a higher risk of developing BD over time [9]. A complicating factor is that individuals, especially in hypomanic, but also in manic states, are likely to be less motivated to seek treatment. Therefore, they are less likely to be seen and diagnosed by a mental health professional. Furthermore, currently depressed individuals are focused on their current distress and are less likely to remember and report previous (hypo)manic symptoms in this situation [5,10]. However, missing a diagnosis of BD in depressed individuals has severe consequences such as under-prescribing mood stabilizers or over-prescribing monotherapy with antidepressant medication, potentially increasing the risk of inducing manic symptoms [11].

As pointed out, reliably assessing psychiatric diagnoses using structured interviews is time-consuming and costly; therefore, self-reported screening tools are recommended as a first step to facilitate and improve the diagnostic process (e.g., [12]). Only if a screening is positive will a detailed, more time-consuming diagnostic assessment be indicated. Therefore, an accurate screening aims at reducing the rate of missed diagnoses by identifying as many potential cases as possible [13]. However, trying to avoid missing any cases bears the risk of identifying a high number of false-positive cases. As a result, a sufficiently detailed diagnostic assessment following a positive screen is essential [14].

In statistical terms, this is captured by sensitivity (SE; i.e., describing the proportion of individuals who truly have the disorder and have had a positive result). For example, an SE of 90% indicates that a test correctly identifies 90% of the people who have the disorder. It also means that 10% of the people who have the disorder are still being missed. The SE for psychiatric screenings should ideally be at least 80% [15,16]. Another important parameter is the specificity (SP), which indicates the proportion of individuals who screen negative and truly do not have the disorder. Recommended cut-offs are mostly found by balancing SE and SP. While highly relevant for screening purposes, the positive predictive value (PPV) and the negative predictive value (NPV) are rarely reported. The PPV is the probability that a person who screens positive actually has the disorder. A PPV of 20% indicates that an individual who screens positive has a 20% chance of being ill. Similarly, an NPV reflects the probability that a negative test result truly means that the person does not have the disorder (Figure 5.1).

In clinical practice, often one or two questions are used to screen for conditions such as mood disorders ([17,18]; e.g., often following an algorithm, outlined in Figure 5.2, to rule out BD). However, there is not much systematic research in the literature identifying how valid and reliable these are compared to self-rated screening tools or even structured clinical

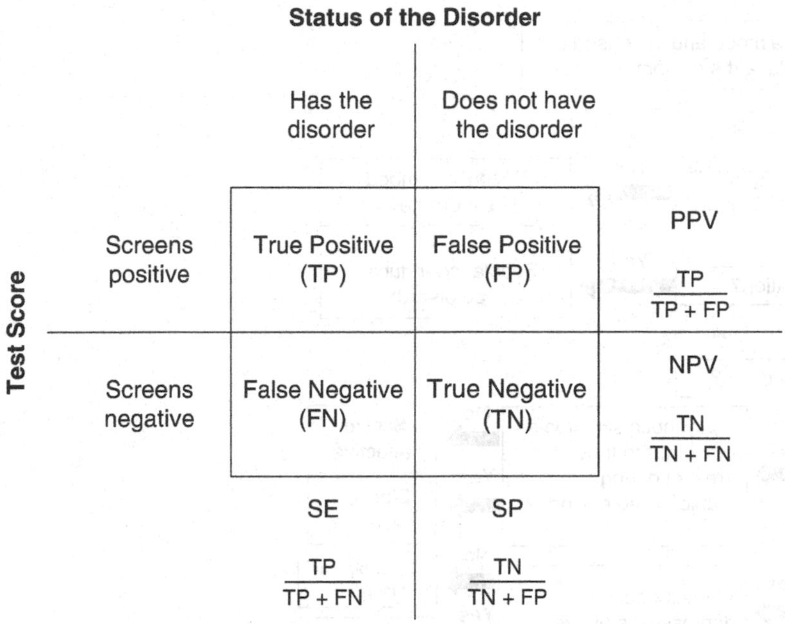

Status of the Disorder

	Has the disorder	Does not have the disorder
Screens positive	True Positive (TP)	False Positive (FP)
Screens negative	False Negative (FN)	True Negative (TN)

Test Score

PPV

$$\frac{TP}{TP + FP}$$

NPV

$$\frac{TN}{TN + FN}$$

SE

$$\frac{TP}{TP + FN}$$

SP

$$\frac{TN}{TN + FP}$$

Figure 5.1 Indicators of diagnostic accuracy: sensitivity, specificity, positive predictive value, and negative predictive value (adapted from [126]).
NPV = Negative Predictive Value, PPV = Positive Predictive Value, SE = Sensitivity, SP = Specificity.

interviews. Therefore, in this chapter we focused on self-reported screening tools, as they can be easily and quickly applied, scored, and interpreted in routine evaluations. For this reason, they are especially useful for primary and specialized care. The screenings for UD and BD reviewed in detail were included if evidence for their diagnostic accuracy were available, for example, through several empirical studies, reviews, or meta-analyses. In addition, we list some screenings that might be of interest but that are used for specific populations or have limited data about their validity. At the end, we discuss recent developments of e-health screenings. An overview of the self-rated screening measures for mood disorders is presented in Table 5.1.

Screening Tools for Depression

On one hand, screening for current depressive symptoms seems to be beneficial to individuals when appropriate follow-up resources are available [19]. One of these resources would be the availability of an appropriate psychiatric or psychological diagnostic assessment after a positive screening to confirm or dismiss a diagnosis [20]. However, this is sometimes difficult to implement, especially when thinking of primary healthcare providers outside specialized clinics and research settings [21]. On the other hand, there are professionals questioning the screening for depression, and national guideline recommendations

vary substantially [22]. It is, at times, argued that rates of depression diagnoses and antidepressant prescription have already increased over the past few years and that an enhanced screening might result in even more over-diagnoses and potential misdiagnoses of major depression [23,24].

Looking at quantitative evaluations, there are a number of studies that evaluate the screening quality of specific instruments. However, there is a lack of reviews or meta-analyses that merge this evidence or that compare screening abilities of the different tools and point out their strengths and weaknesses such as Williams [21] or El-Den [25]. Some studies are not easy to interpret because they do not differentiate between screening, assessment tools, and severity measures. Furthermore, some researchers criticize the employed statistical procedures and reporting from such studies [26].

As far as we know, except for one measure, the Inventory to Diagnose Depression (IDD; [27]), which focuses on a potential history of major depression, all widely used measures focus on current symptoms of depression. Below we start with the description of the Patient Health Questionnaire (PHQ; [28]) because it seems to be the most evaluated tool according to a recent systematic review [25]. Then, we focus on the Centre for Epidemiological Studies Depression Scale (CES-D; [29]) and the five-item World Health Organisation Well-Being Index (WHO-5; [30]),

55

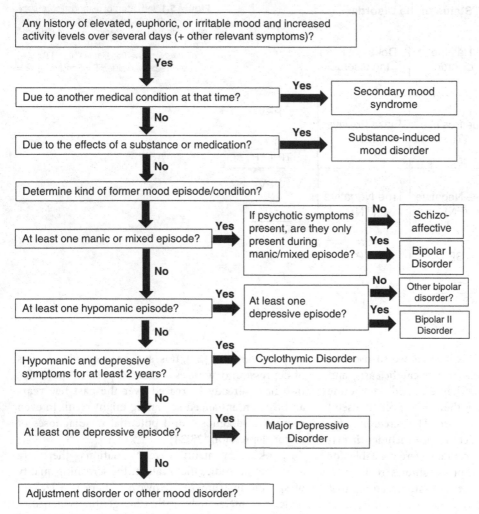

Figure 5.2 Flow chart for ruling out any bipolar disorder at screening.

which are both used internationally and have been validated in several studies. Lastly, we attend to some measures that have only been validated in a few studies or are used for special populations. We do not review severity measures and observer-rated tools.

Patient Health Questionnaire (PHQ-9)

The PHQ-9 [28] is, according to the authors, 'an instrument for making criteria-based diagnoses of depressive and other mental disorders commonly encountered in primary care' (pg. 606). The original version contains nine items that cover current depressive symptoms, for example, 'Little interest or pleasure in doing things' or 'Feeling down, depressed, or hopeless'. Individuals are asked to rate the presence and frequency of these symptoms within the last 2 weeks on a scale ranging from

'0 – not at all' to '3 – nearly every day'. The recommended cut-off to identify clinically relevant depressive symptoms as $\geq$ 10. In addition, a diagnostic algorithm was suggested that requires a minimum of five items with ratings $\geq$ 2 with at least one of the items endorsed including depressed mood or anhedonia.

There are many different versions of the PHQ available. For example, the PHQ-2 can be used as a pre-screening tool before administering the PHQ-9 [31], and the PHQ-4 is an ultra-brief screening scale for anxiety and depression [32]. The Whooley Questions use the same two items as the PHQ-2 but it is observer-rated, and both the time frame and cut-off are different. Additionally, the rating is dichotomous (yes/no) as compared to the 4-point scale of the PHQ-2 [33,34]. The PHQ-9 has been translated and

Table 5.1 Overview of self-rated screening measures for mood disorders

	PHQ-9	CES-D	WHO-5	MDQ	HCL-32	BSDS
Name	Patient Health Questionnaire	Centre for Epidemiological Studies – Depression Scale	World Health Organisation Well-Being Index	Mood Disorder Questionnaire	Hypomania Checklist	Bipolar Spectrum Diagnostic Scale
First publication	Kroenke et al. (2001)[28]	Radloff (1977)[29]	WHO (1998)[30]	Hirschfeld et al. (2000)[76]	Angst et al. (2005) [74]	Ghaemi et al. (2005)[99]
Number of Items	9	20	5	13 items plus 2 questions	32 items plus 7 questions	19 items (sentences) plus 1 question
Range of score	0–27	0–60	0–100	0–13	0–32	0–25
Recommended cut-off	> 10 and algorithm possible	≥ 16	≥ 50	≥ 7 and algorithm	≥ 14	≥ 13
Scale	4-point Likert Scale (0–3)	4-point Likert Scale (1–4)	6-point Likert Scale (0–5)	Dichotomous Yes/No	Dichotomous Yes/No	Dichotomous Yes/No and 4-point Likert scale for one item
Time frame	Last 2 weeks	Past week	Last 2 weeks	Lifetime	Lifetime	Lifetime
Symptom focus	Depression	Depression	Well-being	Hypomania and Mania	Hypomania and Mania	Hypomania, Mania, and Depression
Reading Level*	8.0	3.3	8.0	7.3	7.2	10.0
Diagnostic accuracy in first publication for recommended cut-off	Primary care: SE = 88%, SP = 88% PPV ranges between 31% for cut-off 9 and 51% for cut-off 15, no specific PPV for ≥ 10 reported, NPV is not reported	Household survey: 21% scored ≥ 16 Inpatient psychiatric setting: 70% scored ≥ 16 SE, SP, PPV, or NPV are not reported	Across different medical disciplines: Mean SE = 86%, SP = 81%, PPV and NPV not reported [56]	Used in specialized psychiatric outpatient setting to distinguish BD from other psychiatric diagnoses: SE = 73%, SP = 90% PPV and NPV not reported	Used in specialized psychiatric inpatient and outpatient settings to distinguish BD from UD: SE = 80%, SP = 51%, PPV = 73% and NPV = 61%	Used in specialized and community psychiatric outpatient settings to distinguish BD from UD: SE = 76%, SP = 85% PPV and NPV not reported
Diagnostic criteria applied in first publication	DSM-IV	Clinical and severity measures, diagnostic criteria not specified	DSM-IV, ICD-10, PHQ, and CES-D [56]	DSM-IV	DSM-IV	DSM-IV and bipolar spectrum symptoms (Akiskal and Pinto, 1999)[127]

* Flesch–Kincaid Grade Level that corresponds to US school grades according to [1], [123], [124], and [125].

Abbreviations: BD: bipolar disorders; NPV: negative predictive value; PPV: positive predictive value; SE: sensitivity; SP: specificity; UD: unipolar depression.

validated in a variety of languages including Chinese [35], Spanish [36], French [37], and Arabic [38].

A meta-analysis across 29 studies that used semi-structured interviews to verify the diagnosis of UD in the general population estimated the average SE and SP of the PHQ-9 to be 0.88 and 0.85, respectively, when using the cut-off of 10 or greater [39]. Furthermore, administering the PHQ-9 only after a positive PHQ-2 pre-screening resulted in similar SE but significantly higher SP compared to using the PHQ-9 alone (i.e., it increased the rate of correctly identifying individuals without depression [40]). One study found a high rate of false-positive cases at 34% in a psychiatric setting corresponding to a low SP of 50%, a low PPV of 47%, an SE of 94%, and an NPV of 94% [41]. Therefore, this adds to the evidence that the PHQ-9 screening might work better in primary care than in secondary care [42]. Lastly, it might be that a higher cut-off level of $\geq$ 14, combined with the diagnostic algorithm, will more accurately reflect the prevalence of major depression according to DSM criteria [40].

Nevertheless, since its first publication, the PHQ has been widely used in various medical and some national (e.g., S3 [43]) settings. The ICSI Health Care Guideline [44] and international [45] guidelines on unipolar depression recommend its use.

Centre for Epidemiological Studies – Depression Scale (CES-D)

The CES-D [29] was originally developed to measure current depressive symptomatology in the general population. It contains 20 items that focus on the affective component of depressive disorder and is a structured self-report measure. Respondents are asked to rate the frequency of symptoms within the past week on a 4-point Likert scale. Examples of items included are 'During the past week I felt depressed' and 'During the past week I felt that everything I did was an effort.' In the original study [29], the internal consistencies were high in both the general population (α = .85) and the patient sample (α = .90), and it provided good discriminant and convergent validity. Some items are reverse scored, and scores can range between 0 and 60. The scale has been translated and validated in many languages such as Chinese [46], Japanese [47], Italian [48], Spanish [49], Dutch [50], and German [51]. It has been used with adults, adolescents [52], and elderly individuals with and without cognitive impairments [53].

The recommended cut-off to identify individuals with clinically relevant depression is $\geq$ 16. At this cut-off, a meta-analysis [54] reported a mean SE of 87% and a mean SP of 87% in primary care and in the general population; however, a higher mean SE and SP (0.83 and 0.78, respectively) was reached if a higher cut-off of $\geq$ 20 was applied. In addition, different cut-offs have been discussed for different populations (e.g., a cut-off of $\geq$ 14 for nursing home residents and patients of general hospitals [55]).

In sum, the CES-D is an acceptable screening instrument in the general population and in primary care settings but should not be used as a sole diagnostic tool to assess depressive symptomatology [54]. Depending on the context and the aims of the assessment, it is important to know that it does not match ICD or DSM criteria, and it does not directly ask for suicidality (i.e., it only probes for hopelessness). Therefore, if it is essential to know if the individual has suicidal ideation, the CES-D is not the most appropriate measure.

World Health Organization – Five-Item Well-Being Index (WHO-5)

Although the WHO-5 is a short self-report measure of current mental well-being, it has also been used to screen for depression by defining depression as an absence of well-being. It was developed by the WHO regional office in Europe as part of the DEPCARE project dealing with well-being measures in primary healthcare [30]. It can be used as a measure of well-being with both healthy and mentally/physically ill persons [56]. The project group that developed the WHO-5 deliberately chose only positively phrased items and avoided symptom-related language. The WHO-5 includes 5 items regarding individuals' affective states over the past 14 days (e.g., 'Over the past 2 weeks I have felt cheerful and in good spirits'). The rating scale ranges from '0 – at no time' to '5 – all of the time', and the sum score is multiplied by 4 to result in a final score between 0, indicating the worst well-being, and 100, indicating the best imaginable well-being. When the WHO-5 is used to screen for depression, a cut-off score of $\leq$ 50 is recommended. In the instance of a positive screening, a trained clinician should conduct a diagnostic interview to evaluate if the criteria for a major depressive episode is fulfilled [30]. The WHO-5 is available in 31 languages that can be downloaded from a WHO-5 webpage (www.psykiatri-r egionh.dk/who-5/Pages/default.aspx, April 26, 2021).

A systematic review found an overall SE of .86 and an SP of .81 when the WHO-5 was used to screen for depression using the recommended cut-off [56]. However, some argue that the WHO-5 items are too broad and general to specifically screen for depression [57] and that different cut-off scores may apply more appropriately to different countries [58].

Additional Instruments for Depression

There are several instruments that either have sparse validation data, weak evidence as a screening tool, were primarily designed as severity measures, or are only used in very specific populations. As these tools could still be of use for specific aims and/or settings, we decided at least to refer to some of them briefly in this review.

The Inventory to Diagnose Depression (IDD [27]) uses DSM-III criteria and was previously described as the only instrument specifically asking for a prior history of major depression. The Major Depression Inventory (MDI) consists of 12 items, assesses depressive symptoms according to DSM-IV and ICD-10 criteria, and provides cut-off scores for different severity levels of depression [59]. In the original study, the MDI demonstrated good internal consistency (Cronbach α = .94). Its SE and SP were .90, and SP was .82 for DSM-IV diagnoses, and both indices were .86 for ICD-10 diagnoses [59]. However, there is evidence that the MDI might be a rather conservative measure with restricted screening qualities because the rate of false positives can be low. For example, Cuijpers et al. [60] found an SE of .66 and SP of .65. Using a web-based version Nielsen et al [61] found an even slightly lower SE and SP with .62. The Zung Self-Rating Depression Scale [62] is one of the oldest assessments still in use. It contains 20 items that attend to affective and somatic symptoms of depression. The scale was published before DSM-III criteria were specified, but a more recent study found that it still has good screening properties with an SE of 93% and SP of 69% [63].

One of the most widely known and used depression measures that is sometimes used as a screening measure as well is the Beck Depression Inventory (BDI-II [64]). It has an SE of .86 and SP of .78 at a cut-off of ≤ 14 across different settings; however, in psychiatric settings, a higher cut-off of 19 can differentiate between remission and depression [65]. A seven-item self-rated version for detecting major depression in medical patients also exists (BDI-PC [66,67]), although despite its promising diagnostic accuracy (i.e., SE of 97% and SP of 99% [66]), the BDI-PC has yet to be used widely.

Additionally, there are also self-rating instruments for special populations. For instance, the Geriatric Depression Scale (GDS [68]) can be used as a 30-item, 15-item, 10-item, or 4-item self-rated screening for depressive symptoms amongst older adults. All of these different versions have demonstrated good screening quality and high diagnostic accuracy [69]. The Edinburgh Postnatal Depression Scale (EPDS [70]) has 10 items and is specifically designed to detect postnatal depression. It is validated and translated into a variety of languages and provides high screening accuracy for major depression in pregnant and postpartum women [71]. Finally, there have been attempts to develop instruments that assess and screen for major depression in special medical conditions while accounting for overlapping physical symptoms such as the Neurological Disorders Depression Inventory for Epilepsy (NDDI-E [72]) screening for depression in individuals with epilepsy or the ALS-Depression Inventory 12 (ADI-12 [73]) for patients with amyotrophic lateral sclerosis.

Screening for Bipolar Disorder, Hypomania, and Mania

Throughout the late 1990s and early 2000s some experts raised the issue that the prevalence of BD might be underestimated and that a significant number of cases were left undiagnosed, leading to individuals not receiving the most adequate treatment (e.g., [74,75]). Therefore, several attempts have been made to develop screening tools specifically for BD, such as the Hypomania Checklist-32 (HCL-32 [74]) and the Mood Disorder Questionnaire (MDQ [76]). Since the beginning, test developers were very explicit about a two-step process whereby the screening tool would be the first step. As such, a positive screening does not imply a confirmed diagnosis, and must be succeeded by a thorough diagnostic assessment (ideally a structured clinical interview). Therefore, a higher false-positive rate, which is reflected by a low SP of the screening tool, is not considered the most pressing problem per se, as further assessments are still required.

As (1) the presence of hypomanic or manic symptoms is the main differentiating feature between UD and BD and (2) hypomanic and manic symptoms are often not spontaneously reported (especially when consulting clinicians for current depressive symptoms

[5,10]), the screening tools for BD focus almost exclusively on a lifetime history of hypomanic or manic episodes. As Meyer and colleagues [77] point out in their review, self-ratings for current (hypo)mania exist, but they are typically only used to monitor symptom fluctuations in individuals with an established diagnosis of BD and not to screen for any current manic-like states in primary or secondary care.

Mood Disorder Questionnaire (MDQ)

The MDQ [76] was originally developed to estimate the rate of bipolar disorder I (BD-I) and II (BD-II) in the general population. It consists of three parts: in part one, individuals are screened for a lifetime history of manic/hypomanic symptoms using 13 yes/no items (e.g., 'Has there ever been a period of time when you were not your usual self and you were so irritable that you shouted at people or started fights or arguments?'); in part two, individuals are asked whether two or more of these symptoms have been experienced within the same period; and in part three, individuals are asked to rate the level of impact of the symptoms on a 4-point scale from 'no problems' to 'serious problems'. If the person has a score of > 7 in part one and endorses both experiencing two or more symptoms at the same time and that the symptoms caused moderate or serious problems, then the screening is positive and further assessment for BD is recommended. The MDQ has been translated in Spanish [78], Chinese [79], Arabic [80], French [81], German [82], and Thai [83].

Using the recommended cut-off of > 7, combined with the time and functional impairment criteria, the overall SE was 62% and the SP was 85% in a meta-analysis [84]. Another review reported similar rates, but also noted that the MDQ has more potential to detect BD-I than BD-II because the equivalent SE were 66% and 39% respectively [85]. Thus, the MDQ identifies only two-thirds of true positive cases, which some would consider too low for a screening instrument. In addition, the PPV is 43% in the general population and 39% in psychiatric patients [85]. Which means that more than half of the individuals with a positive screening do not have BD. To address these limitations, it might be beneficial to focus on a modified scoring strategy using only the cut-off score > 7 based on the first part of the questionnaire and ignoring the second and third parts. This approach has shown to improve SE when used to screen for BD in patients already diagnosed with unipolar depression [1,84]. Unfortunately, some publications are not sufficiently specific about the

approach they chose for scoring. Lee and colleagues [86] suggest combining the MDQ with other measures that are more sensitive for BD-II to increase SE, but this would compromise having brief screening tools that can be easily used in clinical practice. Paterniti and Bisserbe [87] hypothesize that the MDQ could be used to screen for a more general psychopathology in primary care settings because the covered symptoms might not be specific enough for BD (e.g., irritability) and can be found in other psychiatric conditions as well [88]. Due to its higher SP; however, the MDQ could be used to rule out bipolarity [89].

Hypomania Checklist (HCL-32)

Originally, the HCL-32 was developed to screen for BD or bipolar spectrum disorders by identifying hypomanic symptoms in patients already diagnosed with major depressive disorder [74] and the measure includes 32 self-rated hypomanic symptoms (e.g., 'I need less sleep', 'I feel more energetic and more active'). The patients are also asked to rate their current emotional state, the consequences of the 'highs' on family, friends, work, and leisure, and the time spent in 'high states'. As it may be easily and quickly administered, scored, and interpreted, it is recommended for psychiatric and general medical practices [74]. A total score of 14 or more indicates suspected BD and a more elaborated assessment should be conducted following. While there is the option of obtaining two subscale scores (i.e., active/elated and risk taking/irritable hypomania), they are hardly ever used or validated for screening purposes. The HCL-32 has been translated and validated in many languages such as English, Swedish, German, and Italian [74], Chinese [90], Korean [91], Spanish [92], and Russian [93]. There are also longer and shorter versions available; for example, revisions with 33 or 34 items include items related to overeating, gambling, or additional hypomanic symptoms (e.g., [94]), and validated shorter versions with 16 or 20 items can be used with clinical and nonclinical samples [95,96,97]. Most validation studies, however, have used the 32-item version.

The cut-off score > 14 showed an SE of 80%, an SP of 51%, a PPV of 73%, and an NPV of 61% in the original sample [74], and a systematic review found similar rates (i.e., estimated overall SE and SP were 80% and 65% respectively [15], indicating that the HCL-32 can help to distinguish BD from major depressive disorder). The HCL-32 may be less adequate to distinguish patients with BD from other clinical adult populations such as adults with substance use problems [15,98], or BD-I from BD-II [74]. The measure does have good internal consistencies ranging between Cronbach α = .83 and .94 and seems to be unrelated to current mood symptoms [15].

Bipolar Spectrum Diagnostic Scale (BSDS)

The BSDS [99] is specifically designed to assess bipolar spectrum conditions including clinically subthreshold conditions, depressive mixed states, cyclothymia, irritable states, and bipolar spectrum disorders. The BSDS uses a prototype matching method instead of a score summation approach [100]. Patients are asked to read a short text that describes hypomanic and depressive symptoms and the episodic character of the mood episodes. Afterwards, the text as a whole as well as each single sentence are self-rated on how well the description applies to the individual. The range of possible scores is 0 to 25, and cut-offs are provided for unlikelihood as well as low, moderate, and high likelihood of BD. The optimum threshold for a positive screening is a score of 13 and above. The BSDS was originally published in English [99] and has since been translated in other languages such as Spanish [101], Persian [102], and Chinese [103].

Originally, Ghaemi and colleagues [99] used the BSDS to differentiate between patients with bipolar spectrum disorders and UD. With a cut-off score ≥ 13, the SE for all BD diagnoses was 76%, the SE for bipolar spectrum conditions was 79%, and the SP in both cases was 85%. When the BSDS is used in routine psychiatric outpatient settings, applying the cut-off ≥ 13, SE was 77% for BD-I, 67% for BD-II, and 69% for BD not otherwise specified or cyclothymia, while the SP was 67% [104]. The authors discuss different cut-off scores and point out that the BSDS works well in identifying 'milder' forms of BD. They also conclude that the BSDS is helpful to rule out certain conditions but might be less adequate in identifying a specific diagnosis.

Finally, a meta-analysis that examined the HCL-32, the MDQ, and the BSDS reported estimated SEs of .81, .66, and .69 and SPs of .67, .79, and .86, respectively, for the detection of any type of BD diagnosis in mental health settings [14]. Therefore, the tools are differently useful depending on whether it is more important not to miss any potential cases or to rule out BD.

Additional Instruments for BD

There are several additional screening instruments that could be useful for special populations and aims but have some weaknesses regarding evidence, accessibility, or formal characteristics. The Mood Swings Survey (MSS [105]), later renamed the Mood Swing Questionnaire (MSQ [106]), aims at distinguishing (hypo)manic episodes from periods of 'normal' happiness in patients diagnosed with UD. The MSQ is embedded into the digital diagnostic system of the Black Dog Institute, which is a specialized mood clinic in Australia [107]. Studies conducted at this clinic revealed similar SE and SP for the MSQ and the previously described MDQ [106]. The items of the MSQ seem not to be published, which limits access and use internationally. The General Behavior Inventory (GBI [108]) was the first self-rating ever designed to identify depressive and hypomanic/cyclic symptoms that does not only focus on the past few weeks. While it has often been used to identify individuals at (future) risk for BD (e.g., [109,110]), it has been criticized due to its high reading level and its length (i.e., 73 items [1]). Furthermore, a shorter, 15-item version showed rather weak screening quality in young adults [10]. However, it might be more useful to discriminate bipolar from non-bipolar cases in child and adolescent samples [111]. Finally, the Workplace Bipolar Inventory (WBI [112]) is designed to specifically screen for symptoms of BD at the workplace. It is available in its original Japanese version and showed good screening efficacy, although some items might be too specific for the work environment to be used more generally [112]. There is an English translation but it has not been validated yet (Imamura personal communication, April 2021).

Gaps and the Future

Several screening measures do exist for current depressive symptoms and a potential lifetime history of (hypo)mania. Our clinical impression is that screening for current depressive symptoms is much more implemented in clinical practice, even in primary care, than in screening for BD. However, the need to screen for BD might be even more essential, as individuals are more likely to consult a clinician for symptoms of low energy, fatigue, or feeling blue (and to spontaneously disclose such symptoms) as opposed to feelings of self-confidence and over-activity. Nevertheless, it is important to consider that one of the problems with screening for hypomania is that its presentations (e.g., feeling very confident, feeling elated) are not clinically relevant per se. To some extent, they will be present in many individuals, leading to high rates of false-positive cases if used in the general population.

In this chapter, we solely focused on screening for diagnosable mood disorders and did not discuss the validity, practicality, and ethical considerations of screenings for individuals at-risk for mental health problems (e.g., [113,114,115]).

Recently, there has been an increase in the use of digital approaches for the management of psychiatric disorders. Such online tools, and computerized algorithms are applied for assessment, treatment, and psychoeducation but can also be used for screening (e.g., the Black Dog Institute's computerized Mood Assessment Program; MAP [107]). National health authorities also employ such digital screenings, for example, Good Thinking, a digital platform for common mental health problems that offers an initial assessment of sleep problems, stress, low mood, and anxiety, and is provided by the UK National Health Service (NHS; www.good-thinking.uk/self-assessments). Another method involves self-screenings for depression and bipolar disorder through apps. While apps have several advantages including high usability and acceptability [116], apps related to affective mood disorders have some weaknesses, such as privacy and safety issues, the use of non-validated screening tools, and exposure to potential triggers for negative mood and thinking patterns [117,118]. It is unclear what consequences an online positive screening has on an individual without easily accessible professional support. While individuals could read the disclaimer that the positive screening does not imply a diagnosis and needs verification by a health professional, they may not contact a clinician to discuss further for a variety of reasons. Finally, there are some machine learning approaches to promote diagnostic precision that use algorithms fed with information provided by an electronic medical file or by patients via their smartphones (e.g., activity, sleep patterns, amount of talking [119,120]). However, at present, studies for all these methods are still scarce and more research is needed to examine their validity, privacy, ethical questions, and, more generally, the pros and cons of digital and virtual screening [121].

Conclusions

At the very least, each patient who presents with depression should also be screened for a history of manic or hypomanic symptoms to inform treatment. To address the concerns of over-diagnosis, a detailed diagnostic assessment should always follow a positive screening. The screening for UD remains an important but also controversial topic (e.g., [122]) and this might be partially because the two-step diagnostic process (i.e., full diagnostic assessment after a positive screening) has not been clearly required until recently. However, it is essential for identifying the best evidence-based treatment for these individuals.

As the different screening instruments have both strengths and weaknesses, the choice of the tool depends on the specific setting and goals of the clinician or researcher. Finally, since evidence is mixed, more studies are highly awaited to evaluate the outcome and cost-effectiveness of such approaches.

References

1. E. A. Youngstrom, G. A. Egerton, J. Genzlinger, et al. Improving the global identification of bipolar spectrum disorders: meta-analysis of the diagnostic accuracy of checklists. *Psychol Bull* 2018;**144**:315–42.

2. M. Cepoiu, J. McCusker, M. G. Cole, et al. Recognition of depression by non-psychiatric physicians – a systematic literature review and meta-analysis. *J Gen Intern Med* 2008;**23**:25–36.

3. A. J. Mitchell, A. Vaze, S. Rao. Clinical diagnosis of depression in primary care: a meta-analysis. *Lancet* 2009;**374**:609–19.

4. K. Bruchmüller, T. D. Meyer. Diagnostically irrelevant information can affect the likelihood of a diagnosis of bipolar disorder. *J Affect Disord* 2009;**116**:148–51.

5. L. Wolkenstein, K. Bruchmüller, P. Schmid, et al. Misdiagnosing bipolar disorder–do clinicians show heuristic biases? *J Affect Disord* 2011;**130**:405–12.

6. L. Ghio, S. Gotelli, M. Marcenaro, et al. (2014). Duration of untreated illness and outcomes in unipolar depression: a systematic review and meta-analysis. *J Affect Disord* 2014;**152**:45–51.

7. N. Drancourt, B. Etain, M. Lajnef, et al. Duration of untreated bipolar disorder: missed opportunities on the long road to optimal treatment. *Acta Psychiatr Scand* 2013;**127**:136–44.

8. C. O'Donovan, M. Alda. Depression preceding diagnosis of bipolar disorder. *Front Psychiatry* 2020;**11**:500.

9. L. V. Kessing. The effect of the first manic episode in affective disorder: a case register study of hospitalised episodes. *J Affect Disord* 1999;**53**:233–9.

10. C. J. Miller, S. L. Johnson, T. R. Kwapil, et al. Three studies on self-report scales to detect bipolar disorder. *J Affect Disord* 2011;**128**:199–210.

11. R. S. McIntyre, M. Berk, E. Brietzke, et al. Bipolar disorders. *Lancet* 2020;**396**:1841–56.

12. A. L. Siu, US Preventive Services Task Force (USPSTF), K. Bibbins-Domingo, et al. Screening for depression in adults: US Preventive Services Task Force Recommendation Statement. *JAMA* 2016;**315**:380–7.

13. M. Zimmerman, C. G. Holst. Screening for psychiatric disorders with self-administered questionnaires. *Psychiatry Res* 2018;**270**:1068–73.

14. A. F. Carvalho, Y. Takwoingi, P. M. Sales, et al. Screening for bipolar spectrum disorders: A comprehensive meta-analysis of accuracy studies. *J Affect Disord* 2015;**172**:337–46.

15. T. D. Meyer, J. Schrader, M. Ridley, et al. The Hypomania Checklist (HCL) – systematic review of its properties to screen for bipolar disorders. *Compr Psychiatry* 2014;**55**:1310–21.

16. M. Zimmerman, J. N. Galione, C. J. Ruggero, et al. Are screening scales for bipolar disorder good enough to be used in clinical practice? *Compr Psychiatry* 2011;**52**:600–6.

17. K. Bosanquet, D. Bailey, S. Gilbody, et al. Diagnostic accuracy of the Whooley questions for the identification of depression: a diagnostic meta-analysis. *BMJ Open* 2015:5.12.

18. I. M. Anderson, P. M. Haddad, J. Scott. Bipolar disorder. *BMJ* 2012;**345**:e8508.

19. S. Smithson, M. P. Pignone. Screening adults for depression in primary care. *Med Clin North Am* 2017;**101**:807–21.

20. R. Alexandrowicz, M. Weiss, B. Marquart, et al. Zur Validität eines zweistufigen Screenings am Beispiel des Depressionsscreening [The validity of a two-step-screening procedure for depression]. *Psychiatr Prax* 2008;**35**:294–301.

21. J. W. Williams Jr, M. Pignone, G. Ramirez, et al. Identifying depression in primary care: a literature synthesis of case-finding instruments. *Gen Hosp Psychiatry* 2002;**24**:225–37.

22. B. D. Thombs, N. Saadat, K. E. Riehm, et al. Consistency and sources of divergence in recommendations on screening with questionnaires for presently experienced health problems or symptoms: a comparison of recommendations from the Canadian Task Force on Preventive Health Care, UK National Screening Committee, and US Preventive Services Task Force. *BMC Med* 2017;**15**:150.

23. A. V. Horwitz, J. C. Wakefield. *The Loss of Sadness: How Psychiatry Transformed Normal Sorrow into Depressive Disorder*. Oxford: Oxford University Press, 2007.

24. B. D. Thombs, J. C. Coyne, P. Cuijpers, et al. Rethinking recommendations for screening for depression in primary care. *Can Med Assoc J* 2012;**184**:413–18.

25. S. El-Den, T. F. Chen, Y. L. Gan, et al. The psychometric properties of depression screening tools in primary healthcare settings: a systematic review. *J Affect Disord* 2018;**225**:503–22.

26. B. D. Thombs, D. B. Rice. Sample sizes and precision of estimates of sensitivity and specificity from primary studies on the diagnostic accuracy of depression screening tools: a survey of recently published studies. *Int J Methods Psychiatr Res* 2016;**25**:145–52.

27. M. Zimmerman, W. Coryell. The Inventory to Diagnose Depression, lifetime version. *Acta Psychiatr Scand* 1987;**75**:495–9.

28. K. Kroenke, R. L. Spitzer, J. B. Williams. The PHQ-9: validity of a brief depression severity measure. *J Gen Intern Med* 2001;**16**:606–13.

29. L. S. Radloff. The CES-D scale: A self-report depression scale for research in the general population. *Appl Psychol Meas* 1977;**1**:385–401.

30. World Health Organisation. *Wellbeing Measures in Primary Health Care/The Depcare Project*. Copenhagen: WHO Regional Office for Europe, 1998.

31. D. S. Brody, S. R. Hahn, R. L. Spitzer, et al. Identifying patients with depression in the primary care setting: a more efficient method. *Arch Intern Med* 1998;**158**:2469–75.

32. K. Kroenke, R. L. Spitzer, J. B. W. Williams, et al. (2009). An ultra-brief screening scale for anxiety and depression: the PHQ-4. *Psychosomatics* 2009;**50**:613–21.

33. M. A. Whooley, A. L. Avins, J. Miranda, et al. Case-finding instruments for depression. Two questions are as good as many. *J Gen Intern Med* 1997;**12**:439–45.

34. M. A. Whooley. Screening for depression – a tale of two questions. *JAMA Intern Med* 2016;**176**:436–7.

35. W. Wang, Q. Bian, Y. Zhao, et al. Reliability and validity of the Chinese version of the Patient Health Questionnaire (PHQ-9) in the general population. *Gen Hosp Psychiatry* 2014;**36**:539–44.

36. C. Diez-Quevedo, T. Rangil. L. Sanchez-Planell, et al. Validation and utility of the patient health questionnaire in diagnosing mental disorders in 1003 general hospital Spanish inpatients. *Psychosom Med* 2001;**63**:679–86.

37. Y. Carballeira, P. Dumont, S. Borgacci, et al. Criterion validity of the French version of Patient Health Questionnaire (PHQ) in a hospital department of internal medicine. *Psychol Psychother* 2007;**80**:69–77.

38. A. N. AlHadi, D. A. AlAteeq, E. Al-Sharif et al. An aRabic translation, reliability, and validation of Patient Health Questionnaire in a Saudi sample. *Ann Gen Psychiatry* 2017;**16**:32.

39. B. Levis, A. Benedetti, B. D. Thombs, et al. Accuracy of Patient Health Questionnaire-9 (PHQ-9) for screening to detect major depression: individual participant data meta-analysis. *BMJ* 2019;**365**:l1476.

40. B. Levis, Y. Sun, C. He, et al. Accuracy of the PHQ-2 alone and in combination with the PHQ-9 for screening to detect major depression: systematic review and meta-analysis. *JAMA* 2020;**323**:2290–2300.

41. T. Inoue, T. Tanaka, S. Nakagawa, et al. Utility and limitations of PHQ-9 in a clinic specializing in psychiatric care. *BMC Psychiatry* 2012;**12**:73.

42. A. S. Moriarty, S. Gilbody, D. McMillan, et al. Screening and case finding for major depressive disorder using the Patient Health Questionnaire (PHQ-9): a meta-analysis. *Gen Hosp Psychiatry* 2015;**37**:567–76.

43. DGPPN, BÄK, KBV, et al., eds. S3-Leitlinie/Nationale VersorgungsLeitlinie Unipolare Depression – Langfassung [S3 Guidelines Unipolar Depression – Long Version]. 2015. Available at: www.depression.v ersorgungsleitlinien.de

44. M. Trangle, J. Gursky, R. Haight, et al. Institute for Clinical Systems Improvement. Adult depression in primary care. Updated March 2016. Available at: www.icsi.org/wp-content/uploads/2019/01/Depr.pdf

45. A. Cleare, C. M. Pariante, A. H. Young, et al. A revision of the 2008 British Association for Psychopharmacology guidelines. *J Psychopharmacol* 2015;**29**:459–525.

46. W. Y. Chin, E. P. H. Choi, K. T. Y. Chan, et al. The psychometric properties of the Center for Epidemiologic Studies Depression Scale in Chinese primary care patients: factor structure, construct validity, reliability, sensitivity and responsiveness. *PLoS One* 2015;**10**:e0135131.

47. S. Shima, T. Shikano, T. Kitamura, et al. New self-rating scale for depression. *Clin Psychiatry* 1985;**27**:717–23.

48. G. A. Fava. Assessing depressive symptoms across cultures: Italian validation of the CES-D self-rating scale. *J Clin Psychol* 1983;**39**:249–51.

49. J. Soler, V. Perez-Sola, D. Puigdemont, et al. [Validation study of the Center for Epidemiological Studies-Depression of a Spanish population of patients with affective disorders]. [Article in Spanish] *Actas Luso Esp Neurol Psiquiatr Cienc Afines* 1997;**25**:243–9.

50. L. Kwakkenbos, W. G. van Lankveld, M. C. Vonk, et al. Disease-related and psychosocial factors associated with depressive symptoms in patients with systemic sclerosis, including fear of progression and appearance self-esteem. *J Psychosom Res* 2012;**72**:199–204.

51. R. Jahn, J. S. Baumgartner, M. van den Nest, et al. Kriteriumsvalidität der deutschsprachigen Version der CES-D in der Allgemeinbevölkerung [Criterion validity of the German version of the CES-D in the general population]. *Psychiatr Prax* 2018;**45**:434–42.

52. E. Stockings, L. Degenhardt, Y. Y. Lee, et al. Symptom screening scales for detecting major depressive disorder in children and adolescents: a systematic review and meta-analysis of reliability, validity and diagnostic utility. *J Affect Disord* 2015;**174**:447–63.

53. L. Ros, J. M. Latorre, M. J. Aguilar, et al. Factor structure and psychometric properties of the center for epidemiologic studies depression scale (CES-D) in older populations with and without cognitive impairment. *Int J Aging Hum Dev* 2011;**72**:83–110.

54. G. Vilagut, C. G. Forero, G. Barbaglia, et al. Screening for depression in the general population with the Center for Epidemiologic Studies Depression (CES-D): a systematic review with meta-analysis. *PLoS One* 2016;**11**:e0155431.

55. K. Blank, C. Gruman, J. T. Robison. Case-finding for depression in elderly people: balancing ease of administration with validity in varied treatment settings. *J Gerontol A Biol Sci Med Sci* 2004;**59**:378–84.

56. C. W. Topp, S. D. Østergaard, S. Søndergaard, et al. The WHO-5 Well-Being Index: a systematic review of the literature. *Psychother Psychosom* 2015;**84**:167–76.

57. B. A. Primack. The WHO-5 Wellbeing Index performed the best in screening for depression in primary care/Commentary. *ACP journal club* 2003;**139**:48.

58. P. E. Sischka, A. P. Costa, G. Steffgen, et al. (2020). The WHO-5 well-being index–validation based on item response theory and the analysis of measurement invariance across 35 countries. *J Affect Disord Reports* 2020;**1**:100020.

59. P. Bech, N. A. Rasmussen, L. R. Olsen, et al. The sensitivity and specificity of the Major Depression Inventory, using the Present State Examination as the index of diagnostic validity. *J Affect Disord* 2001;**66**:159–64.

60. P. Cuijpers, J. Dekker, A. Noteboom, et al. Sensitivity and specificity of the Major Depression Inventory in outpatients. *BMC Psychiatry* 2007;**7**:39.

61. M. G. Nielsen, E. Ørnbøl, P. Bech, et al. The criterion validity of the web-based Major Depression Inventory when used on clinical suspicion of depression in primary care. *Clin Epidemiol* 2017;**9**:355–65.

62. W. W. K. Zung. A self-rating depression scale. *Arch Gen Psychiatry* 1965;**12**:63–70.

63. D. A. Dunstan, N. Scott, A. K. Todd. Screening for anxiety and depression: reassessing the utility of the Zung scales. *BMC Psychiatry* 2017;**17**:329.

64. A. T. Beck, R. A. Steer, G. K. Brown. *Manual for the Beck Depression Inventory-II*. San Antonio: Psychological Corporation. 1996.

65. M. von Glischinski, R. von Brachel, G. Hirschfeld. How depressed is 'depressed'? A systematic review and diagnostic meta-analysis of optimal cut points for the Beck Depression Inventory revised (BDI-II). *Qual Life Res* 2019;**28**:1111–18.

66. A. T. Beck, D. Guth, R. A. Steer, et al. Screening for major depression disorders in medical inpatients with the Beck Depression Inventory for Primary Care. *Behav Res Ther* 1997;**35**:785–91.

67. R. A. Steer, T. A. Cavalieri, D. M. Leonard, et al. Use of the Beck Depression Inventory for Primary Care to screen for major depression disorders. *Gen Hosp Psychiatry* 1999;**21**:106–11.

68. J. A. Yesavage, T. L. Brink, T. L. Rose, et al. Development and validation of a Geriatric Depression Screening Scale: a preliminary report. *J Psychiatr Res* 1983;**17**:37–49.

69. Y. Krishnamoorthy, S. Rajaa, T. Rehman. Diagnostic accuracy of various forms of geriatric depression scale for screening of depression among older adults: Systematic review and meta-analysis. *Arch Gerontol Geriatr* 2020;**87**:104002.

70. J. L. Cox, J. M. Holden, R. Sagovsky. Detection of postnatal depression. Development of the 10-item Edinburgh Postnatal Depression Scale. *Br J Psychiatry* 1987;**150**:782–6.

71. B. Levis, Z. Negeri, Y. Sun, et al. Accuracy of the Edinburgh Postnatal Depression Scale (EPDS) for screening to detect major depression among pregnant and postpartum women: systematic review and meta-analysis of individual participant data. *BMJ* 2020;**371**:m4022.

72. F. G. Gilliam, J. J. Barry, B. P. Hermann, et al. Rapid detection of major depression in epilepsy: a multicentre study. *Lancet Neurol* 2006;**5**:399-405.

73. E. M. Hammer, S. Häcker, M. Hautzinger, et al. Validity of the ALS-Depression-Inventory (ADI-12)– a new screening instrument for depressive disorders in patients with amyotrophic lateral sclerosis. *J Affect Disord* 2008;**109**:213–19.

74. J. Angst, R. Adolfsson, F. Benazzi, et al. The HCL-32: towards a self-assessment tool for hypomanic symptoms in outpatients. *J Affect Disord* 2005;**88**:217–33.

75. M. Zimmerman, M. A. Posternak, I. Chelminski, et al. Using questionnaires to screen for psychiatric disorders: a comment on a study of screening for bipolar disorder in the community. *J Clin Psychiatry* 2004;**65**:605–10.

76. R. M. Hirschfeld, J. B. Williams, R. L. Spitzer, et al. (2000). Development and validation of a screening instrument for bipolar spectrum disorder: the Mood Disorder Questionnaire. *Am J Psychiatry* 2000;**157**:1873–1875.

77. T. D. Meyer, N. Crist, N. La Rosa, et al. Are existing self-ratings of acute manic symptoms in adults reliable and valid? A systematic review. *Bipolar Disord* 2020;**22**:558–68.

78. J. Sanchez-Moreno, J. M. Villagran, J. R. Gutierrez, et al. Adaptation and validation of the Spanish version of the Mood Disorder Questionnaire for the detection of bipolar disorder. *Bipolar Disord* 2008;**10**:400–12.

79. Z. Gan, Z. Han, K. Li, et al. Validation of the Chinese version of the 'Mood Disorder Questionnaire' for screening bipolar disorder among patients with a current depressive episode. *BMC Psychiatry* 2012;**12**:8.

80. U. Ouali, L. Jouini, Y. Zgueb, et al. The factor structure of the Mood Disorder Questionnaire in Tunisian patients. *Clin Pract Epidemiol Ment Health* 2020;**16(Suppl-1)**:82–92.

81. B. Weber Rouget, N. Gervasoni, V. Dubuis, et al. Screening for bipolar disorders using a French version of the Mood Disorder Questionnaire (MDQ). *J Affect Disord* 2005;**88**:103–8.

82. M. Hautzinger, T. D. Meyer. *Diagnostik affektiver Störungen* [Diagnostics of Affective Disorders]. Göttingen: Hogrefe, 2002.

83. P. Waleeprakhon, P. Ittasakul, M. Lotrakul, et al. Development and validation of a screening instrument for bipolar spectrum disorder: the Mood Disorder Questionnaire Thai version. *Neuropsychiatr Dis Treat* 2014;**10**:1497–1502.

84. H. R. Wang, Y. S. Woo, H. S. Ahn, et al. The validity of the Mood Disorder Questionnaire for screening bipolar disorder: a meta-analysis. *Depress Anxiety* 2015;**32**:527–38.

85. M. Zimmerman, J. N. Galione. Screening for bipolar disorder with the Mood Disorders Questionnaire: a review. *Harv Rev Psychiatry* 2011;**19**:219–28.

86. D. Lee, B. Cha, C. S. Park, et al. Usefulness of the combined application of the Mood Disorder Questionnaire and Bipolar Spectrum Diagnostic Scale in screening for bipolar disorder. *Compr Psychiatry* 2013;**54**:334–40.

87. S. Paterniti, J. C. Bisserbe. Factors associated with false positives in MDQ screening for bipolar disorder: Insight into the construct validity of the scale. *J Affect Disord* 2018;**238**:79–86.

88. A. Knackfuss, E. Leibenluft, M. A. Brotman, et al. (2020). Differentiating irritable mood and disruptive behavior in adults. *Trends Psychiatry Psychoth* 2020;**42**:375–86.

89. J. R. Phelps, S. N. Ghaemi. Improving the diagnosis of bipolar disorder: predictive value of screening tests. *J Affect Disord* 2006;**92**:141–8.

90. Y. S. Wu, J. Angst, C. S. Ou, et al. Validation of the Chinese version of the hypomania checklist (HCL-32) as an instrument for detecting hypo(mania) in patients with mood disorders. *J Affect Disord* 2008;**106**:133–43.

91. M. Oh, J. Angst, T. Sung, et al. Reliability and validity of the hypomania symptom checklist-32 in Korea. *Korean J Clin Psychol* 2009;**28**:321–38.

92. E. Vieta, J. Sánchez-Moreno, A. Bulbena, et al. Cross validation with the mood disorder questionnaire (MDQ) of an instrument for the detection of hypomania in Spanish: the 32 item hypomania symptom check list (HCL-32). *J Affect Disord* 2007;**101**:43–55.

93. S. N. Mosolov, A. V. Ushkalova, E. G. Kostukova, et al. Validation of the Russian version of the Hypomania Checklist (HCL-32) for the detection of Bipolar II disorder in patients with a current diagnosis of recurrent depression. *J Affect Disord* 2014;**155**:90–5.

94. A. Gamma, J. Angst, J. M. Azorin, et al. Transcultural validity of the Hypomania Checklist-32 (HCL-32) in patients with major depressive episodes. *Bipolar Disord* 2013;**15**:701–12.

95. L. Forty, M. Kelly, L. Jones, et al. Reducing the Hypomania Checklist (HCL-32) to a 16-item version. *J Affect Disord* 2010;**124**:351–6.

96. P. Bech, E. M. Christensen, M. Vinberg, et al. From items to syndromes in the Hypomania Checklist (HCL-32): psychometric validation and clinical validity analysis. *J Affect Disord* 2011;**132**:48–54.

97. T. D. Meyer, E. Castelao, M. Gholamrezaee, et al. Hypomania Checklist-32 – cross-validation of shorter versions screening for bipolar disorders in an epidemiological study. *Acta Psychiatr Scand* 2017;**135**:539–47.

98. K. Lee H. Oh E. H. Lee, et al. Investigation of the clinical utility of the hypomania checklist 32 (HCL-32) for the screening of bipolar disorders in the non-clinical adult population. *BMC Psychiatry* 2016;**16**:124.

99. S. N. Ghaemi, C. J. Miller, D. A. Berv, et al. Sensitivity and specificity of a new bipolar spectrum diagnostic scale. *J Affect Disord* 2005;**84**:273–7.

100. M. Zimmerman, J. N. Galione, C. J. Ruggero, et al. A different approach toward screening for bipolar disorder: the prototype matching method. *Compr Psychiatry* 2010;**51**:340–6.

101. G. H. Vázquez, E. Romero, F. Fabregues, et al. Screening for bipolar disorders in Spanish-speaking populations: sensitivity and specificity of the Bipolar Spectrum Diagnostic Scale-Spanish Version. *Compr Psychiatry* 2010;**51**:552–6.

102. A. Shabani, M. Mirzaei Khoshalani, S. Mahdavi, et al. Screening bipolar disorders in a general hospital: psychometric findings for the Persian version of mood disorder questionnaire and bipolar spectrum diagnostic scale. *Med J Islam Repub Iran* 2019;**33**:48.

103. H. Chu, C. J. Lin, K. J. Chiang, et al. Psychometric properties of the Chinese version of the Bipolar Spectrum Diagnostic Scale. *J Clin Nurs* 2010;**19**:2787–94.

104. M. Zimmerman, J. N. Galione, I. Chelminski, et al. Performance of the Bipolar Spectrum Diagnostic Scale in psychiatric outpatients. *Bipolar Disord* 2010;**12**:528–38.

105. G. Parker, D. Hadzi-Pavlovic, L. Tully. Distinguishing bipolar and unipolar disorders: an isomer model. *J Affect Disord* 2006;**96**:67–73.

106. G. Parker, R. Graham, D. Hadzi-Pavlovic, et al. Further examination of the utility and comparative properties of the MSQ and MDQ bipolar screening measures. *J Affect Disord* 2012;**138**:104–9.

107. G. Parker, K. Fletcher, M. P. Hyett. The Mood Assessment Program: a computerised diagnostic tool for deriving management plans for mood disorders. *Med J Aust* 2008;**188**:126–8.

108. R. A. Depue, J. F. Slater, H. Wolfstetter-Kausch, et al. A behavioral paradigm for identifying persons at risk for bipolar depressive disorder: a conceptual framework and five validation studies. *J Abnorm Psychol* 1981;**90**:381–437.

109. L. B. Alloy, L. Y. Abramson, P. D. Walshaw, et al. Behavioral approach system (BAS)-relevant cognitive styles and bipolar spectrum disorders: concurrent and prospective associations. *J Abnorm Psychol* 2009;**118**:459–71.

110. M. Hautzinger, T. D. Meyer, B. L. Pheasant. (2002). Cyclothymic but not depressive temperament influences the mood of another person in social interactions. In W. P. Kaschka, editor. *Perspectives in Affective Disorders*. Karger Publishers, 2002; 178–87.

111. E. Youngstrom, O. Meyers, C. Demeter, et al. Comparing diagnostic checklists for pediatric bipolar disorder in academic and community mental health settings. *Bipolar Disord* 2005;**7**:507–17.

112. K. Imamura, N. Kawakami, Y. Naganuma, et al. Development of screening inventories for bipolar disorder at workplace: a diagnostic accuracy study. *J Affect Disord* 2015;**178**:32–8.

113. P. Fusar-Poli, A. De Micheli, M. Rocchetti, et al. Semistructured Interview for Bipolar At Risk States (SIBARS). *Psychiatry Res* 2018;**264**:302–9.

114. S. Moritz, Ł. Gawęda, A. Heinz, et al. Four reasons why early detection centers for psychosis should be renamed and their treatment targets reconsidered: we should not catastrophize a future we can neither reliably predict nor change. *Psychol Med* 2019;**49**:2134–40.

115. M. J. Waugh, T. D. Meyer, E. A. Youngstrom, et al. A review of self-rating instruments to identify young people at risk of bipolar spectrum disorders. *J Affect Disord* 2014;**160**:113–21.

116. M. M. Ng, J. Firth, M. Minen, et al. User engagement in mental health apps: a review of measurement, reporting, and validity. *Psychiatr Serv* 2019;**70**:538–44.

117. J. Nicholas, M. E. Larsen, J. Proudfoot, et al. Mobile apps for bipolar disorder: a systematic review of features and content quality. *J Med Internet Res* 2015;**17**:e198.

118. C. Qu, C. Sas, C. Daudén Roquet, et al. Functionality of top-rated mobile apps for depression: systematic search and evaluation. *JMIR Ment Health* 2020;**7**: e15321. Erratum in: *JMIR Ment Health* 2020;**7**: e18042.

119. G. Parker, M. J. Spoelma, G. Tavella, et al. Differentiating mania/hypomania from happiness using a machine learning analytic approach. *J Affect Disord* 2021;**281**:505–9.

120. C. H. Cho, T. Lee, M. G. Kim, et al. Mood prediction of patients with mood disorders by machine learning using passive digital phenotypes based on the circadian rhythm: prospective observational cohort study. *J Med Internet Res* 2019;**21**:e11029. Erratum in: *J Med Internet Res* 2019;**21**: e15966.

121. G. Andersson, N. Titov. Advantages and limitations of Internet-based interventions for common mental disorders. *World Psychiatry* 2014;**13**: 4–11.

122. R. Mojtabai. universal depression screening to improve depression outcomes in primary care: sounds good, but where is the evidence? *Psychiatr Serv* 2017;**68**:724–6.

123. M. de Wit, F. Pouwer, R. J. Gemke, et al. Validation of the WHO-5 Well-Being Index in adolescents with type 1 diabetes. *Diabetes Care* 2007;**30**:2003–26.

124. C. J. Nelson, C. Cho, A. R. Berk, et al. Are gold standard depression measures appropriate for use in geriatric cancer patients? A systematic evaluation of self-report depression instruments used with geriatric, cancer, and geriatric cancer samples. *J Clin Oncol* 2010;**28**:348–56.

125. K. L. Smarr, A. L. Keefer. Measures of depression and depressive symptoms: Beck Depression Inventory-II (BDI-II), Center for Epidemiologic Studies Depression Scale (CES-D), Geriatric Depression Scale (GDS), Hospital Anxiety and Depression Scale (HADS), and Patient Health Questionnaire-9 (PHQ-9). *Arthritis Care Res* 2011;**63**:S454–S466.

126. R. Trevethan. sensitivity, specificity, and predictive values: foundations, probabilities, and pitfalls in research and practice. *Front Public Health* 2017;**5**:307.

127. Akiskal HS, Pinto O. The evolving bipolar spectrum. Prototypes I, II, III, and IV. *Psychiatr Clin North Am*. 1999;**22**:517–34; vii.

The Socioeconomic Costs of Mood Disorders

Paul McCrone

Introduction

Mood disorders include depression and bipolar disorder and are widespread in terms of numbers and region. They affect people across the life course and may have a biological cause but are frequently linked to key life events [1]. Mood disorders rank highly in terms of burden of disease. The 2019 Global Burden of Disease Study shows that depressive disorders and bipolar disorder were the 2nd and 28th greatest contributors, respectively, to years lived with disability globally [2]. Mood disorders have a substantial impact on the lives of those experiencing them in terms of symptoms, disability, poor quality of life, low well-being, and reduced life opportunities. Sometimes depression or an episode of mania may be transient and so these impacts can be short term. However, mood disorders can be episodic and long term. While there are available evidence-based treatment options for depression and bipolar disorder, there are many who are resistant to treatment, and gaps in provision are common [3].

The human cost of mental illness is also reflected in impacts on the economy. Provision of support and care requires the use of resources that could in principle be used to support those with other health problems or could indeed be used for entirely different purposes such as education, defence, or transport. The consequences of living with a mood disorder can also be expressed in monetary terms. This chapter will provide a discussion of some of the key concepts we need to consider when discussing economic impacts and costs and then summarise some key findings related to depression and bipolar disorder.

What Do We Mean by Cost and Where Does It Fall?

Most people will have some understanding of cost. From an economic perspective, we can categorise costs into those that (i) arise in supporting someone

with a particular condition or illness through treatment and care, (ii) occur as consequences of the condition or illness to the wider economy, and (iii) impact on social and recreational activities. Figure 6.1 provides a conceptual model that identifies the different areas of cost.

The first category is often considered to be direct costs and the economic concept of opportunity cost is helpful here. This indicates that cost occurs when the resources used to address the illness could in principle be used for other purposes. If someone with a mood disorder spends time with a psychiatrists, psychologist, or other clinician then that clearly represents a cost as that clinician could be using their time in other ways (for example, with another patient or in research activities). Other support can come in the form of medication, and again the funds required in its production and administration could be put to other purposes.

Practically all types of service provision that require professional time or financial outlay are costs. However, what about time of patients and family members and friends? While patients will often need to spend time with a professional, this time could also be used in other ways (work, leisure, etc.) and so also has an opportunity cost. The same goes for informal care provided by family and friends. If this care was not provided, then the carer could potentially use the time in other ways. (An alternative way to think about informal care is that in its absence it may need to be replaced by professional input).

The second category of cost reflects the impact of a mood disorder on the wider economy. Lost work is a common impact of mental health problems. Many cost of illness studies have attempted to assess the magnitude of lost work in monetary terms but this is fraught with challenges regarding both measurement and valuation [4]. Different methods exist for valuing lost work time and these are discussed elsewhere [4,5],

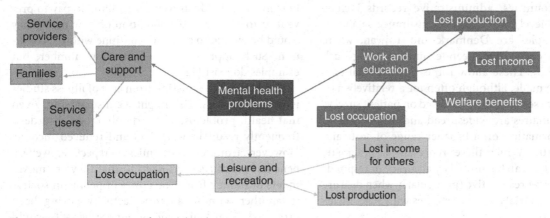

Figure 6.1 Economic impact of mood disorders.

and in most situations the productivity costs associated with mental health problems are substantial.

While most of the debate around productivity costs has concerned methods, much less discussion has been had about issues of equity. Productivity costs generally occur for those of working age and so conditions that affect mainly children or those beyond usual working age will appear disproportionately less costly. This then has serious consequences for the interpretation of economic evaluations with interventions that improve the chances of work more likely to be shown to be cost-effective and therefore prioritised. Indeed, one of the key 'selling points' of some treatments and therapies for mood disorders is that the extra investments required will be offset by increased production if people recover and remain in, or return to, work [6]. There is here a belief that employment outcomes are required and that work is even therapeutic. For many, this may of course be the case but there are other forms of 'occupation' (leisure, voluntary work, etc.), and formal employment might even be the precursor of some mental health problems. It is something of a neoclassical economic idea that work is the ultimate objective.

The third category of cost is usually focussed on less than the previous ones and relates to the impact of a health condition on the ability to engage in social, leisure, and recreational activities. This may be neglect and caused by a desire to concentrate on those more 'productive' activities such as work and education, which provide income for employees and surplus value for employers. However, it may also be because in many assessments of the impact of health problems, these non-work-related activities are covered by measures of quality of life and well-being. In Figure 6.1 it is noted that lost occupation and lost production appear in both the categories relating to reduced productive activities and reduced leisure/recreational activities. This is intentional. If someone with bipolar disorder or depression does not engage in everyday activities such as going to a pub or sporting event, then as well as a personal cost there is also reduced economic activity overall.

Measurement of Cost

Estimating the socioeconomic costs of mood disorders can be achieved using various approaches, perspectives, and methodologies. A consideration is whether we wish to estimate the lifetime costs of a mood disorder from the time it appears (incidence-based approach) or the average annual cost of a mood disorder (prevalence-based approach). Incidence-based studies are arguably more sophisticated and informative from an epidemiological point of view and allow costs over the course of an illness to be tracked. They are particularly useful for public health interventions that aim to reduce the likelihood of a mood disorder emerging. Prevalence-based studies estimate service needs and indirect impacts for a particular year and so only require data covering this period. Such studies are more common and require obtaining data for the period in question and combining these with appropriate cost information.

The data for both incidence- and prevalence-based studies can come from three main sources: administrative records (e.g., hospital records for a given year), surveys of those affected, and mathematical models.

In some countries, administrative records include population-level case registers or insurance databases. Good examples are Denmark and Taiwan, where depression costs have been estimated using such registers [7,8]. These allow robust longitudinal estimates to be made, although often for a relatively narrow range of services. Studies based on patient surveys or questionnaires are widespread and can be used to obtain information on a broader range of costs and effects [9,10]. While these represent a pragmatic approach, they can be limited by accuracy of respondent recall or representative (particularly when data are obtained from trials or other studies with strict inclusion criteria).

It will be apparent that some consequences of mood disorders (e.g., the need for treatment or therapy and the impact on work) are particularly amenable to monetary measurement. For other consequences, it is less straightforward. Very few studies, for example, attach monetary values to lost leisure time associated with mood disorders and yet we know that opportunities to engage in such activities can be hindered by these conditions. A neoclassical economic perspective suggests that such lost time be valued the same as lost work, assuming that individuals choose between work time and leisure time. There are all sorts of reasons why this is not realistic, but what should be clear is that if people have their leisure time adversely affected by a mood disorder, then that is a cost to them. Similarly, mood disorders are likely to impact on general quality of life and again this is not straightforward to value. There are, though, methods for attempting such valuation and examples of where this has been done. Some countries explicitly use health-related quality-of-life measures to assist in the prioritisation of healthcare funds and to do this a value needs to be attached to improved quality of life. In England and Wales, the National Institute for Health and Care Excellence (NICE) values a 'quality-adjusted life year' (or QALY) at £20,000 to £30,000. If the QALY impact of mood disorders can be estimated, then by using such a threshold the impact can also be valued monetarily. A similar approach can be used to value 'disability adjusted life years' (DALYs), although it is usually a proportion of gross domestic product (GDP) that is used in these valuations. This approach was used by McDaid and Park and colleagues in estimating the overall costs of mental health problems in the UK [11]. Alternative approaches to comprehensively valuing the impacts of a mood disorder is to ask (or infer)

how much individuals would be willing to pay to prevent or to fully cure the condition or how much they would be willing to accept to continue with the condition. Such approaches are limited in number, but examples do exist [12].

One common omission from cost of illness studies is welfare benefits. This might seem surprising, given that health problems, and certainly mood disorders, frequently result in work loss and reduced income. However, from an economics perspective, welfare benefits are *transfer payments* in that they are movements of money from one group of people in society to another without anything actually having been produced. That being said, to ignore benefits would be a mistake because funds used in this way could be put to other purposes.

Evidence on the Costs of Mood Disorders

A key European-wide study has estimated the total costs of brain disorders across the continent [13]. It indicated that in 2010 there were 178.5 million people with a brain disorder (psychiatric and neurological) with 33.3 million of these being a mood disorder. The total costs were calculated to be €477 billion and mood disorders had the highest cost at €113 billion.

The impact of mood disorders on work has been investigated in a number of studies. Kessler et al. compared lost workdays in the United States as a result of bipolar disorders and depression [14]. They found that those with bipolar disorder had on average 65.5 days off work while for those with depression it was 27.2 days. They make the point that while depression receives much attention due to the numbers involved, bipolar disorder still has a major impact on the economy.

Costs of Major Depressive Disorder

Depression is common but varied in its impact. For some, depression may not result in the seeking of treatment, and even when diagnosed it may be considered mild and outcomes can be good. For others, it will be longer term and require specialist support including pharmacotherapy and psychological therapy. While outcomes can be positive, up to 20% of people may have poor responses and be considered treatment resistant [15,16]. Not surprisingly, the economic costs associated with depression will depend on its course and severity.

Numerous studies have assessed the economic costs of depression. The findings differ substantially, and this reflects the lack of a common approach. McCrone et al. estimated the costs of depression in 2007 to be £6.3 billion [17]. The majority of this cost was due to lost employment. In the UK, total annual costs of mental health problems have been estimated by McDaid and Park and colleagues at £117.9 billion [11]. This includes the costs due to service provision lots work and disability. Depression accounted for 23% (£27 billion) of this total.

Many studies measure the use of services by people with depression but with the recognition that some of these costs are actually due to other conditions or events. Studies that assessed the *extra* costs due to depression were reviewed by König et al. [18]. They identified 48 studies and found depression in adults to be associated with cost increases of 158%, in adolescents of 179%, in elderly adults of 73%, and those with a physical comorbidity of 39%. In another review, Johnston et al. found that costs increase in line with the extent of resistance to treatment [19]. In a UK study of treatment-resistant depression, the annual costs were £22,124 per person [10]. Of this, lost work accounted for 54% and care from families another 26%. A more recent study estimated the treatment costs at £992 per month [20]. There is much less information on the costs associated with dysthymia, although one study found that these were higher if the condition emerged later [21].

Costs of Bipolar Disorder

Fewer studies have estimated the economic costs of bipolar disorder. The aforementioned study by McDaid and Park and colleagues found that the UK annual cost of bipolar disorder was £19.7 billion [11]. Previous studies used different methods with a more restricted range of costs [22,23]. In the UK, Das-Gupta and Guest estimated that the total costs of bipolar in 1998 were £2.1 billion (around £3.3 billion in 2021 prices) [24]. Of this amount, 86% was due to productivity costs. McCrone et al. estimated costs for 2007 of £5.2 billion (£7.1 billion in 2021 prices) with 69% due to lost production [17]. In another study, Young et al. estimated the healthcare costs of bipolar to be £342 million in 2009/10 prices (around £441 million in 2021 prices) [25]. In the United States, a review of 56 studies published from 2008 to 2018 was conducted by Bessonova et al. and on the basis of this they estimated the annual cost to be $196 billion [26].

Again, direct costs were relatively low compared to indirect costs, accounting for 25% of the total.

The healthcare cost for someone who has had a relapse has been estimated by Hong et al. at £4,083 over 6 months compared to £1,298 for someone without a relapse [27]. These are 2007/8 figures and inflate to £5,553 and £1,765 now (so an excess of £3,788. At least 50% of people with a bipolar diagnosis relapse each year, costing the NHS an estimated additional £1 billion per year.

In 2022, a survey of people with bipolar disorder was conducted as part of a commission led by the charity Bipolar UK (www.bipolaruk.org/bipolar-commission-findings). The survey included questions on the financial and economic impacts of bipolar disorder and the use of health and social care services. Responses from 865 people were included with people on average having been diagnosed around 10 years previously. The types of bipolar disorder included type 1 (28%) and type 2 (34%), with the remainder being unknown or other types. Key findings related to the impact on work were that: 63% had experienced job loss, 72% had not applied for a particular job, 44% hadn't applied for a promotion, and 35% felt that they had been overlooked for promotion. In addition, 82% reported that there earning potential was adversely affected by bipolar disorder and 20% that they currently had out-of-control debt.

The majority of the sample had seen a GP during the past year and the average number of contacts was four. Over half had seen a psychiatrist and around one-fifth had seen another doctor. Less than one-fifth had seen a psychologist, although one-quarter had seen a counsellor. One-third were in contact with a community mental health team and one-third were also in contact with a mental health nurse. Inpatient care was received at some time by 11.6% of respondents. The total cost of care over the year was on average £3,907. The most expensive service was inpatient care (despite its relatively low use), accounting for 37.6% of costs. By comparison, GP costs accounted for 3.6% despite the high use of this service.

The survey also asked respondents to state what services were most desired. These were desired GP care and support from psychiatrists. The level of GP care provided and desired was similar, but there appears to be a gap in the provision of psychiatrist care. Other services that were seemingly underprovided were psychologist support, complementary healthcare, group therapy, weight loss clinic, day centre, and physiotherapist. Although actual use was not reported, contact with a personal trainer was desired by 40% of the respondents.

Interpretation and Use of Findings from Cost of Illness Studies

Establishing the socioeconomic costs of mood disorders (or indeed any condition) can draw much attention to the conditions. Given this, it is not surprising that cost of illness studies are often funded both by charities, who wish to emphasise the impact that those they represent are experiencing, and industry, which can use such findings when promoting the potential effectiveness of their products. As well as these promotional and commercial uses, cost of illness studies can serve as a baseline on which future studies can be based. Cost of illness studies do, though, have important limitations [28]. Chief among these is the fact that they do not in themselves tell us how health and social care funds should be allocated. They also suggest that cost is a negative concept. This seems reasonable when considering the cost of lost work or opportunities, but high service costs may be entirely justified. Service costs are simply a monetary representation of care inputs, and for some conditions it can be argued that costs should be even higher.

To address how the impact of mood disorders can be addressed, we need to conduct economic evaluations. These involve combining information on costs with that on outcomes. Outcomes may be condition specific (e.g., changes in symptoms associated with mania or depression) or generic (e.g., using quality adjusted life years). Condition-specific outcomes are used in cost-effectiveness analyses, whereas generic measures are used in cost-utility analyses. (Confusingly, both types are sometimes referred to as cost-effectiveness analyses). Alternatively, outcomes might be measured in monetary units in the form of a cost–benefit analysis. These studies are, though, rare given the challenges in expressing clinical and quality-of-life changes monetarily.

Cost of illness studies and economic evaluations serve different purposes. The former are used to highlight the overall impact of a condition, while the latter inform us as to what we should do about it. Cost of illness studies can serve as a baseline for subsequent evaluations and can provide much-needed data for simulation models. Therefore, the two types of study can be seen as complementary.

Conclusions and Future Work

This chapter has summarised some of the widespread evidence on the cost of mood disorders. While findings differ substantially, even within countries, what is clear is that the costs are vast and the bulk of these are due to lost work and other opportunities rather than health-care received. What is not directly apparent is that care costs are likely to be quite different for people with depression and those with bipolar disorder. It is also important to point out that when discussing indirect costs, studies do generally mean lost work. Other impacts that are also costs, such as lost leisure time, are generally ignored. Future work should explore these costs so that attention is not just focussed on work and with interventions designed or funded on the basis of improving vocational outcomes. These are certainly important, but other uses of time are valuable and should ideally be included when considering the socioeconomic impact of mood disorders.

Studies have also tended to assess costs over a limited period of time. If the samples are representative, then this can still enable robust estimates to be made. However, it may be more informative to estimate lifetime costs and to address the way in which mood disorders affect people across the life course. There will often be precursors to the emergence of diagnosed problems, and these too will have economic impacts.

References

1. Brown GW, Harris TO, editors. *Life Events and Illness*. New York: Guilford Press, 1989.

2. GBD 2019 Mental Disorders Collaborators. Global, regional, and national burden of 12 mental disorders in 204 countries and territories, 1990–2019: a systematic analysis for the Global Burden of Disease Study 2019. *Lancet Psychiatry*. 2022;**9**:137–50.

3. Kohn R, Saxena S, Levav I, Saraceno B. The treatment gap in mental health care. *Bull World Health Organ*. 2004;**82**:858–66.

4. Pritchard Clive, Sculpher MJ, *Productivity Costs: Principles and Practice in Economic Evaluation*. London: Centre for Health Economics, 2000.

5. Pike J, Grosse SD. Friction cost estimates of productivity costs in cost-of-illness studies in comparison with human capital estimates: a review. *Appl Health Econ. Health Policy* 2018;**16**:765–78.

6. Layard R, Clark DM. Why more psychological therapy would cost nothing. *Front Psychol*. 2015;**6**. doi: 10.3389/fpsyg.2015.01713.

7. Jensen KJ, Gronemann FH, Ankarfeldt MZ, et al. Healthcare resource utilization in patients with treatment-resistant depression – a Danish national registry study. *PLoS One* 2022;**17**. doi: 10.1371/journal.pone.0275299.

8. Pan YJ, Knapp M, McCrone P. Impact of initial treatment outcome on long-term costs of depression: a 3-year nationwide follow-up study in Taiwan. *Psychol Med* 2014;**44**:1147–58.

9. Simon J, Pari AAA, Wolstenholme J, et al. The costs of bipolar disorder in the United Kingdom. *Brain Behav.* 2021;**11**:e2351–e2351.

10. McCrone P, Rost F, Koeser L, et al. The economic cost of treatment-resistant depression in patients referred to a specialist service. *J Ment Health.* 2018;**27**:567–73.

11. McDaid D, Park A-L, Davidson G, et al. The economic case for investing in the prevention of mental health conditions in the UK. London School of Economics and Political Science/Mental Health Foundation, 2022.

12. Morey E, Thacher JA, Craighead WE. Patient preferences for depression treatment programs and willingness to pay for treatment. *J MentHealth Policy Econ.* 2007;**10**:73–85.

13. Olesen J, Gustavsson A, Svensson M, Wittchen HU, Jönsson B. The economic cost of brain disorders in Europe. *Eur J Neurol.* 2012;**19**:155–62.

14. Kessler RC, Akiskal HS, Ames M, et al. Prevalence and effects of mood disorders on work performance in a nationally representative sample of U.S. workers. *Am J Psychiatry.* 2006;**163**:1561–8.

15. Kessler RC, Berglund P, Demler O, et al. The epidemiology of major depressive disorder. *JAMA.* 2003;**289**:3095.

16. Kubitz N, Mehra M, Potluri RC, Garg N, Cossrow N. Characterization of treatment resistant depression episodes in a cohort of patients from a US commercial claims database. *PLoS One.* 2013;**8**:e76882–e76882.

17. McCrone P, Dhanasiri S, Patel A, Knapp M, Lawton-Smith S. Paying the price: the cost of mental health care in England to 2026. London: King's Fund, 2008.

18. König H, König H-H, Konnopka A. The excess costs of depression: a systematic review and meta-analysis. *Epidemiol Psychiatr Sci.* 2019;**29**:e30–e30.

19. Johnston KM, Powell LC, Anderson IM, Szabo S, Cline S. The burden of treatment-resistant depression: a systematic review of the economic and quality of life literature. *J Affect Disord.* 2019;**242**:195–210.

20. Denee T, Ming T, Waller J, et al. A retrospective chart review study to quantify the monthly medical resource use and costs of treating patients with treatment resistant depression in the United Kingdom. *Curr Med Res Opin.* 2021;**37**:311–19.

21. Barbui C, Motterlini N, Garattini L. Health status, resource consumption, and costs of dysthymia. A multi-center two-year longitudinal study. *J Affect Disord.* 2006;**90**:181–6.

22. Sabes-Figuera R, Razzouk D, Mccrone PE. Economics of bipolar disorder. In LN Yatham, M Maj, editors. *Bipolar Disorder: Clinical and Neurobiological Foundations.* New York: Wiley, 2010; 90–5.

23. Jin H, McCrone P. Cost-of-illness studies for bipolar disorder: systematic review of international studies. *Pharmacoeconomics.* 2015;**33**:341–53.

24. Das Gupta R, Guest JF. Annual cost of bipolar disorder to UK society. *Br J Psychiatry.* 2002;**180**:227–33.

25. Young AH, Rigney U, Shaw S, Emmas C, Thompson JM. Annual cost of managing bipolar disorder to the UK healthcare system. *J Affect Disord.* 2011;**133**:450–6.

26. Bessonova L, Ogden K, Doane MJ, O'Sullivan AK, Tohen M. The economic burden of bipolar disorder in the United States: a systematic literature review. *Clinicoecon Outcomes Res.* 2020;**12**:481–97.

27. Hong J, Reed C, Novick D, et al. The cost of relapse for patients with a manic/mixed episode of bipolar disorder in the EMBLEM Study. *Pharmacoeconomics.* 2010;**28**:555–66.

28. Byford S, Torgerson DJ, Raftery J. Cost of illness studies. *BMJ.* 2000;**320**:1335.

Mood Disorders and Suicide

Rina Dutta and Joanna Hook

Introduction

Classed as one of the 20 leading causes of death worldwide with over 800,000 deaths globally per annum, suicide is a global public health challenge faced internationally [1]. This challenge is amplified when considering the spectrum in which completed suicide falls, ranging from thoughts or ruminations, to intention, to planning and making an attempt which can be fatal [2].

The human experience of dealing with all or part of this spectrum is devastating and unquantifiable for family and friends. The consequences for any professionals involved is also poorly understood, although preliminary research suggests a high proportion of mental health professionals report an adverse effect on work and many consider an alternative career following a patient suicide [3]. Some countries have estimated direct and indirect costs of a suicide – including healthcare and funeral costs, and loss of productivity in terms of, for example, employment and childcare – to equate to over £1 million [4], highlighting a significant economic impact. Such is the recognition of suicide as a global epidemiological concern that suicide prevention strategies have become an integral part of national and international public health plans.

It is widely acknowledged that population-based prevention strategies are most effective [5], with less convincing evidence for specifically targeting high-risk groups [6], although exploring the latter remains an important part of strategic planning. While suicide itself remains a rare event for the majority of the population, over 90% of those who do complete suicide have a diagnosis of a mental disorder at the time of death [7]. A significant proportion of those individuals have a mood disorder diagnosis, with a major depressive episode being the most frequently documented.

Nevertheless, it is important to acknowledge that the majority of those with a mood disorder do not attempt or complete suicide. As such, it is imperative when examining this particular 'at risk' group to consider what factors may influence suicidality. This in turn may help guide management of suicidal behaviour.

Epidemiology

Up to 90% of those who complete suicide in high-income countries are found, during the process of psychological autopsy, to have been suffering a mental disorder at the time of their death [8].

Suicide Risk in Mood Disorders

Half of all completed suicides are linked to a mood disorder [7], with a 20-fold increased standardised mortality ratio compared to the general population [9]. Within this spectrum of diagnoses, the most frequently reported rates of both attempts and completed suicides are amongst individuals with bipolar disorder and major depressive disorder [10]. With regard to suicidality, clinical reporting has a notable impact on incidence estimates [11].

Lifetime Risk of Suicide in Mood Disorders

Lifetime risk of suicide was originally quoted to be in the region of 15% for affective disorders, following a seminal meta-analysis published in 1970 [12]. However, this was concluded to be an overestimate, as high suicide rates early in the illness inflate the estimate if proportionate mortality (the percentage of those who die within the follow-up period who end their life by suicide) is used as a proxy [13].

Some of the most recent data quantifying the lifetime risk of suicide in mood disorders indicates the absolute lifetime risk for men with bipolar disorder to be 7.77% (95% confidence interval (CI): 6.01% to 10.05%) and with major depressive disorder, 6.67% (95% CI: 5.72% to 7.78%). For females with bipolar disorder, absolute lifetime risk was calculated as 4.78% (95% CI: 3.48% to 6.56%) and major depressive disorder, 3.77% (95% CI: 3.05% to 4.66%) [14].

Suicide in Major Depressive Disorder versus Bipolar Disorder

The figures above suggest the risk of suicide is higher in patients with a diagnosis of bipolar disorder compared to major depressive disorder, although studies comparing the rates between the two have shown inconsistent results [15]. Several studies do suggest that risk of suicide and attempts is greater in bipolar disorder, with one-third of bipolar patients attempting suicide at least once in their lifetime and that this is most prevalent in patients with mixed or psychotic features [10]. However a comprehensive meta-analysis of observational surveys of suicide attempts in individuals with major depressive disorder calculated a pooled lifetime prevalence of suicide attempt of 31% (95% CI: 27–34%) [16].

Aetiologic Factors

Many patients with a diagnosis of a mood disorder do not plan, attempt or complete suicide, and there are many potential aetiologic factors which drive suicidal behaviour.

Heritability

Genetic heritability of suicidality is suggested from the broad spectrum of twin and adoption studies, with higher concordance rates for suicide in monozygotic than dizygotic twins (24.1% versus 2.8%) [17]. Heritability is estimated to be between 30% and 50% for the range of suicidality that extends from ideation to attempts and, importantly, is thought to be largely separate from the inheritance of a psychiatric disorder [18].

Genetics and Neurobiology

Several candidate genes have been explored for their potential influence on suicidal behaviour including genes within the serotonergic, noradrenergic and dopaminergic systems, largely with inconsistent results [18]. A large treatment trial of major depression reported associations between emerging suicidal ideation and genes encoding glutamate and interleukin receptors [19].

Hypothalamic–Pituitary–Adrenal (HPA) Axis Dysfunction

Dysregulation of the HPA axis has an established association with suicide, although the mechanisms involved are not clear [20]. An abnormal HPA axis has commonly been linked to depressed patients who are often found to have excess cortisol levels [21]. Similar findings have been ascertained amongst bipolar patients, with positive associations during the manic phase in particular [22].

Although one meta-analysis found an inverse correlation between suicide attempts in older age groups and cortisol levels, whereas in younger patients suicide attempts were associated with high levels. The reduction in cortisol levels in those attempting suicide in older age groups was found to be in keeping with studies looking at patients with a major depressive disorder, with possible speculation being that longevity of illness may lead to a fatigued HPA feedback process, such that cortisol release experiences a 'rebound' and returns to normal [23]. When considering suicide in mood disorders specifically, consideration of the exposure to stress overtime, which can be understood in the context of the chronicity of severe depression, may be pertinent.

Impulsive/Aggressive Traits

Impulsivity and aggressive traits have often been linked to suicidality in general, with psychological autopsy studies following suicide identifying higher levels of aggression compared to psychiatric controls. These traits have also been linked more specifically to suicidal behaviour in major depressive disorder, with a specific case control study focused on male patients [24].

Impulsivity itself is often a characteristic of bipolar disorder, particularly in manic or hypomanic phases of the illness, although often described qualitatively. Using memory tasks, impulsivity has been demonstrated as an objective measurable trait associated with a history of medically severe suicide attempts [25].

Environmental

Acknowledging that suicide is a multifactorial phenomenon, the influence of environmental factors, particularly negative life events, cannot be over-looked. Certainly, factors such as economic loss have been identified as key factors amongst suicide cases [26]. Many models exploring the aetiology of suicide consider mental disorder as a more chronic factor, with environmental factors acting as triggers, increasing the propensity for suicide in those with increased vulnerability. O'Connor et al. provide an example of such within their Integrated Motivational-Volitional Model of Suicidal Behaviour, suggesting that suicidality may emerge as a combination of factors which may increase suicidal intention and behaviour [27].

Sociocultural

Clear epidemiological disparities have been found when looking at suicide globally, with Asian countries less likely to attribute the event to mental disorder than the West [28]. Other factors such as isolation, conflict within families and financial loss are proposed to be more predominant factors. Influence of the availability and uptake of mental health support in these populations has also been considered a factor, suggesting that under detection of mood and other mental disorders may occur in certain populations.

Risk Factors Associated with Suicide in Mood Disorders

Risk factors in the context of suicide in general have been extensively researched. This section aims to highlight the differences in risk factors associated with suicide in mood disorders.

Previous Suicide Attempts

Previous suicide attempts are a strong predictor for suicide in general but should be considered particularly pertinent amongst patients with mood disorders. A history of previous attempts occurs in at least half of patients with bipolar disorder [29].

Highlighting past attempts as an important predictor of future risk is perhaps best done by the ratio of attempts to completion. One such study examining this 'lethality index' reported the ratio as 3:1 in patients with a diagnosis of bipolar disorder, compared to 35:1 in the general population [30]. Lower attempt to completion ratios have also been found amongst patients with other psychiatric diagnoses, including depression [31].

Sociodemographic Factors

There appear to be differences in sociodemographic risk factors for suicide depending on the type of mood disorder subtype. Multiple studies suggest that suicide attempts occur at younger ages and earlier in the course of the illness in bipolar disorder [10]. Men with bipolar disorder are at higher risk of death through suicide than their female counterparts [29].

Depression appears to have a less clear pattern of correlation, but studies suggest that suicides occur more in the elderly [7]. One large Australian study identified higher numbers of suicide attempts amongst women with a younger onset of illness [32].

Severity, Type and Duration of Illness

Given the high prevalence of mental disorders found on psychological autopsy, the presence of a diagnosis alone can be viewed as a risk factor for suicidality. With this in mind, it follows that severity of the illness, delays in diagnosis and periods of sub optimal treatment are found to increase the likelihood of suicidal behaviour and acts [10].

Suicide rates appear to vary with the type of illness phase in patients with bipolar disorder. Depressive and mixed affective episodes appear to account for the highest risk of suicide in many studies [2].

A longitudinal study exploring the occurrence of attempted suicide in patients with major depressive disorder over a 5-year period found that three quarters of suicides took place during a depressive episode, a 21-fold increase compared to the those that occurred during the time spent in full remission [33].

Comorbid Disorders

Psychiatric comorbidity is high amongst patients with mood disorder diagnoses who die by suicide, with alcohol or substance abuse and cluster B personality disorders associated with suicide in depression [2]. History of alcohol abuse is shared as a risk factor for suicide in bipolar patients [34].

Mishara and Chagnon's Six-Model Proposal of the Relationship between Mental Disorders and Suicide

Theorising the relationship between mental illness and suicide, Mishara and Chagnon propose six models. Within these is Model 1, which suggests that biological vulnerability and adversity are commonalities that can lead to both. Model 2 suggests that some people may develop an alternative to suicidal thoughts or impulses, for example, a substance use disorder. Under Model 3, it is suggested that suicide can be a consequence of negative cognitions, such as hopelessness in depression. Model 4 postulates that negative experiences that can accompany mental disorders (e.g., discrimination, stigma and social exclusion) contribute to suicide risk. Model 5 describes suicide as iatrogenic, occurring due to sub-optimal treatment of mental disorders. Model 6 is a combined model that incorporates features of the other five but overlays these with a crisis situation [35].

Assessing Suicide Risk

Risk Assessment Tools

Despite the proportion of completed suicides being attributed to patients with a diagnosable mental disorder, the actual prevalence and incidence rates remain low and predicting suicide continues to raise challenges. In fact, structured risk assessments for suicide are deemed to be inaccurate in predicting mortality [36].

Biological Testing

Exploring the option of biological testing as a quantifiable measure in suicide prediction has been questioned in view of the biogenetic theories involving the serotonergic system and HPA axis dysfunction. Prediction models that apply these theories, including measuring cerebral spinal fluid (CSF) and the dexamethasone suppression test, vary widely in performance, making it difficult to integrate into clinical practice [37].

Machine Learning

The advancement of electronic data collection and record keeping has meant that understanding suicide and suicidal behaviours is more research accessible. Systems such as the Clinical Records Interactive Search (CRIS), designed as a database for epidemiological and clinical research within the South London and Maudsley NHS Foundation Trust, allows researchers and clinicians to analyse anonymised data in a variety of ways including free text searches, so that language related to different types of suicidal behaviour can be identified [38].

Data mining and machine learning methods have been applied to automatically learn patterns and rules from large databases on a scale that is impossible for humans. Clinical databases such as electronic health records typically contain a variety of data, of which structured data entries lend themselves well to computational analysis and free text data to natural language processing. Suicidal behaviour is a complex phenomenon that is contextually dependent and can shift rapidly from one day to the next. Capturing the effect of these dynamic risks requires sophisticated measurement and statistical modelling [39].

Machine learning techniques are methods that learn from large datasets using statistical and algorithmic approaches. They can be used to model risk factors, patterns of illness evolution and outcomes. The two key types are predictive models and explanatory models. Both models use features to provide information on future events, such as the likelihood that a patient will attempt suicide within a given time interval, and can model complex relations between features and outcomes [40].

Pharmacological Considerations in Managing Suicide

Lithium

Patients

There is more compelling evidence for lithium providing substantial protection against suicide than any other pharmacological treatment provided for patients with mood disorders [41]. Despite some methodological concerns and heterogeneity in terms of patients, diagnoses, comparators, durations and phase of illness, the evidence from epidemiological and naturalistic data is overwhelmingly in favour of lithium as an anti-suicidal agent. This is so even when balanced against potential long-term deterioration in renal function, which can be checked in clinical practice with regular plasma monitoring [42].

However, a recent randomised controlled trial (RCT) [43] adding in lithium or placebo to existing medication regimes for bipolar disorder or depression in those with substantial comorbidities in a veterans population was stopped for futility after $n = 519$ veterans were randomised, so it may not hold for every patient sub-group.

Lithium Post–Electroconvulsive Therapy (ECT)

There has been a resurgence in interest in the role of lithium to prevent suicide post-ECT as well as maintain well-being [44]. Of 7,000 patients treated with ECT for major depressive disorder identified from a large Swedish cohort register-based study, it was found that at 12 months post-ECT there were no suicides amongst those patients who had been treated with lithium compared to 56 suicides in the non-lithium group [45]. The readmission rate for the lithium group was significantly lower than the non-lithium group. These findings suggest an important role for lithium as part of maintenance therapy following ECT [46].

Population Level

A synthesis of ecological studies, which are, of course, subject to the ecological bias, supports the hypothesis that there is a protective (or inverse) association between lithium intake from public drinking water and suicide mortality at the population level. Naturally occurring lithium in drinking water may have the potential to reduce the risk of suicide and may possibly help in mood stabilisation, particularly in populations with relatively high suicide rates and geographic areas with a greater range of lithium concentration in the drinking water [47].

Antidepressants

Based largely on anecdotal reports from the 1990s of increased suicidal behaviour amongst young patients exposed to selective serotonin reuptake inhibitors (SSRIs) [48], in 2004, the US Food and Drug Administration (FDA) made the decision that there should be a boxed warning on antidepressants regarding the risk of suicidality in young adults. The clinical and public health implications of this have been major, with a decline in the prescription of antidepressant drugs associated with an increase in the rate of suicidal events amongst people with severe depression [49]. Moreover, recent evidence on the overall benefits from the use of antidepressants in the treatment of depression are not so pessimistic and in fact strongly suggest reduced risk of suicide over time [50].

Anxiolytics and Sedatives

Research evidence does not provide strong support for anti-anxiety medications, in particular benzodiazepines being helpful in reducing suicidal risk in mood disorder patients [51]. The behavioural disinhibition associated with benzodiazepine use might increase impulsive and aggressive behaviours, especially in combination with alcohol and thereby increase risk of suicidal behaviours. However, in patients with predominantly anxiety symptoms and concomitant antidepressant treatment or psychotherapy, short duration use of benzodiazepines may reduce odds of suicide [52].

Antipsychotics

Of the antipsychotics, reduction of suicide and suicide attempts is seen consistently and uniquely with clozapine, but trials predominantly involve patients diagnosed with schizophrenia-like disorders. Only 5 of 18 studies included in a recent (2021) systematic review of research reports related to potential effects on suicidal behaviour of clozapine and other modern antipsychotic drugs for psychosis (aripiprazole, olanzapine, risperidone, quetiapine and ziprasidone) included patients with mood disorders rather than psychotic disorders [53]. Therefore, the possible implications for suicide risk for patients with major depression or bipolar disorder cannot be concluded and further studies are needed to test and quantify more specifically the anti-suicidal effect of modern drugs for psychosis effective in treating bipolar depression and mixed episodes in particular.

Ketamine

There is growing evidence supporting use of short-term intravenous ketamine to reduce suicidal ideation compared with placebo or midazolam [54]. More recently, intranasal esketamine has been shown to rapidly treat depression and acute severe suicidality [55].

Nonpharmacological Treatments

Psychological Therapies

When focused on suicidal cognitions and behaviours, cognitive behavioural therapy (CBT) has been found to be effective in adults independent of a focus on treatment of the affective disorder [56]. It has been shown to reduce suicide attempts when compared to treatment as usual. In a secondary analysis of a large RCT sample, Scott and colleagues showed that adjunctive use of CBT was beneficial for individuals diagnosed with bipolar depression, who make up the majority of patients seen in routine clinical practice [57]. Although this does require replicating in larger scale independent studies.

Dialectical behaviour therapy (DBT), which has a greater focus on the emotional and social aspects of behaviours and is more well known for its use in personality disorder, has also been shown to reduce suicidal ideation compared with control samples [58]. The skills-based approach with routine monitoring of suicidal thoughts and urges leads to reductions in suicidal behaviours, particularly in adolescents [59].

Physical Treatments

There is solid evidence that for severely depressed patients with expressed suicidal intent, ECT is rapidly effective. Considering the delayed efficacy of medications, it is prudent to consider ECT earlier in those with a high degree of expressed suicidal intent or plans [60].

There is preliminary evidence that repetitive transcranial magnetic stimulation (rTMS) may decrease suicidal ideation [61]. Of course, from the patient perspective this can be preferable because a general anaesthetic is not required (as with ECT) and rTMS does not normally cause a seizure, which can be associated with memory loss.

In severe treatment-resistant depression, vagus nerve stimulation produced a statistically lower relative risk of suicidal ideation, and treatment with adjunctive vagus nerve stimulation can potentially lower the risk of all-cause mortality, suicide and suicide attempts [62].

With each of these physical treatments, the key is appropriate selection of patients who have found other treatments unsuccessful, unhelpful or unacceptable, and the assessed positive benefit:risk ratio of trying one of these less-used strategies.

References

1. World Health Organisation. Preventing suicide: a global imperative. 2014.

2. Isometsa E. Suicidal behaviour in mood disorders – who, when, and why? *Can J Psychiatry*. 2014;**59** (3):120–30.

3. Rytterstrom P, Ovox SM, Wardig R, Hultsjo S. Impact of suicide on health professionals in psychiatric care mental healthcare professionals' perceptions of suicide during ongoing psychiatric care and its impacts on their continued care work. *Int J Ment Health Nurs*. 2020;**29** (5):982–91.

4. Royal College of Psychiatrists. Self-harm and suicide in adults: final report of the Patient Safety Group. CR229. College Report. 2020.

5. Lewis G, Hawton K, Jones P. Strategies for preventing suicide. *Br J Psychiatry*. 1997;**171**(4):351–4.

6. Schaffer A, Sinyor M, Kurdyak P, et al. Population-based analysis of health care contacts among suicide decedents: identifying opportunities for more targeted suicide prevention strategies. *World Psychiatry*. 2016;**15**(2):135–45.

7. Bachmann S. Epidemiology of suicide and the psychiatric perspective. *Int J Environ Res Public Health*. 2018;**15**(7)

8. Phillips MR. Rethinking the role of mental illness in suicide. *Am J Psychiatry*. 2010;**167**(7):731–3.

9. Tondo L, Pompili M, Forte A, Baldessarini RJ. Suicide attempts in bipolar disorders: comprehensive review of 101 reports. *Acta Psychiatr Scand*. 2016;**133** (3):174–86.

10. Baldessarini RJ, Tondo L. Suicidal risks in 12 DSM-5 psychiatric disorders. *J Affect Disord*. 2020;**271**:66–73.

11. Francis ER, Fonseca de Freitas D, Colling C, et al. Incidence of suicidality in people with depression over a 10-year period treated by a large UK mental health service provider. *BJPsych Open*. 2021;**7**(6):e223.

12. Guze SB, Robins E. Suicide and primary affective disorders. *Br J Psychiatry*. 1970;**117**(539):437–8.

13. Dutta R, Murray RM, Hotopf M, et al. Reassessing the long-term risk of suicide after a first episode of psychosis. *Arch Gen Psychiatry*. 2010;**67**(12):1230–7.

14. Nordentoft M, Mortensen PB, Pedersen CB. Absolute risk of suicide after first hospital contact in mental disorder. *Arch Gen Psychiatry*. 2011;**68**(10):1058–64.

15. Schaffer A, Isometsa ET, Tondo L, et al. Epidemiology, neurobiology and pharmacological interventions related to suicide deaths and suicide attempts in bipolar disorder: part I of a report of the International Society for Bipolar Disorders Task Force on Suicide in Bipolar Disorder. *Aust N Z J Psychiatry*. 2015;**49**(9):785–802.

16. Dong M, Zeng LN, Lu L, et al. Prevalence of suicide attempt in individuals with major depressive disorder: a meta-analysis of observational surveys. *Psychol Med*. 2019;**49**(10):1691–704.

17. Voracek M, Loibl LM. Genetics of suicide: a systematic review of twin studies. *Wien Klin Wochenschr*. 2007;**119**(15–16):463–75.

18. Mann JJ, Arango VA, Avenevoli S, et al. Candidate endophenotypes for genetic studies of suicidal behavior. *Biol Psychiatry*. 2009;**65**(7):556–63.

19. Laje G, Paddock S, Manji H, et al. Genetic markers of suicidal ideation emerging during citalopram treatment of major depression. *Am J Psychiatry*. 2007;**164**(10):1530–8.

20. van Heeringen K, Mann JJ. The neurobiology of suicide. *Lancet Psychiatry*. 2014;**1**(1):63–72.

21. Pandey GN. Biological basis of suicide and suicidal behavior. *Bipolar Disord*. 2013;**15**(5):524–41.

22. Belvederi Murri M, Prestia D, Mondelli V, et al. The HPA axis in bipolar disorder: systematic review and meta-analysis. *Psychoneuroendocrinology*. 2016;**63**:327–42.

23. O'Connor DB, Green JA, Ferguson E, O'Carroll RE, O'Connor RC. Cortisol reactivity and suicidal behavior: investigating the role of hypothalamic-pituitary-adrenal axis responses to stress in suicide attempters and ideators. *Psychoneuroendocrinology*. 2017;**75**:183–91.

24. Dumais A, Lesage AD, Alda M, et al. Risk factors for suicide completion in major depression: a case-control study of impulsive and aggressive behaviors in men. *Am J Psychiatry*. 2005;**162**(11):2116–24.

25. Swann AC, Dougherty DM, Pazzaglia PJ, et al. Increased impulsivity associated with severity of suicide attempt history in patients with bipolar disorder. *Am J Psychiatry*. 2005;**162**(9):1680–7.

26. Oyesanya M, Lopez-Morinigo J, Dutta R. Systematic review of suicide in economic recession. *World J Psychiatry*. 2015;**5**(2):243–54.

27. O'Connor RC, Kirtley OJ. The Integrated Motivational-Volitional Model of Suicidal Behaviour. *Philos Trans R Soc Lond B Biol Sci*. 2018;**373**:20170268.

28. Cho SE, Na KS, Cho SJ, Im JS, Kang SG. Geographical and temporal variations in the prevalence of mental disorders in suicide: systematic review and meta-analysis. *J Affect Disord*. 2016;**190**:704–13.

29. Plans L, Barrot C, Nieto E, et al. Association between completed suicide and bipolar disorder: a systematic review of the literature. *J Affect Disord*. 2019;**242**:111–22.

30. Simon GE, Hunkeler E, Fireman B, Lee JY, Savarino J. Risk of suicide attempt and suicide death in patients treated for bipolar disorder. *Bipolar Disord*. 2007;**9**(5):526–30.

31. Dome P, Rihmer Z, Gonda X. Suicide risk in bipolar disorder: a brief review. *Medicina (Kaunas)*. 2019;55(8]

32. Bradvik L. Suicide risk and mental disorders. *Int J Environ Res Public Health*. 2018;**15**(9]

33. Holma KM, Melartin TK, Haukka J, et al. Incidence and predictors of suicide attempts in DSM-IV major depressive disorder: a five-year prospective study. *Am J Psychiatry*. 2010;**167**(7):801–8.

34. Dutta R, Boydell J, Kennedy N, et al. Suicide and other causes of mortality in bipolar disorder: a longitudinal study. *Psychol Med*. 2007;**37**(6):839–47.

35. Mishara BL, Chagnon F. Why mental illness is a risk factor for suicide: implications for suicide prevention. In RC O'Connor, J Pirkis, editors. *The International Handbook of Suicide Prevention*. 2nd ed. Hoboken: Wiley, 2016; 594–608.

36. Lopez-Morinigo JD, Ayesa-Arriola R, Torres-Romano B, et al. Risk assessment and suicide by patients with schizophrenia in secondary mental healthcare: a case-control study. *BMJ Open*. 2016;**6**(9):e011929.

37. Mann JJ, Currier D, Stanley B, et al. Can biological tests assist prediction of suicide in mood disorders? *Int J Neuropsychopharmacol*. 2006;**9**(4):465–74.

38. Bittar A, Velupillai S, Downs J, Sedgwick R, Dutta R. Reviewing a decade of research into suicide and related behaviour using the South London and Maudsley NHS Foundation Trust Clinical Record Interactive Search (CRIS) system. *Front Psychiatry*. 2020;**11**:553463.

39. Velupillai S, Hadlaczky G, Baca-Garcia E, et al. Risk assessment tools and data-driven approaches for predicting and preventing suicidal behavior. *Front Psychiatry*. 2019;**10**:36.

40. Boudreaux ED, Rundensteiner E, Liu F, et al. Applying machine learning approaches to suicide prediction using healthcare data: overview and future directions. *Front Psychiatry*. 2021;**12**:707916.

41. Baldessarini RJ, Tondo L, Hennen J. Treating the suicidal patient with bipolar disorder. Reducing suicide risk with lithium. *Ann N Y Acad Sci*. 2001;**932**:24–38; discussion 9–43.

42. Smith KA, Cipriani A. Lithium and suicide in mood disorders: updated meta-review of the scientific literature. *Bipolar Disord*. 2017;**19**(7):575–86.

43. Katz IR, Rogers MP, Lew R, et al. Lithium treatment in the prevention of repeat suicide-related outcomes in veterans with major depression or bipolar disorder: a randomized clinical trial. *JAMA Psychiatry*. 2022;**79**(1):24–32.

44. Rasmussen KG. Lithium for post-electroconvulsive therapy depressive relapse prevention: a consideration of the evidence. *J ECT*. 2015;**31**(2):87–90.

45. Brus O, Cao Y, Hammar A, et al. Lithium for suicide and readmission prevention after electroconvulsive therapy for unipolar depression: population-based register study. *BJPsych Open*. 2019;**5**(3):e46.

46. Malhi GS, Bell E, Boyce P, et al. The 2020 mood disorders clinical practice guidelines: Translating

evidence into practice with both style and substance. *Aust N Z J Psychiatry*. 2021;**55**(9):919–20.

47. Memon A, Rogers I, Fitzsimmons S, et al. Association between naturally occurring lithium in drinking water and suicide rates: systematic review and meta-analysis of ecological studies. *Br J Psychiatry*. 2020;**217**(6):667–78.

48. Teicher MH, Glod C, Cole JO. Emergence of intense suicidal preoccupation during fluoxetine treatment. *Am J Psychiatry*. 1990;**147**(2):207–10.

49. Lu CY, Zhang F, Lakoma MD, et al. Changes in antidepressant use by young people and suicidal behavior after FDA warnings and media coverage: quasi-experimental study. *BMJ*. 2014;**348**:g3596.

50. Cipriani A, Furukawa TA, Salanti G, et al. Comparative efficacy and acceptability of 21 antidepressant drugs for the acute treatment of adults with major depressive disorder: a systematic review and network meta-analysis. *Lancet*. 2018;**391**(10128):1357–66.

51. Dodds TJ. Prescribed benzodiazepines and suicide risk: a review of the literature. *Prim Care Companion CNS Disord*. 2017;**19**(2]

52. Boggs JM, Lindroth RC, Battaglia C, et al. Association between suicide death and concordance with benzodiazepine treatment guidelines for anxiety and sleep disorders. *Gen Hosp Psychiatry*. 2020;**62**:21–7.

53. Forte A, Pompili M, Imbastaro B, et al. Effects on suicidal risk: comparison of clozapine to other newer medicines indicated to treat schizophrenia or bipolar disorder. *J Psychopharmacol*. 2021;**35**(9):1074–80.

54. Wilkinson T, Ballard ED, Bloch, MH, et al. The effect of a single dose of intravenous ketamine on suicidal ideation: a systematic review and individual participant data meta-analysis. *Am J Psychiatry*. 2018;**175**(2):150–8.

55. Kritzer MD, Mischel NA, Young JR, et al. Ketamine for treatment of mood disorders and suicidality: a narrative review of recent progress. *Ann Clin Psychiatry*. 2022;**34**(1):33–43.

56. Mewton L, Andrews G. Cognitive behavioral therapy for suicidal behaviors: improving patient outcomes. *Psychol Res Behav Manag*. 2016;**9**:21–9.

57. Scott J, Bentall R, Kinderman P, Morriss R. Is cognitive behaviour therapy applicable to individuals diagnosed with bipolar depression or suboptimal mood stabilizer treatment: a secondary analysis of a large pragmatic effectiveness trial. *Int J Bipolar Disord*. 2022;**10**(1):13.

58. D'Anci KE, Uhl S, Giradi G, Martin C. Treatments for the prevention and management of suicide: a systematic review. *Ann Intern Med*. 2019;**171**(5):334–42.

59. Goldstein TR, Axelson DA, Birmaher B, Brent DA. Dialectical behavior therapy for adolescents with bipolar disorder: a 1-year open trial. *J Am Acad Child Adolesc Psychiatry*. 2007;**46**(7):820–30.

60. Kellner CH, Fink M, Knapp R, et al. Relief of expressed suicidal intent by ECT: a consortium for research in ECT study. *Am J Psychiatry*. 2005;**162**(5):977–82.

61. Bozzay ML, Primack J, Barredo J, Philip NS. Transcranial magnetic stimulation to reduce suicidality – a review and naturalistic outcomes. *J Psychiatr Res*. 2020;**125**:106–12.

62. Olin B, Jayewardene AK, Bunker M, Moreno F. Mortality and suicide risk in treatment-resistant depression: an observational study of the long-term impact of intervention. *PLoS One*. 2012;**7**(10):e48002.

8 Mood and Psychosis: Limits and Overlapping between Psychotic Disorders and Mood Disorders

Fiona Gaughran

Introduction

Although debates continue as to what constitutes its 'heartland' [1], few would argue that schizophrenia and bipolar disorder together contribute a great part of the disease burden in psychiatry. The demarcation of the boundaries of mood and psychotic disorders continue to be contentious, in terms of classification, aetiology and treatment. In this chapter we evaluate the current evidence pertaining to the constructs of schizophrenia, bipolar disorder, schizoaffective disorder and psychotic depression.

Epidemiology

Using DSM-IV classification, the most thorough population study of the lifetime prevalence of psychotic disorders remains that of Perälä et al. [2]. They screened and then conducted diagnostic interviews using the Structured Clinical Interview for DSM-IV with approximately 8,000 people from Finland, finding a lifetime prevalence of psychotic disorders of around 3%, increasing to around 3.5% when registered diagnoses from non-responders were included. These broke down as follows: 0.87% for schizophrenia, 0.32% for schizoaffective disorder, 0.07% for schizophreniform disorder, 0.18% for delusional disorder, 1.0% for bipolar I disorder, 1.5% for bipolar II disorder, 0.35% for major depressive disorder with psychotic features, 0.42% for substance-induced psychotic disorders and 0.21% for psychotic disorders due to a general medical condition.

Diagnosis and Classification

Classifying psychiatric disorders, while necessary from a practical perspective, is difficult, and has historically rested on clinical data on symptoms, course and outcome. This still relies on the Robins and Guze criteria which look to establish validity [3], covering:

a. Clinical description; psychopathology and natural history
b. Laboratory studies
c. Distinguishing homogenous cases
d. Follow-up study
e. Family study

Here we focus on clinical descriptions and follow-up studies (see later chapters for a discussion of laboratory, family and genetics studies).

Clinical Descriptions

The historical roots of the classification of mood and psychotic disorders (and psychiatric classification itself) lie with the German school of the late 1800s. Kahlbaum is credited as the first person to postulate a nosological basis to psychosis, linking together aetiology, pathology and symptoms to a unitary psychosis [4].

This was followed by the father of modern psychiatric classification, Emil Kraepelin, who made the distinction between manic depressive insanity and dementia praecox, based on observations of his own clinical cohort, notably focusing on natural history and outcome [5]. The classification of manic depressive insanity rested on changes in activity, mood and thinking, with emphasis on recurrence and episodic course. Dementia praecox described a deteriorating course in a high proportion of people, though it is sometimes forgotten that around 15% of this cohort had only one episode, and a good outcome [6]. The distinction between the affective psychoses and schizophrenia has continued since then, though it is worth noting the change in nomenclature of manic depressive disorder to bipolar affective disorder in

DSM-III, reflecting not all those with this disorder would experience psychosis (DSM-III itself is acknowledged for focusing on presence and absence of symptoms, reflecting prominence of the so-called Neo-Kraepelinians).

Although most would ascribe psychotic symptoms to schizophrenia, it is striking that the prevalence of psychotic symptoms in bipolar disorder (especially bipolar I) is quite high compared to bipolar II. Using the SCID in a population of 1,342 people with Bipolar 1 disorder, van Bergen et al. [7] showed 73.8% of people had a lifetime history of psychotic symptoms, with delusions in 68.9% and hallucinations in 42.6%. One would assume that, in a clinical study of people with acute mania, this figure would be higher, if one was to include thought disorder (legitimately) as a psychotic symptom.

The term schizoaffective disorder was coined by Kasanin in 1933 for cases that were precipitated by life stressors, with resolution of symptoms [8]. It has been suggested that these cases would now probably be classified as acute and transient psychotic disorders (previously described as cycloid psychosis). Kraepelin probably gave some of the first descriptions of what we would now class as schizoaffective disorder, that is, co-occurrence of mood and psychotic symptoms. He described four subtypes of mania (hypomania, acute mania, delirious mania and delusional mania) and five subgroups for depression (melancholia simplex, melancholia gravis, fantastic melancholia, paranoid melancholia and delirious melancholia). Fish also described co-occurrence of affective symptoms in people with schizophrenia [9], specifically people with established 'chronic' schizophrenia with hypomanic symptoms, without the classical features of bipolar disorder, such as infectious enthusiasm of mania. Schizoaffective disorder is classified in DSM-5 with an emphasis on illness course, and resembles a good outcome form of schizophrenia, hence its place within this group of disorders.

The co-occurrence of depression syndrome has been quantified using OPCRIT criteria in a sample of around 350 people with a diagnosis of schizophrenia. Depression syndrome (defined as four or more symptoms) was identified in around a quarter, indicating a significant degree of comorbidity [10].

In discussing comorbid psychosis and depression, one cannot ignore psychotic depression-which has been relatively understudied. Notwithstanding this, around 10% of people classified with major depressive disorder (MDD) will have positive psychotic symptoms [11]. Psychotic depression is generally viewed as a severe form of depression, the emphasis on severity dating back to DSM-II, where this was the classifier, as opposed to the presence of delusions or hallucinations, though this changed in DSM-III. ICD-10 retains some of this reliance on severity. ICD-11 takes a similar approach to DSM-5, which separates specifiers, that is, one can have psychotic depression without necessarily having a severe form of depression.

Modern attempts to classify psychosis based on symptoms and other outcomes date back to the 1970s and include the use of multivariate statistical techniques. The best examples of these are the studies conducted by Kendell, who used data from the International Pilot Study of Schizophrenia to examine whether a 'point of rarity' existed between the two constructs of affective psychoses and schizophrenia. The initial examination of symptoms data, using discriminant function analysis, failed to show a distinction [12], though the addition of outcome data did indicate a difference [13]. To this literature should be added other analyses of symptoms, using cohorts such as Kraepelin's original cohort [14] and that of the Northwick Park Functional Psychosis Study, finding a symptomatic distinction between the affective psychoses and schizophrenia, though a small number of people with schizoaffective disorder were excluded from analysis [15].

This reliance on symptoms does not sit easily with observations of shared aetiological factors amongst these disorders, and led the ex-head of the National Institute for Mental Health (NIMH), Thomas Insel, to propose the Research Domain Criteria (RDoC) as a framework for the development of a classification system based on pathophysiology, as opposed to symptoms [16]. The RDoC system provides a framework; this excludes categorical diagnoses, instead adopting dimensional evaluations based on genetic, neural and behavioural indicators, consisting of six research and eight analysis domains taking in to account genes, molecules, cells, circuits, physiology, behaviour, self-reports and paradigms [16,17].

Aetiology: Genetic Factors

The genetics of mood disorders are discussed in detail in Chapter 17; a full description of the genetic antecedents of schizophrenia is beyond the scope of this chapter. Some studies have, however, looked at the overlap between mood and psychotic disorders. Like schizophrenia and bipolar disorder, the inheritance of schizoaffective disorder is unclear and it certainly appears to 'run in families', with the risk being greater if a first-degree relative also has the condition [18]. Similarly, twin studies show concordance of around 40% for monozygotic and around 5% in dizygotic twins for schizoaffective disorder (both manic and depressive subtypes) [19]. Twin studies also provided evidence for the existence of some genes with a relative specificity for either schizophrenia or bipolar disorder as well as genes that conferred risk across the Kraeplinian extremes, affecting risk of schizophrenia, bipolar disorder and cases in which both mood and psychotic symptoms were prominent [19]. Potential flaws in these studies have included misclassification of schizoaffective disorder (as it has at times had unknown validity in the classification systems) with poor inter-rater reliability [20] and instability of the diagnosis [18].

Although less investigated than schizophrenia or bipolar disorder, genetic studies of schizoaffective disorder have shown it to be highly heritable (~80%) [21] and polygenic with variations in many genes, each with a small effect size, combining to increase the risk of developing the condition. In this regard it shows substantial overlap with both schizophrenia and bipolar disorder [22]. There may also be genetic variations with larger effects in some affected individuals or families, but these variants are rare in the general population. Genes thus far implicated in schizoaffective disorder have diverse functions in the brain, ranging from those that regulate circadian rhythms [23], neuronal migration during brain development and in neurotransmission [24,25].

Early genome-wide linkage studies in schizoaffective disorder supported the existence of loci on chromosome 1q42, which had previously been implicated in both schizophrenia and bipolar disorder, similar to 22q11 [22]. Similarly, subsequent studies have shown that many of the genetic variations associated with schizoaffective disorder appear also to be involved in schizophrenia or bipolar disorder, whereas some variations seem to be specific to schizoaffective disorder. For example, genome-wide association studies (GWAS) have identified several genes associated with the risk of schizoaffective disorder with one single-nucleotide polymorphism (SNP) in particular (rs7680321) having the strongest association with

schizoaffective disorder, bipolar type. This SNP resides in part of a receptor for gamma-amino butyric acid (GABA), specifically the $GABA_A$ receptor b1 subunit, GABRB [23,24], GABA's primary role as an inhibitory neurotransmitter is to block or inhibit certain brain signals and decrease activity in the nervous system, preventing it being overloaded with too many signals. Altered GABA signalling in the prefrontal cortex (PFC) has been associated with cognitive dysfunction in schizophrenia and schizoaffective disorder [25]. Interestingly however, the GABA-synthesising enzyme glutamic acid decarboxylase 67kD (GAD67) has been reported to be lower in the prefrontal cortex in schizoaffective disorder but not in schizophrenia or age-matched controls [26,27]. This has led to the proposal that some variants may be common across the full bipolar disorder–schizophrenia spectrum whereas others (e.g., rs7680321) may be specific to a distinct clinical phenotype of schizoaffective disorder [24].

Overall, polygenic risk scores (PRSs) also appear to support the psychosis spectrum continuum model [25]. More precisely, the Cardiff group examined schizoaffective disorder depressive-type (SA-D) using polygenic risk scores [28] to determine whether SA-D should be considered a form of schizophrenia or a distinct disorder. They found that, compared to people with schizophrenia, those with SA-D had higher rates of both environmental and genetic risk factors for depression along with a similar genetic liability to schizophrenia, suggesting that SA-D may be a subtype of schizophrenia resulting from elevated liability to both schizophrenia and depression.

Copy number variants (CNVs), which have of course been consistently implicated in risk for schizophrenia [29], but less so in bipolar disorder [30], appear also to contribute in schizoaffective disorder [31]. Rare variant analysis has been possible in large pedigrees from northern Sweden, allowing identification of further rare variants [32] while sporadic cases of schizoaffective disorder have been identified as a subtype for genetic studies [33].

The same challenges apply to transcriptomic differences [34]. Transcriptional changes in the stress pathway have been shown to be related to symptoms in schizophrenia as well as to mood in schizoaffective disorder [35]. Similarly, methylation of glucocorticoid receptor, BDNF and oxytocin receptor genes have been found associated with schizophrenia and schizoaffective disorder, in a small study where childhood maltreatment has been a feature [36].

It is challenging to study the genetics of schizoaffective disorder in isolation because the disorder has such significant overlap with these other mental health conditions, as mentioned above. As a result, in some studies, people with schizoaffective disorder are analysed in the same group as those with schizophrenia or bipolar disorder, making it difficult to determine which genetic variations influence each of these specific diagnoses [37]. Evidence from genetics and neuroscience have informed the development of the operational diagnostic criteria in the latest *Diagnostic and Statistical Manual of Mental Disorders* (DSM-5) such that existing boundaries between bipolar I, schizoaffective disorder and schizophrenia have been retained [38]. However, just as Kraeplin introduced the concept of schizoaffective disorder to recognise the overlap of symptoms, it is clearly challenging to distinguish between schizophrenia, bipolar disorder and schizoaffective disorders solely on a phenomenological basis, highlighting the need to identify biomarkers for these disorders and the importance of systems such as the RDoC framework.

Aetiology: Environmental Factors

From the results of both twin and GWAS studies, it is clear that while genetic factors play a major role in the aetiology of schizophrenia, bipolar disorder and schizoaffective disorder, there are other important factors in determining whether an individual develops a mental disorder. Just as substantial genetic overlap exists between affective and non-affective psychosis, many environmental risk factors have been associated with both bipolar disorder and schizophrenia.

Ethnic minority status is one of the strongest environmental risk factors for psychosis [39]. Much of the research here has focused on the increased incidence rates of psychosis in African- and Caribbean-born migrants and their descendants in the United Kingdom. Meta-analyses have suggested that incidence rates are markedly increased in individuals of Black Caribbean or African origin in both bipolar disorder and schizophrenia compared to the White British population [39–41]. In terms of differences between affective and non-affective psychoses, there is some evidence that social factors such as deprivation, social cohesion and ethnic density are more strongly associated with non-affective compared to affective psychoses [41].

The association between pre- and perinatal risk factors has generally focused on the association with the increased risk of subsequent development of schizophrenia [42]. There is a relative paucity in terms of their relation to subsequent risk of schizoaffective or bipolar disorder and the evidence that does exist is not consistent [43,44]. Parental age appears to increase the risk of both affective and non-affective psychosis [45,46]. Childhood adversity meanwhile has been consistently associated with most mental disorders including both affective and non-affective psychosis [39,47]. Cannabis has become increasingly linked to psychosis, with links between exposure and greater incidence, earlier age of onset and increased severity of symptoms [48]. Much of the research has focused on schizophrenia, but there is evidence of similar associations in bipolar disorder [49,50]. Finally, research into incidence rate differences by sex suggests males have increased rates of schizophrenia below the age of 45 with no difference after, while with bipolar disorder rates were higher in women over the age of 45 with no difference prior [41].

The majority of risk factors discussed above appear to show similar associations with affective and non-affective psychosis. The literature is dominated by studies investigating schizophrenia leaving significant gaps in understanding regarding affective psychoses [39,47]. Although differences in the strength of observed associations exist between disorders, it is difficult to draw any firm conclusions from this as there are typically study level differences that may account for this other than the difference in diagnosis. More studies directly comparing disorders will be required to determine the extent to which environmental risk factors separate between the affective and non-affective psychoses.

Pathophysiology: Neuroimaging

Neuroimaging studies of affective and non-affective psychoses have examined both brain structure and function. In vivo assessment of brain structure had been undertaken earlier with pneumoencephalography, but it was the development of computed tomography (CT) that heralded the modern era of neuroimaging in psychiatry. Early studies showed evidence of ventricular enlargement in schizophrenia, although interpretation was complicated by the fact that antipsychotic treatment may also induce reductions in brain volume. Magnetic resonance imaging

(MRI) is now the standard method for assessment of brain volumes in living patients, and meta-analysis of studies do appear to show gray matter reductions in psychosis even in antipsychotic naïve individuals [51]. Recent studies have shown a high degree of similarity in terms of structural abnormalities in both affective psychoses and schizophrenia [52, 53]. There do, however, also appear to be some disorder specific differences with the temporal gyrus in schizophrenia showing greater reductions than that observed in other disorders [52].

In contrast to examining brain structures, positron emission tomography (PET), electroencephalography (EEG) and functional MRI (fMRI) have all been used to investigate potential aberration of brain function. As with the structural studies, there appears to be a high degree of similarity in between diagnoses in terms of abnormalities observed when compared to controls. A recent meta-analysis of fMRI studies examining cognitive control suggested that aberrant brain function in the dorsal anterior cingulate and bilateral insula, key nodes of the salience network, was implicated across disorders [54]. Some differences between disorders was observed with aberrant activation in a left prefrontal cluster and a portion of the mid-cingulate being more characteristic of psychotic compared to non-psychotic disorders. When examining brain regions involved in emotion processing there was again a great deal of overlap between disorders [55] and here psychotic disorders (consisting of schizophrenia and schizoaffective, schizophreniform, and delusional disorders) were distinguished by aberrant activation in the thalamus and fusiform areas, whereas bipolar disorder demonstrated right amygdala and right ventrolateral prefrontal cortex, while unipolar depressive disorders demonstrated no consistent pattern of aberrant activation.

The study of cerebral neurochemistry has been an area of intense research interest given that the majority of pharmacological interventions act by modulating neurotransmitter function. The dopamine hypothesis of schizophrenia, namely that the positive symptoms of the disorder result from overactivity of mesostriatal dopamine neurons is one of the longest standing theories of pathophysiology in psychiatry. Some of the strongest support came from studies demonstrating that the therapeutic effect of antipsychotic medication was tied to its antagonism of the D2 dopamine receptor. Additional evidence came from preclinical work, and studies demonstrating that

pharmacologically induced dopaminergic signalling could cause psychotic symptoms. More recently, PET has directly imaged the dopamine system in the brain of living patients and demonstrated that dopamine synthesis capacity and release are increased in individuals with schizophrenia [56]. A link between bipolar disorder and dopaminergic hyperactivity is likewise supported by the fact that many antipsychotics have evidence for both treating manic symptoms and preventing relapse. While one previous PET study did not find evidence of dopaminergic dysfunction in mania [57], a more recent study in individuals with first episode psychosis found that the magnitude of striatal hyperdopaminergia was greater in individuals with affective compared to non-affective psychosis [58].

The neuroimaging literature highlights significant similarities between affective and non-affective psychoses in terms of observable abnormalities of brain structure and function. Given that even within a single diagnostic group considerable heterogeneity is observed [59], it may be that current diagnostic boundaries are not always helpful for investigating markers of pathology, and at times a bottom-up approach to delineating pathophysiology may be of more use.

Postmortem Studies

Just as schizophrenia has been coined 'the graveyard of neuropathologists' [60], similarly, there are scant postmortem data available for schizoaffective disorder. A recent meta-analysis of schizophrenia [61] set out to also include people with a diagnosis of schizoaffective disorder, but identified only four studies reporting a total of 10 schizoaffective patients. Roeske et al. [61] reported consistent and replicated evidence of reductions in left- but not right-side hippocampal subfield volumes, neuron number and neuron size in postmortem brains of people with schizophrenia, although neuron density was unaffected.

Harrison et al. [62] in their 2020 systematic review on the neuropathology of bipolar disorder highlight that the bulk of published works derive from a limited number of brain collections, many with, as in the schizophrenia literature [63], small sample sizes. There have been few attempts to replicate postmortem findings in bipolar disorder, precluding substantial meta-analyses. The few replicated [62] postmortem findings in bipolar disorder include reduced cortical thickness and glial density in the subgenual anterior cingulate cortex, reduced neuronal density in some nuclei in the amygdala, along with decreased calbindin-positive neuron density in the prefrontal cortex. Additionally, few studies provide data on clinical features, the mood state at time of death or comorbid conditions [62].

The most consistent finding in the Harrison meta-analysis is that gliosis, that is, increased density, number or size of glial cells, is not a feature of bipolar disorder, which is also the case in schizophrenia. This is relevant as astrocytic gliosis would have suggested neurodegenerative processes, and increased microglia would suggest underlying neuroinflammation. However, functional [64] microglial activation may play a role in schizophrenia, and evidence of microglial activation and elevated cytokine levels have also been found in postmortem brain samples of bipolar disorder patients [65]. While the postmortem studies identifying increased neuronal nuclear antigen and GABAergic interstitial white matter neuron densities in schizophrenia have traditionally been interpreted as suggesting developmental pathology, they could also represent a restorative or protective mechanism, with the brain attempting to mount a repair response to inflammatory damage via neurogenesis [66].

No reviews were identified directly comparing neuropathological findings between schizophrenia and bipolar disorder, although many studies derive from consortia that contain samples from both. Harrison et al., however, note no consistent pattern of similarities or differences between these diagnostic groups other than the absence of gliosis, with some findings specific to each diagnosis and some shared. Nor are such neuropathological findings [67] necessarily core to either disorder; they may reflect differences in brain structure and connectivity either pre-existing or consequential to the disorder.

In neuropathological studies in both schizophrenia and bipolar disorder, psychotropic medications are confounding factors, with antipsychotics, mood stabilisers, and antidepressants having potential impact on brain volume as well as neuronal and glial measures. Evolving methodologies over time [68] further increase the challenge of replication, as does the evidence that people may be given different diagnoses within that spectrum during their lifespan. In future, initiatives such as the PsychENCODE Consortium have the potential to accelerate our understanding of the pathophysiology of psychiatric disorders, in PsychENCODE's case at a molecular level, with large sample sizes allowing examination of non-coding functional genomic elements in human brain tissue.

Peripheral Markers

People with schizophrenia, schizoaffective disorder, bipolar disorder and major depression are at a greater risk of early death, particularly from natural causes, with cardiometabolic disease a major contributor [69]. This is a multi-factorial problem, affected by the wider determinants of health, with input from poor diet and sedentary behaviours, along with effects of illness and adverse effects of medication. Most marked is the effect of tobacco smoking. This is much more common in these groups than in the general population and, although rates vary across diagnostic groups with 65% of people with a diagnosis of schizophrenia and 43.6% of those with bipolar disorder having tobacco use/nicotine dependence, smoking remains the single most important modifiable risk factor [70].

The presence of active mood and psychotic symptoms can compromise one's ability to succinctly communicate health needs, while executive function impairments, again common across mood and psychotic conditions, can result in difficulty in executing health management plans. There is also evidence that negative symptoms of schizophrenia may reduce the response to lifestyle interventions, although no such effect is seen for comorbid depressive symptoms [71].

While some studies compare mood to psychotic disorders in terms of metabolic load, many of the factors are either common to both or vary with the phase of the affective disorder, so findings are difficult to interpret. It is however possible that affective symptoms may have an effect; a recent secondary analysis showed that people with psychotic disorders who experience more severe symptoms of depression have larger waist circumferences [72], with those depressive symptoms also predicting more severe psychotic symptoms and a worse quality of life 12 months later.

The effect of medication is complex and some elements are bidirectional. The main classes of medication include antipsychotics, antidepressants and mood stabilisers with much overlap in prescribing patterns across diagnostic groups. All can impact metabolic risk through factors such as weight gain, dysglycaemia or dyslipidaemia, with individual drugs having different adverse effect profiles. Teasing out exact relationships is difficult, as the physical and metabolic health impact of medications are long-term and vary somewhat between medications. Additionally, people often change medications over time, meaning that data collected cross-sectionally will not reflect lifetime exposure. Large observational studies from Scandinavian databases suggest that effective treatment of the relevant mental disorder conveys a longevity advantage. In people with schizophrenia, being prescribed an antipsychotic, (especially long-acting injections or clozapine [73]), or antidepressant [74] medication is associated with half the mortality risk observed in those not prescribed antipsychotics. The same study found that longer term prescription of benzodiazepines increases the risk of earlier death, which is interesting as benzodiazepines tend to be used when the underlying disorder is inadequately responding to treatment. Similarly, in bipolar disorder, lithium, the most effective treatment [75], is associated with a reduction in all-cause mortality.

Glucose dysregulation may however be core to schizophrenia [76]. In first-episode schizophrenia patients with no or minimal antipsychotic exposure, glucose levels are higher than controls, although total and LDL cholesterol levels [77] in first episode psychosis studies, including people with both schizophrenia and bipolar disorder, are lower than controls. This suggests that the lipid abnormalities, so commonly seen in people with both affective and psychotic disorders, are secondary to emergent illness and medication related factors.

Meta-analytic evidence from first episode psychosis studies shows that non-CNS factors [78] including immune, cardiometabolic and hypothalamic-pituitary-adrenal axis abnormalities exhibit levels of abnormalities that are comparable in degree to those of CNS factors such as brain structure, neurophysiology, and neurochemistry. This raises the possibility that psychosis is a multi-system disorder. However in bipolar disorder, factors such as immune abnormalities have an added degree of complexity; for example, evidence suggests chemokine alterations in bipolar disorder might be related to mood state [79]. Comorbidities add further intricacy; obesity is associated with raised C-reactive protein (CRP), as are mood disorders [80] and psychosis [81], with co-occurrence increasing CRP levels [82]. Similarly [83], life events, such

as childhood trauma [83], are associated with both mood [84] and psychotic disorders but are also associated with higher body mass index, and increased CRP.

Treatment

Treatment of comorbid mood and psychotic symptoms will broadly be based on established treatments for each, and full discussion of this is outwith the remit of this Chapter. Here, we will focus on the use of pharmacotherapy across disorders.

Echoing the themes underpinning the shared aetiologies discussed above, there have been changes in the nomenclature of psychotropic medicines, with the introduction of Neuroscience-Based Nomenclature (NbN), in which medicines are classified according to their effects on systems and receptor subtypes, as opposed to terms such as antidepressant, antipsychotic and mood stabiliser [85]. A good example of this are the antipsychotics (see below).

In terms of evidence, as noted throughout this chapter, there is a lack of clear literature to guide thinking. One of the earliest studies to address the question of dimensional treatment of mood and psychotic symptoms was the Northwick Park Functional Psychosis Study [86], in which people with psychosis (with elevated, depressed mood or no mood symptoms) received 4 weeks' treatment with lithium, pimozide, a combination of both or placebo, that is, treatment for symptoms as opposed to disorder. Though the numbers were not large by today's standards ($n = 120$), there was a clear response of positive psychotic symptoms to pimozide (a strong D2 antagonist), with lithium only exerting an effect on symptoms of elevated mood. This has been borne out by a Cochrane review of lithium in schizophrenia and schizoaffective disorder, which failed to show any significant benefit in schizophrenia, once the participants schizoaffective disorder were excluded [87].

This dimensional view of treatment is echoed by the existing evidence for antipsychotics across a range of mood and psychotic disorders, though they are still predominantly associated with the treatment of schizophrenia [88].

Their use in mania and the maintenance treatment of bipolar disorder is at times underestimated, though the effect size in mania is as high as any other pharmacotherapy [89, 90], and descriptions of the classic original studies of chlorpromazine indicate that a significant proportion of people in the original studies may well have had mania [91]. This also translates to maintenance therapy, where a number of antipsychotics are licensed in bipolar disorder, and bipolar depression (with predominantly D_2 acting antipsychotics demonstrating efficacy in mania prophylaxis, as opposed to those with efficacy in depression prophylaxis). Some antipsychotics, such as aripiprazole and quetiapine, have an evidence base for treatment-resistant depression [92], though have not been studied in great depth in people with comorbid mood and psychotic symptoms.

As stated above, lithium does not appear to have major effects on psychotic symptoms, though it has clear effects in mania, both acutely and prophylaxis [93]. Its evidence in MDD is mainly as adjunctive therapy, with some observational studies indicating some benefits in psychotic depression- though the evidence is of poor quality.

Antidepressants have been trialled in psychotic disorders, notably for negative symptoms, with some evidence to suggest benefit of SSRIs, albeit with a lower effect size than that seen in MDD. Their use in bipolar disorder is still controversial, with most groups suggesting a lack of efficacy and detrimental effects in terms of mixed states and switching, though trial evidence suggests a possible benefit in a small subsample of patients.

A reasonable addition to this literature is 'real-world' data on treatment for schizoaffective disorder, which consists of observational data from registry cohorts. A recent example of this used data from Finland and Sweden, examining adjunctive use of antidepressants, mood stabilisers and benzodiazepines in people diagnosed with schizoaffective disorder. It found decreased hospitalisations in people prescribed clozapine, long-acting injection antipsychotics (AIs), no effect of quetiapine and decreased hospitalisations in people taking adjunctive mood stabilisers, compared to antipsychotic monotherapy. Combination antidepressant use was associated with a small decrease in hospitalisations in one of the cohorts [94].

For the common comorbidity of depression in schizophrenia, the British Association for Psychopharmacology (BAP) recommend discussing a trial of an antidepressant, but suggest discontinuing if it's of no benefit, noting little evidence-based guidance thereafter. Given that response rates to a single antidepressant in major depressive disorder would only be expected to be in the order of 50–60%, this emphasises the need for more research in this area. For psychotic depression, the BAP recommend combining an antidepressant with an antipsychotic initially, over giving an antidepressant or an antipsychotic alone, and note that electroconvulsive therapy (ECT) may be helpful in this context. As an intervention, ECT was originally found to be therapeutic in psychosis, and it has an evidence base not only in depression [95] but also in mania and schizophrenia [96].

Summary

Classifying and differentiating aetiology, associations and evidence for management strategies across schizophrenia, schizoaffective disorder, bipolar disorder and either comorbid depression or psychotic depression remain challenging for a number of reasons. Most research has focused on the more common conditions of schizophrenia and bipolar disorder, with schizoaffective disorder, if specified at all, often subsumed within the other psychosis group. Further, in over 40% of people, psychotic spectrum diagnoses at first episode do not remain static over time [97], so when examining childhood antecedents or postmortem findings, it is not clear which diagnosis non-contemporaneous findings should be associated with. Regarding treatments, there have been few drug trials targeted primarily at psychotic depression, comorbid depression in schizophrenia or schizoaffective disorder, and fewer still which target a particular current mood state within a schizoaffective disorder trial.

The use of newer approaches to characterising populations, such as the Research Domain Criteria (RDoC) framework and the PsychENCODE Consortium, and the adoption of Neuroscience Based Nomenclature (NbN) to categorise pharmacological treatments has the potential to allow more targeted clinical trials in the future and unlock individualised therapeutic avenues for patient benefit.

References

1. Goodwin GM, Geddes JR. What is the heartland of psychiatry? *Br J Psychiatry*. 2007;**191**(3):189–91. doi:10.1192/bjp.bp.107.036343.

2. Perälä J, Suvisaari J, Saarni S I, et al. Lifetime prevalence of psychotic and bipolar I disorders in a general population. *Arch Gen Psychiatry*. 2007;**64** (1):19–28. doi: 10.1001/archpsyc.64.1.19

3. Robins E, Guze SB. Establishment of diagnostic validity in psychiatric illness application to schizophrenia. *Am J Psychiatry*. 1970;**126**(7):983–7. doi: 10.1176/ajp.126.7.983

4. Kahlbaum K. *Die Katatonie oder das Spannnungsirresein*. 1874

5. Kraepelin E. *Dementia Praecox*. Cambridge: Cambridge University Press. 1987

6. Taylor M. Are we getting any better at staying better? The long view on relapse and recovery in first episode nonaffective psychosis and schizophrenia. *Ther Adv Psychopharmacol*. 2019;**9**:2045125319870033. doi: 10.1177/2045125319870033.

7. Van Bergen AH, Verkooijen S, Vreeker A, et al. The characteristics of psychotic features in bipolar disorder. *Psychol Med*. 2019;**49**(12):2036–48. doi: 10.1017/S0033291718002854

8. Kasanin J. The acute schizoaffective psychoses. *Am J Psychiatry*. 1933;**151**(6 Suppl):144–54. doi: 10.1176/ajp.151.6.144

9. Fish FJ, Hamilton M. *Fish's Clinical Psychopathology: Signs and Symptoms in Psychiatry*. Bristol: Wright, 1985

10. Serretti A, Mandelli L, Lattuada E, Smeraldi E. Depressive syndrome in major psychoses: a study on 1351 subjects. *Psychiatry Res*. 2004;**127**(1–2):85–99. doi: 10.1016/j.psychres.2003.12.025

11. Dold M, Bartova L, Kautzky A, et al. Psychotic features in patients with major depressive disorder: a report from the European Group for the Study of Resistant Depression. *J Clin Psychiatry*. 2019;**80**(1):17m12090, doi: 10.4088/JCP.17m12090

12. Kendell RE, Gourlay J. The clinical distinction between the affective psychoses and schizophrenia. *Br J Psychiatry*. 1970;**117**(538):261–6. doi: 10.1192/bjp.117.538.261

13. Brockington IF, Roper A, Copas J, et al. Schizophrenia, bipolar disorder and depression a discriminant analysis, using 'lifetime' psychopathology ratings. *Br J Psychiatry*. 2018;**135**(3):243–8. doi: 10.1192/bjp.135.3.243.

14. Jablensky A, Woodbury MA. Dementia praecox and manic-depressive insanity in 1908: a grade of membership analysis of the Kraepelinian dichotomy. *Eur Arch Psychiatry Clin Neurosci*. 1995;**245**(4–5):202–9. doi: 10.1007/BF02191798

15. Jauhar S, Krishnadas R, Nour MM, et al. Is there a symptomatic distinction between the affective psychoses and schizophrenia? A machine learning approach. *Schizophr Res*. 2018;**202**:241–7, doi: 10.1016/j.schres.2018.06.070

16. Insel TR, Cuthbert B, Garvey M, et al. P. Research Domain Criteria (RDoC): toward a new classification framework for research on mental disorders. *Am J Psychiatry*. 2010;**167**(7):748–51. doi: 10.1176/appi.ajp.2010.09091379

17. Insel TR, Cuthbert BN. Endophenotypes: bridging genomic complexity and disorder hetereogeneity. *Biol Psychiatry*. 2009;**66**:988–9. doi: 10.1016/j.biopsych.2009.10.008

18. Laursen TM, Labouriau R, Licht RW, et al. Family history of psychiatric illness as a risk factor for schizoaffective disorder: a Danish register-based cohort study. *Arch Gen Psychiatry*. 2005;**62**(8):841–8. doi: 10.1001/archpsyc.62.8.841

19. Cardno, AG, Marshall EJ, Coid B, et al. Heritability estimates for psychotic disorders: the Maudsley twin psychosis series. *Arch Gen Psychiatry*. 1999;**56**:162–8. doi: 10.1001/archpsyc.56.2.162

20. Mansour HA, Talkowski ME, Wood J, et al. Association study of 21 circadian genes with bipolar 1 disorder, schizoaffective disorder, and schizophrenia. *Bipolar Disord*. 2009;**11**(7):701–10. doi: 10.1111/j.1399-5618.2009.00756.x

21. Licinio J. Messages from hypothesis-driven genotyping: the case of schizoaffective disorder, bipolar type. *Mol Psychiatry*. 2010;**15**(2):113–14. doi: 10.1038/mp.2009.153

22. Hamshere M, Bennett P, Williams N, et al. Genome-wide linkage scan in schizoaffective disorder: significant evidence for linkage (LOD + 3.54) at 1q42 close to DISC1, and suggestive evidence at 22q11 and 19p13. *Arch Gen Psychiatry*. 2005;**62**:1081–8. doi: 10.1001/archpsyc.62.10.1081

23. Green EK, Grozeva D, Moskvina V, et al. Variation at the GABAA receptor gene, Rho 1 (GABRR1) associated with susceptibility to bipolar schizoaffective disorder. *Am J Med Genet B Neuropsychiatr Genet*. 2010;**153B**(7):1347–9, doi: doi.org/10.1002/ajmg.b.31108

24. Craddock N, Jones L, Jones IR, et al. Strong genetic evidence for a selective influence of GABAA receptors on a component of the bipolar disorder phenotype. *Mol Psychiatry*. 2008;**15**(2):146–53. doi: 10.1038/mp.2008.66

25. Smigielski L, Papiol S, Theodoridou A, et al. Polygenic risk scores across the extended psychosis spectrum. *Transl Psychiatry*. 2021;**11**(1):600. doi: 10.1038/s41398-021-01720-0.

26. Gonzalez-Burgos G, Fish KN, Lewis DA. GABA neuron alterations, cortical circuit dysfunction and cognitive deficits in schizophrenia. *Neural Plast*. 2011;**723184**. doi: 10.1155/2011/723184

27. Glausier JR, Kimoto S, Fish KN, Lewis DA. Lower glutamic acid decarboxylase 650-kDa isoform messenger RNA and protein levels in the prefrontal cortex in schizoaffective disorder but not

schizophrenia. *Biolog Psychiatry*. 2015;**77**:167–76. doi: 10.1016/j.biopsych.2014.05.010

28. Dennison CA, Legge SE, Hubbard L, et al. Risk factors, clinical features, and polygenic risk scores in schizophrenia and schizoaffective disorder depressive-type. *Schizopher Bull*. 2021;**47**(5):1375–84. doi: 10.1093/schbul/sbab036

29. Marshall CR, Howrigan DP, Merico D, et al. Contribution of copy number variants to schizophrenia from a genome-wide study of 41,321 subjects. *Nat Genet*. 2017;**49**(1):27–35. doi: 10.1038/ng.3725

30. Green EK, Rees E, Walters JTR, et al. Copy number variation in bipolar disorder. *Mol Psychiatry*. 2016;**21**(1):89–93. doi: 10.1038/mp.2014.174

31. Charney AW, Stahl EA, Green EK, et al. Contribution of rare copy number variants to bipolar disorder risk is limited to schizoaffective cases. *Biol Psychiatry*. 2019;**86**:110–19. doi: 10.1016/j.biopsych.2018

32. Szatkiewicz J, Crowley JJ, Adolfsson AN, et al. The genomics of major psychiatric disorders in a large pedigree from northern Sweden. *Transl Psychiatry*. 2019;**9**;60. doi: 10.1038/s41398-019-0414-9

33. Van der Merwe NJ, Karayoirgou M, Ehlers R, Roos JL. Family history identifies sporadic schizoaffective disorder as a subtype for genetic studies. *S Afr J Psychiatry*. 2020;**26**;1393. doi: 10.4102/sajpsychiatry.v26i0.1393

34. Lewandowski KE, McCarthy JM, Öngür D, et al. Functional connectivity in distinct cognitive subtypes in psychosis. *Schizophr Res*. 2019;**204**:120–6. doi: 10.1016/j.schres.2018.08.013

35. Lee CH, Sinclair D, O'Donnell M, et al. Transcriptional changes in the stress pathway are related to symptoms in schizophrenia and to mood in schizoaffective disorder. *Schizophr Res*. 2019;**213**:87–95. doi: 10.1016/j.schres.2019.06.026

36. Barker V, Walker RM, Evans KL, Lawrie SM. Methylation of glucocorticoid receptor (NR3C1), BDNF and oxytocin receptor genes in association with childhood maltreatment in schizophrenia and schizoaffective disorder. *Schizophr Res*. 2020;**216**:529–31. doi: 10.1016/j.schres.2019.11.050

37. Dwyer DB, Kalman JL, Budde M, et al. An investigation of psychosis subgroups with prognostic validation and exploration of genetic underpinnings: the PsyCourse Study. *JAMA Psychiatry*. 2020;**1**(77):523–33. doi: 10.1001/jamapsychiatry.2019.4910

38. Cosgrove VE, Suppes T. Informing DSM-5: biological boundaries between bipolar I disorder, schizoaffective disorder, and schizophrenia. *BMC Med*. 2013;**11**:127. doi: 10.1186/1741-7015-11-127

39. Radua J, Ramella-Cravaro V, Ioannidis JPA, et al. What causes psychosis? An umbrella review of risk and protective factors. *World Psychiatry*. 2018;**17**(1):49–66. doi: 10.1002/wps.20490

40. Tortelli A, Errazuriz A, Croudace T, et al. Schizophrenia and other psychotic disorders in Caribbean-born migrants and their descendants in England: systematic review and meta-analysis of incidence rates, 1950–2013. *Soc Psychiatry Psychiatri Epidemiol*. 2015;**50**:1039–55. doi: 10.1007/s00127-015-1021-6

41. Kirkbride JB, Errazuriz A, Croudance TJ, et al. Incidence of schizophrenia and other psychoses in England 1950–2009: a systematic review and meta-analysis. *PLoS One*. 2012;**7**(3);e31660. doi: 10.1371/journal.pone.0031660

42. Davies C, Segre G, Estradé A, et al. Prenatal and perinatal risk and protective factors for psychosis: a systematic review and meta-analysis. *Lancet Psychiatry*. 2020;**7**(5):399–410. doi: 10.1016/S2215-0366(20)30057-2

43. Kinney DK, Yurgelun-Todd DA, Levy DL, et al. Obstetrical complications in patients with bipolar disorder and their siblings. *Psychiatry Res*. 1993;**48**(1):47–56. doi: 10.1016/0165-1781(93)90112-T

44. Serati M, Bertino V, Merlarba MR, et al. Obstetric complications and subsequent risk of mood disorders for offspring in adulthood: a comprehensive overview. *Nord J Psychiatry*. 2020;**74**(7):470–8. doi: 10.1080/08039488.2020.1751878

45. Frans EM, Sandin S, Reichenberg A, et al. Advancing paternal age and bipolar disorder. *Arch Gen Psychiatry*. 2008;**65**(9):1034–40. doi: 10.1001/archpsyc.65.9.1034

46. Torrey EF, Buka S, Cannon TD, et al. Paternal age as a risk factor for schizophrenia: How important is it? *Schizophr Res*. 2009;**114**(1–3);1–5. doi: 10.1016/j.schres.2009.06.017

47. Rodriguez V, Alameda L, Trotta G, et al. Environmental risk factors in bipolar disorder and psychotic depression: a systematic review and meta-analysis of prospective studies. *Schizophr Bull*. 2021;**47**(4):959974. doi: 10.1093/schbul/sbaa197

48. Marconi A, Di Forti M, Lewis CM, Murray RM, Vassos E. Meta-analysis of the association between the level of cannabis use and risk of psychosis. *Schizophr Bull*. 2016;**42**(5):1262–9. doi: 10.1093/schbul/sbw003

49. Gibbs M, Winsper C, Marwaha S, et al. Cannabis use and mania symptoms: a systematic review and meta-analysis. *J Affect Disord*. 2014;**171**:39–47. doi: 10.1016/j.jad.2014.09.016

50. Bally N, Zullino D, Aubry JM. Cannabis use and first manic episode. *J Affect Disord*. 2014;**165**:103–8. doi: 10.1016/j.jad.2014.04.038

51. Fusar-Poli P, Radua J, McGuire P, Borgwardt S. Neuroanatomical maps of psychosis onset: Voxel-wise meta-analysis of antipsychotic-naïve VBM studies. *Schizophr Bull*. 2012;**38**(6):1297–1307. doi: 10.1093/schbul/sbr134

52. Opel N, Goltermann J, Hermesdorf M, et al. Cross-disorder analysis of brain structure abnormalities in six major psychiatric disorders: a secondary analysis of mega- and meta-analytical findings from the ENIGMA Consortium. *Biol Psychiatry*. 2020;**88**(9):678–86. doi: 10.1016 /j.biopsych.2020.04.027

53. Goodkind M, Eickhoff SB, Oathes DJ, et al. Identification of a common neurological substate for mental illness. *JAMA Psychiatry*. 2015;**72**(4):305. doi: 10.1001/jamapsychiatry.2014.2206

54. McTeague LM, Huemer J, Carreon DM, et al. Identification of common neural circuit disruptions in cognitive control across psychiatric disorders. *Am J Psychiatry*. 2017;**174**(7):676–85. doi: 10.1176/appi .ajp.2017.16040400

55. McTeague LM, Rosenberg BM, Lopez JW, et al. Identification of common neural circuit disruptions in emotional processing across psychiatric disorders. *Am J Psychiatry*. 2020;**177**(5):411–21. doi: 10.1176/ appi.ajp.2019.18111271

56. McCutcheon R, Beck K, Jauhar S, Howes OD. Defining the locus of dopaminergic dysfunction in schizophrenia: a meta-analysis and test of the mesolimbic hypothesis. *Schizophr Bull*. 2018;**44** (6):1301–11. doi: 10.1093/schbul/sbx180

57. Yatham LN, Liddle PF, Shiah IS, et al. PET study of [18 F]6-fluoro-L-dopa uptake in neuroleptic and mood-stabilizer-naive first-episode nonpsychotic mania: effects of treatment with divalproex sodium. *Am J Psychiatry*. 2002;**159**(5):768–74. doi: 10.1176/ appi.ajp.159.5.768

58. Jauhar S, Nour MM, Veronese M, et al. A test of the transdiagnostic dopamine hypothesis of psychosis using positron emission tomographic imaging in bipolar affective disorder and schizophrenia. *JAMA Psychiatry*. 2017;**74**(12):1206–13. doi: 10.1001/ jamapsychiatry.2017.2943

59. Brugger SP, Howes OD. Heterogeneity and homogeneity of regional brain structure in schizophrenia. *JAMA Psychiatry*. 2017;**74**(11); 1104. doi:10.1001/jamapsychiatry.2017.2663

60. Plum F. Prospects for research on schizophrenia. 3. Neurophysiology. Neuropathological findings. *Neurosci Res Program Bull*. 1972;**10**(4):384–8. PMID: 4663816

61. Roeske MJ, Konradi C, Heckers S, Lewis AS. Hippocampal volume and hippocampal neuron density, number and size in schizophrenia: a systematic review and meta-analysis of postmortem studies. *Mol Psychiatry*. 2021;**26**:3524–35. doi: 10.1038/s41380-020-0853-y

62. Harrison PJ, Colbourne L, Harrison CH. The neuropathology of bipolar disorder: systematic review and meta-analysis. *Mol Psychiatry*. 2020;**25** (8):1787–1808. doi: 10.1038/s41380-018-0213-3

63. Bakhshi K, Chance SA. The neuropathology of schizophrenia: a selective review of past studies and emerging themes in brain structure and cytoarchitecture. *Neuroscience*. 2015;**303**:82–102. doi: 10.1016/j.neuroscience.2015.06.028

64. Howes OD, McCutcheon R. Inflammation and the neural diathesis-stress hypothesis of schizophrenia: a reconceptualization. *Transl Psychiatry*. 2017;**7**(2); e1024. doi: 10.1038/tp.2016.278

65. Giridharan VV, Sayana P, Pinjari OF, et al. Postmortem evidence of brain inflammatory markers in bipolar disorder: a systematic review. *Mol Psychiatry*. 2019;**25**:94–113. doi: doi.org/10.1038/ s41380-019-0448-7

66. Duchatel RJ, Weickert CS, Tooney PA. White matter neuron biology and neuropathology in schizophrenia. *NPJ Schizophr*. 2019;**5**(1);10. doi: 10.1038/s41537-019-0078-8

67. Harrison PJ, Colbourne L, Harrison CH. The neuropathology of bipolar disorder: systematic review and meta-analysis. *Mol Psychiatry*. 2020;**25** (8):1787–1808. doi: 10.1038/s41380-018-0213-3

68. Bakhshi K, Chance SA. The neuropathology of schizophrenia: a selective review of past studies and emerging themes in brain structure and cytoarchitecture. *Neuroscience*. 2015;**303**:82–102. doi: 10.1016/j.neuroscience.2015.06.028

69. Walker ER, McGee RE, Druss BG. Mortality in mental disorders and global disease burden implications: a systematic review and meta-analysis. *JAMA Psychiatry*. 2015;**72**(4):334–41. doi: 10.1001/ jamapsychiatry.2014.2502. Erratum in: *JAMA Psychiatry*. 2015;72(7);736. Erratum in: *JAMA Psychiatry*. 2015;72(12);1259.

70. Fornaro M, Carvalho AF, De Prisco M, et al. The prevalence, odds, predictors, and management of tobacco use disorder or nicotine dependence among people with severe mental illness: systematic review and meta-analysis. *Neurosci Biobehav Rev*. 2021;**132**:289–303. doi: 10.1016/j.neubiorev .2021.11.039

71. Martland R, Teasdale S, Murray RM, et al. Dietary intake, physical activity and sedentary behaviour patterns in a sample with established psychosis and

associations with mental health symptomatology. *Psychol Med*. 2021;**23**:1–11. doi: 10.1017/S0033291721003147

72. Perez CSH, Ciufolini S, Sood PG, et al. Predictive value of cardiometabolic biomarkers and depressive symptoms for symptom severity and quality of life in patients with psychotic disorders. *J Affect Disord*. 2022;**298** (Pt A):95–103. doi: 10.1016/j.jad.2021.10.038

73. Taipale H, Tanskanen A, Mehtälä J, et al. 20-year follow-up study of physical morbidity and mortality in relationship to antipsychotic treatment in a nationwide cohort of 62,250 patients with schizophrenia (FIN20). *World Psychiatry*. 2020;**19** (1):61–8. doi: 10.1002/wps.20699

74. Tiihonen J, Mittendorfer-Rutz E, Torniainen M, Alexanderson K, Tanskanen A. Mortality and cumulative exposure to antipsychotics, antidepressants, and benzodiazepines in patients with schizophrenia: an observational follow-up study. *Am J Psychiatry*. 2016;**173**(6):600–6. doi: 10.1176/appi.ajp.2015.15050618

75. Toffol E, Hätönen T, Tanskanen A, et al. Lithium is associated with decrease in all-cause and suicide mortality in high-risk bipolar patients: a nationwide registry-based prospective cohort study. *J Affect Disord*. 2015;**183**:159–65. doi: 10.1016/j.jad.2015.04.055

76. Pillinger T, Beck K, Gobjila C, et al. Impaired glucose homeostasis in first-episode schizophrenia: a systematic review and meta-analysis. *JAMA Psychiatry*. 2017;**74**(3):261–9. doi: 10.1001/jamapsychiatry.2016.3803

77. Pillinger T, Beck K, Stubbs B, Howes OD. Cholesterol and triglyceride levels in first-episode psychosis: systematic review and meta-analysis. *Br J Psychiatry*. 2017;**211**(6):339–49. doi: 10.1192/bjp.bp.117.200907

78. Pillinger T, D'Ambrosio E, McCutcheon R, Howes OD. Is psychosis a multisystem disorder? A meta-review of central nervous system, immune, cardiometabolic, and endocrine alterations in first-episode psychosis and perspective on potential models. *Mol Psychiatry*. 2019;**24**(6):776–94. doi: 10.1038/s41380-018-0058-9. Erratum in: Mol Psychiatry. 2018.

79. Misiak B, Bartoli F, Carrà G, et al. Chemokine alterations in bipolar disorder: a systematic review and meta-analysis. *Brain Behav Immun*. 2020;**88**:870–7. doi: 10.1016/j.bbi.2020.04.013

80. Marshe VS, Pira S, Mantere O, et al. C-reactive protein and cardiovascular risk in bipolar disorder patients: a systematic review. *Prog Neuropsychopharmacol Biol Psychiatry*. 2017;**79**(Pt B):442–51. doi: 10.1016/j.pnpbp.2017.07.026

81. Kose M, Pariante CM, Dazzan P, Mondelli V. The role of peripheral inflammation in clinical outcome and brain imaging abnormalities in psychosis: a systematic review. *Front Psychiatry*. 2021;**12**;612471. doi: 10.3389/fpsyt.2021.612471

82. McLaughlin AP, Nikkheslat N, Hastings C, et al. The influence of comorbid depression and overweight status on peripheral inflammation and cortisol levels. *Psychol Med*. 2021;**18**:1–8. doi: 10.1017/S0033291721000088

83. Hepgul N, Pariante CM, Dipasquale S, et al. Childhood maltreatment is associated with increased body mass index and increased C-reactive protein levels in first-episode psychosis patients. *Psychol Med*. 2012;**42**(9):1893–1901. doi: 10.1017/S0033291711002947

84. Kuzminskaite E, Penninx BWJH, van Harmelen AL, et al. Childhood trauma in adult depressive and anxiety disorders: an integrated review on psychological and biological mechanisms in the NESDA Cohort. *J Affect Disord*. 2021;**283**:179–91. doi: 10.1016/j.jad.2021.01.054

85. Nutt DJ, Blier P. Neuroscience-based Nomenclature (NbN) for Journal of Psychopharmacology. *J Psychopharmacol*. 2016;**30**(5):413–15. doi: 10.1177/0269881116642903

86. Johnstone E, Frith C, Crow T, et al. The Northwick Park 'Functional' Psychosis Study: diagnosis and outcome. *Psychol Med*. 1992;**22**(2):331–46. doi: 10.1017/s0033291700030270

87. Leucht S, Helfer B, Dold M, Kissling W, McGrath JJ. Lithium for schizophrenia. *Cochrane Database Syst Rev*. 2015;**2015**(10);CD003834. doi: 10.1002/14651858.CD003834.pub3

88. Young AH, Jauhar S. Antipsychotics, the heartland of clinical psychopharmacology? *J Psychopharmacol*. 2021;**35**(9):1027–9. doi: 10.1177/02698811211043599.

89. Cipriani A, Barbui C, Salanti G, et al. Comparative efficacy and acceptability of antimani drugs in acute mania: a multiple-treatments meta-analysis. *Lancet*. 2011;**378**(9799):1306–15.

90. Baldessarini RJ, Tondo L, Vázquez GH. Pharmacological treatment of adult bipolar disorder. *Mol Psychiatry*. 2019;**24**(2):198–217. doi: 10.1038/s41380-018-0044-2.

91. Delay J, Deniker P, Harl JM. [Therapeutic method derived from hiberno-therapy in excitation and agitations states]. *Ann Med Psychol (Paris)*. 1952;**110**(22):267–73.

92. Strawbridge R, Carter B, Marwood L, et al. Augmentation therapies for treatment-resistant depression: systematic review and meta-analysis. *Br J*

Psychiatry. 2019;**214**(1):42–51. doi: 10.1192/
bjp.2018.233

93. Goodwin GM, Haddad PM, Ferrier IN, et al.
Evidence-based guidelines for treating bipolar
disorder: revised third edition recommendations
from the British Association for
Psychopharmacology. *J Psychopharmacol*. 2016;**30**
(6):495–553. doi: 10.1177/0269881116636545.

94. Lintunen J, Taipale H, Tanskanen A, et al. Long-term
real-world effectiveness of pharmacotherapies for
schizoaffective disorder. *Schizophr Bull*. 2021;**47**
(4):1099–1107. doi: 10.1093/schbul/sbab004.

95. Kirov G, Jauhar S, Sienaert P, Kellner CH,
McLoughlin DM. Electoconvulsive therapy for
depression: 80 years of progress. *Br J Psychiatry*.
2021;**219**(5):594–7. doi: 10.1192/bjp.2021.37

96. Sinclair DJM, Zhao S, Qi F, Nyakyoma K, Kwong
JSW, Adams CE. Electroconvulsive therapy for
treatment-resistant schizophrenia. *Cochrane
Database Syst Rev*. 2019;**2019**:CD011847.

97. Gale-Grant O, Dazzan P, Lappin JM, et al. Diagnostic
stability and outcome after first episode psychosis. *J
Ment Health*. 2021;**30**(1):104–12. doi: 10.1080/
09638237.2020.1818191.

Transcultural Issues in Mood Disorders

Shanaya Rathod, Elizabeth Graves, and Peter Phiri

Culture

Culture can be understood as a set of guidelines, implicit and explicit, that members of a particular society or community learn and inherit, reflected in shared beliefs, values, attitudes and behaviours [1,2]. It is a dynamic concept and has an impact on every individual. It determines what constitutes normality in society and deviation from it. Culture can influence the causal beliefs around health and illness, understanding and expression of symptoms, use of language, coping with emotional traumas and help-seeking behaviour of those experiencing mental health disorders [3,4], thereby impacting on access to interventions and outcomes of treatment. Cultural aspects of social interaction and contexts, including what is acceptable and commonplace, may influence both the experience and the expression of emotional distress, shaped by the language, literature, religion and theology that has informed thinking, and the development of concepts across centuries [5]. Culture-bound syndromes, more commonly seen in some societies than in others, are another example of the impact of culture on illness.

It is easy to use the words 'race', 'ethnicity' and 'culture' synonymously. Race and ethnicity tend to be relatively fixed and enduring, whereas culture can be more flexible and dynamic, changing with circumstances. Ethnic identity can contribute to the cause and course of psychiatric disorders [6]. While similarities in broad regions may therefore occur, smaller emic perspectives will also shape each individual's experience, meaning that every individual has their own unique culture.

Incidence and Prevalence of Mood Disorders across Cultures

Mood disorders are a global phenomenon, although prevalence rates are thought to vary across countries. The World Health Organisation (WHO) has ranked depression the fourth leading cause of disability worldwide [7], and there are predictions that by 2030, depression alone is likely to be the third leading cause of disease burden in low-income countries and the second highest cause of disease burden in middle-income countries [8]. Discussions around prevalence of mood disorders in different cultures remain complex. Social factors, such as poverty, urbanisation, internal migration and lifestyle changes, are moderators of the high burden of mental illness in many low- and middle-income countries [9]. Issues surrounding presentation of mood disorders, help-seeking behaviours, diagnoses, measurements used and research methodologies are important to consider when interpreting prevalence rates.

Ferrari et al. [10] conducted a systematic review to summarise the incidence and prevalence of Major Depressive Disorder (MDD) at a global level, where the majority of the data included was from Western Europe and North America and a meta-regression was used to account for methodological and ecological variables on the prevalence rates found. A higher prevalence of MDD in developing compared to developed regions is reported. Fewer sources on incident data were found ($n = 4$), giving global incidence rates of 2.7% in males and 3.4% in females. The authors noted that heterogeneity in the data, from both naturally occurring differences and methodological differences utilised in capturing the data, meant that interpretation of the data was not simple. Differences in global prevalence rates therefore need to take into account not only variations in naturally occurring rates but also the methodology and measures used to collect this data, and perhaps most importantly, how culturally sensitive the measures used are.

Moreno-Agostino et al. [11] conducted a meta-analysis on global data and found a paucity of useable studies from Africa, Latin America and Asia as well as low- and middle-income countries, making equitable comparisons of prevalence rates difficult. The need for comparable methodologies and data sets to allow for meaningful meta-analyses may mean that the body of research informed by ethnography is also important to consider [5]. This would allow for in-depth exploration of context-specific variations not amenable to study when global descriptions are required.

The prevalence rates of mood disorders in different cultures are also heavily dependent on attributions of illness that define help-seeking behaviours and diagnoses. Due to the complex interplay of various factors like stigma, attributes to mood disorders and somatic or other presentations in many cultures, the diagnosis may vary. The 5th edition of the *Diagnostic and Statistical Manual of Mental Disorders* (DSM-5) [12] and the 11th revision of the *International Statistical Classification of Diseases and Related Health Problems* (ICD-11) [13] are used in many countries across the world. However, there is criticism of their relevance to legitimate remuneration to practitioners from private medical insurance and government programs in local nations due to cultural differences [14]. The DSM-5 has endeavoured to incorporate cultural sensitivity by updating criteria to reflect cross-cultural variations in presentations with some description of cultural concepts of distress and a clinical interview tool, rather than just a simple list of culture-bound syndromes [12]. For example, the criteria for social anxiety now includes the fear of 'offending others' to reflect the phenomenon in Japanese culture in which avoiding harm to others is emphasised rather than harm to oneself [15].

The ICD-11 [13], developed by WHO, interestingly seems to be more suited to transcultural uniformities and convergence but less helpful for variations in presentation. It also provides a brief presentation of culture specific disorders. Guidance for considering culture when using the ICD-11 was developed by a panel of experts after extensive review of the literature and the relevant cultural formulations in the ICD-10 [16].

There are some localised classification systems including the Chinese Classification of Mental Disorders (CCMD-3), the Cubian Glossary of Psychiatry (GC-3) and the Latin American Guide for Psychiatric Diagnosis (GLGP).

Therefore, it is important that the cultural context is recognised in classification systems to develop a common language across countries when measuring prevalence rates.

Culture and Socio-Demographic Profiles of Mood Disorders

Social constructs, political landscapes and policies and differences in life experiences, beliefs systems and customs are associated with differences in rates, presentation and help-seeking pathways in mood disorders. They also contribute to outcomes (e.g., low education, high teen child-bearing, marital disruption, unstable employment), reduced role functioning (e.g., low marital quality, low work performance, low earnings), and elevated risk of onset, persistence, and severity of a wide range of secondary disorders, often with increased risk of early mortality due to physical illness and suicide [17].

Practical considerations of policy and social changes, like rapid urbanisation in many countries leading to large cities with high levels of overpopulation, poor working conditions, gender discrimination, hunger and unemployment, human rights violations and breakup of the large joint family units with high levels of stress, are a possible causal factor for higher rates of urban mood disorders [18]. As an example, almost half of the women in a slum in Brazil reported mental illness [6]. The conflict in countries such as Afghanistan, Iraq and Sudan may account for higher prevalence rates of mood disorders in these regions [10]. Migration is a source of psychological distress, due to trauma prior to migration, separation from friends and family and the need to adjust to a new environment. The level of acculturation is implicated. Ahmed and Bhugra [4] cite studies showing that immigrants from both Mexico and Cuba experienced lower levels of depression than US-born Mexican and Cuban Americans. They hypothesise that higher levels of acculturation may be associated with depression, whereas retaining strong protective cultural values such as family orientation may protect against depression.

Evidence shows that demographic factors such as gender, age, and marital status are associated with depression [19]. In many studies, women are shown to have a twofold increased risk of major depression compared to men; individuals who are separated or divorced have significantly higher rates of major depression than those currently married, and prevalence of major depression generally decreases with age [17,19,20]. Societal and cultural expectations of gender roles and caregiving responsibilities, variations in gender- and age-related financial independence, overall autonomy and education levels, gender-based violence, cultural status of hormone-based gender- and age-related changes and individualistic versus collectivistic orientation are factors that influence these variations.

Conversely, Mohammadi et al. [18] in a large cluster, randomised survey of over 25,000 participants in Iran found a 3.1% lifetime prevalence rate for MDD and 0.1% and 0.7% rates for bipolar disorder types I and II, respectively. They found associations between mood disorders and being female, having lower levels of education, being married, being middle aged, living in cities and not being a homemaker. Commenting on the difference of married and middle-aged people in Iran experiencing more depression as opposed to single and young adults in the West, the authors highlight the low rates of divorce as a possible contributing factor (0.4% in Iran compared to over 50% in the West). This is an interesting finding and reflection as many cultures take pride in family units that can also be protective and support individuals through times of distress [4]. It may also reflect changing social values and cultural constructs.

In summary, there are complexities of exploring the impact of cultural issues at a global and regional level. Even within regions and countries, individuals can have very different social and psychological experiences that may impact on their wellbeing, emphasising the reality that culture is dynamic, affects every individual in a unique way and, therefore, every individual carries their own culture.

Culture and Presentation of Mood Disorders

Presentations of mood disorders can be shaped by cultural factors, impacting on diagnosis and choice of treatment pathways. Some symptoms are universal, for example agitation and reduced need for sleep in bipolar affective disorder manic episodes, whereas symptoms such as grandiosity and hyperactivity may be masked by certain cultural expectations and norms. As an example, overly inflated self-esteem would be considered a sin among Amish individuals [21]. Similarly, phenomenological peculiarities have been documented in different cultures, such as a low occurrence of flight of ideas and a relatively high proportion of persecutory and self-blaming delusions in eastern India [22], possibly in response to the use of shame and guilt as forms of social control in some cultures.

Differences in cultural etiquette and cultural acknowledgement of an individual's position in society places emphasis on social interactions and worry about another's discomfort above one's own. This has been related to a worry seen in social anxiety in Japan: an improper eye gaze could make the viewer distressed, compared with Western cultures where poor eye gaze may depict thoughts of embarrassment. Similarly, Western portrayals of interpersonal conflict and disagreements are commonplace in everyday life, making it possible that people may talk more openly about feelings of distress with healthcare providers [5], compared with cultures where distress is more usually contained in families.

Lack of availability of a universal emotional language can be argued to be a cause for the different presentations of mood disorders across cultures. 'Depression' as a term is absent from some cultures and used very infrequently in others [6]. In the 1980s about four-fifths of Chinese psychiatric outpatients were being treated for neurasthenia, with many seeking treatment for self-diagnosed neurasthenia. The diagnosis includes many somatic, emotional and cognitive symptoms, which may fit with the traditional epistemological ideas of disease causation in China [6]. Commentary at the time, proposed that neurasthenia was a Chinese-specific presentation of depression, also included in Chinese and international classification systems as a separate disorder [23]. Many cultures, for example, in India or China, use somatic metaphors for emotions and emotional experiences [23]. In India, many distress disorders are acknowledged as depression. Expressions of illness can range from aches and pains, autonomic symptoms, weakness and tiredness and behavioural symptoms, to gynaecological symptoms and 'tension as an idiom of distress' [24]. Elderly Korean immigrants in the USA were found to use descriptions of symptoms that incorporated symbolic as well as physical attributes such as 'melancholy has been absorbed into the body' [6]. This highlights the need to understand cultural idioms in presentation during transcultural assessments. Lack of cultural knowledge and understanding of these idioms could potentially lead to misdiagnosis. There is potential for descriptions relating to bodily feelings such as 'heat' or 'peppery' feelings in the head, 'weight on my heart' and 'feelings of heat' to be misdiagnosed as psychosis [4–6]. In Punjabi women in England, such descriptions have been seen to fit with traditional ayurvedic models of hot and cold [6]. However such somatic idioms are also commonly found in the West, such as 'I feel gutted' [6], thereby endorsing the need to understand culture as being unique to each individual.

Somatisation, or the experiencing of psychological distress in a physical, bodily manifestation, has often been referred to as a form of cultural presentation of a mood disorder. Such a theory has been linked to the lack of dichotomisation and distinct separation of the mind and body in many non-Western cultures [6]. Therefore, somatisation of symptoms is common in many Chinese, Japanese, Malayan, Tahitian, Indian and other cultural groups [23]. The symptoms can be linked to specific body parts, such as the abdomen, liver, intestines or heart; as in traditional medicine, body parts are associated with emotions such as the lungs being associated with worry in traditional Korean medicine and imbalances in bodily energy or qi in traditional Chinese medicine [4,6]. Somatisation can be viewed and understood as an expression of distress in cultures where the norm is stress conformity and verbal expressiveness is discouraged [25]. Another explanation for somatisation as a presentation of depression in some cultures is the level of stigma. In cultures where stigma of mental illness remains more pronounced, it may be easier to seek help for physical symptoms and avoid negative consequences for the individual [23].

Kirmayer [5] has argued that somatisation is not unique to one culture and is found in both Western and non-Western populations, especially musculoskeletal pain and fatigue. There is discussion that reporting of somatic symptoms is associated with the method of data collection. If asked to self-report symptoms, Western patients report primarily somatic symptoms, but if asked directly, psychological symptoms are reported [23]. When exploring the validity of cross-cultural differences in somatisation in depression, Ryder et al. [23] found no difference in the type of symptoms clinicians rated during a structured clinical interview. However, Chinese participants did report higher levels of stigma and alexithymia, a difficulty in expressing emotional states, when compared to Canadian participants. Alexithymia has been considered to be a culturally bound difficulty, with Eastern individuals having more externally orientated thinking and Ryder et al. [23] report findings suggesting that such externally orientated thinking may mediate relationship between culture and the reporting of somatic symptoms. In summary, cross-cultural

research methodology for somatisation may require a review.

Guilt and worry can also be a presentation of depression in many cultures, especially where social hierarchy is strong and defines expectations of roles and responsibilities. As an example, around 50% of depressed patients in India reported feelings of guilt. Terms for guilt in Arabic may vary, and it may be more often shown as a behavioural expression rather than a conscious feeling [6]. Therefore, a greater level of clinician understanding and probing of the subtle dynamics to uncover these presentations is required [6].

Suicide rates can vary based on cultural influences. Some cultures, for example Hispanic cultures with their emphasis on close relationships and expectations of adversity, may provide a protective factor against suicide [6]. *Seppuku*, ritual suicide by disembowelment, vulgarised in the West as *harakiri*, has been a popular theme in Japanese literature and theatre for years, and a time-honoured traditional form of suicide among the samurai class in Japan for centuries. While rare in contemporary Japan, it highlights the role of culture in role performance [26].

In summary, understanding the cultural expressions and societal constructs of mood disorders is important for clinicians to enable accurate diagnosis and treatment options.

Culture and Attributions to Mood Disorders

Cultural influences on how individuals view themselves, their place in society, norms and expectations of roles, autonomy and acceptability of life adversities influence attributions to mood disorders. Cultural determinants of acceptable norms in society and family dynamics define how individuals experience shame, guilt and stigma. An example is masturbation, a common sexual behaviour in humans, though viewed negatively in many cultures and therefore implicated in severe depression [27]. We have already discussed many cultural socio-demographic factors implicated in causation of mood disorders earlier in the chapter.

Attributions to mood disorders vary across cultures. Social and situational explanations of mood disorders are often more common in some cultures compared to others that provide biological explanations [28]. Hagmayer and Engelmann [29] conducted a systematic review on causal beliefs about depression. Thirty-six studies investigating 13 non-Western and 32 Western cultural groups were analysed by classifying assumed causes and preferred forms of treatment into common categories. Substantial agreement between cultural groups was found with respect to the impact of observable causes. Stress was generally rated as most important. Less agreement resulted for hidden, especially supernatural, causes. Causal beliefs were related to treatment preferences in Western groups, while evidence was mostly lacking for non-Western groups. There were limitations in the studies.

Understanding the cultural nuances of presentation helps recognition and accurate diagnosis, and knowledge of attributions of illness helps clinicians engage individuals with depression in treatment more effectively. The attributions to illness determine help-seeking behaviours and pathways. As an example, when witchcraft is suspected as the cause of a person's depression, the help of traditional healers is sought, while Western medicine is preferred to address somatic causes and symptoms of depression [30]. Pakriev et al. [31] found in rural Russia that only 4 out of 366 participants who met criteria for depression on an international measure had seen a psychiatrist, and the majority of participants had been untreated. The authors concluded that their participants did not realise there was a need to seek help. They also discussed various barriers to seeking help, including social anxiety.

Culture, Engagement, Treatments and Outcomes

Western medicine, based on evidence-based research, is considered the universal cornerstone for health. The premise is dependence on identification, accurate diagnosis and classification of the mental health disorder. The formal diagnosis of a mental disorder hinges upon several components: a patient's description of their symptoms in terms of intensity and duration, mental state examination and the clinician's observation and interpretation of the signs and behaviours [32]. Clinicians must skilfully conclude whether the patient's behaviour and symptoms significantly impair certain aspects of their life, and this judgement needs to be based on divergence from what is deemed acceptable behaviour in the particular culture and the salient variations in presentation. Culture therefore

plays an important role in understanding behaviours that could be construed as a mental health disorder in Western medicine. Kirmayer [5] has eloquently suggested that it is best to frame cultural differences as 'inter-cultural encounters' that consider the cultural concepts on both sides of the interaction.

Most mood disorders present in primary care settings, and evidence suggests that non-White individuals such as those from South Asian, African American and Hispanic origins are less likely to have depression identified, especially if the doctor and patient are of differing ethnicities [4,6]. Language barriers can prevent recognition of depression, and while translators are beneficial, there can be limitations [33]. Stigma, level of acculturation in migrants and attributions to mood disorders are other factors to consider in engaging individuals from different cultures.

Prescribing a treatment, that is not congruent with an individual's understanding of the cause of their symptoms has little impact due to high levels of self-discontinuation, especially in intercultural settings [6] and also sometimes leading to less use of services voluntarily [28]. Therefore open discussion and education, in a way that is understood and acceptable is needed to develop a collaborative plan of care which may include members of the individual's family and sometimes local community.

There has been a growing body of research to highlight the racial disparity in antidepressant treatment outcomes with generally poorer results for African Americans compared with Caucasians [34]. The majority of this research has found that several environmental factors such as lower socioeconomic status, greater medical and/or psychiatric comorbidity all contribute to the poorer outcomes among African Americans [35,36], with some evidence that biological or genetic factors could also play a role [37,38]. Gene studies on the pharmacodynamics components of SSRI response, including that of the serotonin transporter gene, SLC6A4, and the variants in the serotonin receptor genes, HTR1A and HTR2A, have shown there to be differences in the allele frequencies among ethnic and racial groups [38,39]. Another proposed mechanism is that of dietary differences affecting the metabolism of medications such as Clomipramine, as well as possible interactions with traditional medicines, environmental, social and genetic factors [6]. However, early results remain inconclusive. Pharmacogenomics and personalised medicine is now a fast growing field of research [40] and with the majority of pharmacological development and research being conducted in the West, it will be very important to ensure that individuals from different ethnic and cultural groups are represented in research studies.

Cognitive Behaviour Therapy (CBT), recommended by the National Institute for Health and Care Excellence (NICE), is based on Western philosophies. The Improving Access to Psychological Therapies (IAPT) programme was launched in 2008 in UK to improve the quality and accessibility of mental health services for mild to moderate mental health conditions. Evidence suggests general practitioners are less likely to refer individuals from minority communities due to cultural differences in manifestation of mental health symptoms, cultural stereotypes or beliefs against talking therapies as a treatment option [41]. To overcome this, self-referrals are now accepted that have improved the referral rate but the core problem of understanding remains [42].

In recent years, there has been an emerging interest in ancient Eastern therapies like yoga and mindfulness, but research to establish effectiveness is lacking. Even when language is not an issue, clinical trials on psychological interventions generally enrol few minority individuals, and analysis of trial results is usually not done separately based on the ethnic group [43]. There are, therefore, few studies of the effectiveness of evidence-based interventions in minority groups. Generalisation of results and understanding of whether the principles of Western evidence-based interventions apply to culture based presentations and attributes to illness is therefore limited.

Culture and Implications for Services

Despite societies being multicultural, reports from high-income countries continue to demonstrate health inequalities, with disparity in quality of care and low rates of satisfaction in minority groups [44]. Cultural relevance, while essential, carries its challenges and should follow a multifaceted evidence-based methodology [45]. Cultural competence training shows promise as a strategy for improving the knowledge, attitudes, and skills of health professionals. However, evidence that it improves patient adherence to therapy, health outcomes, or equity of services across cultural groups is debated [46]. Ethnic matching of individuals with clinicians may enable

shared understanding and experiences to enhance care, but this does not guarantee engagement due to issues of assumed knowledge and subcultures within cultures.

Rathod and colleagues have led the development of an evidence based adaptation framework that has been evaluated for use in diverse populations. The framework has four core domains of adaptation [2,33,47]:

Philosophical Orientation: Worldview or life perspective differs for every individual, community, and culture. These perspectives affect perceptions of health and illness, relationships with services and professionals, and treatment goals. Understanding an individual's philosophical orientation helps clinicians to engage with them.

Practical Considerations: The relationship between religion, politics, culture, values and beliefs, expression of sexuality, and relationship with health services is complex in any community. Clinicians should understand this dynamic and how employment, housing, justice and social care policies affect integration of individuals from diverse backgrounds, and provide holistic mental health services that supporting engagement.

Technical Adjustments of Methods and Skills: Within diverse populations, the mode and manner of interactions or interventions, the setting, and the development of the therapeutic relationship may need to be modified to support engagement.

Theoretical Modifications of Concepts: Changes in the description of theoretical concepts may be needed to best fit the individual and their culture. This can involve different ways of explaining specialist concepts, with the use of appropriate metaphors.

Given the varied and individual nature that culture can affect both patients and clinicians, an individual-centred approach to exploring underlying difficulties and presentations is needed. Recognition that each individual has their own culture that derives from the larger group culture and evolves over time and through experiences allows person-centred care.

Cultural strengths like close-knit families and communities are enablers and should be harnessed by services to maximise engagement and outcomes. Alternative pathways into care like places of worship can be strategically used to engage people with mood disorders.

Conclusion

Culture influences every aspect of mood disorders from causation, presentation, attributions to illness, help seeking pathways into care, engagement with services, treatments and outcomes. Health services need to be responsive to the needs of communities they serve and scale up the programme of delivering culturally relevant services.

References

1. Helman C. *Culture, Health and Illness*. 2nd ed. London: Wright, 1990.

2. Mason B, Sawyer, A. *Exploring the Unsaid: Creativity, Risks and Dilemmas in Working Cross-Culturally*. London: Karnac, 2002.

3. Rathod S, Kingdon D, Pinninti N, Turkington D, Phiri P. *Cultural Adaptation of CBT for Serious Mental Illness: A Guide for Training and Practice*. West Sussex: John Wiley & Sons, 2015.

4. Ahmed K, Bhugra, D. Depression across ethnic minority cultures: diagnostic issues. *World Cult Psychiatry Res Rev*. 2007;2:47–56.

5. Kirmayer LJ. Cultural variations in the clinical presentation of depression and anxiety: implications for diagnosis and treatment. *J Clin Psychiatry*. 2001;**62** (suppl 13):22–8.

6. Bhugra D, Mastrogianni, A. Globalisation and mental disorders: overview with relation to depression. *Br J Psychiatry*. 2004;**184**:10–20.

7. Murray CJ, Lopez, A.D. Evidence-based health policy – lessons from the Global Burden of Disease Study. *Science*. 1996;**274**:740–3.

8. Mathers DL. Projections of global mortality and burden of disease from 2002 to 2030. *PLoS Med*. 2006;**3**:e442.

9. Rathod, S, Irfan, M., Gorczynski, P., et al. Mental health service provision in low and middle income countries. *Health Serv Insights*. 2017;**10**.

10. Ferrari AJ, Somerville AJ, Baxter AJ, et al. Global variation in the prevalence and incidence of major depressive disorder: a systematic review of the epidemiological literature. *Psychol Med*. 2013;**43** (3):471–81.

11. Moreno-Agostino D, Wu YT, Daskalopoulou C, et al. Global trends in the prevalence and incidence of depression: a systematic review and meta-analysis. *J Affect Disord*. 2021;**281**:235–43.

12. American Psychiatric Association. *Diagnostic and Statistical Manual of Mental Disorders: DSM-5*. 5th ed. Washington, DC: American Psychiatric Associaiton, 2013.

13. World Health Organisation. *International Statistical Classification of Diseases and Related Health Problems (ICD)*. 11th revision ed. Available at: www.who.int/s tandards/classifications/classification-of-diseases

14. Lee S. From diversity to unity. The classification of mental disorders in 21st-century China. *Psychiatr Clin N Am*. 2001; Sep. **24**(3):421–31.

15. American Psychiatric Association. Cultural concepts in DSM-5. American Psychiatric Association, 2013.

16. Gureje O, Lewis-Fernandez R, Hall BJ, Reed GM. Cultural considerations in the classification of mental disorders: why and how in ICD-11. *BMC Med*. 2020;**18**(1):25.

17. Kessler RC, Bromet EJ. The epidemiology of depression across cultures. *Annu Rev Public Health*. 2013;**34**:119–38.

18. Mohammadi MR, Ghanizadeh A, Davidian H, et al. Prevalence of mood disorders in Iran. *Iran J Psychiatry*. 2006;**1**:59–64.

19. Van de Velde S, Bracke P, Levecque K. Gender differences in depression in 23 European countries. Cross-national variation in the gender gap in depression. *Soc Sci Med*. 2010;**71**(2):305–13.

20. Andrade L, Caraveo-Anduaga JJ, Berglund P, et al. The epidemiology of major depressive episodes: results from the International Consortium of Psychiatric Epidemiology (ICPE) Surveys. *Int J Methods Psychiatr Rese*. 2003;**12**(1):3–21.

21. Egeland JA, Hostetter AM, Eshleman SK. Amish Study: III. The impact of cultural factors on diagnosis of bipolar illness. *Am J Psychiatry*. 1983;**140**(1):67–71.

22. Sethi S, Khanna R. Phenomenology of mania in eastern India. *Psychopathology*. 1993;**26**(5–6):274–8.

23. Ryder AG, Yang J, Zhu X, et al. The cultural shaping of depression: somatic symptoms in China, psychological symptoms in North America? *J Abnorm Psychol*. 2008;**117**(2):300–13.

24. Bhattacharya A, Camacho D, Kimberly LL, Lukens EP. Women's experiences and perceptions of depression in India: a metaethnography. *QualHealth Res*. 2019;**29**(1):80–95.

25. Lee S. A Chinese perspective of somatoform disorders. *J Psychosom Res*. 1997;**43**(2):115–19.

26. Fusé T. Suicide and culture in Japan: a study of seppuku as an institutionalized form of suicide. *Soc Psychiatry*. 1980;**15**(2):57–63.

27. Albobali Y, Madi MY. Masturbatory guilt leading to severe depression. *Cureus*. 2021;**13**(3):e13626.

28. Karasz A. Cultural differences in conceptual models of depression. *Soc Sci Med*. 2005;**60**(7):1625–35.

29. Hagmayer Y, Engelmann N. Causal beliefs about depression in different cultural groups – what do cognitive psychological theories of causal learning and reasoning predict? *Front Psychol*. 2014;**5**:1303.

30. Okello ES, Ekblad S. Lay concepts of depression among the Baganda of Uganda: a pilot study. *Transcult Psychiatry*. 2006;**43**(2):287–313.

31. Pakriev S, Vasar V, Aluoja A, Saarma M, Shlik J. Prevalence of mood disorders in the rural population of Udmurtia. *Acta Psychiatr Scand*. 1998;97:169–74.

32. Office of the Surgeon General, Center for Mental Health Services, National Institute of Mental Health. Introduction. In *Mental Health: Culture, Race, and Ethnicity: A Supplement to Mental Health: A Report of the Surgeon General*. Rockville, MD: Substance Abuse and Mental Health Services Administration (US), 2001.

33. Rathod S, Naeem F, Kingdon D. Can you do meaningful CBT through interpreters? In K Bhui, editor, *Elements of Culture and Mental Health: Critical Questions for Clinicians*. London: RCPsych Publications, 2013.

34. Lesser IM, Castro DB, Gaynes BN, et al. Ethnicity/race and outcome in the treatment of depression: results from STAR*D. *Medi Care*. 2007;**45**(11):1043–51.

35. Lesser IM, Myers, H.F., Lin, K.M., et al. Ethnic differences in antidepressant response: a prospective multi-site clinical trial. *Depress Anxiety*. 2010;**27**(1):56–62.

36. Lesser IM, Zisook, S., Gaynes, B.N., et al. Effects of race and ethnicity on depression treatment outcomes: the CO-MED trial. *Psychiatr Serv*. 2011;**62**(10):1167–79.

37. Luo HR, Poland RE, Lin KM, Wan YJ. Genetic polymorphism of cytochrome P450 2C19 in Mexican Americans: a cross-ethnic comparative study. *Clin Pharmacol Ther*. 2006;80:33–40.

38. McMahon FJ, Charney D, Lipsky R, et al. Variation in the gene encoding the serotonin 2A receptor as associated with outcome of antidepressant treatment. *Am J Hum Genet*. 2006;**78**:804–14.

39. Lotrich FE, Pollock BG, Ferrell RE. Serotonin transporter promoter polymorphism in African Americans. *Am J Pharmacogenomics*. 2003;3(2):145–7.

40. Roden DM, Wilke RA, Kroemer HK, Stein CM. Pharmacogenomics: the genetics of variable drug responses. *Circulation*. 2011;**123**(15):1661–70.

41. Khan S, Lovell K, Lunat F, et al. Culturally-adapted cognitive behavioural therapy based intervention for maternal depression: a mixed-methods feasibility study. *BMC Womens Health*. 2019;**19**(1):21.

42. Rathod S, Phiri P, Naeem F, Halvorsrud K, Bhui K. The importance of cultural adaptation of psychological interventions: learning from UK experiences of IAPT and CBT services. Briefing paper. The Synergi Collaborative Centre. 2020.

43. Carroll KM, Martino S, Ball SA, et al. A multisite randomized effectiveness trial of motivational enhancement therapy for Spanish-Speaking substance users. *J Consult Clin Psychol*. 2009;**77**(5):993–9.

44. Schouler-Ocak M, Graef-Calliess IT, Tarricone I, et al. EPA guidance on cultural competence training. *Eur Psychiatry*. 2015;**30**:431–40.

45. Rathod S, Kingdon D. Case for cultural adaptation of psychological interventions for mental healthcare in low and middle income countries. *BMJ* (Clinical research ed). 2014;**349**:g7636.

46. Beach MC, Price EG, Gary TL, et al. Cultural competence: A systematic review of health care provider educational interventions. *Med Care*. 2005;**43**(4):356–73.

47. Rathod S, Phiri P, Harris S, et al. Cognitive behaviour therapy for psychosis can be adapted for minority ethnic groups: a randomised controlled trial. *Schizophrenia Res*. 2013;**143**(2–3):319–26.

Chapter 10

Mood Disorders and Stress-Related Disorders

Romayne Gadelrab and Mario Juruena

Stress

The concept of stress has been the subject of debate since its creation in the mid-nineteenth century as a fundamental concept in physics. Initially, the definition of the term 'stress' referred to the force, or set of forces, that two pieces of matter exerted reciprocally on each other in order to reach a state of equilibrium [1]. In 1936, Hans Seyle, a Hungarian neuroendocrinologist, incorporated the word 'stress' into the field of physiology, using it to define an organism's non-specific response to an insult [2,3].

In the field of stress research, 'stress' has been used to define different phenomena and situations that range from the reference to stimulation by milder challenges to very severe aversive conditions [4,5]. In order to delimit a more precise definition, a group of researchers recently revised the application of the term 'stress' and proposed that it should be considered as a cognitive perception of uncontrollability and/or unpredictability that would be expressed in a behavioural and physiological response [6]. According to these authors, this definition would be restricted to conditions in which an environmental demand exceeds the regulatory capacity of an organism, particularly in situations where there is no anticipatory response, and which are characterized by a delay in the recovery of the stress response.

Neural, immune, and endocrine mechanisms have been identified as underlying biological mechanisms of chronic stress and its adverse health consequences [7]. More specifically, the hypothalamic–pituitary–adrenal (HPA) axis and immune system are activated by stress and the production of neurotrophic factors reduced [8]. If the stress experienced is chronic, it can lead to the dysfunction of these biological pathways involved in the stress response and ultimately contribute to the development of psychiatric disorders [9,10].

In addition to the neuroendocrine system, the immune system is impacted by the body's response to chronic stress. The stress-related disruption of the immune system has been found to lead to slower wound healing [11,12]. The HPA axis modulates the release of cytokines, which alter the monoamine metabolism, increase excitotoxicity, and decrease the production of trophic factors [13]. These cytokines lead to glucocorticoid resistance [14]. This results in a decreased immune activation in response to stress [15], a mechanism that works similarly to the increased cortisol levels in chronic stress. This suppression of immune functioning has been linked to inflammatory disease [13]. Stress-related immune abnormalities have also been linked to several psychiatric disorders, such as depression [16], bipolar disorder and schizophrenia [17]. This effect is significantly amplified in individuals that have experienced childhood trauma; a meta-analysis found correlations between childhood trauma and adulthood inflammation [18].

Hypothalamic–Pituitary–Adrenal (HPA) Axis

The stress response of an organism is mostly modulated by the HPA system and by the sympathetic adrenomedullary (SAM) system. In a coordinated way, these two systems act in the metabolism, promoting energy mobilization and redistribution of resources (e.g., oxygen and nutrients) to organs and tissues in order to prepare the body to respond to the stressful stimulus and return to a state of equilibrium [19,20,21]. Activation in the HPA axis begins with the secretion of corticotrophin-releasing hormone (CRH) and vasopressin by the paraventricular nucleus of the hypothalamus (PVN) stimulating the production and release of adrenocorticotropic hormone (ACTH) from the anterior part of the pituitary. ACTH then stimulates the adrenal cortex to secrete glucocorticoids into the circulation, the main one being cortisol (the endogenous glucocorticoid in humans). The body's homeostasis is re-established with a feedback signal from cortisol that inhibits further release of ACTH from the pituitary and of CRH from the hypothalamus terminating the action of the HPA axis [22,23,24]. This feedback mechanism occurs through the binding of cortisol to its mineralocorticoid and glucocorticoid receptors (MR and GR, respectively) [25,26,27]; see Figure 10.1.

The activity of the HPA axis follows a circadian secretion pattern. Under normal conditions, cortisol has a pulsatile secretion that follows an endogenous circadian rhythm (CR) pattern. The cortisol circadian rhythm is characterized by a peak that occurs just before awakening and declines for the remainder of the 24 hours of the day. Baseline concentrations of adrenocorticotropic hormone (ACTH) and cortisol are highest in the morning (6–9 h), with a progressive decline throughout the day and night (23–3 h) [28]. Evidence demonstrates that morning awakening is followed by an activation of the HPA axis with elevation of ACTH secretion and salivary cortisol concentrations, by about 50 to 75%, within 30 minutes after waking up in the morning, a phenomenon called cortisol response on waking up (CAR) [29,30,31].

The stress response results in the activation of the HPA axis, which must be acute and limited in time, resulting in anti-growth, anti-reproductive, catabolic, and immunosuppressive effects, which, in a short space of time, are beneficial and prepare the body for an adequate response to stress, for example, a 'flight' reaction in the face of danger. However, chronic activation of the HPA axis induces damage and pathological responses. Chronic stress situations are almost always associated with important deleterious effects related to chronic and degenerative clinical conditions, such as increased insulin resistance, atherosclerosis, increased visceral fat deposition, osteoporosis, immunity alterations and psychiatric disorders [33]. Stress responses are the result of body adjustments and control mechanisms of various functions and the inadequate response to a stressful stimulus can represent a risk of disease and/or threat to life [34]. Therefore, an organism's ability to defend or adapt to stress depends on the magnitude and duration of the stressor, sensitivity to the stressor, as well as the interaction of individual characteristics such as genetic factors, biological development (previous experiences, memories of situations), social support, and physical and mental health conditions, which lead individuals to face stressful situations in different ways. Thus, the inability to deal with stress and the consequent hypersecretion of corticosteroids results in detrimental effects of stress on the body [22,35,36].

The HPA axis plays a fundamental role in the response to external and internal stimuli, including psychological stressors. Furthermore, the fundamental role of stress in precipitating episodes of psychiatric disorders in predisposed individuals is well known. Abnormalities in HPA axis function have been described in people with psychiatric disorders [37]. Evidence suggests that behavioural, neurochemical, and molecular alterations induced by stressful situations trigger changes in the HPA axis that are associated with depression. Findings from multiple lines of research have provided evidence that during depression, dysfunction of limbic structures, including the hypothalamus and hippocampus, results in hypersecretion of CRH, dehydroepiandrosterone (DHEA), and arginine vasopressin (AVP), leading to pituitary–adrenal activation. A failure in this system, caused by factors such as excessive stress, high levels of glucocorticoids, social isolation, and depressive symptoms, would make it difficult to adapt to stress and predispose to the onset of depression by impairing hippocampal serotonergic neurotransmission [33,35]. In melancholic depression, there is evidence of increased activation of the HPA axis, increased release of ACTH and CRH, and increased cortisol levels, mainly in post-challenge tests. On the other hand, the first studies with patients in a depressive episode with atypical features with inverted vegetative symptoms demonstrated reduced cortisol and lower HPA activity when compared with controls. However, most of the studies have not differentiated this depressive subtype from healthy controls [38]. The same dysfunction observed in one or recurrent melancholic depressive episodes may also be present in bipolar patients in mixed, manic, hypomanic, and/or depressive episodes [39,40], see Figure 10.2.

Depression

Stressful life events play an important role in the pathogenesis of mood disorders, particularly in triggering depressive episodes, and are well established as acute precipitants of psychiatric illness [43]. Hyperactivity of the HPA axis in patients with major depression is one of the most frequently reported

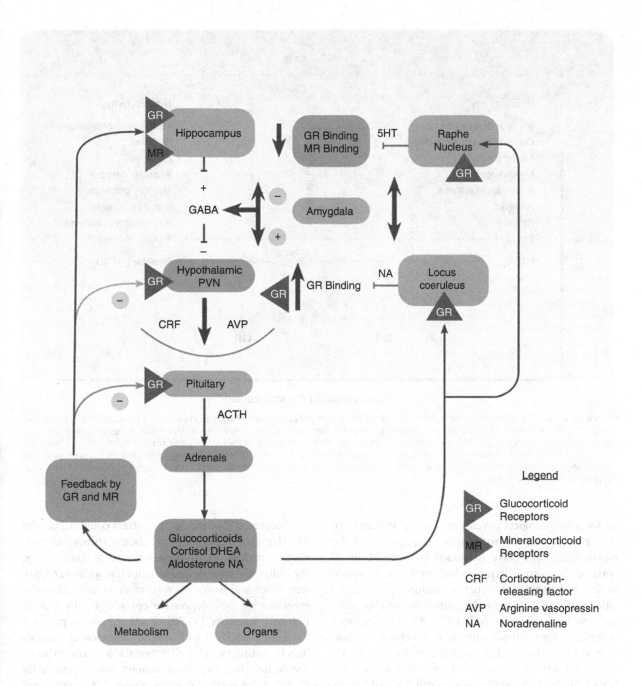

Figure 10.1 Representation of the HPA axis. It summarizes the negative (–) feedback of hormones binding in GR and MR. The system includes essential areas of the limbic system, amygdala, hippocampus, locus coeruleus, raphe nucleus, and their relation via noradrenaline (NA) and serotonin (5HT), with adrenal hormones and GR/MR. Adapted from [32].

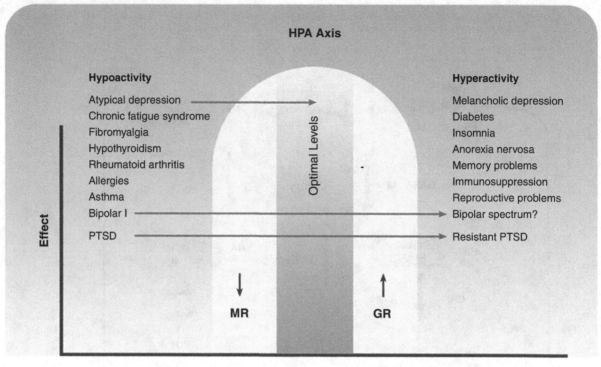

Figure 10.2 The HPA axis dysfunction induces changes in the activity of GCs on the MR and GR and in the (–) feedback impacting on the release of HPA axis hormones. An impaired (–) feedback, leading to increased GCs, as in melancholic depression, diabetes (mainly type II), eating disorders (e.g., anorexia), and sleep disorders (e.g., insomnia). The hypoactivation of the HPA axis may increase the negative (–) feedback, in subjects with atypical depression (or normal activation), seasonal affective disorders, post-traumatic stress disorder (PTSD), fibromyalgia, and chronic fatigue syndrome. Bipolar disorder and PTSD depending on the course could be related to lower or higher activity of the HPA axis. Adapted from [22,32,37,41,42].

findings in biological psychiatry. Several studies have shown that patients with major depression of the melancholic type have increased concentrations of cortisol in plasma, urine, saliva, and cerebrospinal fluid (CSF), exaggerated cortisol response after stimulation with ACTH, and enlargement of both the pituitary and adrenal glands [44,45]. As some authors describe, hypercortisolemia in melancholic depression occurs due to dysregulation of the HPA axis negative feedback [24,38,46]. However, the mechanisms underlying these changes are still not well understood [47]. In addition, other disorders may be associated with increased and prolonged activation of the HPA axis, including anorexia nervosa with or without malnutrition, obsessive-compulsive disorder, panic disorder, chronic alcoholism, alcohol and narcotic withdrawal, excessive exercise, poorly controlled diabetes mellitus, childhood sexual abuse, and hyperthyroidism [8,48].

According to some authors, stress could trigger the first depressive episode in genetically vulnerable individuals, making them more sensitive to stress. Thus, the individual would need less and less stress to trigger new crises and would become more vulnerable to the repetition of new depressive episodes in the face of different stressors [49,50]. Furthermore, depression has been associated with several biological abnormalities including vascular alterations, alterations in autonomic function, hypercoagulability, and hyperactivity of the HPA axis. Evidence shows that depression in adulthood is linked to a high risk of developing cardiovascular disease, diabetes, metabolic disorders, obesity, dyslipidaemia, hypertension, and dementia, and these clinical conditions are associated with a worse prognosis and worse response to treatment [51].

However, it should be taken into account that depression is a heterogeneous disorder that involves a wide range of depressive subtypes that have distinct clinical manifestations and distinct pathophysiological mechanisms. In this regard, there is another group of diseases that is characterized by under-activation of the stress system, rather than permanent activation, in which chronically reduced secretion of CRH can result in pathological hyporeactivity and intensified negative feedback from the HPA axis. Patients with seasonal depression, atypical depression, PTSD, and chronic fatigue syndrome fall into this category [38,52].

Data confirming the notion that glucocorticoid-mediated feedback inhibition is impaired in major depression come from several studies, many developed in the 1970s and 1980s. The dexamethasone depression test (DST) had become a widely used research tool for assessing the function of the HPA axis in depression [53]. At that time, Carroll et al. [53] found that severely depressed patients had decreased HPA axis suppression on the dexamethasone test. However, despite its usefulness in predicting clinical outcome in some patients, the widespread use of DST as a diagnostic tool was limited by the low sensitivity of the test, ranging between 20% and 50%, that is, low ability to distinguish patients with major depression in patients with other psychiatric disorders or in healthy individuals [54]. Furthermore, dexamethasone has pharmacodynamic and pharmacokinetic characteristics that are very different from cortisol, for example, dexamethasone, unlike cortisol, binds preferentially to GR [55,47].

Approximately 10 years after the development of DST, von Bardeleben and Holsboer [56] developed a more sensitive neuroendocrine function test to detect HPA axis imbalance. They combined the DST and the CRH stimulation test and called it the Dex/CRH challenge test. This test involves the oral administration of a single 1.5 mg dose of dexamethasone at 11 pm, followed at 3 am the next day with an intravenous bolus of 100 µg of CRH [56]. Some early literature related to the Dex/CRH test describes increases in cortisol and ACTH in depressed patients compared to controls [56,57]. In healthy individuals, cortisol secretion after dexamethasone continues to be suppressed after CRH injection; however, in depressed patients, HPA axis suppression fails and patients have elevated cortisol concentrations in response to the test. This occurs due to reduced GR sensitivity, which leads to an attenuation of the suppressive effects of dexamethasone in the pituitary and inhibition of CRH and AVP secretion by the hypothalamus, resulting in an increased stimulatory effect of exogenous

CRH in the Dex/CRH test in depressed patients [57]. Perhaps one of the most consistent findings in the literature related to the Dex/CRH test is the association between hypercortisolemia and recurrence of depressive episodes, as well as a reduction in the time to relapse. Zobel et al. [58] investigated a group of patients at two different times: at the beginning of treatment and a few days before discharge. These authors found that patients who showed increased cortisol levels after the Dex/CRH test between admission and discharge tended to relapse during the follow-up period, whereas those who showed decreased cortisol levels on the test of Dex/CRH tended to remain clinically stable in the follow-up period [58].

Although, according to Heuser et al. [57], the Dex/CRH test has a sensitivity greater than 80%, depending on age and sex, findings of HPA axis hyperactivity to the test have not been consistently confirmed in a number of studies investigating a variety of subpopulations of depressive disorders. Furthermore, the Dex/CRH test has limitations due to the pharmacokinetic profile and the low affinity of dexamethasone to MR receptors.

Recently, a suppression test using another synthetic glucocorticoid, prednisolone, with greater affinity for the MR receptor, was developed by Pariante et al [55]. Prednisolone is a synthetic glucocorticoid similar to cortisol in its pharmacokinetic and pharmacodynamic characteristics. In particular, it binds to cortisol-carrying globulin and its half-life is similar to that of cortisol. However, most importantly, prednisolone and cortisol are similar in their abilities to bind and activate GR and MR receptors, especially when compared to dexamethasone [55,59]. Prednisolone has an affinity that is twice that of cortisol, while dexamethasone has an affinity that is seven times that of cortisol. Studies in rats with GR demonstrate that prednisolone has cortisol-like potency in activating GRs, whereas dexamethasone has four times the potency of cortisol [59,60]. Thus, the prednisolone suppression test has been shown to be a promising tool for the assessment of the HPA axis, as it allows investigating both the functioning of the GR and the MR. According to the findings by Juruena et al. [47], in a study where cortisol responses in depressed patients and controls were compared after suppression with prednisolone and dexamethasone, controls suppressed cortisol in both challenges, while depressed patients suppressed cortisol only in the prednisolone challenge. These data suggest that controls were equally sensitive to both glucocorticoids.

On the other hand, such correlation was not observed in depressed patients. Thus, the dissociation between sensitivity to prednisolone and dexamethasone in depression suggests the existence of a selective impairment of GR sensitivity while MR sensitivity is maintained [60].

Bipolar Disorder

Bipolar disorder (BD) is associated with periodic mood episodes, often alternating from a depressive prolonged episode to a manic episode. Manic episodes come with a decreased need for sleep, and often individuals sleep substantially less than during their euthymic phases [61], whereas depression can often lead to a decreased level of energy, and therefore an increased need for sleep [62]. Evidence shows these alterations in the sleep–wake cycle, and moreover in the peripheral circadian clocks, can correlate with cortisol secretion and melatonin levels of patients diagnosed with BD [63].

When dealing with disorders that have overlapping symptomatology, it can become challenging to formulate a primary diagnosis, and eventually administer the most efficient treatment [64]. Clinicians can question if pharmacological treatment is indeed failing or if the characteristics of the maladaptive behaviours of a BD are influencing the course of treatment, and still struggle to find a conclusion [65].

Despite the flexibility of diagnostic criteria, BD is still one of the most challenging disorders to diagnose and, therefore, understanding if certain biomarkers could indicate the presence of the disorder would be very helpful [66].

Low levels of cortisol have also been found in bipolar depressive patients. According to the study published by Maripuu et al. [67], the results show that more than 70% of patients with bipolar disorder had hypocortisolaemia and this was associated with a higher frequency of depression among these patients, worse quality of life, and impairment in global functioning.

Considering the high correlation of BD with stress and how stress influences the development or progression of symptoms [32,49], understanding how stress influences patients from a biological standpoint could potentially help the formulation of a more suitable treatment [68]. Furthermore, the presence of a potential biomarker able to portray an elevated level of stress through a simple blood test could prevent relapses [69,70].

Ultimately, evidence shows that hyper-responsiveness of the HPA axis activity in cases of sustained stress is highly correlated with a persistent depressive mood, particularly in recurrent in BD patients [71,72]. Nonetheless, when considering patients who might be affected by both a PD and BD, understanding how the interaction between oxidative stress [72], HPA axis alteration [73], and rapid cycling between depressive episodes and hypomanic/manic episodes [74], could really be impactful in providing the adequate treatment [75]. Ultimately it would also help to address the interaction between the disorders, since stress particularly triggers HPA responsiveness in PDs, and then HPA responsiveness can trigger the rapid cycling between one mood episode and the other [76].

Steen and colleagues [77] recruited 81 patients with BD and 70 patients with schizophrenia (SCZ) spectrum disorder and compared them with 98 healthy controls (HC). Salivary samples were collected before and an hour after participants performed a neuropsychological test on logical memory, digital memory, working memory, coding, and visual cognition. The authors did not find a significant baseline difference in cortisol levels between all the groups, neither between BD nor SCZ patients, but they found that male patients had a suppressed cortisol release after the mental test compared to HC. Fang et al. [78] collected salivary samples from 16 BD (1 manic, 11 depressives, 4 in remission) and 15 HC. Results showed that cortisol levels were significantly suppressed in depressed BD patients compared to HC, whereas patients in remission showed similar cortisol levels as controls [78]. Watson and colleagues [79] demonstrated that patients with BD showed an increased serum cortisol response to Dex/CRH test compared with control ($p = 0.001$). Fifty-three patients with BD, 27 of whom were in full remission, and 28 HC received orally 1.5 mg DST the night before being tested. The following day, repeated measures were taken every 15 minutes after receiving 100 mg of human CRH. Furthermore, post hoc analysis showed that cortisol was significantly lower in non-remitted patients compared to patients who were in remission.

An article addressed potential differences in HPA axis activity between patients with borderline personality disorder (BPD) versus BD [80]. Patients were screened for comorbidities and other medical conditions before having their blood samples taken. Morning plasma cortisol levels were found to be significantly different between the three groups, both BPD and BD patients having lower cortisol levels than controls, with no significant difference found between BD and BPD. However, BD patients had the lowest cortisol levels among all the groups [80].

Early Life Stress

Adverse experiences in early life have been associated with significant increases in the risk of developing depression in adulthood, particularly in response to additional stressors [81,82]. Among the factors associated with depression in adulthood are exposure to stressors in childhood, such as abuse and neglect, death of parents or surrogates, maternal or paternal deprivation due to abandonment, parental separation or divorce, caregivers with psychiatric disorders, illnesses in children, family violence, and lack of basic care, among others. Early stress, defined by Bernstein et al. [83] as emotional, physical and sexual abuse, physical and emotional neglect, is a global social problem and is associated with a number of psychiatric consequences [83, 84]. In addition, early stress affects the health of the individual as a whole, and because of that, physical and clinical consequences can also be observed. In a recent study on the role of childhood adversities in the development of medical comorbidities in psychiatric patients, Post [50] demonstrated that early stress is associated with the occurrence of multiple clinical medical conditions in adult bipolar patients, such as asthma, arthritis, allergy, chronic fatigue syndrome, chronic menstrual irregularities, fibromyalgia, hypertension, hypotension, irritable bowel syndrome, and headache [85]. Magnetic resonance studies show that early stress can result in several neurostructural changes, such as a reduction in the hippocampus and corpus callosum, which lead to an alteration in performance and cognitive functioning in individuals who suffered early stress, thus generating an increase in the risk of developing mental disorders in adult life. In this sense, growing evidence indicates that early stress can be a risk factor for the development of depression, anxiety, and mood disorders, both in childhood and adulthood [43,82].

During childhood and adolescence, important brain structures are being formed and the occurrence of traumatic events at this stage can be perceived as disturbing agents of neurological

development and, depending on when they occur, can cause serious neurological 'scars' in some brain structures, such as the amygdala, prefrontal cortex, and hippocampus, whose development is complete during childhood and adolescence [86]. Thus, adverse events occurring early can interrupt or impair the brain maturation process, causing changes in neurotransmitters, neuroendocrine hormones, and neurotrophic factors that are crucial for normal brain development [87], which could make individuals more vulnerable to certain types of psychopathology, especially depression, PTSD, and substance abuse [81,88]. According to Heim and Nemeroff [89], children exposed to adverse experiences in early childhood are at increased risk for developing depression. Persistent sensitization of the central nervous system (CNS) circuits, which are integrally involved in the regulation of tension and emotion, as a consequence of early stress may represent the underlying biological substrates for greater vulnerability to subsequent stress, predisposing these individuals to develop a wide range of physical and mental disorders that are known to manifest or worsen with acute stress [89]. These patients present with symptoms that are resistant to treatment with antidepressants, but that benefit from concomitant treatment with psychotherapy [90]. However, it is important to emphasize that not every individual exposed to early stress will necessarily develop a psychiatric disorder, and not every adult with a psychiatric disorder necessarily suffered some experience of abuse or neglect in childhood, which demonstrates the importance of the genetic character and individual vulnerability in the development of depressive disorders.

Furthermore, as the HPA axis is activated in response to stressors, stressful events in early life may also play a significant etiological role in the HPA axis abnormalities found in people with psychiatric disorders [88,91,92]. Studies carried out in both animals and humans suggest that stress in the early stages of development can induce persistent changes in the ability of the HPA axis to respond to stress in adulthood and that this mechanism could lead to an increased susceptibility to depression [91,93]. Evidence indicates that early adverse experiences combined with genetic background culminate in the sensitization of certain brain circuits to an acute stressor. As a result, changes in HPA axis reactivity occur which, when persistent, result in axis modulation imbalance [60,86]. Furthermore, data indicate that CRH may play an important role in early stress susceptibility. According to the findings of Chen et al. [94], these authors observed that in the immature hippocampus there is a special population of cells capable of releasing CRH in response to stress, but this does not occur in the adult hippocampus. Exposure of the immature hippocampus to excessive levels of CRH would result in a delayed and progressive effect on cell survival and the dendritic branching that shapes the effects of early stress [94,95]. For Faravelli et al. [96], the effect of childhood trauma on psychopathology during adulthood is attributed to the HPA axis, which, once overactivated during developmental processes, would remain permanently unstable, overstimulated, vulnerable, or dysfunctional. Recent studies demonstrate that depressed patients with a history of childhood trauma and chronic forms of depression are more likely to have abnormal HPA axis functioning and that factors such as age at maltreatment, repeated exposure to stressors, and type of maltreatment can influence the degree and pattern of HPA axis disturbance [88].

One of the mechanisms that could be involved in this dysregulation of the HPA axis is the alteration in the capacity of circulating glucocorticoids to exert negative feedback from the HPA axis. The activity of the HPA axis stimulates the production of glucocorticoids by the adrenal cortex (cortisol in humans and corticosterone in rodents), which intercede their actions through two subtypes of intracellular receptors: type I receptors or mineralocorticoid receptors (MR) and type II receptors or glucocorticoid receptors (GR). These receptors differ in their affinity for endogenous glucocorticoids. While MR receptors have high affinity for cortisol, GR receptors have low affinity [32]. Their distributions in the CNS of rodents also differ, with MR predominating in limbic areas, mainly the hippocampus, whereas GR are more widely distributed among all brain regions [97]. In primates, MRs are also preferentially located in cortical and subcortical structures [98]. MRs are believed to play an essential role in regulating the hormonal fluctuation of the circadian cycle, cortisol response on awakening, and in the early stages of stress, whereas GR are only activated when endogenous glucocorticoid levels are high; being thus, GR is believed to be more important in regulating the stress response [22,99].

Post-Traumatic Stress Disorder (PTSD)

In patients with post-traumatic stress disorder (PTSD), hypoactivity and low hormone levels have been reported despite high central nervous system corticotropin-releasing factor (CRF) activity [100]. An increase of GR mediated negative feedback in the pituitary of PTSD patients, as demonstrated with the DST [101]. Furthermore, the correlation between PTSD, high dissociation, high impulsiveness and aggressiveness, high levels of testosterone, and high levels of cortisol should probably be studied. If the stress sensitivity is causing a cortisol reaction rather than the disorder itself, as some studies showed, the psychological treatment of BPD can target cognitive association to stress in order to desensitize the response to stressful stimuli. Considering that hypervigilance during conflicts could potentially trigger a delayed response to stress, working on stress sensitivity could change the entire HPA axis activity.

However, hippocampal MR, which have a higher affinity for cortisol than do GR, exert an inhibitory influence on HPA axis activity [102]. The possibility of dynamic regulation of MR was demonstrated in a preclinical study showing an increase in hippocampal MR density after psychological stress [103]. However, so far no investigation has characterized the role of MR in PTSD. Based on our hypothesis that PTSD patients exhibit an elevated MR function, we predicted an amplified cortisol response in PTSD patients compared to healthy subjects after administration of the mineralocorticoid receptor antagonist spironolactone, and enhanced cortisol secretion after subsequent stimulation with CRH.

Conclusion

Understanding the role of stress in psychiatric disorders will improve our knowledge of the pathophysiology of mood disorders and provide opportunity to recognize predisposing factors and could potentially help the formulation of a more suitable treatment. In this chapter we have presented current research on the stress response and how chronic stress can lead to the dysfunction of neuroendocrine and immune responses involved in the stress response and ultimately contribute to the development of psychiatric disorders.

Understanding the pathways involved in the stress response, in particular the HPA system and the role of cortisol in the stress response and also in maintaining the body's homeostasis through negative feedback loops, helps us to understand the impact of chronic stress and how hyperactivity of the HPA axis can contribute to major depressive disorder.

We have reviewed the impact of early life stress and the association with increased risk of developing depression in adulthood; however, it is important to emphasize that not every individual exposed to early stress will necessarily develop a psychiatric disorder, and not every adult with a psychiatric disorder experienced stress in childhood. It must be noted that despite strong evidence suggesting that early stress is associated with abnormalities in the HPA axis that lead to depression, there is still no consensus on whether early stress leads to hypo- or hyperactivation of this axis.

It is important that other factors including genetics, the impact of the individual's environment, and an individual's capacity for resilience are taken into consideration when considering the role of stress in mood disorders.

References

1. Muirhead RF. Stress – its definition. *Nature*. 1901;**64** (1652).

2. Seyle H. A syndrome produced by diverse nocuous agents. *Nature*. 1936.

3 Seyle H. *The Physiology and Pathology of Exposures to Stress*. Montreal: Acta Medica, 1950.

4. Chrousos GP. Stress and disorders of the stress system. *Nat Rev Endocrinol*. 2009;**5**:374–81.

5. Levine S, Ursin H. What is stress? In MR Brown, GF Koob, C Rivier, editors. *Stress: Neurobiology and Neuroendocrinology*. New York: Marcel Dekker, 1991;3–21

6. Koolhaas JM, Bartolomucci A, Buwalda B, et al. Stress revisited: a critical evaluation of the stress concept. *Neurosci Biobehav Rev*. 2011;**35**(5):1291–1301.

7. Chapman CR, Tuckett RP, Song CW. Pain and stress in a systems perspective: reciprocal neural, endocrine, and immune interactions. *J Pain*. 2008;**9**(2):122–45.

8. Tsigos C, Chrousos GP. Hypothalamic-pituitary-adrenal axis, neuroendocrine factors and stress. *J Psychosom Res*. 2002;**53**(4):865–71.

9. van Winkel R, Stefanis NC, Myin-Germeys I. Psychosocial stress and psychosis. A review of the neurobiological mechanisms and the evidence for gene-stress interaction. *Schizophr Bull*. 2008;**34** (6):1095–105.

10. Carr CP, Martins CMS, Stingel AM. Lemgruber V, Juruena MF. The role of early life stress in adult psychiatric disorders. *J Nerv Ment Dis*. 2013;**201** (12):1007–20

11. Marucha PT, Kiecolt-Glaser JK, Favagehi M. Mucosal wound healing is impaired by examination stress. *Psychosom Med*. 1998;**60**(3):362–5.

12. Walburn J, Vedhara K, Hankins M, Rixon L, Weinman J. Psychological stress and wound healing in humans: a systematic review and meta-analysis. *J Psychosom Res*. 2009;**67**(3):253–71.

13. Miller GE, Cohen S, Ritchey AK. Chronic psychological stress and the regulation of pro-inflammatory cytokines: a glucocorticoid-resistance model. *Health Psychol*. 2002;**21**(6):531–41.

14. Raison CL, Miller AH. When not enough is too much: the role of insufficient glucocorticoid signaling in the pathophysiology of stress-related disorders. 2003;**160** (9):1554–65

15. Miller AH, Maletic V, Raison, CL. Inflammation and its discontents: the role of cytokines in the pathophysiology of major depression. *Biol Psychiatry*. 2009;**65**(9), 732–41.

16. Valkanova V, Ebmeier KP, Allan CL. CRP, IL-6 and depression: a systematic review and meta-analysis of longitudinal studies. *J Affect Disord*. 2013;**150**(3), 736–44.

17. Mondelli V, Dazzan P, Pariante CM. Immune abnormalities across psychiatric disorders: clinical relevance. *BJPsych Advances*. 2015;**21**(3):150–6.

18. Baumeister D, Ciufolini S, Mondelli V. Effects of psychotropic drugs on inflammation: consequence or mediator of therapeutic effects in psychiatric treatment?. *Psychopharmacology*. 2016;**233** (9),1575–89.

19. Joëls M, Baram TZ. The neuro-symphony of stress. *Nat Rev Neurosci*. 2009;**10**(6), 459–66.

20. McEwen BS. Physiology and neurobiology of stress and adaptation: central role of the brain. *Physiol Rev*. 2007;**87**(3):873–904.

21. Sapolsky, R. M. The possibility of neurotoxicity in the hippocampus in major depression: a primer on neuron death. *Biol Psychiatry*. 2000;**48**(8):755–65.

22. De Kloet ER, Vreugdenhil E, Oitzl MS, Joëls, M. Brain corticosteroid receptor balance in health and disease. *Endocr Rev*. 1998;**19**(3):269–301.

23. Kalafatakis,K, Russell GM, Zarros A, Lightman SL. Temporal control of glucocorticoid neurodynamics and its relevance for brain homeostasis, neuropathology and glucocorticoid-based therapeutics. *Neurosci Biobehav Rev*. 2016;**61**:12–25.

24. Nemeroff, CB. The corticotropin-releasing factor: CRF hypothesis of depression: new findings and new directions. *Mol Psychiatry*. 1996;**1**(4):336.

25. Juruena MF, Baes CVW, Menezes IC, Guilherme F. Early life stress in depressive patients: role of glucocorticoid and mineralocorticoid receptors and of hypothalamic-pituitary-adrenal axis activity. *Curr PharmDes*. 2015;**21**(11):1369–78.

26. Reul JM, de Kloet ER. Two receptor systems for corticosterone in rat brain: microdistribution and differential occupation. *Endocrinology*. 1985;**117**:2505–11.

27. Spijker AT, van Rossum EFC. Glucocorticoid receptor polymorphisms in major depression. Focus on glucocorticoid sensitivity and neurocognitive functioning. *Ann N Y Acad Sci*. 2009;**1179**:199–215.

28. Elder G, Wetherell MA, Barclay NL, Ellis JG. The cortisol awakening response – applications and implications for sleep medicine. *Sleep Med Rev*. 2014;**18**:215e224.

29. Pruessner JC, Kirschbaum C, Meinlschmid G, Hellhammer D. Two formulas for computation of the area under the curve represent measures of total hormone concentration versus time-dependent change. *Psychoneuroendocrinology*. 2003;**28**:916–31.

30. Ruiz Roa SL, Elias PCL, Castro M, Moreira AC. The cortisol awakening response is blunted in patients with active Cushing's disease. *Eur J Endocrinology*. 2013;**168**:657–64.

31. Stalder T, Kirschbaum C, Kudielka BM, et al. Assessment of the cortisol awakening response: expert consensus guidelines. *Psychoneuroendocrinology*. 2016;**63**:414–32.

32. Juruena MF, Cleare AJ, Young AH. Neuroendocrine stress system in bipolar disorder. *Curr Top Behav Neurosci*. 2021;**48**:149–71.

33. Juruena MF. Early-life stress and HPA axis trigger recurrent adulthood depression. *Epilepsy Behav*. 2014;**38**:148–59.

34. Tofoli SMC, Baes CVW, Martins CMS, Juruena M. Early life stress, HPA axis, and depression. *Psychol Neurosci*. 2011;**4**(2):229–34.

35. Holsboer F. The corticosteroid receptor hypothesis of depression. *Neuropsychopharmacology*. 2000;**23**(5):477–501.

36. Roozendaal B, McEwan BS, Chattarj S. Stress, memory and the amygdala. *Nat Rev Neurosci*. 2009;**10**:423–33.

37. Gold PW, Chrousos GP. Organization of the stress system and its dysregulation in melancholic and atypical depression: high vs low CRH/NE states. *Mol Psychiatry*. 2002;**7**(3):254–75.

38. Juruena MF, Bocharova M, Agustini B, Young AH. Atypical and non-atypical depression: is HPA axis function a biomarker? *J Affect Disord*. 2018;**233**:45–67.

39. Juruena MF, Calil HM, Fleck MP, Del Porto JA. Melancholia in Latin American studies: a distinct mood disorder for the ICD-11. *Braz J Psychiatry*. 2011;**33**:S37≠S58.

40. Valiengo LL, Soeiro-de-Souza, MG, Andreazza AC, et al. Plasma cortisol in first episode drug-naïve mania: differential levels in euphoric versus irritable mood. *J Affect Disord*. 2012;**138**:149–52.

41. Palma BD, Tiba P, Machado RB, Tufik S, Suchecki D. Immune outcomes of sleep disorders: the hypothalamic-pituitary-adrenal axis as a modulatory factor. *Braz J Psychiatr*. 2007;**29**(Suppl 1):s33–s38

42. Young AH, Juruena MF. The neurobiology of bipolar disorder. *Curr Top Behav Neurosci*. 2021;**48**:1–20.

43. Kendler KS, Sheth K, Gardner CO, Prescott CA. Childhood parental loss and risk or first-onset of major depression and alcohol dependence: the time-decay of risk and sex differences. *Psychol Med*. 2002;**32**(7):1187–94.

44. Parker KJ, Schatzberg AF, Lyons DM. Neuroendocrine aspects of hypercortisolism in major depression. *Horm Behav*. 2003;**43**:60–66.

45. Carroll BJ, Cassidy F, Naftolowitz D, et al. Pathophysiology of hypercortisolism in depression. *Acta Psychiatr Scand Suppl*. 2007;**433**:90–103.

46. Gold PW, Goodwin FK, Chrousos GP. Clinical and biochemical manifestations of depression. Relation to the neurobiology of stress. *N Engl J Med*. 1988;**319**:413–20.

47. Juruena MF, Cleare AJ, Papadopoulos AS, et al. Different responses to dexamethasone and prednisolone in the same depressed patients. *Psychopharmacology*. 2006;**189**(2):225–35.

48. Gold PW, Wong M-L, Goldstein DS, et al. Cardiac implications of increased arterial entry and reversible 24-h central and peripheral norepinephrine levels in melancholia. *Proc Natl Acad Sci U S A*. 2005:**102**(23):8303–8.

49. Post RM Transduction of psychosocial stress into the neurobiology of recurrent affective disorder. *Am J Psychiatry*. 1992;**149**:999–1010.

50. Post RM. The kindling/sensitization model and early life stress. *Curr Top Behav Neurosci*. 2021;**48**:255–75.

51. Danese A, Moffitt TE, Harrington H, et al. Adverse childhood experiences and adult risk factors for age-related disease: depression, inflammation, and clustering of metabolic rick markers. *Arch Pedratr Adolesc Med*. 2009;**163**(12):1135–43.

52. Juruena MF, Cleare AJ. Overlap between atypical depression, seasonal affective disorder and chronic fatigue syndrome. *Rev Bras Psiquiatr*. 2007; **29** (Suppl I):S19–26.

53. Carroll BJ, Curtis GC, Mendels J. Neuroendocrine regulation in depression. II. Discrimination of depressed from nondepressed patients. *Arch Gen Psychiatry*. 1976; **33**(9):1051–8.

54. Ribeiro SC, Tandon R, Grunhaus L, Greden JF. The DST as a predictor of outcome in depression: a meta-analysis. *Am J Psychiatry*. 1993;**150**(11):1618–29.

55. Pariante CM, Papadopoulos AS, Poon L, et al. A novel prednisolone suppression test for the hypothalamic-pituitary-adrenal axis. *Biol Psychiatry*. 2002; **51** (11):922–30.

56. Von Bardeleben U, Holsboer F. Effect of age on the cortisol response to human corticotropin-releasing hormone in depressed patients pretreated with dexamethasone. *Biol Psychiatry*. 1991; **29**(10):1042–50.

57. Heuser I, Yassouridis A, Holsboer F. The combined dexamethasone/CRH test: a refined laboratory test for psychiatric disorders. *J Psychiatr Res*. 1994;**28**:341–56.

58. Zobel AW, Nickel T, Sonntag A, et al. Cortisol response in the combined dexamethasone/CRH test as predictor of relapse in patients with remitted depression. a prospective study. *J Psychiatr Res*. 2001;**35**:83–94.

59. Grossmann C, Scholz T, Rochel M, et al. Transactivation via the human glucocorticoid and mineralocorticoid receptor by therapeutically used steroids in CV-1 cells: A comparison of their glucocorticoid and mineralocorticoid properties. *Eur J Endocrinol*. 2004;**151**(3):397–406.

60. Juruena MF, Pariante CM, Papadoulos AS, et al. Prednisolone suppression test in depression: prospective study of the role of HPA axis dysfunction in treatment resistance. *Br J Psychiatry*. 2009;**194** (4):342–9.

61. Valvassori SS, Resende WR, Dal-Pont G, et al. Lithium ameliorates sleep deprivation-induced mania-like behavior, hypothalamic-pituitary-adrenal (HPA) axis alterations, oxidative stress and elevations of cytokine concentrations in the brain and serum of mice. *Bipolar Disord*. 2017;**19**(4):246–58

62. Mukherjee D. Weissenkampen JD. Wasserman E, et al. Dysregulated diurnal cortisol pattern and heightened night-time cortisol in individuals with bipolar disorder. *Neuropsychobiology*. 2021;**81**(1):1–9.

63. Yang S, Van Dongen HPA, Wang K, Berrettini W, Bućan M. Assessment of circadian function in fibroblasts of patients with bipolar disorder. *Mol Psychiatry*. 2009;**14**(2):143–55

64. Freeman AJ, Youngstrom EA, Youngstrom JK, Findling RL. Disruptive mood dysregulation disorder in a community mental health clinic: prevalence, comorbidity and correlates. *J Child Adolesc Psychopharmacol*. 2016;**26**(2):123–30.

65. Muran JC, Safran JD, Eubanks CF, Gorman BS. The effect of alliance-focused training on a cognitive-behavioral therapy for personality disorders. *J Consult Clin Psychol*. 2018;**86**(4):384.

66. Lomholt LH, Andersen DV, Sejrsgaard-Jacobsen C, et al. Mortality rate trends in patients diagnosed with schizophrenia or bipolar disorder: a nationwide study with 20 years of follow-up. *Int J Bipolar Disord*. 2019;**7** (1):1–8.

67. Maripuu M, Wikgren M, Karling P, Adolfsson R, Norrback KF. Relative hypo- and hypercortisolism are both associated with depression and lower quality of life in bipolar disorder: a cross-sectional study. *PLoS One*. 2014;**9**(6):e98682

68. Maes M, Landucci Bonifacio K, Morelli NR, et al. Major differences in neurooxidative and neuronitrosative stress pathways between major depressive disorder and types I and II bipolar disorder. *Mol Neurobiol*. 2019;**56**(1):141–56.

69. Maripuu M, Wikgren M, Karling P, Adolfsson R, Norrback KF. Hyper- and hypocortisolism in bipolar disorder – a beneficial influence of lithium on the HPA-axis? *J Affect Disord*. 2017;**213**:161–7.

70. Quidé Y, Girshkin L, Watkeys OJ, et al. The relationship between cortisol reactivity and emotional brain function is differently moderated by childhood trauma, in bipolar disorder, schizophrenia and health individuals. *Eur Arch Psychiatry Clin Neurosci*. 2021;**271**(6),1089–1109.

71. Steinberg LJ, Mann JJ. Abnormal stress responsiveness and suicidal behavior: a risk phenotype. *Biomark Neuropsychiatry*. 2020;**2**:100011.

72. Steullet P, Cabungcal JH, Bukhari SA, et al. The thalamic reticular nucleus in schizophrenia and bipolar disorder: role of parvalbumin-expressing neuron networks and oxidative stress. *Mol Psychiatry*. 2018;**23**(10):2057–65.

73. Markopoulou K, Fischer S, Papadopoulos A, et al. Comparison of hypothalamo-pituitary-adrenal function in treatment resistant unipolar and bipolar depression. *Transl Psychiatry*. 2021;**11**(1):1–8.

74. Michael UE, Oyesanya MO. Relating the effect of HPA axis to the emotional state of bipolar II disorder patient. *Asian Res J Math*. 2018;**11**(1):1–19.

75. Lightman SL, Birnie, MT, Conway-Campbell BL. Dynamics of ACTH and cortisol secretion and implications for disease. *Endocrine Rev*. 2020;**41** (3):470–90.

113

76. Wehr TA. Bipolar mood cycles and lunar tidal cycles. *Mol Psychiatry*. 2018;**23**(4):923–31.

77. Steen, N. E., Lorentzen, S., Barrett, E. A., et al. Sex-specific cortisol levels in bipolar disorder and schizophrenia during mental challenge – relationship to clinical characteristics and medication. *Prog Neuropsychopharmacology Biol Psychiatry*. 2011;**35**(4):1100–7.

78. Fang L, Yu Q, Yin F, et al. Combined cortisol and melatonin measurements with detailed parameter analysis can assess the circadian rhythms in bipolar disorder patients. *Brain Behav*. 2021;**11**(7):e02186.

79. Watson S, Gallagher P, Ritchie JC, Ferrier IN, Young AH. Hypothalamic-pituitary-adrenal axis function in patients with bipolar disorder. *Br J Psychiatry*. 2004;**184**(6):496–502.

80. Mazer AK, Cleare AJ, Young AH, Juruena MF. Bipolar affective disorder and borderline personality disorder: differentiation based on the history of early life stress and psychoneuroendocrine measures. *Behav Brain Res*. 2019;**357**:48–56.

81. Heim C, Newport DJ, Heit S, et al. Pituitary-adrenal and autonomic responses to stress in women after sexual and physical abuse in childhood. *JAMA*. 2000;**284**(5):592–7.

82. Fergusson DM, Swain-Campbell NR, Horwood LJ. Does sexual violence contribute to elevated rates of anxiety and depression in females? *Psychol Med*. 2002;**32**(6):991–6.

83. Bernstein DP, Fink L, Handelsman L, et al. Initial reliability and validity of a new retrospective measure of child abuse and neglect. *Am J Psychiatry*. 1994;**151**(8):1132–6.

84. Bernstein DP, Stein JA, Newcomb MD, et al. Development and validation of a brief screening version of the childhood trauma questionnaire. *Child Abuse Negl*. 2003;**27**(2):169–90.

85. Post RM, Altshuler LL, Leverich GS, et al. Role of childhood adversity in the development of medical co-morbidities associated with bipolar disorder. *J Affect Disord*. 2013;**147**:288–94.

86. Lupien SJ, McEwen BS, Gunnar MR, et al. Effects of stress throughout the lifespan on the brain, behaviour and cognition. *Nat Rev Neurosci*. 2009;**10**(6):434–45.

87. Andersen SL. Trajectories of brain development: point of vulnerability or window of opportunity? *Neurosci Biobehav Rev*. 2003;**27**:3–18.

88. Juruena MF, Bourne M, Young AH, Cleare AJ. Hypothalamic-pituitary-adrenal axis dysfunction by early life stress. *Neurosci Lett*. 2021;**759**:136037.

89. Heim C, Nemeroff CB. The role of childhood trauma in the neurobiology of mood and anxiety disorders: preclinical and clinical studies. *Biol Psychiatry*. 2001;**49**:1023–39.

90. Nemeroff CB, Heim CM, Thase ME, et al. Differential responses to psychotherapy versus pharmacotherapy in patients with chronic forms of major depression and childhood trauma. *Proc Natl Acad Sci U S A*. 2003;**100**(24):14293–6.

91. Shea A, Walsh C, Macmillan H, Steiner M. Child maltreatment and HPA axis dysregulation: relationship to major depressive disorder and post traumatic stress disorder in females. *Psychoneuroendocrinology*. 2005;**30**:162–78.

92. Tyrka AR, Wier L, Price LH, et al. Childhood parental loss and adult hypothalamic-pituitary-adrenal function. *Biol Psychiatry*. 2008;**63**:1147–54.

93. Juruena MF, Gadelrab R, Cleare AJ, Young AH. Epigenetics: a missing link between early life stress and depression. *Prog Neuropsychopharmacol Biol Psychiatry*. 2021;**109**:110231.

94. Chen Y, Brunson KL, Adelmann G, et al. Hippocampal corticotropin releasing hormone: pre- and postsynaptic location and release by stress. *Neuroscience*. 2004;**126**(3): 533–40.

95. Brunson KL, Eghbal-Ahmadi M, Bender R, et al. Long-term, progressive hippocampal cell loss and dysfunction induced by early-life administration of corticotropin-releasing hormone reproduce the effects of early-life stress. *Proc Natl Acad Sci U S A*. 2001;**98**(15):8856–61.

96. Faravelli C, Amedei SG, Rotella F, et al. Childhood traumata, Dexamethasone Suppression Test and psychiatric symptoms: a trans-diagnostic approach. *Psychol Med*. 2010;**40**:2037–48.

97. Herman JP, Patel PD, Akil H, Watson S. Localization and regulation of glucocorticoid and mineralocorticoid receptor messenger RNAs in the hippocampal formation of the rat. *Mol Endocrinol*. 1989;**3**:1886–94.

98. Patel PD, Lopez JF, Lyons DM, et al. Glucocorticoid and mineralocorticoid receptor mRNA expression in squirrel monkey brain. *J Psychiatr Res*. 2000;**34**:383–92.

99. Young EA, Lopez JF, Murphy-Weinberg V, Watson SJ, Akil H. Normal pituitary response to metyrapone in the morning in depressed patients: implications for circadian regulation of CRH secretion. *Biol Psychiatry*. 1997; **41**:1149–55.

100. Kellner M, Yehuda R. Do panic disorder and posttraumatic stress disorder share a common psychoneuroendocrinology? *Psychoneuroendocrinology*. 1999;**24**:485–504

101. Yehuda R, Boisoneau D, Lowy MT, Giller EL Jr, Dose-response changes in plasma cortisol and

lymphocyte glucocorticoid receptors following dexamethasone administration in combat veterans with and without posttraumatic stress disorder. *Arch Gen Psychiatry.* 1995;52:583–93

102. Spencer RL, Kim PJ, Kalman BA, Cole MA. Evidence for mineralocorticoid receptor facilitation of glucocorticoid receptor-dependent regulation of hypothalamic-pituitary-adrenal axis activity. *Endocrinology.* 1998;139(6):2718–26

103. Gesing A, Bilang-Bleuel A, Droste SK, et al. Psychological stress increases hippocampal mineralocorticoid receptor levels: involvement of corticotropin-releasing hormone. *J Neurosci.* 2001;21:4822–9.

The Common Ancestors of Anxiety and Depression: Comorbidity as a Cognitive, Behavioural, Neural and Cellular Phenotype, and Current Evidence for Photobiomodulation as a Novel Treatment

Gabriel Barg, Julia N. Lukacs, and Guillermo Perez Algorta

As of June 2021, the COVID-19 pandemic had threatened the physical and mental health of individuals for over a year. The capacity for resilience both as individuals and as a global community had been and continues to be tested. Billions of people may be experiencing sustained emotional stress. This has been brought about or exacerbated by increased levels of sadness, fear of illness or their own death or that of a loved one, and hopelessness due to the personal and material losses associated with the pandemic.

Different groups – older adults, healthcare front-line workers, and children – have faced a range of common and specific challenges. Those with pre-existing mental health conditions, such as depression and/or anxiety, are confronting new situations of daily life disruptions, such as longer periods of isolation or lack of access to health support. Preliminary evidence comparing mental health experiences before and after COVID-19 indicates an increase in levels of psychological distress in US adults [1] and adults from the United Kingdom [2].

In the Netherlands, people with more severe chronic mental health problems reported more fear of COVID-19 and less coping with the pandemic than people with less severe or no mental health issues [3]. However, this same research shows that the relative increase in depressive symptoms, anxiety, worry, and loneliness is greater in people with no or less severe problems than those with more severe or already existing problems, foreshadowing the impact of COVID-19 on mental wellness of the general population.

Now that vaccination programs have been initiated and have shown signs of success around the world, albeit inequalities between low- and high-income countries, the resolution of the acute COVID-19 crisis is within view. Nevertheless, even in high-income countries such as England, first models forecast the impact of COVID-19 on mental health to be long-lasting. It is safe to anticipate significant increments in demand (referrals) of mental health services over the next years throughout the world. It would be premature to despair, however, as crises are often a time of ample opportunity.

The information we have gleaned from the COVID-19 crisis will allow us, as a field, to examine our conceptualisation of mental health issues, their treatment and limitations, and whether there are new treatment alternatives that require further evaluation. This chapter intends to be a response to this opportunity, where we review epidemiological and clinical data concerning the problem of anxiety and depression comorbidity. This is followed by the description of novel theoretical models of this comorbidity, which integrate psychopathological and neuroscientific evidence in different dimensions: cognition, behaviour, neural circuits, and cellular mechanisms. Finally, with a focus on recent key findings on intracellular processes involving the mitochondria shared by anxiety and depression, the last section of the chapter provides a review of the evidence of photobiomodulation (PBM); a promising non-invasive, low-cost intervention for anxiety and depression.

Evidence on Comorbidity: Epidemiological and Clinical Data

Before COVID-19, the estimated lifetime prevalence of anxiety disorders was between 25% and 29%. For unipolar major depression alone this number was

17% [4]. Regarding the prevalence of comorbid depression and anxiety, in the United States, 58% of those with lifetime depression also had a lifetime anxiety disorder diagnosis, and for those with major depressive disorder (MDD) in the past 12 month, 51% had an anxiety disorder [5]. Data from the same study also showed that 68% of people with secondary depression presented with a primary anxiety disorder (contrasting, for example, with 19% with primary substance use disorder). The types of anxiety in descending order of frequency observed with depression are generalised anxiety disorder, panic disorder, and post-traumatic stress disorder (PTSD) [6].

Adding to the epidemiological evidence about the co-occurrence of these anxiety disorders and depression, clinical data tell us that first-line treatment recommendations for these problems are similar if not identical (e.g., selective serotonin reuptake inhibitrs [SSRI], cognitive behavioural therapy [CBT]). They also share the same challenges regarding treatment response. Current treatments are still suboptimal, resulting in limited remission rate efficiency for depression (approximately 50% in adults) [7], while more than a third of anxiety disorder patients are treatment-resistant [8].

These observations imply that the commonalities between depression and anxiety need special attention. Comparing similarities between mood and anxiety at a cognitive, behavioural, and neurobiological level may elucidate our understanding of their comorbidity. Considering comorbidity in this manner may advance both theoretical conceptualisation and treatment.

The Cognitive Dimension

At a cognitive level, different hypotheses involving higher-order cognitive schemes for processing information have been proposed. One classic proposal comes from Beck [9], who suggested that anxiety disorders are characterised by vulnerability schemes, while mood disorders would be characterised by schemes of self-depreciation. *Schemes*, as defined by Beck, are internally stored representations of stimuli, ideas, or experiences, capable of controlling information processing systems [10]. The cognitive similarities between depression and anxiety are observed at basic, automatic levels of processing, rather than at content levels. In these automatic levels, shared cognitive biases have been found, especially in attention and memory.

People experiencing anxiety tend to allocate more attentional resources to threatening stimuli, ignoring non-threatening stimuli. This observation has been replicated in diverse populations using different experimental paradigms, such as emotional stroop, dot probe, and flanker tasks [11,12]. A similar type of processing has been observed in people experiencing depression, where the ability to disengage from negative stimuli to allocate resources in the environment is compromised [13,14].

Attentional disengagement is a key coping mechanism to counter negative or threatening situations. COVID-19 is an example of a real-world test of attentional disengagement capacity, as social networks and media are constantly offering information about disease, danger, and loss. In fact, to respond to this challenging situation, one of the recommendations during the lockdowns was to "take breaks from the news" to facilitate people disengaging from negative events and focusing on other things [15].

Similar shared mechanisms have also been identified regarding memory in anxiety and depression [16]. For example, selective retrieval of negative information is a maintenance factor of worry and depressed mood [17]. People recognise items related to experiences (familiarity) but have trouble retrieving the contextual information related to that element (recollection). In the context of COVID-19, selective retrieval may occur when watching news related to the pandemic. Familiarity is demonstrated when people later remember precise verbatim information only (e.g., number of deaths per day) instead of contextual details (recollection).

From an adaptive point of view, however, the recovery of contextual cues (e.g., information about location and time, sanitary conditions) may be considered a better resource to cope with challenges such as COVID-19. An individual who recalls only familiarity-based specific experiences reinforces the feeling of having seen something negative, but is unable to recollect specific details of past news to palliate negative experiences. This selective retrieval in favour of familiarity (versus recollection) impairs coping and promotes generalisation of fear [18]. In anxiety, the familiarity bias is evidenced when the anxious subject recognises negative stimuli with accuracy but might have difficulty recovering contextual information, necessary to effectively cope with the situation. Consequently, they develop increasing avoidance of such stimuli. In depression, this bias towards familiarity manifests in the over-generalisation of autobiographical memory, preventing a reality-based correction of global negative self-referent thoughts [19].

In summary, both anxiety and depression manifest memory biases in their faulty retrieval of items without contextual information. The difference between the posited processes in both conditions is that familiarity recognition is oriented towards future stimuli in anxiety and overgeneralisation is oriented towards the past stimuli in depression [20]. These basic cognitive biases in attention and memory constitute some of the basis of common clinical observations of repetitive negative thinking in people with anxiety (worry, "what if?") and depression (rumination, "why?") [21].

The Behavioural Domain

At a behavioural level, the inhibition of functional behaviour is characteristic of anxiety and depression. In the former case, inhibition is linked to the avoidance of stimuli, while in the latter it is due to a lack of motivation [22,23]. These two aspects of inhibition have been explained through two propositions of cognitive functioning: by the action of a behavioural inhibition system [24] and by the withdrawal-approach complex [25].

Excessive activation of the behavioural inhibition system, triggered by increased punishment or the absence of reward expectations, has often been observed in anxiety and depression [26,27]. The functions impaired in people experiencing depression and anxiety extend to the capacity to stop ongoing behaviours to avoid harm and the search for other adaptive goals. Attention needs to be biased towards negative information to recognise negative feedback and stop an ongoing action. Furthermore, to ensure that new goals are associated with positive outcomes in personal experience, memory retrieval must also be biased towards negative content to screen any potential negative outcomes.

During the COVID-19 health crisis, a study corroborated the impact of behavioural inhibition system activation. Specifically, young adults with a stable pattern of excessive activation of the behavioural inhibition system in childhood (measured using behavioural observations of children's response to novel toys and interactions with unfamiliar adults) had problems with worry regulation in adolescence and developed more anxiety symptoms during the pandemic [28]. Broadly (beyond COVID-19), this kind of worry dysregulation has been considered a developmental pathway to depression in youth [29].

The Neurobiological Domain

At a neurobiological level, people with high trait anxiety (a phenotype associated with anxiety and mood disorders risk [30]) tend to present enhanced activation of the amygdala in response to emotional stimuli, mainly in the basolateral area. In addition, concomitant hyper-reactivity of the hypothalamic–pituitary–adrenal (HPA) axis, present in individuals with high trait anxiety, potentiates a "fight or flight" physiological response not only to negative stimuli, but also to neutral stimuli perceived as threatening [31].

Individuals with high trait anxiety may also show disruptions between the amygdala and other brain regions. For example, it has been proposed that the prefrontal cortex may have limited capacity to down-regulate hyperactivation of the amygdala caused by negative stimuli, and the integration of contextual information via hippocampal connections may be compromised and restricted. Evidence on these processes was assessed and summarised in a recent meta-analysis of 226 functional magnetic resonance imaging (fMRI) studies of people with both anxiety and mood disorders [32]. Three right-sided clusters of hypoactivation were identified centred in the inferior prefrontal cortex/insula, the inferior parietal lobule, and the putamen, while the dorsal anterior cingulate cortex, the left amygdala/parahippocampal gyrus, and the left thalamus were hyperactivated across the reviewed studies.

In sum, when individuals with high trait anxiety are exposed to major stressful life events, the hyper-reactivity of the amygdala to threats is strengthened and reinforced by a loop of sympathetic activation produced by HPA dysfunction [30].

Meanwhile, attention and memory bias are consolidated in a mood-congruent bias, oriented to negative thoughts. Intense negative affect would activate the behavioural inhibition system and interfere with higher-order cognitive processes, such as executive functions, social cognition, and learning. Behavioural and neurophysiological changes reinforce each other, for the better or for the worse.

The person experiencing intense negative affect and cognitive biases about their own abilities will avoid interactions with other individuals, decreasing social reinforcement. The lack of motivation for social interactions could lead to learned helplessness [33]. According to the tripartite model [22,23], the prevalence of each dimension of the process (distress, low positive affect [anhedonia] and/or physiological hyperarousal) will determine the development of anxiety problems (i.e., worry, hyper-arousal) [34,28], mood problems (loss of motivation), or a combination of both, comorbidity [35].

The Cellular Domain: Mitochondrial Function

Several single nucleotide polymorphisms (SNPs) associated with the serotonergic, dopaminergic, and GABAergic system have been associated with trait anxiety. These SNPs are posted to act through the modification of proteins that alter behavioural outcomes, such as reactivity to emotional stimuli [36,37]. These findings have informed the development and refinement of pharmacological interventions where monoamine depletion plays a role as a mechanistic model. However, the delay observed between pharmacological action and clinical relief (e.g., antidepressants act within minutes to hours of administration, contrasting with the alleviation of symptoms that usually happens after two weeks of chronic administration) unveil the presence of a more complex pathogenic model. In fact, new ideas have been proposed about the role of the downstream cascade resulting from cellular events and adaptive brain processes beyond monoamine transmission as an underlying element shared by anxiety and depression [38,39]. In particular, mitochondrial function has been linked to the pathophysiology and treatment of these problems [40].

The complex intracellular cascades upregulated in stress-related conditions such as anxiety and depression may be associated with mitochondrial capacity for resilience to sustain resources and provide stability at a cellular level [41]. For example, elevated levels of glucocorticoids can compromise cellular energy capacity and facilitate neurotoxicity [40,42,43]. Also, downregulation of brain-derived neurotrophic factor (BDNF) during stress [44], and disruptions in the regulation of intracellular calcium – a critical mediator of apoptosis – can generate reactive oxygen species (ROS) via the electron transport chain [45].

These are examples of mitochondrial function affected by glucocorticoids and other stress mediators. However, it is notable that stress hormone glucocorticoids are produced and metabolised by mitochondria, determining the magnitude of stress response and regulating the cellular homeostasis during response to stress. Mitochondria may be at the core of the mechanisms of stress adaptation and regulation [46]. Mitochondrial function is fundamental for neuronal growth and sprouting, synaptic transmission, neuronal plasticity, and connectivity, supporting complex cognitive and behavioural functions that are common to anxiety and depression [46,47].

Unsurprisingly, new treatments informed by the role of mitochondria have been developed to target varied medical conditions. Well-known limitations with current mental health treatments, such as side effects of pharmacological treatments [48] or lack of access to evidence-based psychological interventions, have stimulated new treatment alternatives informed by these mechanistic models. Photobiomodulation (PBM), an intervention based on light as energy to support biological changes, is one example of a recent mechanism-targeting intervention. The next section offers an introduction to photobiomodulation and summarises preliminary findings of studies with non-responsive groups of patients suffering from mood and anxiety problems.

Photobiomodulation: A New Light in Treatment Options?

With appropriate wavelengths and light dosing parameters, all eukaryotic cells and tissues should be responsive to PBM via mitochondria [49–51]. Two mechanisms have been proposed to explain this mitochondrial response and the production of ATP. The most popular model refers to the absorption of the photons by cytochrome C oxidase (CCO), leading to high levels of adenosine triphosphate (ATP) [52]. A second novel model [53] suggests that PBM targets the interfacial water layer (IWL) viscosity on hydrophilic surfaces, associated with ATP-level restoration. In this model, the target for photons absorbed by cells will be H_2O molecules constituting the IWL on intracellular surfaces, whose physical properties can be modulated by light.

To reach its target, the photons need to cross barriers, and different strategies are under evaluation to obtain better stimulation of different brain areas [54].

In transcranial PBM (t-PBM), the most prevalent modality, the light must cross tissues and the skull to reach the cortex, and it is estimated that near infrared radiation (NIR) coming from low-level lasers or light-emitting diodes (LED) has a penetration rate of 2–3% at target prefrontal cortex regions [50]. This small percentage fluence (or energy density) on the human brain has been considered equivalent to the energy density capable of inducing neurological benefits in animal model studies [55]. Furthermore, different studies are currently testing different parameters such as irradiation wavelengths, continuous or pulse patterns to enhance penetration (for a review relevant to mental health, see [56]).

Photobiomodulation for Anxious and Depressive Symptomatology

Few pioneer animal studies showed positive clinical results for treatment of anxiety and depression problems with t-PBM [57,58]. These results have been replicated by Eshaghi et al. [59], where they delivered t-PBM using animal (mice) models of anxiety and depression (chronic restraint stress). The research indicated noticeable improvement in behavioural results, decreased serum cortisol levels, increased serotonin, and decreased nitric oxide concentrations in the prefrontal cortex and hippocampus.

Caldieraro and Cassano (2019) conducted a systematic review, indicating the growth of literature on PBM in humans [50]. In 2009, Schiffer et al. [60] conducted a within-subjects pilot study, and found that single-session t-PBM (four times 4 minutes, randomised NIR/sham, at 810 nm) delivered at electrode sites F3 and F4 (on the forehead, bilaterally targeting the dorsolateral prefrontal cortex) led to remission (assessed using the Hamilton Depression Rating Scale [HAM-D]) in six of ten patients. Nine of these ten patients had comorbid anxiety, and they found remission in seven of ten subjects for anxiety (using the Hamilton Anxiety Rating Scale [HAM-A]). Greatest changes were observed at the two-week mark.

Of note, two randomised clinical trials of t-PBM and two randomised clinical trials of low-intensity laser acupuncture have been conducted. Adjunctive t-PBM (at 1,064 nm) to attention bias modification (ABM) treatment for elevated depressive symptoms ($n = 51$) at right and left (bilateral) forehead locations demonstrated that t-PBM enhanced improvements.

However, this was specific to right stimulation (not left), and there were no significant differences due solely to t-PBM [61]. These results may be expected given the additive nature of the therapy.

In non-adjunctive trials, Cassano et al. [62] utilised t-PBM (823 nm) to test efficacy in MDD treatment. Twenty-one participants were randomised to a sham or experimental condition and received bilateral stimulation to the forehead. The PBM condition yielded a greater decrease in scores than the sham condition on the HAM-D, and response to treatment was higher in the active treatment condition than the sham condition (50% and 27%, respectively).

The team of Quah-Smith et al. ([63], $n = 30$); ([64], $n = 47$) took a different approach and tested acupuncture points as targets for laser therapy on limbs and trunks (primary depression acupoints) over up to 12 sessions over 8 weeks. The researchers found significant antidepressant effects in both samples.

While these studies are smaller and may leave something to be desired in terms of sample size, a team of researchers in Russia [65,66] have conducted a series of larger ($n = 180$ and $n = 79$) open studies using a combination of red and NIR intravenously and transcutaneously. The first study included a treatment group who accepted PBM as an add-on to pharmacological treatments, resulting in significant decrease in HAM-D and HAM-A scores (as compared to non-randomised controls). The second compared outcomes in individuals with MDD, bipolar disorder (BD), or mixed diagnoses and notably reported a 23% rate of relapse in study participants as compared to 50% in non-randomised, non-blinded controls.

These results in large part focused on depression (with the exception of [60] and [66]), but case studies in other mood and anxiety disorders corroborate results. One elderly individual saw a 50% improvement in symptoms of anxiety while using intranasal PBM and t-PBM as an adjunctive treatment to pharmaceutical treatment for MDD with anxious distress [67]. Four patients with BD diagnoses who used bilateral t-PBM to address anhedonia residuals also saw improvements in their condition [68].

Overall, PBM is an example of a novel intervention for treatment of mood and anxiety disorders that is simple and cost-effective, with few apparent side effects [50]. Several clinical trials (NCT02959307, NCT02898233, and NCT03420456) have been registered, and results should hopefully be forthcoming.

Conclusions and Future Directions

The COVID-19 pandemic tested our response capacity to address pre-existing and new global mental health issues, in particular prevalent ones such as the comorbidity of anxiety and depression. Different types of health measures are needed, from public health initiatives to novel clinical interventions for those experiencing pervasive negative experiences related to anxiety and depression.

Photobiomodulation may be a promising treatment option that is easily deployable, low cost, and potentially effective as a complement to traditional evidence-based approaches. Through targeting basic cellular processes, PBM generates a positive cascade in the nervous system, improving regulation of behaviour, affect, and cognition. Moreover, some evidence shows a general neuro-protective effect of PBM. Enhancement of learning and memory has been observed in preliminary studies with people with Alzheimer's disease, dementia, or stroke and with healthy subjects [69].

This evidence highlights a general improvement of prefrontal cortex functioning (the most frequent sites in anxiety and depression studies where LEDs are applied in the F3 and F4 positions in the 10–20 international system), as an important mediator for the behavioural effects of PBM therapy. The prefrontal cortex has an important role orienting basic cognitive processes (attention, memory) and emotion regulation. In that sense, PBM can potentiate traditional pharmacological and psychotherapeutic interventions. Ongoing clinical trials will advance our knowledge about PBM, including the time-to-effects of metabolic changes, and should deepen our understanding of these changes using multimodal neuroscience approaches.

For example, MRI can be used to describe functional changes in blood flow (BOLD signal in functional MRI or even functional near-infrared spectroscopy [fNIRS]) and identify cellular biochemical mechanisms (magnetic resonance spectroscopy). At a clinical level, combining PBM with electroencephalography (EEG) could be an excellent avenue for monitoring changes in cortical activity. Moreover, in a setup for evoked-related potentials, experimental tasks could be used to test specific cognitive effects of PBM. Photo stimulation and EEG sensors could be integrated in the same device, at a reasonable cost and with high temporal resolution.

In conclusion, this chapter demonstrates that reviewing important characteristics of the comorbidity of depression and anxiety in the cognitive, behavioural, and neurobiological domains may unearth commonalities pertinent to the improvement of care. This is demonstrated through the comorbidity in neurobiological (mitochondrial) functioning and its cognitive and behavioural correlates, which lend credence to the transdiagnostic treatments such as PBM. This novel treatment may be both appropriate and promising in targeting of shared mechanisms, particularly essential in a post-pandemic world with an increased demand for mental health services.

References

1. McGinty EE, Presskreischer R, Han H, Barry CL. Psychological distress and loneliness reported by US adults in 2018 and April 2020. *JAMA*. 2020;**324**(1):93–4.

2. Pierce M, Hope H, Ford T, et al. Mental health before and during the COVID-19 pandemic: a longitudinal probability sample survey of the UK population. *Lancet Psychiat*. 2020;**7**(10):883–92.

3. Pan K-Y, Kok AAL, Eikelenboom M, et al. The mental health impact of the COVID-19 pandemic on people with and without depressive, anxiety, or obsessive-compulsive disorders: a longitudinal study of three Dutch case-control cohorts. *Lancet Psychiat*. 2021;**8**(2):121–9.

4. Kessler RC, de Jonge P, Shahly V, et al. Epidemiology of depression. In IH Gotlib and CL Hamman, editors. *Handbook of Depression*. New York: Guilford Press, 2014; 7–24.

5. Kessler RC, Berglund P, Demler O, et al. The epidemiology of major depressive disorder: results from the National Comorbidity Survey Replication (NCS-R). *JAMA*. 2003;**289**(23):3095–105.

6. Kessler RC, Berglund P, Demler O, et al. Lifetime prevalence and age-of-onset distributions of DSM-IV disorders in the National Comorbidity Survey Replication. *Arch Gen Psychiatry*. 2005;**62**(6):593–602.

7. Rush AJ, Warden D, Wisniewski SR, et al. STAR*D: revising conventional wisdom. *CNS Drugs*. 2009;**23**(8):627–47.

8. Bystritsky A. Treatment-resistant anxiety disorders. *Mol Psychiatry*. 2006;**11**(9):805–14.

9. Beck AT, Brown G, Steer RA, Eidelson JI, Riskind JH. Differentiating anxiety and depression: a test of the cognitive content-specificity hypothesis. *J Abnorm Psychol*. 1987;**96**(3):179.

10. Beck AT. *Depression Causes and Treatment*. Philadelphia: University of Pennsylvania Press, 1972.

11. Williams JMG. *Cognitive Psychology and Emotional Disorders*. 2nd ed. Chichester: Wiley, 1997; **xii.**

12. Bar-Haim Y, Lamy D, Pergamin L, Bakermans-Kranenburg MJ, Van Ijzendoorn MH. Threat-related attentional bias in anxious and nonanxious individuals: a meta-analytic study. *Psychol Bull.* 2007;**133**(1):1.

13. Armstrong T, Olatunji BO. Eye tracking of attention in the affective disorders: A meta-analytic review and synthesis. *Clin Psychol Rev.* 2012;**32**(8):704–23.

14. Peckham AD, McHugh RK, Otto MW. A meta-analysis of the magnitude of biased attention in depression. *Depress Anxiety.* 2010;**27**(12):1135–42.

15. NIMH. Supporting mental health during the COVID-19 pandemic 2020 Available from: www.nimh.nih.gov/news/science-news/2020/supporting-mental-health-during-the-covid-19-pandemic.

16. Duyser F, van Eijndhoven P, Bergman M, et al. Negative memory bias as a transdiagnostic cognitive marker for depression symptom severity. *J Affect Disord.* 2020;**274**:1165–72.

17. Mathersul DC, Ruscio AM. Forecasting the future, remembering the past: misrepresentations of daily emotional experience in generalized anxiety disorder and major depressive disorder. *Cognit Ther Res.* 2020;**44**(1):73–88.

18. Barg G, Carboni A, Roche T, Nin V, Carretié L. Evaluating the association of high trait anxiety with a bias in familiarity-based recognition of emotional stimuli. *J Psychophysiol.* 2020;**34**(3):179–91.

19. Raes F, Hermans D, Williams JMG, et al. Reduced autobiographical memory specificity and rumination in predicting the course of depression. *J Abnorm Psychol.* 2006;**115**(4):699.

20. Eysenck MW, Fajkowska M. Anxiety and depression: toward overlapping and distinctive features. *Cognit Emot.* 2018;**32**(7):1391–400.

21. McEvoy PM, Watson H, Watkins ER, Nathan P. The relationship between worry, rumination, and comorbidity: evidence for repetitive negative thinking as a transdiagnostic construct. *J Affect Disord.* 2013;**151**(1):313–20.

22. Clark LA, Watson D. Tripartite model of anxiety and depression: psychometric evidence and taxonomic implications. *J Abnorm Psychol.* 1991;**100**(3):316–36.

23. Watson D. Differentiating the mood and anxiety disorders: a quadripartite model. *Annu Rev Clin Psychol.* 2009;**5**:221–47.

24. Gray J, McNaughton N. *The Neuropsychology of Anxiety: An Enquiry into the Functions of the Septohippocampal System*. 2nd ed: Oxford: Oxford University Press, 2003.

25. Davidson RJ, Ekman P, Saron CD, Senulis JA, Friesen WV. Approach-withdrawal and cerebral asymmetry: emotional expression and brain physiology: I. *J Pers Soc Psychol.* 1990;**58**(2):330.

26. Winer ES, Salem T. Reward devaluation: dot-probe meta-analytic evidence of avoidance of positive information in depressed persons. *Psychol Bull.* 2016;**142**(1):18.

27. Larson CL, Nitschke JB, Davidson RJ. Common and distinct patterns of affective response in dimensions of anxiety and depression. *Emotion* (Washington, DC). 2007;**7**(1):182.

28. Zeytinoglu S, Morales S, Lorenzo NE, et al. A developmental pathway from early behavioral inhibition to young adults' anxiety during the COVID-19 pandemic. *J Am Acad Child Adolesc Psychiatry.* 2021;**60**(10):1300–8.

29. Folk JB, Zeman JL, Poon JA, Dallaire DH. A longitudinal examination of emotion regulation: pathways to anxiety and depressive symptoms in urban minority youth. *Child Adolesc Ment Health.* 2014;**19**(4):243–50.

30. Sandi C, Richter-Levin G. From high anxiety trait to depression: a neurocognitive hypothesis. *Trends Neurosci.* 2009;**32**(6):312–20.

31. Rodrigues SM, LeDoux JE, Sapolsky RM. The influence of stress hormones on fear circuitry. *Annu Rev Neurosci.* 2009;**32**:289–313.

32. Janiri D, Moser DA, Doucet GE, et al. Shared neural phenotypes for mood and anxiety disorders: a meta-analysis of 226 task-related functional imaging studies. *JAMA Psychiatry.* 2020;**77**(2):172–9.

33. Chorpita BF, Barlow DH. The development of anxiety: the role of control in the early environment. *Psychol Bull.* 1998;**124**(1):3–21.

34. Ravaldi C, Ricca V, Wilson A, Homer C, Vannacci A. Previous psychopathology predicted severe COVID-19 concern, anxiety, and PTSD symptoms in pregnant women during "lockdown" in Italy. *Arch Womens Ment Health.* 2020;**26**(6):783–6.

35. Fountoulakis KN, Apostolidou MK, Atsiova MB, et al. Self-reported changes in anxiety, depression and suicidality during the COVID-19 lockdown in Greece. *J Affect Disord.* 2021;**279**:624–9.

36. Weger M, Sandi C. High anxiety trait: a vulnerable phenotype for stress-induced depression. *Neurosci Biobehav Rev.* 2018;**87**:27–37.

37. Savage JE, Sawyers C, Roberson-Nay R, Hettema JM. The genetics of anxiety-related negative valence system traits. *Am J Med Genet B Neuropsychiatr Genet.* 2017;**174**(2):156–77.

38. Kalia M. Neurobiological basis of depression: an update. *Metabolism.* 2005;**54**(5):24–7.

39. Manji HK, Drevets WC, Charney DS. The cellular neurobiology of depression. *Nature Med.* 2001;**7** (5):541–7.

40. Einat H, Yuan P, Manji HK. Increased anxiety-like behaviors and mitochondrial dysfunction in mice with targeted mutation of the Bcl-2 gene: further support for the involvement of mitochondrial function in anxiety disorders. *Behav Brain Res.* 2005;**165**(2):172–80.

41. Burroughs S, French D. Depression and anxiety: role of mitochondria. *Curr Anaesth Crit Care.* 2007;**18** (1):34–41.

42. Devane CL, Chiao E, Franklin M, Kruep EJ. Anxiety disorders in the 21st century: status, challenges, opportunities, and comorbidity with depression. *Am J Manag Care.* 2005;**11**(12 Suppl):S344–53.

43. Zhang L, Zhou R, Li X, Ursano RJ, Li H. Stress-induced change of mitochondria membrane potential regulated by genomic and non-genomic GR signaling: a possible mechanism for hippocampus atrophy in PTSD. *Med Hypotheses.* 2006;**66**(6):1205–8.

44. Dwivedi Y, Rizavi HS, Pandey GN. Antidepressants reverse corticosterone-mediated decrease in brain-derived neurotrophic factor expression: differential regulation of specific exons by antidepressants and corticosterone. *Neuroscience.* 2006;**139**(3):1017–29.

45. Duchen MR. Mitochondria in health and disease: perspectives on a new mitochondrial biology. *Mol Aspects Med.* 2004;**25**(4):365–451.

46. Filiou MD, Sandi C. Anxiety and brain mitochondria: a bidirectional crosstalk. *Trends Neurosci.* 2019;**42** (9):573–88.

47. Allen J, Romay-Tallon R, Brymer KJ, Caruncho HJ, Kalynchuk LE. Mitochondria and mood: mitochondrial dysfunction as a key player in the manifestation of depression. *Front Neurosci-Switz.* 2018;**12**:386.

48. Shankman SA, Gorka SM, Katz AC, et al. Side effects to antidepressant treatment in patients with depression and comorbid panic disorder. *J Clin Psychiatry.* 2017;**78**(4):433–40.

49. Lanzafame R. Light dosing and tissue penetration: it is complicated. *Photobiomodul Photomed Laser Surg.* 2020;**38**(7):393–4.

50. Caldieraro MA, Cassano P. Transcranial and systemic photobiomodulation for major depressive disorder: a systematic review of efficacy, tolerability and biological mechanisms. *J Affect Disord.* 2019;**243**:262–73.

51. de Freitas LF, Hamblin MR. Proposed mechanisms of photobiomodulation or low-level light therapy. *IEEE J Sel Top Quantum Electron.* 2016;**22**(3):348–64.

52. Karu TI. Mitochondrial signaling in mammalian cells activated by red and near-IR radiation. *Photochem Photobiol.* 2008;**84**(5):1091–9.

53. Sommer AP. Revisiting the photon/cell interaction mechanism in low-level light therapy. *Photobiomodul Photomed Laser Surg.* 2019;**37**(6):336–41.

54. Salehpour F, Gholipour-Khalili S, Farajdokht F, et al. Therapeutic potential of intranasal photobiomodulation therapy for neurological and neuropsychiatric disorders: a narrative review. *Rev Neurosci.* 2020;**31**(3):269–86.

55. Chung H, Dai T, Sharma SK, et al. The nuts and bolts of low-level laser (light) therapy. *Ann Biomed Eng.* 2012;**40**(2):516–33.

56. Askalsky P, Iosifescu DV. Transcranial photobiomodulation for the management of depression: current perspectives. *Neuropsych Dis Treat.* 2019;**15**:3255–72.

57. Wu X, Alberico SL, Moges H, et al. Pulsed light irradiation improves behavioral outcome in a rat model of chronic mild stress. *Lasers Surg Med.* 2012;**44**(3):227–32.

58. Salehpour F, Rasta SH, Mohaddes G, Sadigh-Eteghad S, Salarirad S. Therapeutic effects of 10-HzPulsed wave lasers in rat depression model: a comparison between near-infrared and red wavelengths. *Lasers Surg Med.* 2016;**48**(7):695–705.

59. Eshaghi E, Sadigh-Eteghad S, Mohaddes G, Rasta SH. Transcranial photobiomodulation prevents anxiety and depression via changing serotonin and nitric oxide levels in brain of depression model mice: a study of three different doses of 810 nm laser. *Lasers Surg Med.* 2019;**51**(7):634–42.

60. Schiffer F, Johnston AL, Ravichandran C, et al. Psychological benefits 2 and 4 weeks after a single treatment with near infrared light to the forehead: a pilot study of 10 patients with major depression and anxiety. *Behav Brain Funct.* 2009;**5**:46.

61. Disner SG, Beevers CG, Gonzalez-Lima F. Transcranial laser stimulation as neuroenhancement for attention bias modification in adults with elevated depression symptoms. *Brain Stimul.* 2016;**9**(5):780–7.

62. Cassano P, Petrie SR, Mischoulon D, et al. Transcranial photobiomodulation for the treatment of major depressive disorder. The ELATED-2 Pilot Trial. *Photomed Laser Surg.* 2018;**36**(12):634–46.

63. Quah-Smith JI, Tang WM, Russell J. Laser acupuncture for mild to moderate depression in a primary care setting – a randomised controlled trial. *Acupunct Med.* 2005;**23**(3):103–11.

64. Quah-Smith I, Smith C, Crawford JD, Russell J. Laser acupuncture for depression: a randomised double

blind controlled trial using low intensity laser intervention. *J Affect Disord*. 2013;**148**(2–3):179–87.

65. Kartelishev AV, Kolupaev GP, Vernekina NS, et al. [Laser technologies used in the complex treatment of psychopharmacotherapy resistant endogenic depression]. *Voen Med Zh*. 2004;**325**(11):37–42.

66. Kolupaev GP, Kartelishev AV, Vernekina NS, Chebotkov AA, Lakosina ND. [Technologies of laser prophylaxis of depressive disorder relapses]. *Voen Med Zh*. 2007;**328**(2):31–4.

67. Caldieraro MA, Sani G, Bui E, Cassano P. Long-term near-infrared photobiomodulation for anxious depression complicated by Takotsubo cardiomyopathy. *J Clin Psychopharmacol*. 2018;**38**(3).

68. Mannu P, Saccaro LF, Spera V, Cassano P. Transcranial photobiomodulation to augment lithium in bipolar-I disorder. *Photobiomodul Photomed Laser Surg*. 2019;**37**(10):577–8.

69. Hennessy M, Hamblin MR. Photobiomodulation and the brain: a new paradigm. *J Opt*. 2016;**19**(1):013003.

Chapter 12

Mood Disorders and Comorbid Substance Use Disorders

Michael Weaver, Angela M. Heads, and Louis A. Faillace

Substance use disorders (SUDs) commonly co-occur with other psychiatric disorders. Mood disorders, including depressive and bipolar disorders, are the most common psychiatric comorbidity for individuals with SUD. Due to symptom overlap and complexity, diagnosis is difficult, effective treatment planning is sometimes delayed, and treatment outcomes tend to be worse for those with co-occurring SUD and mood disorders than for those with either a psychiatric or substance use diagnosis alone. Symptoms of mood disorder can be masked by the physiological effects of some substances, and people with mood disorders commonly report using substances to relieve depression, increase self-confidence, and ease social interactions [1]. Researchers have proposed several explanations for the high level of co-occurrence of mood disorders and SUDs. Proposed explanations include the possibility that the effects of a mood disorder increase the risk for a SUD (e.g., through self-medication) and vice versa (e.g., substance use intensifying symptoms and uncovering a mood disorder), and the possibility that genetic factors contribute to both mood disorders and SUDs [2]. This chapter will provide an overview of drug class effects as they relate to mood disorders, substance-induced mood disorders, co-occurring disorders, and treatment implications.

Drug Class Effects

Although the most commonly cited reasons for using substances include relief of depression, increased self-confidence, and improvement in social abilities, substance use often masks mood disorders symptoms, interfering with diagnosis and treatment and can in many cases worsen symptoms [1].

Alcohol, commonly prescribed sedatives, and opioids are central nervous system depressants and can cause or exacerbate depression. According to some surveys, up to 33% of elderly North American patients are prescribed either a benzodiazepine or similar sedative for a sleep problem [3]. Sleep problems are often a manifestation of a mood disorder, and this may go unrecognized. Older age, female gender, poor perceived health status, and poor actual physical health are associated with long-term use of sedatives, especially benzodiazepines [4]. Older adults (over age 64) are at risk to develop dependence on sedatives prescribed for insomnia or anxiety. Zolpidem and eszopiclone ("z-drugs") misuse is relatively rare when compared with benzodiazepines, but patients with a history of a SUD or psychiatric comorbidity such as mood disorders are at higher risk to misuse these medications [5]. The "high" from sedative medications is described as being very similar to alcohol intoxication. Tolerance, dependence, and withdrawal are all reported with sedatives, though this appears to be less severe and with lower incidence for z-drugs than for benzodiazepines or barbiturates [5]. Problems from misuse and abuse of sedatives have continued to grow with time. Long-term use of benzodiazepines can worsen underlying depression [6]. One study showed that benzodiazepines accounted for nearly 30% of deaths from pharmaceutical agents [7].

A protracted abstinence syndrome can occur after stopping long-term use of alcohol, sedatives, stimulants, or opioids. Patients may go through medical withdrawal treatment and get over the worst withdrawal symptoms quickly, but notice mood and concentration problems over the ensuing weeks, which can look very much like dysthymia. However, this is usually a time-limited problem [8].

Prevalence rates for current major depression among patients in treatment programs for opioid use disorder (OUD) are 10–20% and lifetime rates are 20–50% [9]. Depression interferes with OUD treatment effectiveness, but is also associated with increased retention in methadone maintenance, so may actually help motivate patients with OUD toward treatment [10]. Opioid withdrawal syndrome is associated with activation of the locus coeruleus, leading to autonomic activation and dysphoria with depression, which may be protracted. Treatment entry with reduction or cessation of opioid use results in improvement in depressive symptoms.

Long-term stimulant use can also lead to dopamine depletion, which can bring about long-term depression [8]. The clinical features of chronic stimulant use include depression, fatigue, and poor concentration. Stimulant withdrawal symptoms include anhedonia, irritability, and acute depression. Passive suicidal thoughts may occur, although suicide attempts are rare during withdrawal. If marked depression persists longer than one week after withdrawal, the patient should be evaluated carefully to determine if they are "self-medicating" an underlying depression, which then should be treated with a specific antidepressant [11].

Symptoms of nicotine withdrawal are similar regardless of the route of administration (e.g., combustible cigarettes, e-cigarettes, chewing tobacco, snuff). Withdrawal symptoms include irritability, difficulty concentrating, restlessness, anxiety, depression, and increased appetite. Withdrawal symptoms peak around 48 hours after the last use, then gradually diminish over several weeks. Symptoms of dysphoria, anhedonia, and depression may continue for several months.

There is evidence that cannabis use may increase the risk of depression [12] in a dose–response relationship. According to research, depression may lead to initiation or increase in frequency of cannabis use [13]. Although many patients report that a motivation for cannabis use is to improve mood, there is no evidence of any positive long-term effect on the outcome of depressive symptoms, and there have been no placebo-controlled clinical trials showing that cannabis is useful for treatment of depression. In fact, cannabis use in patients with depression can prevent improvement in depressive symptoms and impair treatment. Early-onset cannabis use predisposes users to suicide [14]. According to twin and family studies, there may even be a common genetic association between cannabis use and depression [15]. Heavy cannabis use for more than three weeks results in a withdrawal syndrome after abrupt cessation [16]. Cannabis withdrawal begins within 10 hours of the last dose and includes irritability, agitation, depression, and insomnia; most symptoms peak in 48 hours and last for five to seven days [17]. Cannabis withdrawal is uncomfortable but not life threatening, so treatment is entirely supportive and nearly always accomplished without adjunctive medications [18].

Adolescents with a hallucinogen use disorder are more likely than those without to have a comorbid SUD or other mental health problems [19], including mood disorders. Hallucinogen use may result in long-term psychiatric consequences, including depression. The risk of a prolonged psychiatric reaction depends upon the user's underlying predisposition to develop psychopathology, the amount of prior hallucinogen use, the use of other drugs, as well as dose and purity of the hallucinogen taken. Patients may present with apathy, formal thought disorder, or dissociative states. Treatment of prolonged depression is the same as when these conditions are not associated with hallucinogen use [20].

SUDs have been implicated in suicidal behavior, especially in women, in multiple studies, and polysubstance use is associated with a significantly greater risk of suicide mortality [21]. Screening for suicide risk in persons with SUD is strongly encouraged.

Substance-Induced Mood Disorder

A substance-induced mood disorder (SIMD) develops within the context of intoxication or withdrawal from an abused substance. SIMDs can be the result of any class of substance for which a SUD diagnosis exists [16].

It can be difficult to determine whether a patient who abuses substances and exhibits symptoms of a mood disorder is experiencing the symptoms of a separate existing mood disorder or is suffering from a substance-induced mood disorder, acute withdrawal, acute intoxication, or a combination [2]. While a mood disorder can persist, a SIMD is usually temporary, with symptoms resolving within one month of onset in most cases.

The presentations of a mood disorder and a substance-induced mood disorder are very similar. Differentiation of a mood disorder from a SIMD requires a thorough assessment which includes a detailed history of psychiatric symptoms and substance use including the timing of such use, and careful consideration of established diagnostic criteria. See Table 12.1 for DSM-5 criteria for SIMD.

Clinicians recommend a methodological approach to diagnosis starting with the initial assessment to identify patients who present with both mood symptoms and substance use and who may require a more

Table 12.1 DSM-5 criteria for substance-induced mood disorder

Criterion	
1	The disorder represents a clinically significant symptomatic presentation of the relevant mood disorder (i.e., a pervasive and noticeable disruption in mood): a) Loss of interest/pleasure or depressed mood for depression b) Elevated or irritable mood for bipolar and related disorders
2	There is evidence from the history, physical examination, or laboratory findings of both of the following: a) The mood disorder developed during or within one month of a substance intoxication or withdrawal; and b) The involved substance/medication is capable of producing the mental disorder.
3	The disorder is not better explained by an independent mood disorder (i.e., one that is not substance or medication induced). Such evidence of an independent mental disorder could include the following: a) The disorder preceded the onset of severe intoxication or withdrawal or exposure to the medication; or b) The mood disorder persisted for a substantial period of time (e.g., at least one month) after the cessation of acute withdrawal or severe intoxication or taking the medication.
4	The disorder does not occur exclusively during the course of a delirium.
5	The disorder causes clinically significant distress or impairment in social, occupational, or other important areas of functioning.

thorough assessment and follow up plan. There are several recommended diagnostic tools to help to identify mood symptoms in the SUD treatment setting. The Symptom Checklist-90-Revised (SCL-90) is a diagnostic tool that is widely used for detecting general distress [22]. Although it is a good indicator of the presence of a psychiatric disorder, it does not provide specific diagnostic information. As a screening tool, the SCL-90 provides good specificity and sensitivity for mood disorders in individuals who abuse substances. The Beck Depression Inventory–II (BDI-II) is a brief self-report instrument with utility in detecting depression in SUD treatment settings [23]. The Addiction Severity Index (ASI) is often used to guide treatment planning in SUD treatment settings and has a subscale that detects general distress [24]. These instruments can be a good first step in mood disorders screening for patients with SUD.

Co-Occurring Disorders

Lifetime prevalence of mood disorders, SUDs, and the co-occurrence of these in the general population is high, with lifetime rates for any SUD with any bipolar disorder at approximately 47% and any SUD with major depressive disorder (MDD) at approximately 40% [25]. There have been several theories proposed to explain the high level of co-occurrence of mood disorders and SUDs including the self-medication hypothesis whereby the effects of a mood disorder increase the risk for a SUD and genetic risk factors that place an individual at risk for both mood disorders and SUD [2]. Furthermore, the confounding of acute intoxication and withdrawal with mood disorders symptoms may also account for the high levels of reported co-occurring disorders [2].

Some patients take controlled substances that have been prescribed for specific conditions, such as sedatives for panic attack disorder or opioids for pain, in order to obtain other benefits: to induce sleep, reduce anxiety from stressful life circumstances, elevate their mood when depressed, or provide additional energy. This behavior is a form of self-medication and has also been termed "chemical coping" [26]. Patients who engage in self-medication may develop tolerance to these other effects of sedatives and opioids more rapidly than to the therapeutic effect for which the medication was prescribed, leading to dose escalation. Increases in emotional stress (disputes with family or friends, professional pressures, or financial worries) can heighten a patient's sensitivity to discomfort from anxiety symptoms, leading to increased consumption of controlled substance medications [27]. However, this is not the same as addiction or intentional malingering. A benzodiazepine or opioid is not an appropriate treatment for depression, especially when the patient may escalate the dose to attempt to achieve some symptom relief despite tolerance to this [28]. Self-medication behavior is challenging for physicians to address. Somatization of psychological distress into physical symptoms is pervasive in medical practice [29], and the boundary between physical and mental distress is not clear and distinct for many patients. Use of prescribed medications or other substances of abuse becomes a reliable coping mechanism, but is maladaptive. The challenge for the treating physician is to help patients identify the underlying (often subconscious) reasons for reliance on other inappropriate effects of the medication, then help the patient begin the process of developing new coping skills for dealing with symptoms of depression. Utilization of specific antidepressant medications can be very effective as a way to shift the focus away from inappropriate use of sedatives or opioids toward treatment of the underlying condition [28]. The selective serotonin reuptake inhibitors (SSRIs) are safe and not prone to misuse, and can be accompanied by cognitive behavioral therapy for long-term treatment of comorbid psychiatric diagnoses.

Assessment of Co-Occurring Disorders

Substance use disorder is more prevalent in patients who have depression or anxiety disorders or other psychiatric comorbidities (including personality disorders) and in those who use tobacco or alcohol [18]. Patients with a dual diagnosis (i.e., both SUD and another major psychiatric disorder) may present with complex clinical histories and symptoms that make diagnosis challenging. Intoxication and withdrawal symptoms may be mistaken for other psychiatric or medical symptoms. It is important to be alert for SUD. However, even careful assessment by clinicians looking for SUD may not identify all current users. A combination of universal questionnaire screening and urine toxicology for those at high risk is more effective than either alone. Findings from physical examination and laboratory studies can provide important clues to SUD. Although many of these findings can be caused by other diseases, the differential diagnosis should include SUD, and additional information can help verify this.

A definitive diagnostic assessment for a co-occurring mood and SUD should be performed after the patient has had a period of abstinence. Commonly clinicians opt to wait several weeks before treating a suspected co-occurring mood disorder because the diagnostic picture is unclear at the start of treatment. However, the period of time of abstinence before solidifying the diagnosis and formulating a comprehensive treatment plan depends on both the mood disorder under consideration and the substance being used. For example, one meta-analysis found that MDD can be reliably diagnosed after one week of abstinence [10]. Delaying treatment of either disorder while clarifying diagnosis can result in poorer outcomes, as substance use exacerbates mood symptoms and vice versa.

Due to the complex nature of diagnosing co-occurring mental health and SUDs, researchers created the Psychiatric Research Interview for Substance and Mental Disorders (PRISM). Originally created for DSM-IV criteria, it has recently been updated for DSM-5 and has demonstrated acceptable test re-test reliability [30]. The PRISM-5 is a semi-structured diagnostic interview specifically created to assess substance use and psychiatric disorders based on DSM 5 criteria.

Patients presenting with a combination of SUDs and mood disorders have a more severe clinical presentation and have worse outcomes than patients with only one of these disorders. Therefore, careful consideration of both disorders is necessary for optimal clinical outcomes.

Treatment Issues

Several studies suggest that depression and substance use outcomes are partially causally related and support concurrently treating both disorders. It is recommended that treatment for SUD be started first. Establishing abstinence or a reduction in substance use prior to diagnosis and treatment of a mood disorder helps to clarify treatment planning. The full range of addiction treatment options should be considered, including different levels of care, evidence-based behavioral interventions, and medications. Behavioral treatment for SUD includes cognitive behavioral interventions that have components focused on managing mood symptoms, so may have inherent antidepressant effects. By helping reduce substance use, behavioral interventions help improve mood. Twelve Step groups such as Alcoholics Anonymous and Narcotics Anonymous contain elements including social support that can benefit both substance problems and depression, and may even reduce suicide risk [31].

Other nonpharmacological options to address mood or SUDs include digital therapeutic applications (apps) for smartphones. There are now nearly 10,000 apps that exist to address mental health [32]. These can provide general information, links to support resources, Twelve Step meeting finders, avoidance of triggers to use, tracking of abstinence or use, and methods for journaling, among other features.

Careful clinical history can establish evidence of independent MDD, especially if it occurred prior to onset of substance use or during previous periods of abstinence. Antidepressant medication has been the most thoroughly studied treatment modality for co-occurring mood and SUDs with numerous placebo-controlled trials [33]. Treatment of a co-occurring depression with antidepressant medication may be helpful in reducing substance use as the depression improves, especially for alcohol use disorders. SSRIs such as sertraline and escitalopram are good choices in terms of minimal side effects and few drug–drug interactions [8]. Serotonin and norepinephrine reuptake inhibitors (SNRIs), mirtazapine, or nefazodone may be good choices if SSRIs are not effective. Finally, prescribers may consider tricyclic antidepressants, but should consider the risks of sedation and overdose.

The prevalence of tobacco use disorder is higher among individuals with psychiatric disorders than the general population, and some medications for tobacco cessation also help to improve mood symptoms [34]. An available pharmacotherapy for tobacco cessation is bupropion (Zyban). Bupropion is a prescribed polycyclic antidepressant in oral tablet form that is started prior to tobacco cessation and continued for three to six months of therapy to achieve tobacco cessation. Randomized controlled trials demonstrate that bupropion increases the long-term success of quit attempts for tobacco smoking [35]. Bupropion can be used for treatment of both depression and tobacco use disorder. The effect of nortriptyline for nicotine use disorder is related to reduction of postquit dysphoria, not depression [36].

Individuals with bipolar disorder and a co-occurring SUD are more likely to experience rapid cycling between depressive and manic symptoms and mixed depression and mania episodes [37]. Pharmacological treatment is the mainstay of treatment of bipolar disorder. Mania is a psychiatric emergency requiring pharmacological management. Mania may be accompanied by substance use, so brief hospitalization can help to establish initial abstinence as well as control the mania. It is important to evaluate the relationship between the manic symptoms and substance use [33]. Patients with bipolar depression may respond better to a mood stabilizer (anticonvulsant or lithium) or combined with a low-dose second-generation antipsychotic. An antidepressant may be helpful if depression symptoms persist despite combination therapy. Medication treatment of bipolar disorder will not adequately or fully treat the SUD, so the SUD must also be treated specifically with behavioral and possibly pharmacological therapy. Patients with bipolar disorder may become impulsive or lose insight, especially during manic phases, or may lose sight of the need to continue treatment during periods when bipolar symptoms are under good control. This may lead to relapse to substance use, so maintaining continuity of care is essential.

Some opioids, including tramadol, meperidine, dextromethorphan, and methadone, are weak serotonin reuptake inhibitors [38]. When given – especially at high doses – with monoamine oxidase inhibitors (MAOIs) or other serotonergic drugs, they can cause serotonin syndrome. Opioids that do not have serotonin activity are morphine, oxycodone, and buprenorphine; these would be better choices for patients taking other serotonergic medications [18]. Diazepam and fluoxetine can elevate methadone serum levels and increase the risk of opioid intoxication. Disulfiram treatment for alcohol use disorder has been associated with psychosis, possibly due to inhibiting dopamine beta-hydroxylase and increasing dopamine levels, so should be used with caution in patients with severe mental illness such as bipolar disorder [39].

Candidate medication studies for pharmacological treatment of methamphetamine addiction have included the commonly prescribed psychiatric medications sertraline, bupropion, mirtazapine, risperidone, aripiprazole, and gabapentin. However, no single medication has demonstrated consistent efficacy and each trial contained a variety of methodological limitations [40]. A clinical trial of duloxetine demonstrated inhibition of effects of 3,4-methylenedioxymethamphetamine (MDMA), including subjective drug effects, so this may be useful for treatment of addiction [41].

Esketamine, an enantiomer of ketamine with higher affinity for the N-methyl-D-aspartate (NMDA) receptor, was recently approved by the US Food and Drug Administration for treatment-resistant depression in adults. It is administered as a nasal spray, which demonstrated rapid onset and persistent efficacy in patients with treatment-resistant depression as well as in depressed patients at imminent risk for suicide. Esketamine can be combined with oral antidepressant medication [42].

Hallucinogens such as lysergic acid diethylamide (LSD or Acid), psilocybin (from certain mushrooms), and N,N-dimethyltryptamine (DMT) are agonists at serotonin 5-HT2A receptors that are being studied as treatments for major depression that has been resistant to other medications and electroconvulsive therapy and for depression associated with bipolar disorder. Single doses are associated with antidepressive effects, with less consistent results regarding SUD due to lack of clinical trials [43]. They have been associated with rapid therapeutic effects that can last for weeks to months. These cannot be recommended yet due to the small number of studies with few subjects and short duration, but may offer a possible future therapeutic option for some patients.

Conclusion

Substance use disorders commonly co-occur with mood disorders and are due to direct effects of substances such as intoxication and withdrawal, or chronic use, including substance-induced mood disorders. Self-medication of mood disorders with legal or illicit substances is highly prevalent. Careful assessment is necessary, and many mood symptoms may resolve with treatment of the SUD. Treat independent mood disorders with behavioral and standard pharmacological therapy. Some mood disorder medications are also effective for SUDs, and some addictive substances are currently being studied as possible treatments for mood disorders.

References

1. Thornton LK, Baker AL, Lewin TJ, et al. Reasons for substance use among people with mental disorders. *Addict Behav.* 2012;**37**(4):427–34.

2. Quello SB, Brady KT, Sonne SC. Mood disorders and substance use disorder: a complex comorbidity. *Sci Pract Perspect.* 2005;**3**(1):13–21.

3. Glass J, Lanctôt KL, Herrmann N, Sproule BA, Busto UE. Sedative hypnotics in older people with insomnia: meta-analysis of risks and benefits. *BMJ.* 2005;**331**(7526):1169.

4. Lader M. Benzodiazepine harm: how can it be reduced? *Br J Clin Pharmacol.* 2014;**77** (2):295–301.

5. Hajak G, Müller W, Wittchen H-U, Pittrow D, Kirch W. Abuse and dependence potential for the non-benzodiazepine hypnotics zolpidem and zopiclone: a review of case reports and epidemiological data. *Addiction.* 2003;**98**(10):1371–8.

6. Rickels K, Lucki I, Schweizer E, Garcia-Espana F, Case WG. Psychomotor performance of long-term benzodiazepine users before, during, and after benzodiazepine discontinuation. *J Clin Psychopharmacol.* 1999;**19**(2):107–13.

7. Jones CM, Mack KA, Paulozzi LJ. Pharmaceutical overdose deaths, United States, 2010. *JAMA.* 2013;**309**(7):657–9.

8. Weaver MF. *Addiction Treatment.* Newburyport, MA: Carlat Publishing, 2017.

9. Nunes EV, Quitkin F, Brady R, Post-Koenig T. Antidepressant treatment in methadone maintenance patients. *J Addict Dis.* 1995;**13**(3):13–24.

10. Nunes EV, Levin FR. Treatment of depression in patients with alcohol or other drug dependence: a meta-analysis. *JAMA.* 2004;**291**(15):1887–96.

11. Weaver MF, Delos Reyes, C., Schnoll, S. H. Club drug addiction. In GO Gabbard, editor. *Gabbard's Treatments of Psychiatric Disorders.* 5th ed. Washington, DC: American Psychiatric Publishing, 2014; 851–8.

12. Patton GC, Coffey C, Carlin JB, et al. Cannabis use and mental health in young people: cohort study. *BMJ.* 2002;**325**(7374):1195–8.

13. Feingold D, Weinstein A. Cannabis and depression. In E Murillo-Rodriguez, SR Pandi-Perumal, JM Monti, editors. *Cannabinoids and Neuropsychiatric Disorders.* Cham: Springer International, 2021; 67–80.

14. Lynskey MT, Glowinski AL, Todorov AA, et al. Major depressive disorder, suicidal ideation, and suicide attempt in twins discordant for cannabis dependence and early-onset cannabis use. *Arch Gen Psychiatry.* 2004;**61**(10):1026–32.

15. Hodgson K, Almasy L, Knowles EE, et al. The genetic basis of the comorbidity between cannabis use and major depression. *Addiction.* 2017;**112**(1):113–23.

16. American Psychiatric Association. *Diagnostic and Statistical Manual of Mental Disorders: DSM-5.* 5th ed. Washington, DC: American Psychiatric Association Publishing, 2013.

17. Budney AJ, Hughes JR, Moore BA, Vandrey R. Review of the validity and significance of cannabis withdrawal syndrome. *Am J Psychiatry.* 2004;**161** (11):1967–77.

18. Weaver M. Substance-related disorders. In JL Levenson, editor. *The American Psychiatric Association Publishing Textbook of Psychosomatic Medicine and Consultation-Liaison Psychiatry.* 3rd ed.

Washington, DC: American Psychiatric Association Publishing, 2019; 435–62.

19. Wu L-T, Ringwalt CL, Weiss RD, Blazer DG. Hallucinogen-related disorders in a national sample of adolescents: the influence of ecstasy/MDMA use. *Drug Alcohol Depend*. 2009;**104**(1–2):156–66.

20. Weaver MF. Hallucinogens. In RJ Levesque, editor. *Encyclopedia of Adolescence*. 2nd edition. New York: Springer, 2016.

21. Lynch FL, Peterson EL, Lu CY, et al. Substance use disorders and risk of suicide in a general US population: a case control study. *Addict Sci Clin Pract*. 2020;**15**(1):1–9.

22. Derogatis LR, Unger R. Symptom Checklist-90-Revised. *The Corsini Encyclopedia of Psychology*. 2010; 1–2.

23. Beck AT, Steer RA, Brown G. Beck Depression Inventory-II (BDI-II) [Database record]. APA PsychTests. 1996.

24. McLellan AT, Kushner H, Metzger D, et al. The fifth edition of the Addiction Severity Index. *J Subst Abuse Treat*. 1992;**9**(3):199–213.

25. Pettinati HM, O'Brien CP, Dundon WD. Current status of co-occurring mood and substance use disorders: a new therapeutic target. *Am J Psychiatry*. 2013;**170**(1):23–30.

26. Weaver M, Schnoll S. Addiction issues in prescribing opioids for chronic nonmalignant pain. *J Addict Med*. 2007;**1**(1):2–10.

27. Weaver M. Prescribing medications with potential for abuse. *J Clin Outcomes Manag*. 2009;**16**(4):171–9.

28. Weaver MF. Focus: addiction: prescription sedative misuse and abuse. *Yale J Biol Med*. 2015;**88**(3):247.

29. Katon W, Sullivan M, Walker E. Medical symptoms without identified pathology: relationship to psychiatric disorders, childhood and adult trauma, and personality traits. *Ann Intern Med*. 2001;**134**(9_Part_2):917–25.

30. Hasin D, Shmulewitz D, Stohl M, et al. Test-retest reliability of DSM-5 substance disorder measures as assessed with the PRISM-5, a clinician-administered diagnostic interview. *Drug Alcohol Depend*. 2020;**216**:108294.

31. Mann RE, Zalcman RF, Smart RG, Rush BR, Suurvali H. Alcohol consumption, Alcoholics Anonymous membership, and homicide mortality rates in Ontario 1968 to 1991. *Alcohol Clin Exp Res*. 2006;**30**(10):1743–51.

32. Chang BP, Kessler RC, Pincus HA, Nock MK. Digital approaches for mental health in the age of COVID-19. *BMJ*. 2020;**369**.

33. Nunes EV, Weiss RD. Co-occurring mood and substance use disorders. In S Miller, D Fiellin, R Saitz, editors. *ASAM Principles of Addiction Medicine*. 6th ed. Chevy Chase, MD: American Society of Addiction Medicine, 2019; 1360–88.

34. Kalman D, Morissette SB, George TP. Co-morbidity of smoking in patients with psychiatric and substance use disorders. *Am J Addict*. 2005;**14**(2):106–23.

35. Hughes JR. How confident should we be that smoking cessation treatments work? *Addiction*. 2009;**104**(10):1637–40.

36. Tulloch HE, Pipe AL, Clyde MJ, Reid RD, Els C. The quit experience and concerns of smokers with psychiatric illness. *Am J Prev Med*. 2016;**50**(6):709–18.

37. Sonne SC, Brady KT. Substance abuse and bipolar comorbidity. *Psychiatr Clin North Am*. 1999;**22**(3):609–27.

38. Gillman P. Monoamine oxidase inhibitors, opioid analgesics and serotonin toxicity. *Br J Anaesth*. 2005;**95**(4):434–41.

39. Nunes E, Quitkin F. Disulfiram and bipolar affective disorder. *J Clin Psychopharmacol*. 1987;**7**(4):284.

40. Brackins T, Brahm NC, Kissack JC. Treatments for methamphetamine abuse: a literature review for the clinician. *J Pharm Pract*. 2011;**24**(6):541–50.

41. Hysek CM, Simmler LD, Nicola VG, et al. Duloxetine inhibits effects of MDMA ("Ecstasy") in vitro and in humans in a randomized placebo-controlled laboratory study. *PLoS One*. 2012;**7**(5):e36476.

42. Popova V, Daly EJ, Trivedi M, et al. Efficacy and safety of flexibly dosed esketamine nasal spray combined with a newly initiated oral antidepressant in treatment-resistant depression: a randomized double-blind active-controlled study. *Am J Psychiatry*. 2019;**176**(6):428–38.

43. Dos Santos RG, Bouso JC, Alcázar-Córcoles MÁ, Hallak JE. Efficacy, tolerability, and safety of serotonergic psychedelics for the management of mood, anxiety, and substance-use disorders: a systematic review of systematic reviews. *Expert Rev Clin Pharmacol*. 2018;**11**(9):889–902.

Chapter 13

Mood Disorders with Attention-Deficit/ Hyperactivity Disorder, Impulse Control Disorders, or Borderline Personality Disorder

Susan L. McElroy, Anna I. Guerdjikova, and Francisco Romo-Nava

Introduction

A hallmark feature of mood disorders is their high comorbidity with other psychiatric disorders. This includes disorders defined by pathological impulsivity. In this chapter, we discuss the epidemiology, clinical features, and management of individuals with mood disorders and co-occurring attention-deficit/ hyperactivity disorder (ADHD), impulse control disorders (ICDs), and borderline personality disorder (BPD).

Attention-Deficit/Hyperactivity Disorder (ADHD)

Present in about 2.5% of the adult general population, ADHD is very common among individuals with mood disorders, with estimates of its prevalence ranging from 9% to 16% among individuals with depressive disorders and from 9% to 90% among those with bipolar disorders (BD) [1–3]. This wide variation in prevalence seems to vary by age and gender – with higher rates in youth and males, and is likely due in part to the phenomenological overlap between hypo/mania and ADHD. Further supporting a relationship between mood disorders and ADHD are longitudinal studies finding the many individuals initially diagnosed with ADHD go on to develop BD [4], controlled family history studies showing BD and ADHD breed true [5], as well as recent genome-wide association studies (GWAS) showing considerable genetic overlap among depression, BD, and ADHD [6,7].

When mood disorder co-occurs with ADHD, there is a greater burden of illness, especially for BD. As compared to BD patients without ADHD, those with ADHD have an earlier onset of BD, shorter periods of wellness and more frequent periods of depression, more suicidality, and greater comorbidity with other psychiatric disorders, including anxiety and substance use disorders [3,8,9].

Treatment of Mood Disorders with ADHD

No medication has regulatory approval for the treatment of individuals with both a mood disorder and ADHD. Moreover, no treatment with regulatory approval for major depressive disorder (MDD) or BD also has approval for treatment of ADHD. Mixed evidence suggests that certain antidepressants with noradrenergic reuptake blocking properties, especially desipramine and bupropion, might have some efficacy in ADHD [10–20]. However, studies of primarily serotonergic antidepressants in ADHD have been negative [21,22] and most standard ADHD treatments, including various formulations of the psychostimulants amphetamine and methylphenidate and the selective norepinephrine-reuptake inhibitor atomoxetine, have typically failed in randomized controlled trials (RCTs) in individuals with MDD [23–26]. A possible exception is the serotonin norepinephrine reuptake (SNRI) viloxazine, which was recently approved for ADHD in children in the United States and used in Europe before that as an antidepressant [27,28].

Of note, ADHD drugs have received limited study in individuals with BD. In the two RCTs of an ADHD medication in patients with mania, there was no difference between methylphenidate and lithium in the first [29] and no difference between methylphenidate and placebo in the second [30]. In the only RCT of a stimulant in BD depression, lisdexamfetamine was not superior to placebo for decreasing depressive symptoms as assessed with the Montgomery–Asberg Depression Scale (MADRS), but was superior to placebo for decreasing self-reported depressive symptoms [31]. All patients were required to be on mood stabilizers and/or antipsychotics and there were no instances of hypo/mania. Importantly, a randomized, placebo-controlled trial of a long-acting formulation of mixed amphetamine salts (Mydayis®) in individuals with patients with BD depression is ongoing (NCT04235686).

Preliminary data suggest BD patients ADHD receiving stimulants should also receive a mood stabilizer and/or a second-generation antipsychotic, as stimulants may worsen BD symptomatology when given as monotherapy. In a large Swedish registry study of 2,307 adults with BD initiating treatment with methylphenidate between 2006 and 2014, those not receiving concomitant mood stabilizer treatment displayed a greater rate of manic episodes than those receiving such treatment [32].

Randomized Controlled Trials in Patients with Co-occurring Mood Disorders and ADHD

One RCT evaluated treatment of individuals with both MDD and ADHD. In this study, 142 youth with MDD and ADHD, ages 12–18 years, were randomized to receive atomoxetine or placebo for nine weeks [33]. ADHD, but not depressive, symptoms were significantly reduced with atomoxetine versus placebo. In a post hoc analysis of an RCT comparing fluoxetine, cognitive behavioral therapy (CBT), fluoxetine plus CBT, and placebo in 439 adolescents with MDD, 62 with co-occurring ADHD, all active treatment arms were superior to placebo and comparable to each other in youth with both disorders [34]. Among youth with MDD but without ADHD, monotherapy with either drug or CBT was inferior to the combination. The authors concluded that comorbid ADHD moderated the treatment response of MDD in adolescents.

Four RCTs have evaluated treatment of BD patients with comorbid ADHD [35–38]. In the first, 47 youth ages 6–17 years with BDI or BDII with manic symptoms (defined as a Young Mania Rating Scale [YMRS] score ≥ 14) and ADHD received eight weeks of open-label valproate treatment, followed by a four-week randomized, placebo-controlled trial of mixed amphetamine salts in those patients whose manic symptoms responded to valproate [35]. While 32 patients had an anti-manic response to valproate, only three had significant improvement in ADHD symptoms. For the 30 participants subsequently randomized to receive mixed amphetamine salts or placebo, mixed amphetamine salts were significantly better than placebo for reducing ADHD symptoms.

In the second study, youth ages 5–17 years with BD and ADHD receiving at least one thymoleptic were randomized to receive methylphenidate or placebo for four weeks [36]. Sixteen youth completed the trial. ADHD scores were lower with methylphenidate compared with placebo with a large effect size (Cohen's $d = 0.90$). In the third study, 46 youth with BD and ADHD who were experiencing an acute manic or mixed episode were randomized to receive aripiprazole or placebo for six weeks [37]. Compared with placebo recipients, aripiprazole recipients showed significantly greater reductions in clinician- and parent-rated mania scores and higher rates of response and remission. There were no significant treatment effects for ADHD (or depressive) symptoms.

The fourth study was a randomized, crossover study of methylphenidate versus placebo (each administered for two weeks) in 16 youth with BD and ADHD who had had a significant mood stabilizing response to aripiprazole [38]. Among the 14 youth who completed the trial, no significant differences between methylphenidate and placebo were found on ADHD or manic symptoms. One methylphenidate recipient had a severe mixed episode.

These findings are supported by clinical reports. For example, Chang et al. described 8 of 12 euthymic youth with BD and ADHD receiving at least one mood stabilizer in which ADHD responded to addition of atomoxetine [39].

These studies suggest that although mood disorders and ADHD are related, patients with both conditions often require treatment for each condition. Regarding pharmacotherapy for individuals with BD and ADHD, these studies further suggest that the treatment of BD be conducted either before or concurrently with the treatment of ADHD.

Impulse Control Disorders (ICDs)

There is some controversy as to what exactly an ICD is. Historically, these conditions were defined as irresistible impulses to do harmful behaviors [40]. Types of ICDs have included intermittent explosive disorder (IED), kleptomania, pathological gambling, pyromania, and trichotillomania, as well as repetitive self-mutilation, compulsive skin picking, compulsive shopping, and compulsive internet use [41]. DSM-IV included IED, kleptomania, pathological gambling, pyromania, and trichotillomania as ICDs Not Elsewhere Classified [42]. With DSM-5, pathological gambling was moved to the substance use disorder section, highlighting the issue that these conditions have also been conceptualized as behavioral addictions [43].

No matter the precise nosological classification of these disorders as ICDs or behavioral addictions, extensive research show they are highly comorbid with mood disorders, especially BD [44–47]. In one study evaluating ICDs in 124 consecutive patients with BD I disorder, 34 (24%) had at least one ICD, with the most common being compulsive skin picking, compulsive shopping, IED, and trichotillomania [48]. In a review evaluating 28 studies of behavioral addictions among individuals with BD, the authors concluded that these conditions were overrepresented in BD patients and vice versa [49]. The most prevalent behavioral addictions were pathological gambling, kleptomania, compulsive buying, compulsive sexual behavior, and internet addiction.

No medication has regulatory approval for the treatment of an ICD. Drugs that have shown promise for individuals with an ICD include opioid antagonists (for pathological gambling and trichotillomania) [50] and N-acetylcysteine (NAC) for trichotillomania [51,52]. Of note, a recent meta-analysis concluded NAC was not efficacious in BD depression [53].

Randomized Controlled Trials in Patients with Co-occurring Mood Disorders and ICDs

To our knowledge, only one RCT has evaluated a treatment in patients with both a mood disorder and an ICD. In this study, 40 patients with a bipolar spectrum disorder and pathological gambling were randomized to receive lithium or placebo for 10 weeks [54]. Patients receiving lithium showed significantly more improvement than those receiving placebo on scores of both mania and pathological gambling. Of note, a randomized, placebo-controlled trial of olanzapine in individuals with pathological

gambling but without BD conducted by our group was negative [55]; we concluded that agents with mood stabilizing properties might work in pathological gambling only when associated with co-occurring BD.

Borderline Personality Disorder (BPD)

Epidemiological and clinical data suggest substantial overlap between mood disorders and BPD [56–61]. Data from the National Epidemiologic Survey on Alcohol and Related Conditions (NESARC) showed that BPD was strongly associated with both MDD and BD [56]. The relationship of BPD with BD remained strong and significant after controlling for comorbidity with other psychiatric disorders. In another analysis of data from the NESARC, lifetime prevalence of BPD was 29% in BDI and 24% in BDII [57]. In a meta-analysis of 42 papers exploring the relationship between BD and BPD, it was estimated that 21.6% of individuals with BD had co-occurring BPD, and conversely, that 18.5% of individuals with BDP had BD [58].

Considerable data show mood disorders and BPD may be related on a pathophysiological level. In an analysis of NESARC data to determine if BD and BPD were alternative expressions of the same disorder, the authors concluded that BD and BPD had overlapping but different psychopathologies [62]. Indeed, a recent GWAS showed BPD had genetic overlap with both MDD and BD (as well as schizophrenia) [63].

Mood disorder patients with BPD have a substantially greater illness burden than those without BPD. In a study of 183 depressed patients randomized to fluoxetine or nortriptyline, the 30 patients with co-occurring BPD had earlier onset of depression, more chronic depression, were more likely to have histories of suicide attempts and self-mutilation, and had greater rates of alcohol and cannabis abuse [64]. In a longitudinal study of individuals with MDD recruited from a community sample, the presence of BPD at baseline predicted persistence of depression three years later [65]. In the above- mentioned NESARC study [57], as compared to BD individuals without BPD, those with BPD had an earlier age of BD onset and more depressive episodes, comorbidity, and childhood trauma. In a study comparing 128 outpatients with BD without BPD and 517 outpatients with BD and BPD, those with BPD had more suicidality, comorbid disorders, childhood trauma, psychopathology in first-degree relatives, and hospitalizations [66]. They also had more time unemployed and were more likely to receive disability payments. In a large comparison of BD inpatients with BPD ($n = 268,232$) and without BPD ($n = 242,379$), the presence of BPD was associated with a longer hospital stay, higher cost, higher suicide risk, and higher use of ECT [67]. Of interest, a retrospective analysis of 139 patients with a unipolar depressive episode receiving ECT showed that those with BPD were more likely to have medication-resistant depression and a less robust antidepressant response to ECT [68].

No medication has regulatory approval for the treatment of BPD. Psychotherapy is generally considered the foundational treatment of BPD [69–73], but most BPD patients also receive psychopharmacology, often with multiple drugs [74,75]. Reviews and meta-analyses on pharmacotherapy of BPD differ in their conclusions, with some saying that medications may be helpful, particularly selective serotonin reuptake inhibitors (SSRIs), second-generation antipsychotics, and mood stabilizers [75–80], while others conclude there is not sufficient evidence to recommend pharmacotherapy let alone one drug over another [69]. Of note, despite initial positive studies for lamotrigine, a recent meta-analysis of lamotrigine trials in BPD was negative [81]. An industry-sponsored, multicenter, pivotal, randomized, placebo-controlled trial of brexpiprazole in combination with sertraline in BPD patients with minimal psychiatric comorbidity is ongoing (NCT03418675).

Randomized Controlled Trials in Patients with Co-Occurring Mood Disorders and BPD

We found RCTs that evaluated treatment options in patients with both a mood disorder and BPD. Four of these studies were in patients with depression and one was in patients with BD.

In the first depression study, 308 patients with MDD were evaluated for co-occurring personality disorder and randomized to receive sertraline or citalopram for 24 weeks [82]. At treatment endpoint, patients were again evaluated for personality disorders. Significant reduction in frequency was seen for BPD, as well as for paranoid, avoidant, and dependent personality disorders. In the second study, 39 outpatients with BPD and a major depressive episode were randomized to

receive fluoxetine 20–40 mg/day alone or to fluoxetine 20–40 mg/day with interpersonal psychotherapy (IPT) [83]. Fluoxetine plus IPT was more effective than fluoxetine alone for reducing depressive symptoms and for improving quality of life and interpersonal functioning.

In the third study, 35 outpatients with BPD and a major depressive episode were randomized to receive fluoxetine with IPT or fluoxetine with CBT for 24 weeks [84]. Both treatments were effective for treating depressive symptoms in BPD. In the fourth study, 30 inpatients with BPD and depression were randomized to receive emotional intelligence training (12 sessions) or a control [85]. Compared with the control group, the group receiving emotional intelligence training showed an increase in emotional intelligence. Depressive symptoms decreased in both groups but decreased more in the group receiving emotional intelligence training.

In the only study of BD plus BPD, 30 women with BD II and BPD were randomly assigned to receive divalproex or placebo in a 2:1 ratio for six months [86]. Divalproex was superior to placebo for decreasing interpersonal sensitivity and anger/hostility assessed by the Symptom Checklist–90 (SCL-90), as well as overall aggression measured with the Modified Overt Aggression Scale (MOAS) scale.

Conclusion

Considerable research indicates that mood disorders often co-occur with other psychiatric disorders characterized by pathological impulsivity, including ADHD, ICDs, and BPD. Such patients often have a greater psychiatric illness burden, with earlier age of mood disorder onset, more severe course of mood disorder, and greater comorbidity with other psychiatric disorders. Though not well studied, treatment of such patients is probably more complex than treatment of mood disorder patients without these comorbidities.

The first step in the treatment of such patients is recognition of this high degree of comorbidity. Thus, any patient with a depressive or bipolar disorder should also be evaluated for co-occurring ADHD, ICDs, and BPD. Just as importantly, patients with ADHD, an ICD, or BPD should be carefully evaluated for a co-occurring mood disorder.

The second step in the management of such patients is the recognition that both the mood

135

disorder and the co-occurring disorder will likely need be addressed – though the temporal relationship in which this is done may vary. In patients with MDD, an antidepressant may be started, such as an agent with noradrenergic properties in patients with ADHD or an agent with serotonergic properties in BPD. Conversely, foundational treatment for ADHD (stimulants) or BPD (psychotherapy) may be initiated and the course of MDD symptoms monitored. If they persist, an appropriate antidepressant may be added.

Treatment of BD patients with these conditions likely differs from that of MDD patients. Based on available RCTs, which are limited, it could be argued that pharmacotherapy of BD should probably be initiated before pharmacotherapy of ADHD, ICDs, or BPD. In contrast, psychotherapy could be started at any time – in part to help educate the patient about the co-occurrence of these disorders. More data are available for BD with ADHD – these studies suggest beginning with a mood stabilizer or second-generation antipsychotic, and once manic symptoms have resolved, adding a standard ADHD medication. In other words, mood stabilization typically is not accompanied by amelioration of ADHD symptoms. By contrast, the only RCT in BD patients with an ICD (pathological gambling) suggests pharmacotherapy begin with a mood stabilizer (in this case, lithium), as there may also be some response of gambling symptoms to stabilization of BD [54]. Of course, the treatment of BD with pathological gambling cannot be generalized to the treatment of BD with other ICDs. Nonetheless, the only RCT in patients with BD and BPD also suggests that treatment with a mood stabilizer (in this case, divalproex) may benefit BPD as well as BD symptoms [86].

Further RCTs of treatments in individuals with mood disorders and ADHD, ICDs, and BPD are greatly needed. Though essential, these studies are difficult to conduct, primarily because of scant funding sources.

Author Conflicts of Interest

SLM is or has been a consultant to or member of the scientific advisory boards of Allergan, Bracket (now Signant Health), F. Hoffmann-La Roche Ltd., Idorsia, Intra-Cellular Therapies, Mitsubishi Tanabe Pharma America, Myriad, Novo Nordisk, Otsuka, Shire (now Takeda), and Sunovion. She has been or is a principal or co-investigator on studies sponsored by the Allergan, Brainsway, Jazz, Marriott Foundation, Myriad, National Institute of Mental Health, Novo Nordisk, Shire (now Takeda), and Sunovion. She is also an inventor on United States Patent No. 6,323,236 B2, Use of Sulfamate Derivatives for Treating Impulse Control Disorders, and along with the patent's assignee, University of Cincinnati, Cincinnati, Ohio, has received payments from Johnson & Johnson, which has exclusive rights under the patent.

AIG is a consultant to Idorsia and Signant Health.

FRN receives grant support from the National Institute of Mental Health K23 Award (K23MH120503) and from a 2017 NARSAD Young Investigator Award from the Brain and Behavior Research Foundation; is an inventor on a U.S. Patent and Trademark Office patent # 10,857,356, Transcutaneous Spinal Cord Stimulation for Treatment of Psychiatric Disorders; and has received non-financial research support from Soterix Medical.

References

1. Katzman MA, Bilkey TS, Chokka PR, Fallu A, Klassen LJ. Adult ADHD and comorbid disorders: clinical implications of a dimensional approach. *BMC Psychiatry*. 2017;**17**(1):302.

2. Wingo AP, Ghaemi SN. A systematic review of rates and diagnostic validity of comorbid adult attention-deficit/hyperactivity disorder and bipolar disorder. *J Clin Psychiatry*. 2007;**68**(11):1776–84.

3. Nierenberg AA, Miyahara S, Spencer T, et al. Clinical and diagnostic implications of lifetime attention-deficit/hyperactivity disorder comorbidity in adults with bipolar disorder: data from the first 1000 STEP-BD participants. *Biol Psychiatry*. 2005;**57**(11):1467–73.

4. Meier SM, Pavlova B, Dalsgaard S, et al. Attention-deficit hyperactivity disorder and anxiety disorders as precursors of bipolar disorder onset in adulthood. *Br J Psychiatry*. 2018;**213**(3):555–60.

5. Biederman J, Faraone SV, Petty C, et al. Further evidence that pediatric-onset bipolar disorder comorbid with ADHD represents a distinct subtype: results from a large controlled family study. *J Psychiatr Res*. 2013;**47**(1):15–22.

6. Brainstorm C, Anttila V, Bulik-Sullivan B, et al. Analysis of shared heritability in common disorders of the brain. *Science*. 2018;**360**(6395).

7. Wu Y, Cao H, Baranova A, et al. Multi-trait analysis for genome-wide association study of five psychiatric disorders. *Transl Psychiatry*. 2020;**10**(1):209.

8. Lan WH, Bai YM, Hsu JW, et al. Comorbidity of ADHD and suicide attempts among adolescents and young adults with bipolar disorder: a nationwide longitudinal study. *J Affect Disord*. 2015;**176**:171–5.

9. Warden D, Riggs PD, Min SJ, et al. Major depression and treatment response in adolescents with ADHD and substance use disorder. *Drug Alcohol Depend*. 2012;**120**(1–3):214–9.

10. Biederman J, Baldessarini RJ, Wright V, Knee D, Harmatz JS. A double-blind placebo controlled study of desipramine in the treatment of ADD: I. *Efficacy. J Am Acad Child Adolesc Psychiatry*. 1989;**28** (5):777–84.

11. Wilens TE, Biederman J, Prince J, et al. Six-week, double-blind, placebo-controlled study of desipramine for adult attention deficit hyperactivity *disorder*. Am J Psychiatry. 1996;**153**(9):1147–53.

12. Biederman J, Baldessarini RJ, Wright V, Keenan K, Faraone S. A double-blind placebo controlled study of desipramine in the treatment of ADD: III. Lack of impact of comorbidity and family history factors on clinical response. *J Am Acad Child Adolesc Psychiatry*. 1993;**32**(1):199–204.

13. Otasowie J, Castells X, Ehimare UP, Smith CH. Tricyclic antidepressants for attention deficit hyperactivity disorder (ADHD) in children and adolescents. *Cochrane Database Syst Rev*. 2014; **9**:CD006997.

14. Wilens TE, Spencer TJ, Biederman J, et al. A controlled clinical trial of bupropion for attention deficit hyperactivity disorder in adults. *Am J Psychiatry*. 2001;**158**(2):282–8.

15. Maneeton N, Maneeton B, Srisurapanont M, Martin SD. Bupropion for adults with attention-deficit hyperactivity disorder: meta-analysis of randomized, placebo-controlled trials. *Psychiatry Clin Neurosci*. 2011;**65**(7):611–17.

16. Ng QX. A systematic review of the use of bupropion for attention-deficit/hyperactivity disorder in children and adolescents. *J Child Adolesc Psychopharmacol*. 2017;**27**(2):112–16.

17. Verbeeck W, Bekkering GE, Van den Noortgate W, Kramers C. Bupropion for attention deficit hyperactivity disorder (ADHD) in adults. *Cochrane Database Syst Rev*. 2017;**10**:CD009504.

18. Amiri S, Farhang S, Ghoreishizadeh MA, Malek A, Mohammadzadeh S. Double-blind controlled trial of venlafaxine for treatment of adults with attention deficit/hyperactivity disorder. *Hum Psychopharmacol*. 2012;**27**(1):76–81.

19. Ghanizadeh A. A systematic review of reboxetine for treating patients with attention deficit hyperactivity disorder. *Nord J Psychiatry*. 2015;**69**(4):241–8.

20. Bilodeau M, Simon T, Beauchamp MH, et al. Duloxetine in adults with ADHD: a randomized, placebo-controlled pilot study. *J Atten Disord*. 2014;**18**(2):169–75.

21. Weiss M, Hechtman L, Adult ARG. A randomized double-blind trial of paroxetine and/or dextroamphetamine and problem-focused therapy for attention-deficit/hyperactivity disorder in adults. *J Clin Psychiatry*. 2006;**67**(4):611–9.

22. Biederman J, Lindsten A, Sluth LB, et al. Vortioxetine for attention deficit hyperactivity disorder in adults: a randomized, double-blind, placebo-controlled, proof-of-concept study. *J Psychopharmacol*. 2019;**33** (4):511–21.

23. Patkar AA, Masand PS, Pae CU, et al. A randomized, double-blind, placebo-controlled trial of augmentation with an extended release formulation of methylphenidate in outpatients with treatment-resistant depression. *J Clin Psychopharmacol*. 2006;**26** (6):653–6.

24. Trivedi MH, Cutler AJ, Richards C et al. A randomized controlled trial of the efficacy and safety of lisdexamfetamine dimesylate as augmentation therapy in adults with residual symptoms of major depressive disorder after treatment with escitalopram. *J Clin Psychiatry*. 2013;**74**(8):802–9.

25. Madhoo M, Keefe RS, Roth RM, et al. Lisdexamfetamine dimesylate augmentation in adults with persistent executive dysfunction after partial or full remission of major depressive disorder. *Neuropsychopharmacology*. 2014;**39** (6):1388–98.

26. Richards C, McIntyre RS, Weisler R, et al. Lisdexamfetamine dimesylate augmentation for adults with major depressive disorder and inadequate response to antidepressant monotherapy: results from 2 phase 3, multicenter, randomized, double-blind, placebo-controlled studies. *J Affect Disord*. 2016;**206**:151–60.

27. Nasser A, Liranso T, Adewole T, et al. Once-daily SPN-812 200 and 400 mg in the treatment of ADHD in school-aged children: a phase III randomized, controlled trial. *Clin Ther*. 2021;**43**(4):684–700.

28. Moller HJ, Fuger J, Kasper S. Efficacy of new generation antidepressants: meta-analysis of imipramine-controlled studies. *Pharmacopsychiatry*. 1994;**27**(6):215–23.

29. Dorrego MF, Canevaro L, Kuzis G, Sabe L, Starkstein SE. A randomized, double-blind, crossover study of methylphenidate and lithium in adults with attention-deficit/hyperactivity disorder: preliminary findings. *J Neuropsychiatry Clin Neurosci*. 2002;**14** (3):289–95.

30. Hegerl U, Mergl R, Sander C, et al. A multi-centre, randomised, double-blind, placebo-controlled clinical trial of methylphenidate in the initial treatment of acute mania (MEMAP study). *Eur Neuropsychopharmacol.* 2018;**28**(1):185–94.

31. McElroy SL, Martens BE, Mori N, et al. Adjunctive lisdexamfetamine in bipolar depression: a preliminary randomized, placebo-controlled trial. *Int Clin Psychopharmacol.* 2015;**30**(1):6–13.

32. Viktorin A, Ryden E, Thase ME, et al. The risk of treatment-emergent mania with methylphenidate in bipolar disorder. *Am J Psychiatry.* 2017;**174**(4):341–8.

33. Atomoxetine ADHD, Comorbid MDD SG, Bangs ME, Emslie GJ, Spencer TJ, et al. Efficacy and safety of atomoxetine in adolescents with attention-deficit/hyperactivity disorder and major depression. *J Child Adolesc Psychopharmacol.* 2007;**17**(4):407–20.

34. Kratochvil CJ, May DE, Silva SG, et al. Treatment response in depressed adolescents with and without co-morbid attention-deficit/hyperactivity disorder in the Treatment for Adolescents with Depression Study. *J Child Adolesc Psychopharmacol.* 2009;**19**(5):519–27.

35. Scheffer RE, Kowatch RA, Carmody T, Rush AJ. Randomized, placebo-controlled trial of mixed amphetamine salts for symptoms of comorbid ADHD in pediatric bipolar disorder after mood stabilization with divalproex sodium. *Am J Psychiatry.* 2005;**162**(1):58–64.

36. Findling RL, Short EJ, McNamara NK et al. Methylphenidate in the treatment of children and adolescents with bipolar disorder and attention-deficit/hyperactivity disorder. *J Am Acad Child Adolesc Psychiatry.* 2007;**46**(11):1445–53.

37. Tramontina S, Zeni CP, Ketzer CR, et al. Aripiprazole in children and adolescents with bipolar disorder comorbid with attention-deficit/hyperactivity disorder: a pilot randomized clinical trial. *J Clin Psychiatry.* 2009;**70**(5):756–64.

38. Zeni CP, Tramontina S, Ketzer CR, Pheula GF, Rohde LA. Methylphenidate combined with aripiprazole in children and adolescents with bipolar disorder and attention-deficit/hyperactivity disorder: a randomized crossover trial. *J Child Adolesc Psychopharmacol.* 2009;**19**(5):553–61.

39. Chang K, Nayar D, Howe M, Rana M. Atomoxetine as an adjunct therapy in the treatment of co-morbid attention-deficit/hyperactivity disorder in children and adolescents with bipolar I or II disorder. *J Child Adolesc Psychopharmacol.* 2009;**19**(5):547–51.

40. Frosch J, Wortis SB. A contribution to the nosology of the impulse disorders. *Am J Psychiatry.* 1954;**111**(2):132–8.

41. Hollander E, Stein DJ (Eds.). *Clinical Manual of Impulse-Control Disorders.* Washington, DC: American Psychiatric Association, 2006.

42. American Psychiatric Association. *Diagnostic and Statistical Manual of Mental Disorders.* 4th ed. Washington, DC: American Psychiatric Association, 1994.

43. American Psychiatric Association. *Diagnostic and Statistical Manual of Mental Disorders: DSM-5.* 5th ed. Washington, DC: American Psychiatric Association, 2013.

44. McElroy SL, Hudson JI, Pope HG, Keck PE. Kleptomania: clinical characteristics and associated psychopathology. *Psychol Med.* 1991;**21**(1):93–108.

45. McIntyre RS, McElroy SL, Konarski JZ, et al. Problem gambling in bipolar disorder: results from the Canadian Community Health Survey. *J Affect Disord.* 2007;**102**(1–3):27–34.

46. Coccaro EF. Psychiatric comorbidity in intermittent explosive disorder. *J Psychiatr Res.* 2019;**118**:38–43.

47. Pereira DCS, Coutinho ESF, Corassa RB, Andrade LH, Viana MC. Prevalence and psychiatric comorbidities of intermittent explosive disorders in Metropolitan Sao Paulo, Brazil. *Soc Psychiatry Psychiatr Epidemiol.* 2021;**56**(4):687–94.

48. Karakus G, Tamam L. Impulse control disorder comorbidity among patients with bipolar I disorder. *Compr Psychiatry.* 2011;**52**(4):378–85.

49. Varo C, Murru A, Salagre E, et al. Behavioral addictions in bipolar disorders: A systematic review. *Eur Neuropsychopharmacol.* 2019;**29**(1):76–97.

50. Mouaffak F, Leite C, Hamzaoui S, et al. Naltrexone in the treatment of broadly defined behavioral addictions: a review and meta-analysis of randomized controlled trials. *Eur Addict Res.* 2017;**23**(4):204–10.

51. Grant JE, Odlaug BL, Kim SW. N-acetylcysteine, a glutamate modulator, in the treatment of trichotillomania: a double-blind, placebo-controlled study. *Arch Gen Psychiatry.* 2009;**66**(7):756–63.

52. Deepmala, Slattery J, Kumar N, et al. Clinical trials of N-acetylcysteine in psychiatry and neurology: a systematic review. *Neurosci Biobehav Rev.* 2015;**55**:294–321.

53. Okamoto Y, Sekine T, Grammer J, Yount RG. The essential light chains constitute part of the active site of smooth muscle myosin. *Nature.* 1986;**324**(6092):78–80.

54. Hollander E, Pallanti S, Allen A, Sood E, Baldini Rossi N. Does sustained-release lithium reduce impulsive gambling and affective instability versus placebo in pathological gamblers with bipolar spectrum disorders? *Am J Psychiatry.* 2005;**162**(1):137–45.

55. McElroy SL, Nelson EB, Welge JA, Kaehler L, Keck PE Jr. Olanzapine in the treatment of pathological gambling: a negative randomized placebo-controlled trial. *J Clin Psychiatry*. 2008;**69**(3):433–40.

56. Grant BF, Stinson FS, Hasin DS, et al. Prevalence, correlates, and comorbidity of bipolar I disorder and axis I and II disorders: results from the National Epidemiologic Survey on Alcohol and Related Conditions. *J Clin Psychiatry*. 2005;**66**(10):1205–15.

57. McDermid J, Sareen J, El-Gabalawy R, et al. Co-morbidity of bipolar disorder and borderline personality disorder: findings from the National Epidemiologic Survey on Alcohol and Related Conditions. *Compr Psychiatry*. 2015;**58**:18–28.

58. Fornaro M, Orsolini L, Marini S, et al. The prevalence and predictors of bipolar and borderline personality disorders comorbidity: systematic review and meta-analysis. *J Affect Disord*. 2016;**195**:105–18.

59. Blanco C, Compton WM, Saha TD, et al. Epidemiology of DSM-5 bipolar I disorder: results from the national epidemiologic survey on alcohol and related conditions – III. *J Psychiatr Res*. 2017;**84**:310–17.

60. Shah R, Zanarini MC. Comorbidity of borderline personality disorder: current status and future directions. *Psychiatr Clin North Am*. 2018;**41**(4):583–93.

61. Zanarini MC, Horz-Sagstetter S, Temes CM, et al. The 24-year course of major depression in patients with borderline personality disorder and personality-disordered comparison subjects. *J Affect Disord*. 2019;**258**:109–14.

62. de la Rosa I, Oquendo MA, Garcia G, et al. Determining if borderline personality disorder and bipolar disorder are alternative expressions of the same disorder: results from the national epidemiologic survey on alcohol and related conditions. *J Clin Psychiatry*. 2017;**78**(8):e994–e999.

63. Witt SH, Streit F, Jungkunz M, et al. Genome-wide association study of borderline personality disorder reveals genetic overlap with bipolar disorder, major depression and schizophrenia. *Transl Psychiatry*. 2017;**7**(6):e1155.

64. Joyce PR, Mulder RT, Luty SE, et al. Borderline personality disorder in major depression: symptomatology, temperament, character, differential drug response, and 6-month outcome. *Compr Psychiatry*. 2003;**44**(1):35–43.

65. Skodol AE, Grilo CM, Keyes KM, et al. Relationship of personality disorders to the course of major depressive disorder in a nationally representative sample. Am J Psychiatry. 2011;**168**(3):257–64.

66. Zimmerman M, Balling C, Chelminski I, Dalrymple K. Patients with borderline personality disorder and bipolar disorder: a descriptive and comparative study. *Psychol Med*. 2021;**51**(9):1479–90.

67. Patel RS, Manikkara G, Chopra A. Bipolar disorder and comorbid borderline personality disorder: patient characteristics and outcomes in US hospitals. *Medicina (Kaunas)*. 2019;**55**(1).

68. Feske U, Mulsant BH, Pilkonis PA, et al. Clinical outcome of ECT in patients with major depression and comorbid borderline personality disorder. Am J Psychiatry. 2004;**161**(11):2073–80.

69. Borderline Personality Disorder: Treatment and Management. National Institute for Health and Clinical Excellence: Guidance. Leicester, 2009.

70. Oldham JM, Gabbard GO, Goin MK, et al. *Practice Guideline for the Treatment of Patients with Borderline Personality Disorder*. Washington, DC: American Psychiatric Association, 2010.

71. Tyrer P, Silk KR. A comparison of UK and US guidelines for drug treatment in borderline personality disorder. *Int Rev Psychiatry*. 2011;**23**(4):388–94.

72. Oud M, Arntz A, Hermens ML, Verhoef R, Kendall T. Specialized psychotherapies for adults with borderline personality disorder: a systematic review and meta-analysis. *Aust N Z J Psychiatry*. 2018;**52**(10):949–61.

73. Stone MH. Borderline personality disorder: clinical guidelines for treatment. *Psychodyn Psychiatry*. 2019;**47**(1):5–26.

74. Riffer F, Farkas M, Streibl L, Kaiser E, Sprung M. Psychopharmacological treatment of patients with borderline personality disorder: comparing data from routine clinical care with recommended guidelines. *Int J Psychiatry Clin Pract*. 2019;**23**(3):178–88.

75. Lieb K, Vollm B, Rucker G, Timmer A, Stoffers JM. Pharmacotherapy for borderline personality disorder: Cochrane systematic review of randomised trials. *Br J Psychiatry*. 2010;**196**(1):4–12.

76. Vita A, De Peri L, Sacchetti E. Antipsychotics, antidepressants, anticonvulsants, and placebo on the symptom dimensions of borderline personality disorder: a meta-analysis of randomized controlled and open-label trials. *J Clin Psychopharmacol*. 2011;**31**(5):613–24.

77. Stoffers JM, Lieb K. Pharmacotherapy for borderline personality disorder – current evidence and recent trends. *Curr Psychiatry Rep*. 2015;**17**(1):534.

78. Hancock-Johnson E, Griffiths C, Picchioni M. A focused systematic review of pharmacological treatment for borderline personality disorder. *CNS Drugs*. 2017;**31**(5):345–56.

79. Stoffers-Winterling J, Storebo OJ, Lieb K. Pharmacotherapy for borderline personality disorder: an update of published, unpublished and ongoing studies. *Curr Psychiatry Rep*. 2020;**22**(8):37.

80. Schulkens J, Bergs N, Ingenhoven T, et al. Selective serotonin reuptake-inhibitors for symptom-based treatment of borderline personality disorders in older adults: an international delphi study. *Clin Psychopharmacol Neurosci*. 2021;**19**(1):53–62.

81. Pahwa M, Nunez NA, Joseph B, et al. Efficacy and tolerability of lamotrigine in borderline personality disorder: a systematic review and meta-analysis. *Psychopharmacol Bull*. 2020;**50**(4):118–36.

82. Ekselius L, von Knorring L. Personality disorder comorbidity with major depression and response to treatment with sertraline or citalopram. *Int Clin Psychopharmacol*. 1998;**13**(5):205–11.

83. Bellino S, Zizza M, Rinaldi C, Bogetto F. Combined treatment of major depression in patients with borderline personality disorder: a comparison with pharmacotherapy. *Can J Psychiatry*. 2006;**51**(7):453–60.

84. Bellino S, Zizza M, Rinaldi C, Bogetto F. Combined therapy of major depression with concomitant borderline personality disorder: comparison of interpersonal and cognitive psychotherapy. *Can J Psychiatry*. 2007;**52**(11):718–25.

85. Jahangard L, Haghighi M, Bajoghli H, et al. Training emotional intelligence improves both emotional intelligence and depressive symptoms in inpatients with borderline personality disorder and depression. *Int J Psychiatry Clin Pract*. 2012;**16**(3):197–204.

86. Frankenburg FR, Zanarini MC. Divalproex sodium treatment of women with borderline personality disorder and bipolar II disorder: a double-blind placebo-controlled pilot study. *J Clin Psychiatry*. 2002;**63**(5):442–6.

Phenomenological Psychopathology of Mood Disorders

Roland Zahn

Introduction

In his book *General Psychopathology*, first published in 1913 [1], Karl Jaspers presented a methodological framework for exploring the phenomenology of symptoms of psychiatric disorders as well as relating experimental psychology and nosology to phenomenology. Jaspers, a philosopher and psychiatrist, was freed from clinical duties to write his book at Heidelberg University's psychiatry department, and most would argue it still remains the deepest description of symptoms to date. He was influenced by philosophers Brentano and Husserl among others who had described the phenomenological method as applied to philosophical psychology [2]. Modern consensus-based diagnostic classification systems [3] would have been sharply criticised by Jaspers, who argued against algorithmic definitions of disorders based on fixed definitions of symptoms that were already developed by some of his contemporaries. Such an algorithmic approach, we would argue, however, does not exclude Jaspers' quest for keeping an open mind when observing our patients' experiences and trying to refine our phenomenological understanding and description for research and future refinements of our classification systems and assessment instruments.

This chapter will briefly introduce the phenomenological approach to symptoms and how this has influenced symptoms as opposed to diagnostic criterion-based assessment instruments. A transcultural and historic perspective will be employed to identify relevant symptoms of mood disorders. Descriptions of these symptoms will be provided, and lastly the contribution of phenomenology to subsyndrome discovery and network-based approaches to the psychopathology of mood disorders will be discussed.

The Phenomenological Approach to Symptoms

In his introductory chapters [1], Jaspers explains his method of empathic understanding as key to the phenomenological approach to symptoms. There has to be empathy and understanding of the external characteristics of the psychic state, or of the conditions under which the phenomena occur so as to determine whether a patient's experience is understandable as a usual consequence of psychosocial events or whether it is qualitatively or quantitatively different and cannot be solely explained on that basis. He writes that the patients' own self-descriptions provide the best-defined and clearest data and this is why one should try to describe symptoms in the patients' own words rather than summarise them in technical terms. The description is solely based on things that are present to the patients' consciousness. We should attend to what exists before us, what we can apprehend, discriminate and describe. We should refuse to prejudge. The phenomenological orientation is something we have to attain to again and again and involves a continual onslaught on our prejudices. This has to be acquired painfully through critical self-reflection and frequent failure, he writes.

In part I of his book [1], "individual psychic phenomena" are studied and these are defined as either our patients' "subjective experiences, vividly represented by us" (i.e., subjective psychopathology = phenomenology) or objective psychopathology based "on observable performances, somatic symptoms or meaningful phenomena found in expressive gesture and in personal worlds and creations". In parts II and III, he attempts at a summary of the knowledge at the time with regard to connections between individual psychic phenomena. He describes the method as containing two steps:

1) "We understand genetically by empathy how one psychic event emerges from another."

2) "We find by repeated experience that a number of phenomena are regularly linked together, and on this basis we explain causally."

This brief summary of the approach to psychopathology proposed by Jaspers in his own words highlights the simplicity and the value of the method in principle, but he acknowledges the difficulty in freeing oneself from prejudices and assumptions when observing and describing our patients' experiences and behaviour. The next section will describe the implications for the assessment instruments used in research and clinical practice.

Symptom-Based versus Diagnostic Criterion-Based Assessment

Although most clinicians would probably agree that an individualised approach to assessment is ideal, there is nevertheless a need to classify observations in some way, to compare observations between different clinicians and provide a framework for collecting evidence on how individual symptoms are connected. To overcome this weakness of the phenomenological approach whilst retaining its general principles, symptom-based assessment instruments have been developed which required operationalising definitions to ensure high inter-rater reliability. The Present State Exam (PSE) was developed by an international consortium, led by John Wing at the Institute of Psychiatry in London [4], incorporating phenomenological traditions and assessing symptoms rather than diagnostic criteria for disorders, as the now more widely used structured clinical interview for the *Diagnostic and Statistical Manual of Mental Disorders* (DSM [5]) does. The PSE has been further developed into the Schedules for Clinical Assessment in Neuropsychiatry (SCAN), which is available in many languages involving field trial centres in 14 countries and has been published by the World Health Organisation (WHO [6]). SCAN includes a computer algorithm that can be used to synthesise symptoms into diagnostic classifications according to ICD-10.

Independently, the Association for Methodology and Documentation in Psychiatry (AMDP) system has been developed, which is widely used to record symptoms using operational criteria in German-speaking countries [7] and was also published in English [8]. We have extended the interview with a freely available moral emotion addendum, showing high inter-rater reliability at a single symptom level [9]. These symptom-based assessment instruments present a compromise between the pure phenomenological approach and the approach chosen in the structured clinical interview for DSM [5] that assesses symptom- and aetiology-based diagnostic criteria rather than the symptoms themselves.

Transcultural and Historical Symptom Identification and Description

Although the threshold of perceiving a phenomenon as bothering or impairing is variable across observers and cultures, there should be some degree of symptom expression that is looked upon as such in most cultures so that this symptom can be considered as a core part of a mood disorder as a valid category of enquiry. It has been pointed out that each culture has its own emotional lexicon that encodes socio-morally significant values and its own idioms of distress [10]. This emphasises why symptom-based assessments should not be fully structured, allowing the assessor to adapt the wording to the cultural context.

Although symptom criteria from DSM-based diagnostic instruments have been used for transcultural comparisons [11], we would argue that the DSM was neither designed for assessing symptoms nor are its diagnostic symptom criteria useful as units of analysis in such studies. This is because several symptoms are combined into one criterion (e.g., hopelessness/low mood or worthlessness/guilt), and these symptoms are rated using different thresholds. For example, being bothered by guilt would not be marked as diagnostically relevant on the DSM if it is related to one's illness being a burden on others [5], whereas in symptom-based assessments one would not define such threshold criteria other than the level of subjective distress and objective impairment [7].

Therefore, probably the most systematic- and symptom-based transcultural comparisons of depressive disorders are still found in the older literature, in particular the WHO Collaborative Study [12]. Tseng [13] reviews these and other studies and summarises that it is not clear whether differences in frequencies of specific symptoms across cultures were due to ethnocultural variations or differences in the levels of severity. Among the symptoms with differences in frequencies were guilt feelings, somatic symptoms and suicidal ideas [13]. The authors of the WHO Collaborative Study conclude [12]: "A common core of depressive symptomatology was present in practically all patients and in every centre of the study. Differences that were found between the groups of patients in the different centres were relatively minor, and they were mainly variations of degree rather than of kind". The core symptoms present in all centres regardless of diagnostic classification were [12] "sadness, joylessness, anxiety and tension, lack of energy, loss of interests, experience of loss of the ability to concentrate, and ideas of insufficiency, inadequacy and worthlessness".

Anxiety and tension were among the most frequently reported symptoms. Differences in symptoms occurred between "endogenous" and "psychogenic" groups, a distinction abandoned in later classification systems, for example "worse in the morning, early awakening, slowness or retardation of thought, psychomotor retardation" was more frequent in the "endogenous" group.

Feelings of inadequacy (including self-worthlessness) was thus a consistent symptom of depression [12], whereas guilt was only found in a subgroup of patients across cultures [10]. We showed that solely asking about "guilt" underestimated the frequency of self-blaming feelings and that self-disgust/loathing was more frequently endorsed, with all self-blaming emotions together reported in over 80% of patients [9].

Transculturally consistent symptoms of depressive disorders can also be traced back historically to earlier nineteenth-century descriptions. A review of 28 influential textbooks from the late nineteenth-century reports the following symptom description of melancholia as highly consistent [14]: low mood, suicidal ideation, psychomotor retardation, change in posture and facial expression, loss of appetite/weight and sleep disturbance (but not the opposite), changes in the content of thoughts ("most commonly: hopelessness, guilt, self-reproach, shame, wickedness, worthlessness, expectation of future calamities and fears of damnation, disgrace, poverty or unremitting suffering"). Melancholic mood was described as "depression, soul-pain, sadness, ill-humor, sorrow, oppression, misery, woe, distress, gloom, despondency, anguish and dejection".

The majority of descriptions also contained anxiety symptoms and loss of interest. "Anxiety was variously described as fears, worries and palpitations with precordial anxiety. Most commonly, loss of interest was described as withdrawal from and/or indifference to work responsibilities and prior social relationships

with friends and family". The changes in cognition were most commonly "general mental inhibition and more specifically slowing of thoughts and impairment of attention and concentration".

Transcultural comparisons of symptoms of bipolar disorder are scarce, possibly, because there is less debate about cultural variability. A large international study of bipolar symptom criteria controlled for transcultural variations and confirmed the widely assumed transcultural stability of key symptoms used in the DSM with >80% consistency (elevated mood, increased activity and goal-directed activities, increased self-esteem, decreased sleep, being more talkative [15]). Historically, Kraepelin's conceptualisation of depressive and manic states as part of the same manic-depressive disorder has been highly influential and provides an elegant way of conceptualising both states as part of shared symptom dimensions. The key part of Kraepelin's concept is that different symptoms have independent temporal dynamics, which he then uses to explain the occurrence of mixed affective states at the transition between mood states (see Figure 14.1).

Psychopathological Description of Mood Disorder Symptoms

Based on the description of symptoms from transcultural and historical studies above and on the definitions used by Kraepelin, Jaspers, the PSE/SCAN, AMDP and my own observations, as well as modern psychological concepts, this section provides brief definitions and descriptions of relevant mood disorder symptoms and aims at stimulating further research and clinical observation.

Attention [7]
Concentration [7]

Concentration difficulties are often reported as "memory" difficulties by patients, but on closer examination recent memory for important events such as family gatherings is intact and depressive memory difficulties are typically linked to less salient information and are often associated with being distracted by depressive thoughts [16].

Formal Thought [7]
Circumstantial Thinking [7] and Flight of Ideas [7]

In circumstantial thinking, someone is not able to distinguish important from seemingly irrelevant information during a conversation and goes off on tangents.

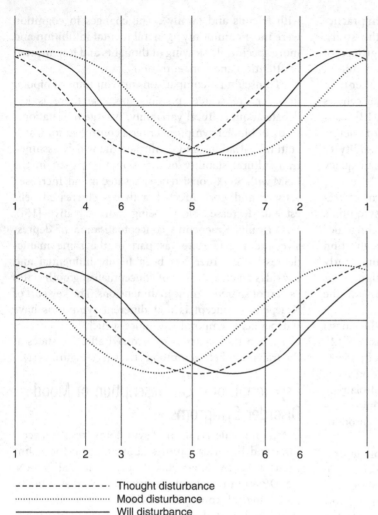

Figure 14.1 Kraepelin's concept of mood symptom dynamics.

Kraepelin's Figure XXIV describes the composition of mixed states in manic-depressive illness [17]. He conceptualises disturbances of mood, thought and will as independent. He describes mood as empty (= "verödet"), thought as inhibited and an inability to decide as an expression of depressive will disturbance. Numbers 1 to 7 describe the composition of different mixed states: 1. Mania with flight of ideas, elated mood and urge to be active, 2. In angry/irritable mania, the elated mood switches into being irritable and sensitive, whilst still having an increased self-esteem; this is accompanied by a mild flight of ideas and restlessness and increased activity, also including excessive smoking or drinking. 3. Depressive agitation is a state when there is a marked impoverishment of thoughts and sad mood, combined with restlessness. 4. A state of an unproductive mania with impoverished thinking. In this state, patients feel elated in mood. 5. Depression with an inhibition of thought, sad mood and an inability to make decisions. 6. Manic stupor: patients do not respond; if they speak, they only speak with a low voice to themselves, smile without reason and are usually calm. They often develop a pressure to talk and a flight of ideas. 7. Within the usual picture of depression, inhibition of thought can be replaced by a flight of ideas. 8. Is not depicted, but Kraepelin notes also an observation of combined symptoms of a flight of ideas together with elated mood and psychomotor inhibition. Sometimes he observed irritability, distractibility, jocularity, flight of ideas and pressure to talk, as well as an increased number of sound associations. At the same time, he observed an absence of motor restlessness.

- - - - - - - - - - Thought disturbance
.... Mood disturbance
————— Will disturbance

This can be observed in people with attention-deficit/hyperactivity disorder (ADHD) syndromes and people with a detail-focussed cognitive style. When not part of someone's usual conversation style, however, it can be an important early sign of transitioning into a hypomanic thought pattern. Flight of ideas is a more pronounced phenomenon where someone's train of thought is accelerated, but rather than finishing one thought, they interrupt themselves often with only superficially related thoughts. These can be triggered by things in the environment or based on sound associations as classically observed [17]. Unlike the incoherence of thought found in schizophrenia, the associative connection between thoughts is still detectable.

Rumination [7]

This common symptom in depressive states is being pre-occupied with recurrent depressive thoughts that are not necessarily experienced as feeling compelled to think in that way, but are hard to stop. These thoughts typically revolve around self-critical themes, and Beck described the phenomenology of characteristic cognitive distortions, such as overgeneralisation, in his seminal work [18].

Inhibited Thinking [7] and Pressured Thinking [7]

Inhibited thinking is defined as a subjective experience of one's thinking feeling blocked or thinking against an inner resistance and is more distinctive of depression than the more ubiquitous concentration difficulties. In pressured thinking, people have lots of ideas coming into their mind, an experience linked with hypomanic/manic states.

Drive and Psychomotor Activity [7]
Inhibition of Drive [7,19]

Inhibition of drive is the experience of having to work against an inner resistance to get started with things and cannot be solely explained by a lack of motivation. We usually ask about things people want or need to do to probe this symptom. It was shown to be a predictor of future development of major mood episodes and thought to be more specific for endogenous depression than a mere lack of drive [19].

Lack of Drive and Increased Drive [7]

A lack of drive or energy and interest is experienced very consistently in depression. Increased drive/energy is a core feature of hypomania and mania. It is closely associated with increased goal-directed and pleasure-related activity, but not necessarily identical to it. One interesting distinction in the modern neuroscience literature is that of the anticipation of versus the experience of pleasure [20]. Lack of drive, mental energy and motivation is usually closely associated with a lack of anticipating pleasure or success; the latter is important, as duty-related motivation is more relevant in people with depressive disorders than in those without [21]. Anticipating pleasure is impaired not only in major depressive disorder, but also in other conditions such as schizophrenia spectrum disorders [22]. A lack of drive can also be found after withdrawing from substances or in people with ADHD in the absence of interesting stimulation.

Motor Restlessness [7]

This observable increase in movement or fidgetiness is a non-specific symptom and can be related to anxiety, increased drive in hypomania or agitated depression.

Talkativeness (Logorrhoe [7])

This observable increase in the flow of verbal utterances, which can occur without affecting the semantic connection between thoughts, is observed commonly in hypomanic states, but its mild forms can be hard to detect without a reference to people's usual states due to cultural and individual variability.

Delusions
Delusional Ideas [7]

Most patients with depressive episodes do not experience delusions, but in the subgroup who do, the content is often distinctive. A delusion is a belief that is immediately evident to the person, cannot be corrected, is objectively untrue and is not shared by the person's socio-cultural community. The so-called synthymic delusions in depressed states are typically related to guilt, impoverishment and hypochondriac concerns or occur as delusions of grandeur in mania, where people can be convinced to have god-like powers. Jaspers would argue that synthymic beliefs such as these need to have a quality that cannot be explained on the basis of the mood state to be classified as delusions [1].

Temporal Experience [23] of Affect
Hopelessness [7], Over-optimism [6,24] and Mood-Congruent Memory [25]

Owen summarises that in "severe depression or mania, anticipation of future outcomes is inflexibly fixed at one end of the value spectrum", with an inability to imagine an alternative outcome [23]. Over-optimism is also likely to play an important role in disregarding likely negative consequences of one's behaviour in mania. Mood-congruent memory biases are not formally described in psychopathology assessments, but there is a rich experimental psychology literature, and one can observe that people with depression usually display enhanced negative and self-critical memories and a difficulty in recalling positive autobiographical events [25] and successes. This can also lead to re-activation of traumatic memories in depression, and I have seen a full post-traumatic stress syndrome developing in someone with old-age depression relating to war experiences, 50 years earlier, which disappeared on treating the depressive episode, with no post-traumatic symptoms prior to the episode.

Current Affective Experience
Mood – Depressed/Euphoric [7]

If one asks people to describe their mood state, they use a variety of emotionally charged terms, but one important characteristic of a mood state in my view is that it represents the internal propensity to respond to a stimulus in a certain way, which may be influenced by the emotional characteristics of the stimulus, but is not determined by it. In contrast, affective lability [7] is typically observed in emotionally unstable personalities and ADHD and is a strong emotional response primarily driven by the external stimulus and occurring immediately in response to it. I would therefore argue that emotional lability is most pronounced in the absence of a mood state that is more stable in duration. Intriguingly though, mixed affective states and people with bipolar disorder show evidence of daily mood instability [26], and one wonders whether this could be the result of co-existing hypomanic and depressive mood states priming mood-congruent stimuli of opposite polarity to result in more pronounced rapid switches in emotions. Patients in mixed states can indeed describe feeling bouts of euphoria for a couple of hours in the midst of a depressed mood state, but this is often uncoupled from obvious psychological stimuli.

Affective Rigidity [7] and Blunted Affect [7]

Affective rigidity is defined as a diminished amplitude of emotional response to stimuli, which is not necessarily confined to pleasurable things only (i.e., anhedonia). This corresponds to the consummatory aspects of pleasurable experiences. People with atypical depression lack affective rigidity. The AMDP concept of blunted affect is misleading in that it refers to a diminished range of emotions being experienced rather than the more common understanding of it as a reduced emotional intensity.

Feeling of Loss of Feeling [7]

This is a distressing and often painfully diminished ability to experience feelings. Jaspers quotes a patient [1]: "I no longer feel gladness or pain. I no longer love my relatives. I feel indifferent to everything", and contrasts this symptom against apathy, where there is an absence of feeling without being bothered by it, which brings about aboulia (i.e. an inability to act), because there is no incentive to act. Whereas a feeling of loss of feeling is a common symptom in depression [9], whenever I have observed apathy, it was in the context of an organic affective disorder such as frontotemporal dementia [16].

Feelings of Inadequacy / Exaggerated Self-Esteem [7]

Self-esteem / worth is a core aspect of depressed or elated mood states. Self-esteem for some people is more strongly linked to professional achievements and for others more to interpersonal functioning, but consistently entails social comparisons. It is interesting to observe that people with depression typically think that others are better able to do certain things or are worth more in general than themselves, whereas the opposite can be observed in mania.

Self-Blaming Feelings [9]

Our study in the UK found that most people with fully remitting forms of depression prefer the labels "self-loathing" to describe self-disgust, a self-blame-related feeling which was more common than "guilt", which was also found in a high proportion of people. Shame and guilt were distinguishable by most people, and shame is more prominent in people whose concern is primarily with how others perceive them. Self-directed anger was less frequent but associated with self-harming impulses (e.g., hitting oneself) in my experience.

Other-Blaming Feelings [9] / Irritability [7]

Although, in the fully remitting sample of depression, we found anger and disgust towards others being present only in a minority of patients and it was always accompanied by feelings of inadequacy, there is a description of a so-called anger subtype of depression [27]. My observation was that rejection sensitivity can be linked with irritability and anger in unipolar depression. The other source of irritability and anger towards others is often linked to traumatic experiences and anxiety more generally. Irritability and anger are a common symptom in people with mixed affective states, hypomania and mania, even when their primary mood state is euphoric. My observation is that when you challenge someone's increased self-esteem in a manic state and restrict some of their actions, this usually provokes marked anger.

Anxious [14]

Historically, anxiety has been thought of as being more typical of "neurotic" rather than "endogenous" depression [28] or "melancholia", but has been included in some melancholia descriptions [14]. In my observation, anxiety in depressive episodes of otherwise non-anxious patients is often linked to feelings of inadequacy, but more generalised and somatic anxiety can also be seen [14], and all the themes which occur in delusions can also occur as themes of depressive anxiety.

Obsessive Thoughts [7]

Obsessive thoughts are distinguished from rumination in that they are experienced as unreasonable or exaggerated and the person tries to resist or dismiss them [8]. This puristic definition, however, is often blurred in that people with chronic obsessive thoughts may start to rationalise them and interestingly is also the transition of delusions into obsessive thoughts when delusions improve and people stop being convinced of them [29], but nevertheless worry about them. Although obsessive thoughts are not a classical symptom of depression per se, cases have been described with a full obsessive-compulsive syndrome appearing in a depressive episode and then disappearing on remission and whilst switching into a manic state [30]. Most people with compulsive actions in an episode, however, have a history of these compulsive actions prior to the onset of the episode in my experience.

Affective and Self-Imagery [31,32]

Holmes and colleagues note [31]: "Mental imagery dysfunction in depression include an excess of intrusive mental imagery, impoverished positive imagery, observer perspective imagery, and overgeneral memory (in which specific imagery is lacking)". Related to this is an under-investigated phenomenon of implicit feelings such as acting in a particular way when faced with a difficult social situation (so-called action tendencies [33]). Some action tendencies, such as 'feeling like hiding' have been entailed in the operationalisations of self-blaming feelings such as shame [34] shown to be associated with depressive symptoms, but their systematic investigation in current depression is lacking. We found increased endorsements of questions about feeling like hiding and creating a distance from oneself/withdrawing from oneself in remitted depression [32]. A patient with current depression vividly described this as a combination of a "strong feeling of wanting to stop feeling and stop thinking, hitting one's head, wanting to die, wanting to be obliterated", "wanting to switch myself off (my conscious part)", "sense of floating away from myself into space", "exploding into thin air", "escape my body and feelings", "an astronaut on a rope shooing away from the earth leaving my human body behind". Depersonalisation is a related phenomenon, common in anxious patients, and has been classified as a disturbance of the ego perception in its identity or unity [7] and found in classical descriptions of depression [14].

Felt Loss of Vitality [7]

Jaspers [1] and Schneider [2] placed a great emphasis on bodily or "vital" feelings. A feeling like "misery" is experienced as located in body parts ("limbs", "forehead", "chest", "stomach"). More commonly, one can observe a tiredness, weakness [7], heaviness ("leaden paralysis") or achiness felt in one's body that needs to be separated from a mental lack of energy.

Social Withdrawal [7] / Excessive Social Contact [7] / Over-Familiarity

Social withdrawal is a highly consistent symptom of depression and appears to be often related to wanting to hide one's depression and finding it exhausting to spend time with others. Although not a classically used label, I would postulate that 'social overproximity' is a consistent symptom of hypomania in that not only would people with hypomania/mania typically socialise more, but always appeared to me to show less social distance when conversing. We found that social role definitions play an important part of our way of defining socially appropriate behaviour (supplement [35]), and it appears that linked to increased self-esteem is also an over-familiarity (included under socially embarrassing behaviour in [6]) and a reversal or abolishment of social role hierarchies in interactions with manic patients, which would be important to study in more detail.

Somatic and Circadian Functions

Interrupted Sleep and Early Wakening [7] / Hypersomnia, Decreased/Increased Appetite [7], Worse in the Morning [7]

Feeling worse in the morning, early wakening, interrupted sleep, and decreased appetite were classical symptoms of "endogenous" depression [12]. Kendler found that hypersomnia and increased appetite were absent from classical descriptions of melancholia [14], but these play an important role in defining the current concept of atypical depression.

Decreased Need for Sleep [6]

Markedly decreased need for sleep is a distinctive feature of hypomania/mania, but only if it occurs over several days and patients describe feeling "wired" or energetic when waking up.

Symptom Coherence and the Future of Psychopathology

All our diagnostic categories are based on symptom-complexes (i.e., syndromes) with additional aetiological constraints (e.g., the temporal relationship with changes in medications or medical conditions). Thus, if we define disorders in our classification systems, we always take symptom-complexes as the starting point. As

Jaspers summarises [1], there are different aspects of the relation of symptoms within a symptom-complex:

1) Frequency of symptom co-occurrence
2) Coherence of symptoms by being related to a common aspect or function
3) Primary symptoms caused by the aetio-pathogenetic process and secondary symptoms emerging from these in an understandable way

The second aspect, that of symptom coherence, has been emphasised by Carl Schneider (reviewed in Jaspers) arguing about symptoms: *"Their connectedness must be due to a normal complex of psychic function, which complex has been affected by the illness."*

At the time of Jaspers' writing, he acknowledged the limited knowledge about aetiopathogenetic mechanisms, and he had a very critical attitude towards employing cognitive neuroscience, referring to Wernicke and Meynert's psychopathological models as "brain mythologies" [1]. I would argue that although it is premature to settle on a fixed conceptual framework of cognitive and emotional function domains, as the Research Domain Criteria (RDoC) framework [36] proposes, and link them to specific neuroanatomical and molecular mechanisms, our methods for collecting and analysing such evidence have made remarkable progress.

Among these breakthroughs was the cognitive revolution of the 1980s, which led to major advancements in our understanding of human motivation [37] as not solely relying on simple drives, but also including attributions of human causal agency. This work helped us to understand complex socio-moral feelings such as guilt, shame and moral anger as entailing implicit causal attributions [38]. These attributional models of motivation influenced re-conceptualisations of learned helplessness as a model of depression, primarily developed from animal behavioural experiments of exposure to uncontrollable stress [39].

Indeed, we found frequent co-occurrence of self-blaming feelings, hopelessness and feelings of inadequacy [9] as predicted by these attributional models of motivation. Furthermore, feelings of inadequacy are an excellent primary symptom candidate, as they are a more distinctive feature of depression compared with depressed mood, which can be found across a broad range of conditions, together with its transcultural and historical consistency. We further found an association of highly consistent symptoms in a depressive core subsyndrome in our sample that included feelings of inadequacy, hopelessness, depressed mood, lack of drive, blunted affect, affective rigidity and social withdrawal [9].

Recently, using network analytical approaches [40], there has been a rekindled interest in classical psychopathological questions. A recent application of this method found worthlessness to be closely associated with "blaming yourself for things", "feelings of guilt", "feeling inferior to others" and "thoughts of ending your life" [41]. The research found self-blame and guilt to be associated through a mutual connection with worthlessness, which is in keeping with our findings.

Lack of drive as well as a reduced range of emotional experience, particularly an inability to experience pleasure or success, are part of the core depressive syndrome. This would argue for the anticipation of positive feelings to be a necessary symptom across subtypes, although it also occurs in other conditions. Interestingly, we found that self-blaming feelings and loss of interest/pleasure were negatively associated cross-sectionally in current depression [42]. This is in keeping with the neuroscience evidence for separable mesolimbic reward systems whose disruption is hypothesised to underpin anticipatory anhedonia [20] and the subgenual frontal–anterior temporal lobe networks linked to individual differences in self-blaming biases [43] and overgeneral self-blame [44], as well as self-worth [45].

Many other symptoms of depression, such as somatic symptoms, are unlikely primary symptom candidates, as they are neither necessary nor sufficient for the occurrence of the more distinctive symptoms of depression. Furthermore, the co-occurrence of different symptom directions (e.g., decreased and increased appetite) with the same core syndrome (such as depressed mood, feelings of inadequacy), indicates their accessory nature. These accessory symptoms may, however, play an important role in subtypes of depression, and the aetiological validity of these symptoms is yet to be determined.

In summary, many basic psychopathological questions remain unanswered and will require longitudinal studies to understand the temporal dynamics of symptoms of different polarity, which could employ modern network analytical approaches to identify subsyndromes. For example, it is possible that anxiety is a primary symptom in a subgroup and leads to feelings of inadequacy via avoidance and thereby an objective reduction in psychosocial function (i.e., objective inadequacy). In other cases, perceived feelings of inadequacy could be the primary symptom. Particularly, the study of rapid cycling bipolar disorder could prove to be of immense value in understanding whether core symptoms such as over-optimism and increased self-esteem may dissociate from increased drive and interest. Another important gap in the literature is the study of self-praising feelings in bipolar disorder such as pride that could play an analogous role to self-blaming feelings in depression.

Psychopathological research will be essential for our understanding and stratification of mood disorders in the future and, as we have argued, is essential for "translational cognitive neuroscience" [46], which seeks to link psychopathology with cognitive–anatomical models as an intermediary level of description likely to be more closely associated with molecular mechanisms than diagnostic categories themselves. Psychopathology is thus not just a historical discipline, but one which will be essential for future progress in our understanding, assessment and treatment of mood disorders.

References

1. Jaspers K. *General Psychopathology*. 7th ed. Chicago: University of Chicago Press, 1963/1959.

2. Broome MR. *The Maudsley Reader in Phenomenological Psychiatry*. Cambridge: Cambridge University Press, 2012; xiii, 283 p.

3. Spitzer RL, First MB. Classification of psychiatric disorders. *JAMA*. 2005;**294**(15):1898–9; author reply 1899–900.

4. Wing JK, Cooper JE, Sartorius N. *The Measurement and Classification of Psychiatric Symptoms*. New York: Cambridge University Press, 1974.

5. First MB, Spitzer RL, Gibbon M, Williams JBW. *Structured Clinical Interview for DSM-IV-TR Axis I Disorders, Research Version*. Patient edition. (SCID-I/P). New York: Biometrics Research, New York State Psychiatric Institute, 2002.

6. WHO. *Schedules for Clinical Assessment in Neuropsychiatry – Manual*. Version 2. Geneva: World Health Organisation, Division of Mental Health, 1994.

7. Faehndrich E, Stieglitz RD. *Das AMDP-System: Manual zur Dokumentation psychiatrischer Befunde*. 6th ed. Goettingen: Hogrefe Verlag, 1997.

8. AMDP. *The AMDP-System: Manual for Assessment and Documentation of Psychopathology in Psychiatry*. Boston: Hogrefe Publishing, 2018.

9. Zahn R, Lythe KE, Gethin JA, et al. The role of self-blame and worthlessness in the psychopathology of major depressive disorder. *J Affect Disord*. 2015;**186**:337–41.

10. Bhugra D, Mastrogianni A. Globalisation and mental disorders – overview with relation to depression. *Br J Psychiatry*. 2004;**184**:10–20.

11. Goodmann DR, Daouk S, Sullivan M, et al. Factor analysis of depression symptoms across five broad cultural groups. *J Affect Disord*. 2021;**282**:227–35.

12. Sartorius N, Jablensky A, Gulbinat W, Ernberg G. WHO Collaborative Study – assessment of depressive disorders. *Psychol Med*. 1980;**10**(4):743–9.

13. Tseng W-S. 18 – Disorders of Depression. In W-S Tseng, editor. *Handbook of Cultural Psychiatry*. San Diego: Academic Press, 2001; 335–42.

14. Kendler KS. The genealogy of major depression: symptoms and signs of melancholia from 1880 to 1900. *Mol Psychiatry*. 2017;**22**(11):1539–53.

15. Angst J, Azorin JM, Bowden CL, et al. Prevalence and characteristics of undiagnosed bipolar disorders in patients with a major depressive episode: the BRIDGE Study. *Arch Gen Psychiatry*. 2011;**68**(8):791–9.

16. Zahn R, Burns A. Dementia disorders: an overview. In G Waldemar, A Burns, editors. *Alzheimer's Disease. Oxford Neuropsychiatry Library*. 2nd ed. Oxford: Oxford University Press; 2017; 2–9.

17. Kraepelin E. *Psychiatrie – Ein Lehrbuch für Studierende und Ärzte*. 7th ed. Leipzig: Verlag von Johann Ambrosius Barth, 1904.

18. Beck AT. Thinking and depression. I. Idiosyncratic content and cognitive distortions. *Arch Gen Psychiatry*. 1963;**9**:324–33.

19. Ebert D. Alterations of drive in differential diagnosis of mild depressive disorders – evidence for the spectrum concept of endogenomorphic affective psychosis. *Psychopathology*. 1992;**25**(1):23–8.

20. Berridge KC, Robinson TE. What is the role of dopamine in reward: hedonic impact, reward learning, or incentive salience? *Brain Res Rev*. 1998;**28**(3):309–69.

21. Bhalla G. Duty- and pleasure-related regret – validation of a novel measure and its role in the vulnerability to major depressive disorder. Unpublished master's degree thesis. King's College London; 2020.

22. Hallford DJ, Sharma MK. Anticipatory pleasure for future experiences in schizophrenia spectrum disorders and major depression: a systematic review and meta-analysis. *Br J Clin Psychol*. 2019;**58**(4):357–83.

23. Owen GS, Martin W, Gergel T. Misevaluating the future: affective disorder and decision-making

capacity for treatment – a temporal understanding. *Psychopathology.* 2018;**51**(6):371–9.

24. Schönfelder S, Langer J, Schneider EE, Wessa M. Mania risk is characterized by an aberrant optimistic update bias for positive life events. *J Affect Disord.* 2017;**218**:313–21.

25. Dalgleish T, Werner-Seidler A. Disruptions in autobiographical memory processing in depression and the emergence of memory therapeutics. *Trends Cogn Sci.* 2014;**18**(11):596–604.

26. Holmes EA, Bonsall MB, Hales SA, et al. Applications of time-series analysis to mood fluctuations in bipolar disorder to promote treatment innovation: a case series. *Transl Psychiatry.* 2016;**6**:e720.

27. Fava M. Depression with anger attacks. *J Clin Psychiatry.* 1998;**59**:18–22.

28. Wolpe J. The renascence of neurotic depression: its varied dynamics and implications for outcome research. *J Nerv Ment Dis.* 1988;**176**(10):607–13.

29. Garety PA, Hemsley DR. *Delusions: Investigations into the Psychology of Delusional Reasoning.* Hove: Psychology Press, 1997; xi, 171 p.

30. Zahn HW. Über Zwangsvorstellungen. *Eur Neurol.* 1918;**43**(1):59–75.

31. Holmes EA, Blackwell SE, Heyes SB, Renner F, Raes F. Mental imagery in depression: phenomenology, potential mechanisms, and treatment implications. In TD Cannon, T Widiger, editors. *Annual Review of Clinical Psychology*, Vol. 12. Palo Alto, CA: Annual Reviews, 2016; 249–80.

32. Duan S, Lawrence A, Valmaggia L, Moll J, Zahn R. Maladaptive blame-related action tendencies are associated with vulnerability to major depressive disorder. *J Pasychiatr Res.* 2022;**145**:70–6.

33. Roseman IJ, Wiest C, Swartz TS. Phenomenology, behaviors, and goals differentiate discrete emotions. *J Pers Soc Psychol.* 1994;**67**(2):206–21.

34. Tangney JP, Stuewig J, Mashek DJ. Moral emotions and moral behavior. *Annu Rev Psychol.* 2007;**58**:345–72.

35. Zahn R, Green S, Beaumont H, et al. Frontotemporal lobar degeneration and social behaviour: dissociation between the knowledge of its consequences and its conceptual meaning. *Cortex.* 2017;**93**:107–18.

36. Cuthbert BN, Insel TR. Toward the future of psychiatric diagnosis: the seven pillars of RDoC. BMC Med. 2013;**11**:126.

37. Weiner B. *Human Motivation: Metaphors, Theories, and Research.* Thousand Oaks, CA: Sage, 1992.

38. Weiner B. An attributional theory of achievement-motivation and emotion. *Psychol Rev.* 1985;**92**(4):548–73.

39. Abramson LY, Seligman MEP, Teasdale JD. Learned helplessness in humans – critique and reformulation. *J Abnorm Psychol.* 1978;**87**(1):49–74.

40. Robinaugh DJ, Hoekstra RHA, Toner ER, Borsboom D. The network approach to psychopathology: a review of the literature 2008–2018 and an agenda for future research. *Psychol Med.* 2020;**50**(3):353–66.

41. Blanken TF, Deserno MK, Dalege J, et al. The role of stabilizing and communicating symptoms given overlapping communities in psychopathology networks. *Sci Rep.* 2018;**8**(1):5854.

42. Harrison P, Walton S, Fennema D, et al. Development and validation of the Maudsley Modified Patient Health Questionnaire (MM-PHQ-9). *BJPsych Open.* 2021;**7**(4):e123.

43. Lythe KE, Gethin JA, Workman CI, et al. Subgenual activation and the finger of blame: individual differences and depression vulnerability. *Psychol Med.* 2022;**52**(8):1560–8.

44. Green S, Ralph MAL, Moll J, Deakin JFW, Zahn R. Guilt-selective functional disconnection of anterior temporal and subgenual cortices in major depressive disorder. *Arch Gen Psychiatry.* 2012;**69**(10):1014–21.

45. Zahn R, Weingartner JH, Basilio R, et al. Blame-rebalance fMRI neurofeedback in major depressive disorder: a randomised proof-of-concept trial. *NeuroImage: Clin.* 2019;**24**:101992.

46. Zahn R. The role of neuroimaging in translational cognitive neuroscience. *Top Magn Reson Imaging.* 2009;**20**(5):279–89.

Chapter 15

Brain Imaging in Mood Disorders: Pathophysiological Significance and Clinical Perspectives

Victoria C. Wing, Eilidh Miller, and David Cousins

Introduction

Understanding the brain mechanisms underlying psychiatric conditions, including mood disorders, can aid the identification of biomarkers for an illness, its progression and response to treatment. Ultimately, this has the potential to allow the individualisation of treatment and optimise outcomes for patients. Neuroimaging methods such as structural magnetic resonance imaging (MRI) and diffusion-weighted imaging are powerful tools to investigate the neuroanatomical basis of brain disorders and the effects of treatment. In this chapter we focus on how recent neuroimaging advances have increased our understanding of a key treatment for bipolar disorder, lithium. Further, we discuss how the advent of direct imaging of brain lithium distribution using multinuclear MRI techniques (^{7}Li-MRI) may provide insights into the effects of lithium on the brain, with the potential to develop combined biomarkers or biosignatures of response to treatment.

Lithium has been used as a treatment for bipolar disorder for over 70 years and remains the gold-standard prophylactic treatment, preventing episodes of mania and depression (Severus et al., 2018) as well as reducing suicidal behaviour (Lewitzka et al., 2015) and all-cause mortality (Cipriani et al., 2005). Some people with bipolar disorder have an excellent response to lithium, and the identification such patients may optimise their treatment whilst avoiding the risks of lithium treatment in those less likely to respond. Regrettably, despite the benefits of treatment and the scope to develop stratified interventions, the use of lithium is in decline worldwide (Post, 2018).

The importance of identifying responders to lithium treatment is underlined by the potential long-term benefits, evidenced not only from clinical research in relapse prevention but also from mechanistic studies. For instance, there is an established body of evidence that lithium has neuroprotective properties which may underlie its therapeutic benefit. Preclinical research has elucidated various cellular mechanisms by which lithium may exert these effects (Machado-Vieira et al., 2009), and clinical research generally supports the proposal that lithium has protective effects on the brain. The latter is from imaging-based studies in bipolar disorder (Lucini-Paioni et al., 2021) as well as observational research linking it to reduced rates of dementia (Velosa et al., 2020) and as a potential early intervention in related conditions (Forlenza et al., 2019). Lithium has anti-apoptotic actions, directly and indirectly inhibiting glycogen synthase kinase-3ß (GSK-3ß) (Freland and Beaulieu, 2012), which increases myelination, repair and plasticity (Bartzokis, 2012), as well as reducing tau protein phosphorylation and amyloid production pertinent to the potential use in neurodegenerative disorders (Diniz et al., 2013). Increased expression of anti-apoptotic proteins such as bcl-2, observed in rodent brain studies and in human neuronal cell cultures with lithium administration, as well as the attenuation of excitotoxicity mediated cell death such as that induced by glutamate and N-methyl-D-aspartate receptor-activation (Chen et al., 1999; Manji et al., 2000), underline the neuroprotective actions of lithium. Similarly, lithium has been linked to an increased expression of neurotrophins such as brain-derived neurotrophic factors (BDNF), which have long-term neurotrophic and neuroprotective effects (Hashimoto et al., 2002). Lithium also directly inhibits inositol polyphosphate 1-phosphatase (IPPase) and inositol monophosphatase (IMP), relevant to its short- and long-term therapeutic potential (Quiroz et al., 2010). Studies in humans have begun to link the cellular effects of lithium to its clinical efficacy. For instance, lithium has been shown to increase plasma BDNF in acute bipolar mania (de Sousa et al., 2011), and lithium responders have been found to have normal BDNF and cognitive function (Rybakowski et al., 2010). There is scope to explore the structure and integrity of the brain in bipolar disorder with respect to lithium treatment, using established and advanced neuroimaging techniques. These will be outlined in this chapter.

Magnetic Resonance Imaging (MRI) in Bipolar Disorder

Structural MRI (sMRI) yields high-resolution images based on the behaviour of protons (hydrogen) in applied magnetic fields in combination with specific radiofrequency pulses. In most sMRI studies, images are T1-weighted, providing good contrast between grey and white matter (based largely on the longitudinal relaxation time of protons in the tissues) with common analysis output measures being tissue compartment volume, thickness or area (depending on processing algorithms), globally or regionally defined. Structural MRI studies have compared bipolar disorder subjects with healthy controls, with the finding of smaller brain volumes and larger lateral ventricle volumes consistently reported and emerging as significant in meta-analysis (Kempton et al., 2008). Regional reductions in brain volumes have been reported, including the frontal cortex, anterior cingulate, thalamus, hippocampus and amygdala (Drevets et al., 2008; Lochhead et al., 2004; Lyoo et al., 2004). Recent mega- and meta-analyses have, however, reported widespread alterations in grey and white matter measures (Ching et al., 2022; Favre et al., 2019; Haukvik et al., 2022; Hibar et al., 2018; Hibar et al., 2016). Whils one early meta-analysis found no significant difference in whole brain volume or whole brain grey matter volume in patients compared to controls (McDonald et al., 2004), heterogeneity in the original studies was noted. Heterogeneity can arise from differences in study design and analysis but may also be related to the biological differences in clinical phenotypes, the impact of illness severity or due to direct medication effects (Phillips et al., 2008). Reduced grey matter has been associated with clinical severity in bipolar disorder (Lyoo et al., 2006), and an increased number of episodes is associated with decreased volume of cortical and subcortical structures as well as increased ventricle volume (Ekman

et al., 2010; Moorhead et al., 2007). The effects of lithium treatment on brain structure have been the subject of investigation for over 20 years, initially with respect to grey matter but latterly its effects on white matter volume and integrity.

Lithium and Brain Structure in MRI Studies

Early Exploratory Analyses

The majority of the early sMRI findings reporting lithium's effect on brain structure were obtained from small subgroup secondary analyses of medication effects in studies comparing healthy controls to those with bipolar disorder (Hafeman et al., 2012). For instance, a study designed to compare hippocampal volumes in early- and late-onset bipolar disorder completed an exploratory analysis revealing that lithium therapy alone or in combination with sodium valproate ($n = 27$) was associated with greater hippocampal size compared to the small group treated with sodium valproate monotherapy ($n = 5$) (Beyer et al., 2004). A study in adolescents with bipolar disorder found smaller cortical volumes across a range of regions compared to controls, but a secondary analysis found higher orbitofrontal cortex volumes in patients treated with medication compared to those not, an effect that appeared to be driven by the small subset of patients with lithium ($n = 7$) (Wang et al., 2011). Regional differences in which lithium-treated patients have larger volumes compared to healthy controls have been reported for the hippocampus (Javadapour et al., 2010), and substantially greater volumes have been noted in the right anterior cingulate cortex (ACC) (Javadapour et al., 2007). However, not all secondary analyses have reported effects of current or past lithium exposure on brain structure in bipolar disorder (Chen et al., 2007; Perico et al., 2011).

Exploratory analyses often have limited statistical power, and meta-analyses have been conducted to examine the effects of medication on brain structure in bipolar disorder more robustly. In a meta-regression of 98 studies, lithium use was associated with greater total grey matter volume (Kempton et al., 2008). An international mega-analysis of regional volumetric measurements from patients with bipolar disorder ($n = 321$) and matched health controls ($n = 422$) found that those with bipolar disorder taking lithium ($n = 141$) had significantly greater hippocampal and amygdala volumes compared to those not taking lithium and to healthy controls (Hallahan et al., 2011). Similarly, a meta-analysis focussing on hippocampal volumes in bipolar disorder subdivided patients based on the presence or absence of current lithium treatment from a database of 16 studies – hippocampal volumes (left and right) were significantly larger in the lithium-treated group ($n = 101$) than the non-lithium group ($n = 245$) and healthy controls ($n = 456$) (Hajek et al., 2012).

Despite the increased statistical power conferred by such meta- and mega-analyses, they remain influenced by the heterogeneity in the studies included. For example, confounding factors such as current and past use of antipsychotic and other mood-stabilising medications limit interpretation, as does whether non-lithium-treated groups were naïve to the drug or had taken it in the past. Thus, appraisal of the cross-sectional studies and the findings of longitudinal hypothesis-driven studies are also required to better understand the effects of lithium on brain structure.

Cross-Sectional Studies

One of the first cross-sectional studies examining the effects of lithium on brain structure compared healthy controls ($n = 46$), untreated patients with bipolar disorder ($n = 12$) and lithium-treated patients with bipolar disorder ($n = 17$). Total grey matter volume was significantly greater in the lithium-treated group compared to the other groups, taken as early in vivo evidence for the putative neuroprotective effects of lithium (Sassi et al., 2002). The duration of lithium treatment in this early study was moderate (minimum 2 weeks with a median of 27 weeks), and there were significant differences in mood-state between the groups, with the greater degree of depression in the untreated group potentially contributing to the differences in grey matter volumes. In an extension of this work, reporting on an overlapping patient cohort to specifically examine the effects of lithium treatment on the cingulate cortex, untreated patients with bipolar disorder had smaller left ACC volumes compared to patients on lithium monotherapy and the healthy control group (Sassi et al., 2004). The effects of lithium have also been explored by employing cortical pattern matching methods to map grey matter abnormalities over the entire cortical surface in adults with

bipolar disorder and healthy controls (Bearden et al., 2007). Here, lithium-treated patients ($n = 20$) had greater grey matter volumes compared to those not treated with lithium ($n = 8$) and healthy controls ($n = 28$), specifically in the frontal, temporal and parietal lobes. A secondary region of interest (ROI) analysis identified greater grey matter density in lithium-treated bipolar patients in the right ACC compared to untreated patients, and in the left dorsolateral prefrontal cortex (DLPFC) compared to healthy controls. Bearden and colleagues focussed their attention on hippocampal anatomy, due to the declarative memory impairments seen in bipolar disorder. They found that bipolar patients treated with lithium for at least 2 weeks ($n = 21$) had greater hippocampal volumes than patients not medicated for at least 2 weeks ($n = 12$) and matched healthy controls ($n = 62$) (Bearden et al., 2008). Similarly, larger hippocampal volumes in lithium-treated patients ($n = 10$) were reported in comparison to healthy controls ($n = 32$), but at trend-level significance compared to non-lithium-treated patients ($n = 8$) (van Erp et al., 2012).

The amygdala and hippocampus are involved in emotional processing and so are further implicated in the pathophysiology of bipolar disorder. However, imaging studies are inconclusive regarding their structure in bipolar disorder when compared to healthy controls, with reports of larger, smaller and no difference in volumes. Whilst heterogeneity may be related to neurodevelopment or stage of illness at the time of various studies, the effects of medication (lithium in particular) has attracted attention (Lucini-Paioni et al., 2021). In an ROI sMRI study (Foland et al., 2008), greater left amygdala and bilateral hippocampal volumes were observed in lithium-treated patients ($n = 12$) compared to patients not treated with lithium ($n = 37$). However, the study was not specifically designed to examine the effects of lithium, with a relatively small size and patients in comparator groups having commonalities in other medications such as sodium valproate. Subsequently, Usher et al. (2010) completed a cross-sectional sMRI study specifically designed to examine amygdala volumes in euthymic patients with bipolar I disorder who were either treated with lithium ($n = 15$) or had no current or past treatment with lithium ($n = 24$), both in comparison to matched healthy controls ($n = 41$); lithium treatment in bipolar disorder was associated with larger right amygdala volume. Employing 3T MRI to afford better segmentation of the amygdala compared to 1.5T imaging, Savitz et al. (2010) conducted a similar study with an unmedicated bipolar disorder comparator group. Medicated bipolar patients ($n = 17$), of whom 9 were taking lithium, had greater amygdala volumes compared to unmedicated bipolar patients ($n = 18$; mean medication free period 11 months), and to healthy controls ($n = 17$). A larger cross-sectional sMRI study of adults with bipolar disorder in remission ($n = 74$) compared patients receiving monotherapy with either lithium, anticonvulsants or antipsychotics (Germana et al., 2010). It reported that lithium treatment was associated with greater regional grey matter volumes in limbic and paralimbic brain areas (right subgenual anterior cingulate gyrus, postcentral gyrus, hippocampus/amygdala complex and the left insula) compared to other medications used as prophylaxis in bipolar disorder. Global grey matter volume did not differ between medication groups, but there was an inverted U-shaped relationship between global grey matter and length of lithium treatment. Most studies have investigated working age adults, or adolescents, but Zung et al. (2016) studied patients with bipolar disorder aged over 60 years. In comparing elderly patients treated with lithium long term (> 1 year) ($n = 30$) with patients who had not received lithium in the previous 9 months ($n = 27$) and aged-matched controls ($n = 22$), patients not taking lithium had significantly lower global grey matter volumes. The study reported a voxel-based morphometry (VBM) analysis of the medial temporal region, which revealed a significantly larger left hippocampal volume in patients treated with lithium compared to those not taking lithium. Further, the lithium-treated group had better cognitive function than the other two groups but a correlation with brain structure was not formally examined. Collectively, these studies suggest the effects of lithium on brain structure are regional and may localise to areas involved in emotional processing.

Consortium Analyses

Individually, early studies were relatively small and there has been a move towards large-scale national and international collaborations to yield larger data sets for analysis. The Enhancing Genetics through Meta-Analysis (ENGIMA) Consortium completed a case-control MRI analysis of subcortical brain volume changes including data from 1,710 subjects with bipolar disorder and 2,594 healthy controls (Hibar et al., 2016). Subjects with bipolar disorder had smaller hippocampal, amygdala and thalamic volumes and larger ventricles compared to controls, but those taking lithium did not differ in the volume of the hippocampus compared to the controls. Bipolar disorder subjects taking lithium ($n = 535$) had larger thalamic volumes compared to those not taking lithium ($n = 845$). Analysing cortical thickness in an expanded data set from ENIGMA with 1837 patients with bipolar disorder and 2,582 health controls, bipolar disorder was found to be associated with widespread cortical thinning including in the bilateral frontal, temporal and parietal cortices (Hibar et al., 2018). Within this analysis, a statistical model accounting for different medication combinations across individuals was employed, and lithium treatment ($n = 700$) was found to be associated with increased cortical thickness in the left paracentral gyrus, left paracentral lobule and bilateral superior parietal gyrus compared to those not taking lithium ($n = 892$). Despite the greater power of these large-scale analyses, utilising data from cross-sectional studies has limitations, not least of which is the selection bias for patients taking lithium or other medications prior to enrolment.

Longitudinal Studies

Prospective studies comparing structural images before and after initiation of lithium treatment allow the temporal sequence of effects to be better determined, with various designs, durations and comparator medications employed. In the earliest study, Moore et al. (2000) reported a 3% grey matter volume increase following 4 weeks of lithium treatment in 10 patients with bipolar disorder, subsequently expanding their sample ($n = 28$) to report that the effects were greatest in the prefrontal cortex (Moore et al., 2009). In this larger sample, a correlation between favourable clinical response to lithium and grey matter volume increase was observed and subsequently replicated by others (Lyoo et al., 2010). The study conducted by Lyoo et al. (2010) had notable strengths, examining grey and white matter volumes repeatedly over several weeks before and during treatment in patients with bipolar disorder who were naïve to mood stabilisers and antipsychotic medications and randomised to receive either lithium ($n = 13$) or valproic acid ($n = 9$) treatment, in comparison to a healthy control group ($n = 14$). All participants underwent baseline imaging, with controls completing at least one follow-up scan and patients at least three. Whole brain grey matter but not white matter volumes increased over time in the lithium-treated patients (up to a maximum of 2.56%); no volumetric changes were observed in controls or patients taking valproic acid. Using the available data points, the estimated change in grey matter over time was modelled and yielded a predicted peak effect of lithium of 11.5 weeks. As noted previously, clinical response to lithium correlated with grey matter volume increase.

Yucel et al. longitudinally assessed the effects of short- and long-term lithium use on hippocampal volumes bilaterally. In the long-term study (Yucel et al., 2007), hippocampal volume and recollective memory were assessed over a period of 2 to 4 years in patients with bipolar disorder who were medication naïve before lithium initiation ($n = 12$). Bilateral increases in hippocampus volume (total and head) were observed as well as some improvement in memory performance. In the short-term treatment study (Yucel et al., 2008), patients with bipolar disorder ($n = 36$) who were medication naïve were grouped according to the treatment they received after entering the study: lithium treatment, valproic acid or lamotrigine treatment or no treatment. A comparator group of healthy controls ($n = 30$) was also included. The lithium group received treatment for 1 to 8 weeks and were found to have greater bilateral hippocampal volumes compared to the unmedicated group and healthy controls, whereas the valproic acid/lamotrigine treatment group showed no difference. This study demonstrated that even brief exposure to lithium can result detectable changes in brain structural imaging.

Monkul et al. (2007) conducted a study to examine the effects of lithium administration in healthy controls ($n = 13$) rather than patients with bipolar disorder. A VBM analysis demonstrated increased grey matter volumes in the left ACC and the DLPFC bilaterally after taking lithium for 4 weeks. However, total brain and total grey matter volumes were unchanged whilst total white matter volume increased in this study. It is more challenging to invoke neuroprotection as a cause of volumetric change in healthy volunteers, and changes in hydration status have been proposed as an explanation (Moore et al., 2000; Phatak et al., 2006). Cousins et al. (2013) argued that the ability of lithium to reduce the T1 time of protons (Fabricand and Goldberg, 1967; Rangel-Guerra et al., 1983) may alter MRI tissue contrast, resulting in misclassification of grey and white matter in analysis techniques dependent on voxel intensity such as

VBM. In a longitudinal study of healthy volunteers ($n = 31$), VBM showed a grey matter volume increase in those taking lithium compared to placebo but a paired-edge analysis technique sensitive to boundaries rather than intensities did not detect a difference in brain volumes between the groups. In a subset in which quantitative imaging was conducted, taking lithium reduced the proton T1 time of grey matter (Cousins et al., 2013). Rather than a purely artefactual effect of the drug, the T1 changes may localise the areas in the brain in which lithium either concentrates or has most marked effects on cellular composition.

In summary, numerous cross-sectional and longitudinal sMRI studies indicate that taking lithium is associated with greater grey matter volumes, a finding which is commonly taken as support of its neuroprotective effects. Whilst fewer studies have reported the relationship between lithium use and white matter volume, there is mounting interest and evidence that lithium can have effects on white matter integrity, determined using diffusion magnetic resonance imaging.

Diffusion-Weighted Imaging

Early Exploratory Analyses

There are comparatively fewer studies in bipolar disorder that have focussed specifically on white matter; however, interest in this area is burgeoning in parallel with more advanced imaging techniques. Initial studies investigating white matter in bipolar disorder reported lower than expected total white matter volumes and a greater than normal number of white matter hyperintensities (WMH), of a severity beyond that typical of ageing. These WMH were generally accepted as evidence of white matter damage, though the exact underlying pathology and evolution with respect to the course of the illness remained incompletely elucidated. Intriguingly, a small study observed an association between WMH and better lithium response (Kato et al., 2000).

The development of diffusion-weighted MRI (dMRI) has enabled the examination of white matter on a micro- and macrostructure level. With dMRI, the contrast is determined by the microscopic mobility of water molecules (which is restricted to various degrees in different biological environments) and reported in the derived metrics of fractional anisotropy (FA) and mean diffusivity (MD). FA is a measure that reflects the overall directionality of water diffusion, and in healthy axonal white matter, FA values are high because water diffuses more readily along the axons compared to across them. Low FA values are thought to reflect demyelination and axonal injury (Boretius, 2012; Song, 2002). MD describes the magnitude of water diffusion, reflecting the composition of brain tissues and sensitive to variations or changes in the intra- and extracellular spaces. Greater MD values indicate a reduction in the barriers to movement of water, such as cell membranes, and so many be indicative of altered tissue integrity.

Meta-Analyses

Consistent with initial studies, recent meta-analyses and literature reviews indicate that there are structural changes in white matter in bipolar disorder. In a meta-analysis, there were significantly lower FA values in bipolar disorder localising to clusters in tissues and pathways associated with the regulation of mood and emotional regulation (Marlinge et al., 2014). Employing meta-analyses and mega-analyses techniques to dMRI studies of bipolar disorder, the ENIGMA group (Ching et al., 2022) found lower white matter FA values in patients with bipolar disorder compared to healthy controls, indicative of disrupted tissue integrity. They evaluated the effect of lithium on white matter in their analyses, finding that FA values more closely approximated those of healthy controls compared to those not taking this drug. These findings were supported by a systematic review of the effect of lithium on DTI measures; 11 of 13 studies identified reported a positive effect of lithium on white matter integrity (Espanhol and Vieira-Coehlo, 2022)

Cross-Sectional Studies

Collective interpretation of the dMRI studies in bipolar disorder is hindered by their heterogeneity, but there is consensus supporting widespread white matter abnormalities in the condition (Hafemann et al., 2012). The following sections highlight some key publications demonstrating the major themes and findings in the field. An early study by Regenold et al. (2006) reported greater mean apparent diffusion coefficient values in patients with bipolar disorder, suggesting decreased white matter integrity. McIntosh et al. (2008) similarly found lower FA values in the uncinate fasciculus and anterior thalamic radiations in bipolar disorder, but with no association between lithium use (amongst other medications) and FA values. Likewise, Wang et al. (2008) studied 42 patients with bipolar disorder (11 on lithium treatment) and reported lower FA values in the anterior cingulum compared to healthy controls; no association between medication status and FA values was found. In a further study of 33 patients with bipolar disorder (9 of whom were taking lithium, with or without other medications) compared to 31 healthy controls, Wang et al. (2009) reported lower FA values in the ventral frontal white matter in the patient group, which correlated with decreased amygdala–perigenual anterior cingulate cortex functional connectivity; there was no association between medication status and FA values. Whether the changes in white matter integrity in bipolar disorder are global or localised has attracted interest, though it must be noted that studies have reported widespread changes in conjunction with more significant differences in certain brain regions. Emsell et al. (2013) compared euthymic bipolar disorder patients with control subjects, noting that patients had significantly lower FA, higher MD and greater radial diffusivity in all divisions of the corpus callosum, left fornix and subgenual cingulum. The axial diffusivity was also greater in the fornix bilaterally and the right dorsal–anterior cingulum, collectively suggesting limbic system microstructural disorganisation as a feature of bipolar disorder.

The early dMRI studies require cautious interpretation, as they were conducted when the field was in its relative infancy, using what would now be considered sub-optimal numbers of diffusion directions or less well-established processing pipelines. Whilst lower FA values were generally observed, this was not the case with all studies. Wessa et al. (2009), for instance, reported higher FA values in bipolar disorder in medial frontal, precentral, interior parietal and occipital areas, with no association with lithium treatment. With methodological advances combined with improvements in study design, notably larger samples specifically controlling for mood and/or medication status, an emerging pattern of white matter abnormalities potentially positively influenced by lithium is emerging.

There has been keen interest in the effects of lithium on FA values in bipolar disorder by virtue of its increasingly well evidenced neuroprotective or neurorestorative properties. In a study assessing diffusion parameters in 15 white matter regions in euthymic patients with bipolar disorder ($n = 28$), Macritchie et al. (2010) found higher MD values in all regions and lower FA values in all but two regions, compared to healthy controls ($n = 28$). The differences were most notable in prefrontal and periventricular regions for MD and in occipital and callosal regions for FA. Importantly, this study reported that lithium intake might be an ameliorating factor in the white matter tissue disruption in bipolar disorder. Other studies reveal similar associations. Benedetti et al. (2011) found that patients with bipolar disorder ($n = 40$) had lower FA values in the uncinate fasciculus compared to healthy controls, but this difference was not present in the subgroup of patients treated with lithium ($n = 14$). Likewise, Haarman et al. (2016) studied 21 euthymic patients with bipolar disorder with controls, dividing the bipolar disorder group according to lithium-treatment status and finding those taking lithium had higher FA in the corpus callosum and left anterior corona radiata, areas of importance in mood regulation and cognitive function. In a large study comparing bipolar disorder ($n = 257$) to controls ($n = 167$), Abramovic et al. (2018) found that patients had lower FA and higher MD values in several brain regions, notably the corpus callosum, but consistent with the other studies, they found that FA was higher in those on lithium treatment. Examining older adults (> 50 years), Gildengers et al. (2015) completed a cross-sectional sMRI and dMRI study of bipolar disorder ($n = 58$) and age-matched controls ($n = 21$). The bipolar group was divided into those who had taken lithium ($n = 33$) and those who had minimal lithium exposure (< 1 year; $n = 25$), and in a stepwise regression, longer duration of lithium treatment was related to higher overall white matter FA but not total grey matter.

Cross-sectional studies are limited in their generalisability and prone to selection bias or the challenges of post hoc group determination for comparison medication effects. To examine the potential of lithium to normalise white matter integrity, longitudinal designs are required.

Longitudinal Studies

Berk et al. (2017) undertook a prospective cohort study examining the potential neuroprotective effects of mood stabilisers, using imaging outcomes as a proxy measure. Patients with first episode mania were stabilised on a combination of lithium and quetiapine and then randomised to continue lithium ($n = 20$) or quetiapine ($n = 21$) monotherapy. Using VBM to appraise change over time, a reduction in white matter volume was observed in the left internal capsule at 3 and 12 months compared to baseline. Analysed by treatment status, lithium was found to be more effective than quetiapine in protecting against white matter decreases after a first episode of mania. Regrettably, there is a paucity of longitudinal imaging studies examining dMRI metrics in white matter in bipolar disorder. Kafantaris et al. (2017) investigated the relationship between changes in FA in the cingulum hippocampus and clinical response to lithium in adolescents with bipolar disorder ($n = 18$). Compared to controls at baseline, those with bipolar disorder had lower FA in the cingulum hippocampus, but FA values increased following lithium treatment. Importantly, those with a favourable response to lithium showed the greatest percentage increase in FA, whilst non-responders had, on average, a very slight decline in FA values. This finding adds to the consensus that lithium is associated with improvements or rectification of disruptions to white matter microstructure. However, the Kafantaris et al. (2017) study examined a single region *a priori*, so further work is required to determine whether global effects emerge or if the findings are localised to candidate brain regions.

Direct Lithium Imaging

As noted, structural and diffusion MRI techniques derive imaging contrast from protons, but it is also possible to directly detect lithium (^{7}Li) using multinuclear magnetic resonance techniques. Following Renshaw and Wicklund's (1988) first demonstration of the ability to detect lithium in the human brain in those taking it as a treatment for bipolar disorder, numerous magnetic resonance spectroscopy (MRS) studies have been conducted and reviewed (Komoroski 2000; Soares et al., 2000). From these, with respect to this chapter, two salient issues emerge. First, the relationship between brain lithium concentration, serum concentration and its clinical effects and second, the limited spatial resolution of ^{7}Li MRS.

Early studies used surface coils to localise the concentration of lithium in the brain, generally finding that the brain concentration was lower than that in the serum (Gyulai et al., 1991; Kato et al., 1992, 1993, 1994, 1996; Komoroski et al., 1990, 1993; Kushnir et al., 1993). Following administration, peak brain lithium concentration was found to lag the serum peak (Komoroski 1990), with the brain elimination half-time longer than for serum (Komoroski 1993, Plenge 1994). Although this complicates the interpretation of brain to serum ratios, the initial findings of these studies suggested that there is a correlation between the brain and serum lithium levels and between brain to serum ratio and age (reviewed by Soares et al., 2000), although this latter relationship was not upheld in older subjects (Forester et al., 2008). Other studies have suggested that there is limited correlation between these measures (Gonzalez et al., 1993; Kato et al., 1996) and the relationship between brain concentrations and response to lithium treatment has not been robustly demonstrated. The introduction of whole-head volume coils (Gonzalez 1993) permitted the measurement of lithium concentration across larger brain volumes (Moore et al., 2002; Sachs et al., 1995; Soares et al., 2001). Initial localisation studies suggested a relatively uniform distribution of lithium across the brain (Girard 2001), in contrast to the heterogenous distribution demonstrated in preclinical rodent studies (Komoroski and Pearce 2004; Komoroski 2005). This disparity may have been due to the crude spatial localisation of even more recent ^{7}Li-MRS studies in humans (Lee et al., 2012), limited by clinically determined acquisition times.

Magnetic resonance spectroscopy studies can directly determine the concentration of lithium, but because lithium yields a spectral singlet, it is amenable to true imaging techniques with better spatial encoding. The technique of [7]Li-MRI permits greater spatial resolution in clinically viable scan times, deriving relative signal intensity through efficient MR sequences dependent on lithium concentration and its relaxation properties (Smith et al., 2018). With such techniques, brain lithium distribution has been shown to be heterogenous and to vary between individuals with bipolar disorder despite comparable therapeutic serum concentrations. Harnessing the power of 7 T field strength, it has recently been demonstrated that lithium appears to concentrate in the hippocampus (Stout et al., 2020), pertinent to its proposed neuroprotective properties and likely of importance in the interpretation of its effects on white matter integrity (Kafantaris et al., 2017).

Combining neuroimaging techniques in the same study group allows their different strengths to be harnessed to better understand the pathophysiology underlying bipolar disorder and its treatment. Necus et al. (2019) used dMRI and [7]Li-MRI to explore whether the positive effects of lithium on white matter integrity were related to its regional distribution, comparing FA values in euthymic bipolar patients against healthy control subjects. Mean white matter FA was higher in the healthy control and long-term lithium-treated bipolar groups compared to bipolar patients treated with other maintenance medications (and naïve to lithium). Moreover, mean white matter FA in the lithium-treated bipolar group was no different to the healthy control group, suggesting lithium may normalise white matter changes associated with bipolar disorder. Within the lithium-treated group, a linear mixed effect analysis found a significant association between [7]Li-MRI signal and FA once the white matter content of a [7]Li-MRI exceeded 50%. These data provide evidence to support the theory that lithium directly influences white matter integrity, effectively co-localising the distribution of a psychotropic drug with its tissue level effects.

Conclusion

In this chapter we have illustrated how neuroimaging has progressed our understanding of lithium, one of the key treatments of bipolar disorder. Structural MRI (sMRI) studies suggest that lithium normalises both global and regional reductions in grey matter volume associated with bipolar disorder, and diffusion-weighted MRI (dMRI) has shed light on its potential to rectify abnormalities in white matter integrity. These results support preclinical evidence for lithium's neuroprotective effects. However, structural imaging alone is insufficient to reveal the underlying mechanism of lithium's therapeutic benefits.

Recently, the unique properties of lithium have been exploited by magnetic resonance imaging to demonstrate the first direct non-invasive in vivo imaging of a psychoactive drug in its target organ. The spatially heterogenous distribution of the [7]Li-MR signal may suggest that lithium directly influences brain structure and function based on lithium tissue concentrations and initial work combining [7]Li-MRI and dMRI support this hypothesis. However, multi-modal imaging studies in this area remain in their infancy and there is great scope to further harness the potential of direct lithium imaging.

There are also a variety of established functional neuroimaging methods which could be employed to better understand the effects of bipolar disorder and treatments such as lithium on brain neurochemistry. Functional MRI (fMRI) typically uses blood-oxygen-level-dependent (BOLD) contrast as a proxy for brain activity and can be used to scrutinise regions as well as connectivity between regions. Despite the surge in psychiatric fMRI research, it has tended to focus on disease states with relatively fewer pharmacological-fMRI studies. The downstream effects of medications can also be assessed using proton MRS to detect biochemical changes in tissues, measuring concentrations of γ-aminobutyric acid (GABA) or glutamate levels, for instance, whilst positron emission tomography (PET) involves injection of a radioactive tracer to quantify receptor binding and neurotransmitter release.

Going forward, it will be important for the field to recruit larger cohorts to allow more robust exploration of the relationships between neuroimaging findings and patient outcomes, including clinical response, cognition and side effects. Longitudinal designs can be challenging but are essential to understand lithium's effects over time and to establish causality. The move towards multi-site studies and research consortiums will help meet these goals with the added benefit of bringing together expertise across different imaging modalities, allowing their relative strengths to be harnessed.

While it was beyond the scope of this chapter to review the neuroimaging literature across the field of bipolar disorder, by using lithium as an example we have demonstrated how technological and scientific advances can aid understanding of the pathophysiology of the disease and the mechanism of action its treatment. The continued advancement of this burgeoning area of research will facilitate the development of new therapies and personalised medicine approaches, thus holding great promise to improve the lives of people affected by bipolar disorder.

References

Abramovic, L., Boks, M. P., Vreeker, A., et al. White matter disruptions in patients with bipolar disorder. *Eur Neuropsychopharmacol.* 2018;**28**(6):743–51.

Bartzokis, G. Neuroglialpharmacology: myelination as a shared mechanism of action of psychotropic treatments. *Neuropharmacology.* 2012;**62**:2137–53.

Bearden, C. E., Soares, J. C., Klunder, A. D., et al. Three-dimensional mapping of hippocampal anatomy in adolescents with early-onset bipolar disorder. *Biol Psychiatry.* 2007;**61**:184S.

Bearden, C. E., Thompson, P. M., Dutton, R. A., et al. Three-dimensional mapping of hippocampal anatomy in unmedicated and lithium-treated patients with bipolar disorder. *Neuropsychopharmacology.* 2008;**33**:1229–38.

Benedetti, F., Absinta, M., Rocca, M. A., et al. Tract-specific white matter structural disruption in patients with bipolar disorder. *Bipolar Disord.* 2011;**13**(4):414–24.

Berk, M., Dandash, O., Daglas, R., et al. Neuroprotection after a first episode of mania: a randomized controlled maintenance trial comparing the effects of lithium and quetiapine on grey and white matter volume. *Transl Psychiatry.* 2017;**7**(1):e1011.

Beyer, J. L., Kuchibbatla, M., Payne, M. E., et al. Hippocampal volume measurement in older adults with bipolar disorder. *Am J Geriat Psychiatry.* 2004;**12**, 613–20.

Boretius, S., Escher, A., Dallenga, T., et al. Assessment of lesion pathology in a new animal model of MS by multiparametric MRI and DTI. *Neuroimage.* 2012;**59**(3):2678–88.

Chen, B., Wang, J. F., hill, B. C, Young, L. T. Lithium and valproate differentially regulate brain regional expression of phosphorylated CREB and c-Fos. *Mol Brain Res.* 1999;**70**:45–53.

Chen, X. H., Wen, W., Malhi, G. S., Ivanovski, B, Sachdev, P. S. Regional gray matter changes in bipolar disorder: a voxel-based morphometric study. *Aust N Z J Psychiatry.* 2007;**41**:327–36.

Ching, C. R. K., Hibar, D. P., Gurholt, T. P., et al. What we learn about bipolar disorder from large-scale neuroimaging: findings and future directions from the ENIGMA Bipolar Disorder Working Group. *Hum Brain Mapp.* 2022;**43**:56–82.

Cipriani, A., Pretty, H., Hawton, K, Geddes, J. R. Lithium in the prevention of suicidal behavior and all-cause mortality in patients with mood disorders: a systematic review of randomized trials. *Am J Psychiatry.* 2005;**162**:1805–19.

Cousins, D. A., Aribisala, B., Ferrier, I. N, Blamire, A. M. Lithium, gray matter, and magnetic resonance imaging signal. *Biol Psychiatry.* 2013;**73**:652–7.

De Sousa, R. T., Van de Bilt, M. T., Diniz, B. S., et al. Lithium increases plasma brain-derived neurotrophic factor in acute bipolar mania: a preliminary 4-week study. *Neursci Lett.* 2011;**494**:54–6.

Diniz, B. S., Machado-Vieira, R., Forlenza, O. V. Lithium and neuroprotection: translational evidence and implications for the treatment of neuropsychiatric disorders. *Neuropsychiatr Dis Treat.* 2013;**9**:493–500.

Drevets, W. C., Savitz, J., Trimble, M. The subgenual anterior cingulate cortex in mood disorders. *CNS Spectr.* 2008;**13**:663–81.

Ekman, C. J., Lind, J., Ryden, E., Ingvar, M., Landen, M. Manic episodes are associated with grey matter volume reduction – a voxel-based morphometry brain analysis. *Acta Psychiatr Scand*. 2010;**122**:507–15.

Emsell, L., Leemans, A., Langan, C., et al. Limbic and callosal white matter changes in euthymic bipolar I disorder: an advanced diffusion magnetic resonance imaging tractography study. *Biol Psychiatry*. 2013;**73** (2):194–201.

Espanhol, J.C.L, Vieria-Coehlo, M.A. Effects of lithium use on the white matter of patients with bipolar disorder – a systematic review. *Nord J Psychiatry*. 2022;**76**:1–11.

Fabricand, B. P., Goldberg, S. G. Proton relaxation times in 7LiCl and 6LiCl solutions. *Mol Phys*. 1967;**13**:323–30.

Favre, P., Pauling, M., Stout, J., et al. Widespread white matter microstructural abnormalities in bipolar disorder: evidence from mega- and meta-analyses across 3033 individuals. *Neuropsychopharmacology*. 2019;**44**:2285–93.

Foland, L. C., Altshuler, L. L., Sugar, C. A., et al. Increased volume of the amygdala and hippocampus in bipolar patients treated with lithium. *Neuroreport*. 2008;**19**, 221–224.

Forester, B., Berlow, Y. A., Finn, C. T., et al. Brain lithium, N-acetyl aspartate (NAA) and myo-inositol (m-Ino) levels in older adults with bipolar disorder treated with lithium: a lithium-7 and proton magnetic resonance spectroscopy study *Bipolar Disord*. 2008;**10**:691–700.

Forlenza, O. V., Radanovic, M., Talib, L. L., Gattaz, W. F. Clinical and biological effects of long-term lithium treatment in older adults with amnestic mild cognitive impairment: randomised clinical trial. *Br J Psychiatry*. 2019;**215**:668–74.

Freland, L., Beaulieu, J.-M. Inhibition of GSK3 by lithium, from single molecules to signaling networks. *Front Mol Neurosci*. 2012;**5**.

Germana, C., Kempton, M. J., Sarnicola, A., et al. The effects of lithium and anticonvulsants on brain structure in bipolar disorder. *Acta Psychiatr Scand*. 2010;**122**:481–7.

Gildengers, A. G., Butters, M. A., Aizenstein, H. J., et al. Longer lithium exposure is associated with better white matter integrity in older adults with bipolar disorder. *Bipolar Disord*. 2015;**17**(3):248–56.

Gonzalez, R. G., Guimaraes, A. R., Sachs, G. S., et al. Measurement of human brain lithium in-vivo by MR spectroscopy. *AJNR Am J Neuroradiol*. 1993;**14**:1027–37.

Gyulai, L., Wicklund, S. W., Greenstein, R., et al. Measurement of tissue lithium concentration by lithium magnetic-resonance spectroscopy in patients with bipolar disorder. *Biol Psychiatry*. 1991;**29**:1161–70.

Haarman, B. C. M., Riemersma–van der Lek, R. F., Burger, H., et al. Diffusion tensor imaging in euthymic bipolar disorder – a tract-based spatial statistics study. *J Affect Disord*. 2016;**203**:281–91.

Hafeman, D. M., Chang, K. D., Garrett, A. S., Sanders, E. M., Phillips, M. L. Effects of medication on neuroimaging findings in bipolar disorder: an updated review. *Bipolar Disord*. 2012;**14**:375–410.

Hajek, T., Kopecek, M., Hoeschl, C., Alda, M. Smaller hippocampal volumes in patients with bipolar disorder are masked by exposure to lithium: a meta-analysis. *J Psychiatry Neurosci*. 2012;**37**:333–43.

Hallahan, B., Newell, J., Soares, J. C., et al. Structural magnetic resonance imaging in bipolar disorder: an international collaborative megaanalysis of individual adult patient data. *Biol Psychiatry*. 2011;**69**:326–35.

Hashimoto, R., Takei, N., Shimazu, K., et al. Lithium induces brain-derived neurotrophic factor and activates TrkB in rodent cortical neurons: an essential step for neuroprotection against glutamate excitotoxicity. *Neuropharmacology*. 2002;**43**:1173–9.

Haukvik, U. K., Gurholt, T. P., Nerland, S., et al. In vivo hippocampal subfield volumes in bipolar disorder – a mega-analysis from the Enhancing Neuro Imaging Genetics through Meta-Analysis Bipolar Disorder Working Group. *Hum Brain Mapp*. 2022;**43**:385–98.

Hibar, D. P., Westlye, L. T., Van Erp, T. G. M., et al. Subcortical volumetric abnormalities in bipolar disorder. *Mol Psychiatry*. 2016;**21**:1710–16.

Hibar, D. P., Westlye, L. T., Doan, N. T., et al. Cortical abnormalities in bipolar disorder: an MRI analysis of 6503 individuals from the ENIGMA Bipolar Disorder Working Group. *Mol Psychiatry*. 2018;**23**:932–42.

Javadapour, A., Malhi, G. S., Ivanovski, B., et al. Increased anterior cingulate cortex volume in bipolar I disorder. *Aust N Z J Psychiatry*. 2007;**41**:910–16.

Javadapour, A., Malhi, G. S., Ivanovski, B., et al. Hippocampal volumes in. adults with bipolar disorder. *J Neuropsychiatry Clin Neurosci*. 2010;**22**:55–62.

Kafantaris, V., Spritzer, L., Doshi, V., et al. Changes in white matter microstructure predict lithium response in adolescents with bipolar disorder. *Bipolar Disord*. 2017;**19** (7):587–94.

Kato, T., Takahashi, S., Inubushi, T. Brain lithium concentration by Li-7-magnetic and H-1-magnetic resonance spectroscopy in bipolar disorder. *Psychiatry Res*. 1992;**45**:53–63.

Kato, T., Takahashi, S., Shioiri, T., Inubushi, T. Alterations in brain phosphorus-metabolism in bipolar disorder detected by in vivo P-31 and Li-7 magnetic-resonance spectroscopy. *J Affect Disord*. 1993;**27**:53–9.

Kato, T., Inubushi, T., Takahashi, S. Relationship of lithium concentrations in the brain measured by Li-7 magnetic-resonance spectroscopy to treatment response in mania. *J ClinPsychopharmacol*. 1994;**14**:330–5.

Kato, T., Fujii, K., Shioiri, T., Inubushi, T., Takahashi, S. Lithium side effects in relation to brain lithium concentration measure by lithium-7 magnetic resonance spectroscopy. *Prog Neuropsychopharmacol Biol Psychiatry.* 1996;**20**:87–97.

Kato, T., Fujii, K., Kamiya, A., Kato, N. White matter hyperintensity detected by magnetic resonance imaging and lithium response in bipolar disorder: a preliminary observation. *Psychiatry Clin Neuroscis.* 2000;**54**(1):117–20.

Kempton, M. J., Geddes, J. R., Ettinger, U., et al. Meta-analysis, database, and meta-regression of 98 structural imaging studies in bipolar disorder. *Arch Gen Psychiatry.* 2008.;**65**:1017–32.

Komoroski, R. A., Newton, J. E. O., Walker, E., et al. In vivo NMR-Spectroscopy of Li-7 in Humans. *Magn Reson Med.* 1990;**15**:347–56.

Komoroski, R. A., Newton, J. E. O., Sprigg, J. R., et al. In vivo 7Li nuclear magnetic resonance study of lithium pharmacokinetics and chemical shift imaging in psychiatric patients. *Psychiatry Res.* 1993;**50**:67–76.

Komoroski, R.A. Applications of (7)L NMR in biomedicine. *Magn Reson Imaging.* 2000;**18**:103–16.

Komoroski, R. A., Pearce, J. M. Localized Li-7 MR spectroscopy and spin relaxation in rat brain in vivo. *Magn Reson Med.* 2004;**52**:164–8.

Komoroski, R. A. Biomedical applications of Li-7 NMR. *NMR Biomed.* 2005;**18**:67–73.

Kushnir, T., Itzchak, Y., Valevski, A., et al. Relaxation-times and concentrations of Li-7 in the brain of patients receiving lithium-therapy. *NMR Biomed.* 1993;**6**:39–42.

Lee, J. H., Adler, C., Norris, M., et al. 4-T 7Li 3D MR spectroscopy imaging in the brains of bipolar disorder subjects. *Magn Reson Med.* 2012;**68**:363–8.

Lewitzka, U., Severus, E., Bauer, R., et al. The suicide prevention effect of lithium: more than 20 years of evidence-a narrative review. *Int J Bipolar Disord.* 2015;**3**.

Lochhead, R. A., Parsey, R. V., Oquendo, M. A., Mann, J. J. Regional brain gray matter volume differences in patients with bipolar disorder as assessed by optimized voxel-based morphometry. *Biol Psychiatry.* 2004;**55**:1154–62.

Lucini-Paioni, S., Squarcina, L., Cousins, D., Brambilla, P. Lithium effects on Hippocampus volumes in patients with bipolar disorder. *J Affect Disord.* 2021;**295**:521–6.

Lyoo, I. K., Kim, M. J., Stoll, A. L., et al. Frontal lobe gray matter density decreases in bipolar I disorder. *Biol Psychiatry.* 2004;**55**:648–51.

Lyoo, I. K., Sung, Y. H., Dager, S. R., et al. Regional cerebral cortical thinning in bipolar disorder. *Bipolar Disord.* 2006;**8**:65–74.

Lyoo, I. K., Dager, S. R., Kim, J. E., et al. Lithium-induced gray matter volume increase as a neural correlate of treatment response in bipolar disorder: a longitudinal brain imaging study. *Neuropsychopharmacology.* 2010;**35**:1743–50.

Machado-Vieira, R., Manji, H. K., Zarate, C. A. The role of lithium in the treatment of bipolar disorder: convergent evidence for neurotrophic effects as a unifying hypothesis. *Bipolar Disord.* 2009;**11**:92–109.

Macritchie, K. A., Lloyd, A. J., Bastin, M. E., et al. White matter microstructural abnormalities in euthymic bipolar disorder. *Br J Psychiatry.* 2010;**196**(1):52–8.

Manji, H. K., Moore, G. J., Chen, G. Lithium up-regulates the cytoprotective protein bcl-2 in the CNS in vivo: a role for neurotrophic and neuroprotective effects in manic depressive illness. *J Clin Psychiatry.* 2000;**61**:82–96.

Marlinge, E., Bellivier, F., Houenou, J. White matter alterations in bipolar disorder: potential for drug discovery and development. *Bipolar Disord.* 2014;**16**(2):97–112.

McDonald, C., Zanelli, J., Rabe-Hesketh, S., et al. Meta-analysis of magnetic resonance imaging brain morphometry studies in bipolar disorder. *Biol Psychiatry.* 2004;**56**:411–17.

McIntosh, A. M., Maniega, S. M., Lymer, G. K. S., et al. 2008. White matter tractography in bipolar disorder and schizophrenia. *Biol Psychiatry.* 2008;**64**(12):1088–92.

Monkul, E. S., Matsuo, K., Nicoletti, M. A., et al. Prefrontal gray matter increases in healthy individuals after lithium treatment: a voxel-based morphometry study. *Neursci Lett.* 2007;**429**:7–11.

Moore, C. M., Demopulos, C. M., Henry, M. E., et al. Brain-to-serum lithium ratio and age: an in vivo magnetic resonance spectroscopy study. *Am J Psychiatry.* 2002;**159**:1240–2.

Moore, G. J., Bebchuk, J. M., Wilds, I. B., et al. Lithium-induced increase in human brain grey matter. *Lancet.* 2000;**356**:1241–2.

Moore, G. J., Cortese, B. M., Glitz, D. A., et al. A longitudinal study of the effects of lithium treatment on prefrontal and subgenual prefrontal gray matter volume in treatment-responsive bipolar disorder patients. *J Clin Psychiatry.* 2009;**70**:699–705.

Moorhead, T. W., McKirdy, J., Sussmann, J. E., et al. Progressive gray matter loss in patients with bipolar disorder. *Biol Psychiatry.* 2007;**62**: 894–900.

Necus, J., Sinha, N., Smith, F. E., et al. White matter microstructural properties in bipolar disorder in relationship to the spatial distribution of lithium in the brain. *J Affect Disord.* 2019;**253**:224–31.

Perico, C. D., Duran, F. L. S., Zanetti, M. V., et al. A population-based morphometric MRI study in patients with first-episode psychotic bipolar disorder: comparison with geographically matched healthy controls and major depressive disorder subjects. *Bipolar Disord.* 2011;**13**:28–40.

Phatak, P., Shaldivin, A., King, L. S., Shapiro, P., Regenold, W. T. Lithium and inositol: effects on brain water homeostasis in the rat. *Psychopharmacology.* 2006;**186**:41–7.

Phillips, M. L., Travis, M. J., Fagiolini, A., Kupfer, D. J. Medication effects in neuroimaging studies of bipolar disorder. *Am J Psychiatry*. 2008;**165**:313–20.

Plenge, P., Stensgaard, A., Jensen, H. V., et al. 24-hour lithium concentration in human brain studied by Li-7 magnetic resonance spectroscopy. *Biol Psychiatry*. 1994;**36**:511–16.

Post, R. M. The new news about lithium: an underutilized treatment in the United States. *Neuropsychopharmacology*. 2018;**43**:1174–9.

Quiroz, J. A., Machado-Vieira, R., Zarate, C. A. Jr, Manji, H. K. Novel insights into lithium's mechanism of action: neurotrophic and neuroprotective effects. *Neuropsychobiology*. 2010;**62**:50–60.

Rangel-Guerra, R. A., Perezpayan, H., Minkoff, L., Todd, L. E. Nuclear magnetic-resonance in bipolar affective-disorders. *Am J Neuroradiol*. 1983;**4**:229–31.

Regenold, W. T., D'agostino, C. A., Ramesh, N., et al. Diffusion-weighted magnetic resonance imaging of white matter in bipolar disorder: a pilot study. *Bipolar Disord*. 2006;**8**(2):188–95.

Renshaw, P. F., Wicklund, S. In vivo measurement of lithium in humans by nuclear magnetic resonance spectroscopy. *Biol Psychiatry*. 1988;**23**:465–75.

Rybakowski, J., Permoda-Osip, A., Suwalska, A. The absence of cognitive deficits in prophylactic lithium responders. *Int J Neuropsychopharmacol*. 2010;**13**:132.

Sachs, G. S., Renshaw, P. F., Lafer, B., et al. Variability of brain lithium levels during maintenance treatment – a magnetic resonance spectroscopy study. *Biol Psychiatry*. 1995;**38**:422–8.

Sassi, R. B., Brambilla, P., Hatch, J. P., et al. Reduced left anterior cingulate volumes in untreated bipolar patients. *Biol Psychiatry*. 2004;**56**:467–75.

Sassi, R. B., Brambilla, P., Nicoletti, M., et al. Lithium influences the volume of the cingulate cortex in bipolar mood disorder patients. *Biol Psychiatry*. 2002;**51**:84S.

Savitz, J., Nugent, A. C., Bogers, W., et al. Amygdala volume in depressed patients with bipolar disorder assessed using high resolution 3T MRI: the impact of medication. *Neuroimage*. 2010;**49**:2966–76.

Severus, E., Bauer, M., Geddes, J. Efficacy and effectiveness of lithium in the long-term treatment of bipolar disorder: an update 2018. *Pharmacopsychiatry*. 2018;**51**:173–6.

Smith, F. E., Thelwall, P. E., Necus, J., et al. 3D ^{7}Li magnetic resonance imaging of brain lithium distribution in bipolar disorder. *Mol Psychiatry*. 2018;**23**:2184–91.

Soares, J. C., Boada, F., Keshavan, M.A. Brain lithium measurements with Li-7 magnetic resonance spectroscopy (MRS): a literature review. *Eur Neuropsychopharmacol*. 2000;**10**:151–8.

Soares, J. C., Boada, F., Spencer, S., et al. Brain lithium concentrations in bipolar disorder patients: preliminary 7Li magnetic resonance studies at 3 T. *Biol Psychiatry*. 2001;**49**:437–43.

Song, S. K., Sun, S. W., Ramsbottom, M. J., et al. Dysmyelination revealed through MRI as increased radial (but unchanged axial) diffusion of water. *Neuroimage*. 2002;**17**(3):1429–36.

Stout, J., Hozer, F., Coste, A., et al. Accumulation of lithium in the hippocampus of patients with bipolar disorder: a Lithium-7 magnetic resonance imaging study at 7 Tesla. *Biol Psychiatry*. 2020;**88**(5):426–33.

Usher, J., Menzel, P., Schneider-Axmann, T., et al. Increased right amygdala volume in lithium-treated patients with bipolar I disorder. *Acta Psychiatr Scand*. 2010;**121**:119–24.

Van Erp, T. G. M., Thompson, P. M., Kieseppa, T., et al. Hippocampal morphology in lithium and non-lithium-treated bipolar I disorder patients, non-bipolar co-twins, and control twins. *Hum Brain Mapp*. 2012;**33**:501–10.

Velosa, J., Delgado, A., Finger, E., et al. Risk of dementia in bipolar disorder and the interplay of lithium: a systematic review and meta-analyses. *Acta Psychiatr Scand*. 2020;**141**:510–21.

Wang, F., Jackowski, M., Kalmar, J. H., et al. Abnormal anterior cingulum integrity in bipolar disorder determined through diffusion tensor imaging. *Br J Psychiatry*. 2008;**193**(2):126–9.

Wang, F., Kalmar, J.H., He, Y., et al. Functional and structural connectivity between the perigenual anterior cingulate and amygdala in bipolar disorder. *Biol Psychiatry*. 2009;**66**:515–21.

Wang, F., Kalmar, J. H., Womer, F. Y., et al. Olfactocentric paralimbic cortex morphology in adolescents with bipolar disorder. *Brain*. 2011;**134**(7):2005–12.

Wessa, M., Houenou, J., Leboyer, M., et al. Microstructural white matter changes in euthymic bipolar patients: a whole-brain diffusion tensor imaging study. *Bipolar Disord*. 2009;**11**(5):504–14.

Yucel, K., McKinnon, M. C., Taylor, V. H., et al. Bilateral hippocampal volume increases after long-term lithium treatment in patients with bipolar disorder: a longitudinal MRI study. *Psychopharmacology*. 2007;**195**:357–67.

Yucel, K., Taylor, V. H., McKinnon, M. C., et al. Bilateral hippocampal volume increase in patients with bipolar disorder and short-term lithium treatment. *Neuropsychopharmacology*. 2008;**33**:361–7.

Zung, S., Souza-Duran, F. L., Soeiro-de-Souza, M. G., et al. The influence of lithium on hippocampal volume in elderly bipolar patients: a study using voxel-based morphometry. *Transl Psychiatry*. 2016;**6**:e846.

Chapter 16

Inflammation and Metabolic Issues in Mood Disorders

Marsal Sanches and Jair C. Soares

Introduction

The pathophysiology of mood disorders (depression and bipolar disorders [BD]) remains poorly understood, with available evidence pointing to dysfunctions in the brain circuits involved in the processing of emotions, neurodevelopmental disruptions, and abnormalities in different neurotransmission systems [1–3]. In addition, over the past few decades, the role of systemic process (particularly inflammation) in the development of mood disorders has been the focus of great attention [4,5].

A relationship between inflammatory processes and mood disorders was first proposed in the early 1980s, with the hypothesis that the therapeutic effects of lithium could be related to its modulatory effects on the immune system, in addition to evidence indicating high comorbidity rates between inflammatory illnesses and mood disorders [6,7]. Concomitantly, researchers' phenotypical similarities between the symptoms experienced by patients with mood disorders (particularly during depressive states) and those commonly associated with systemic inflammatory diseases ("sickness behavior"), as well as evidence indicating that exogenous administration of cytokines is able to precipitate depressive-like states [8]. These observations inspired countless numbers of studies focusing on investigating the biological basis of a possible interface between inflammation and mood, as well as numerous trials looking at the inflammation system as a potential therapeutic target in mood disorders. More recently, the role of inflammation in the pathophysiology of mood disorders has been expanded to include possible links with other systemic processes, such as metabolic issues and the renin–angiotensin system [9,10].

The present chapter is composed of three parts. In the first one, we summarize the available evidence on the role of inflammation in the pathophysiology of mood disorders. Next, we discuss the interface between inflammation, metabolic dysfunction, and mood disorders. Last, we critically analyze the clinical implications associated with a better understanding of the role of inflammatory processes in mood disorders.

Inflammation and the Pathophysiology of Mood Disorders: An Overview

A growing amount of evidence supports the hypothesis that disruptions in the immune–inflammatory system play a critical role in the pathophysiology of mood disorders. One of the key methods to explore this role corresponds to the measurement of cytokine levels among patients with mood disorders. Since peripheral cytokines are able to cross the blood–brain barrier [11], these levels can be measured in the peripheral blood or centrally (e.g., in the cerebrospinal fluid). While the latter seem to be more robustly correlated with neuroinflammation, the relative invasiveness of lumbar punctures when compared to venipunctures makes the measurement of peripheral cytokine levels more popular and easier to implement. Some cytokines (e.g., IL-1β, IL-6, IL-8, and TNF-α) have proinflammatory activities, while others (e.g., IL-1Ra, IL-4, IL-10, and TGF-β1) have anti-inflammatory properties and are able to regulate the inflammatory response by decreasing the gene expression associated with the production of proinflammatory cytokines [8,12]. Among patients with unipolar depression, meta-analyses have consistently identified elevations in cytokines among patients with depression compared to non-depressed individuals, particularly C-reactive protein (CRP), IL-1, IL-6, and TNF-α [12–14]. Similarly, patients with BD have been found to display chronically elevated serum levels of cytokines, specially TNF-α, soluble IL-2 receptor, IL-1β, IL-6, soluble receptor of TNF-α type 1 (sTNFR1), and

CRP [7]. Even though the evidence points to a chronic proinflammatory state in BD, some studies indicate different profiles in terms of cytokine levels across different mood states in BD, which might normalize during periods of euthymia and as a result of treatment with mood stabilizers [15–17].

Put together, these findings do support the hypothesis that abnormal immune activation seems to be involved in the development of mood disorders. Nonetheless, from a pathophysiological standpoint, the interaction between this abnormal immune response and other risk factors for mood disorders, as well the downstream effects of inflammation that are of relevance in mood disorders, are complex (Figure 16.1). For example, it has been suggested that a genetically mediated vulnerability of the immune system could interact with other factors, such as stress exposure or other processes able to trigger activation of the immune system not only centrally but also peripherally, such as systemic infections [4,18].

The resulting elevated levels of cytokines have several potential effects at a systemic and central level. For example, proinflammatory cytokines increase leukocyte proliferation and migration across the blood–brain barrier, as well as the overexpression of microglia and other brain macrophages, bringing about the release of proteolytic enzymes, cytotoxicity, and expression of major histocompatibility complex (MHC) antigens responsible for the induction of further inflammatory activity [12]. Under physiological circumstances, these mechanisms aim at eliminating

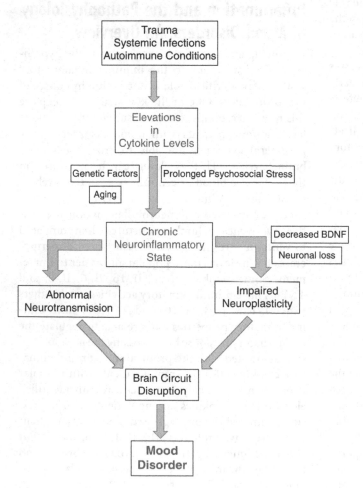

Figure 16.1 Inflammation and mood disorders: pathophysiological mechanisms.

Abbreviation: BDNF: brain-derived neurotrophic factor.

the causative agent responsible for the triggering of the immune response and are self-regulated. On the other hand, the abnormal immune reaction observed among patients with mood disorders, likely mediated by genetic vulnerability, chronic stress exposure, and aging, results in a chronic neuroinflammatory state associated with decreases in *BDNF* gene expression, reduced neuroplasticity, abnormal monoaminergic transmission, and neuronal loss [19]. According to this hypothesis, the consequent disruptions in the brain circuits associated with emotional regulation and processing would be the ultimate common pathway that would result in the development of mood disorders.

Moreover, consider the proposed role of stress exposure in the triggering of inflammatory responses – the interface between hypothalamic–pituitary–adrenal (HPA) axis hyperactivation, inflammation, and mood disorders has been the object of great interest. Adult individuals exposed to childhood trauma have been found to show significantly higher levels of CRP compared to controls, suggesting that early trauma is able to produce a chronic inflammatory state that persists into adulthood and may contribute to the development of mood disorders [20]. The relationship between stress and inflammation is likely bidirectional [4], with hyperactivation of the HPA axis contributing to enhanced inflammatory response and vice versa. Under normal circumstances, the stimulation of glucocorticoid receptors by cortisol, in addition to regulating HPA response, also leads to the up-regulation of genes associated with the production of anti-inflammatory cytokines, such as IL-10 [4,21]. Therefore, decreased expression or sensitivity of these receptors, a putative mechanism associated with the development of mood disorders, may contribute to increases in inflammatory response. In contrast, it has been proposed that chronically elevated levels of cytokines can reduce the number and expression of glucocorticoid receptors, as well as their response to cortisol, ultimately undermining the mechanism associated with regulation of the HPA axis during stress exposure [22]. Ultimately, this would result in chronic hypercortisolism, which can contribute to the development and perpetuation of abnormal mood states, especially depression, as well as to other central and systemic consequences, as explained in the next section.

The Link between Inflammation, Mood Disorders, and Metabolic Disorders

The association between mood disorders and systemic illnesses is well established. Bipolar disorder is associated with high rates of diabetes, obesity, cardiovascular conditions, and shorter life expectancy compared to the general population [23]. Similar associations have been described among patients with major depressive disorder [24]. Even though the reasons behind these high comorbidity rates are likely multiple, inflammation seems to be an important factor in this association.

On the one hand, systemic inflammatory processes may be involved in the development of the systemic illness and, through the mechanisms described in the previous section, of the mood disorder. For example, chronically elevated levels of proinflammatory cytokines, in addition to contributing to neuroinflammation, can have deleterious effects on the cardiovascular system through endothelial dysfunction and abnormal platelet aggregation [25,26]. On the other hand, the proposed chronic inflammatory state associated with mood disorders and stress can have systemic repercussions, bringing about a higher risk for the development of medical illnesses. Chronic activation of the HPA axis, with elevation in serum levels of glucocorticoids, can contribute to obesity, and there are strong associations between stress exposure, elevated cytokines (specially IL-1), and insulin resistance, which seem to be mediated by inflammation and are associated with obesity, type II diabetes, non-alcoholic fatty liver disease, dyslipidemia, and metabolic syndrome [10].

Last, it has been proposed that the relationship between mood disorders, metabolic syndrome, and inflammation is mediated by oxidative stress [10]. Individuals with metabolic syndrome have increased rates of free radical formation, resulting in chronic oxidative stress, which, on its turn, is associated with increased inflammatory activity, as well as microvascular alterations and excessive production of vascular nitride oxide [27]. Some of these microvascular abnormalities, when occurring in the central nervous system, may play a potential role in the development of mood disorders, particularly with regard to its progression and staging (see next section).

Clinical Implications

The clinical implications related to the involvement of inflammation in the pathophysiology of mood disorders are many. While some of the inflammatory abnormalities described in the previous sections seem to reverse with appropriate treatment of the mood disorders with traditional agents, the inflammatory system has been regarded with great interest as a potential target for novel treatments for mood disorders. In addition, it has been proposed that certain clinical features found in patients with mood disorders may be directly related to the presence and severity of ongoing inflammatory processes.

Inflammation, Cognition, and Staging

In patients with BD, several studies found correlations between elevated levels of proinflammatory cytokines and cognitive impairment [7]. In particular, TNFα, IL-6, and IL-1 have been found to be associated with poor cognitive impairment among BD patients with longer illness duration [28]. In contrast, anti-inflammatory cytokines (e.g., IL-4 and IL-10) might attenuate the impact that proinflammatory cytokines have on cognition [29]. In a study looking at cytokine levels as candidate biomarkers of BD staging, proinflammatory cytokines (TNF-α and IL-6) were found to be elevated in both early and late phases of the illness, but the elevations in TNF-α were more pronounced in the late phases, whereas elevations in IL-6 were more pronounced in the early phases of the illness [30]. On the other hand, IL-10 was found to be elevated only in the early phases, what has been interpreted as the result of possible compensatory mechanism-triggered increases in proinflammatory cytokines [30]. These findings support the existence of correlations between inflammatory activity and BD staging, suggesting that inflammatory markers may contribute to the characterization of neuroprogression in BD [31], with consequent therapeutic and prognostic implications.

Although a similar staging model has not yet been described for major depressive disorders, associations between inflammatory activity and cognitive impairment in patients with unipolar depression have been previously described, and in animal models of depression, the administration of IL-10 was able to reverse deficits in novel object recognition, spatial working memory, and hippocampal dendritic spine density [32].

Accelerated Aging

As previously discussed, life expectation among patients with mood disorders is considerably lower than in the general population. While most of the deaths among mood disorder patients are associated with medical comorbidities, which are highly prevalent among patients with mood disorders, it has been proposed that chronic inflammation could be implicated in accelerated aging in mood disorders [33]. Telomere shortening, considered a biological marker of aging, has been described among patients with mood disorders [34]. Given the evidence pointing to associations between chronic inflammation and telomere shortening, it has been proposed that accelerated telomere shortening could correspond to the link between inflammation and accelerated aging [35]. Nevertheless, it is not yet clear whether telomere shortening in mood disorder patients is a predisposing factor for mood disorders or a consequence of telomere attrition secondary to inflammation. In a 2011 study [36], telomere length was found to be inversely correlated with IL-6 levels among major depressive disorder (MDD) patients, and only patients with a chronic illness course were found to have shorter telomere length when compared to controls. On the other hand, in a more recent study [37], decreased telomere length was found among patients with BD and their unaffected siblings compared to controls, while elevated levels of IL-6 were higher among patients (but not among siblings) when compared to controls.

Inflammatory Phenotypes of Mood Disorders

Despite the large amount of evidence linking inflammatory processes to mood disorders, it has been pointed out that these disorders are heterogeneous with respect to the role and importance of inflammation in their pathophysiology. Specifically with regard to depression, there are inconsistencies with respect to the strength and directions of associations with inflammation, suggesting that inflammation likely plays a more critical role in certain depression subtypes than in others. Even though CRP levels are commonly adopted as a clinical measure of inflammation, there is a high degree of intra-individual variability with regard to those levels, suggesting that they should not be used as the sole factor for the characterization of inflammatory depression [38]. Given the fact that inflammation has been extensively regarded as a promising target for the treatment of mood disorders (see next section), the identification of "inflammatory phenotypes" for mood disorders has important potential therapeutic implications. In that sense, studies have identified correlations between elevated inflammation and specific depressive symptoms, such as anhedonia, vegetative symptoms of depression (fatigue, sleep, and appetite disturbances), cognitive impairment, and suicidality [39]. In addition, inflammation among MDD patients has also been found to be associated with elevated body mass index (BMI) levels, anxiety, and negative perceptions about one's own childhood [40].

Furthermore, in a recent paper [38], a model aiming at a better characterization of an inflammatory phenotype was proposed. Rather than relying on specific clinical features of depression, the model in question focuses on "biology-based" elements and lifestyle behaviors that seem to be associated with enhanced inflammation among mood disorder patients, including obesity, decreased high-density lipoprotein (HDL) levels, high triglyceride levels, hypertension, hypothyroidism, migraines, rheumatoid arthritis, diabetes, inflammatory diseases of the bowel and skin, cigarette smoking, and chronic psychosocial stress.

Inflammation and Therapeutic Strategies

Several studies have investigated the potential role of interventions targeting inflammation in the treatment of mood disorders. Attention has also been given to the anti-inflammatory effects of currently available medications for the treatment of mood disorders,

such as lithium, valproate, and ketamine [12,28,41]. Table 16.1 lists the main compounds recently investigated for the treatment of mood disorders with specific effects on inflammatory processes.

For example, our group has previously assessed the potential role of adjunctive treatment with celecoxib, a COX-2 inhibitor, in the treatment of bipolar depression [42]. Results pointed to a positive effect of celecoxib on the reduction of depressive symptoms in the first week of treatment, although differences in improvement between the medication and placebo groups at the end of the 6-week follow-up period were not significant. Celecoxib has also been evaluated in the treatment of MDD. In a 2009 study, the augmentation of fluoxetine with celecoxib was found to be superior to fluoxetine plus placebo in the treatment of MDD patients, over a period of 6 weeks [43].

Another agent with anti-inflammatory and antioxidant properties, N-acetyl-cysteine (NAC) has been investigated as a promising augmentation strategy for the treatment of different psychiatric conditions, including unipolar depression and bipolar disorder [44–46]. In a meta-analysis of five studies (including MDD, bipolar depression, and depressive symptoms in other psychiatric conditions), treatment with NAC was found to produce significant improvement in depressive symptomatology when compared with placebo, even though no impact on participants' quality of life was observed [47]. In another randomized, double-blind study carried out by our group, the combination of aspirin and NAC as an augmentation strategy over a period of 16 weeks was found to

Table 16.1 Pharmacological agents with anti-inflammatory properties investigated for their potential role in the treatment of mood disorders

Agent	Mechanism of action
Naproxen	Cyclooxygenase inhibition
Aspirin	cyclooxygenase inhibition
Celecoxib	Selective cyclooxygenase–2 (COX-2) inhibition
Infliximab	TNF-α antagonism
Omega-3 fatty acids	Multiple
N-acetyl-cysteine	Multiple
Minocycline	Multiple
Pioglitazone	Multiple
Curcumin	Multiple

produce significant improvement in depressive symptoms among patients with BD [48].

Similarly, omega-3 polyunsaturated fatty acids (OM3FA), which have well-demonstrated anti-inflammatory properties, have been extensively studied for their role in the treatment of mood disorders. The mechanisms behind the anti-inflammatory effects of OM3FA are multiple and seem to include changes in cell membrane phospholipid fatty acid composition, decreased activation of pro-inflammatory transcription factors, and binding to the G protein coupled receptors [49]. Results from meta-analyses have been mixed, with a 2015 Cochrane Database systematic review suggesting "small-to-modest, non-clinically beneficial effect" of OM3FA on depressive symptoms when compared to placebo among patients with MDD [50], even though the quality of the evidence available to reach that conclusion was considered low/very low. A significantly smaller number of studies assessed the efficacy of these agents in the treatment of BD, with evidence suggesting OM3FA might have a role in the treatment of bipolar depression but not of manic symptoms [51].

Moreover, in a recent study, infliximab, a monoclonal antibody targeting tumor necrosis factor, was evaluated for its putative efficacy in the treatment of bipolar depression as an augmentation strategy [52]. In the primary analysis, the study medication did not seem to produce improvements in depression when compared to placebo, although a secondary analysis revealed that individuals with a history of childhood trauma (physical and/or sexual abuse) showed significant improvements in their depressive symptoms when compared to placebo.

With regard to nonpharmacological strategies, the impact of physical exercise on mood symptomatology has been extensively studied. Evidence from animal and human research supports the anti-inflammatory effects of exercise, which seems to have the ability to decrease chronic inflammation in the central nervous system [53,54]. Different mechanisms seem to be involved in these anti-inflammatory effects, including decreases in oxidative stress and the enhancement of *PGC1α* gene expression, which in turn reduces the production of pro-inflammatory cytokines and increases anti-inflammatory cytokines [53,55]. Evidence suggests that the response rates associated with exercise may be similar to those observed with well-stablished treatments for MDD, such as antidepressants and cognitive behavioral therapy, and

the Canadian Network for Mood and Anxiety Treatments recommended exercise as a first- or second-line therapy for the treatment of mild to moderate MDD [56,57]. Despite the much more limited amount of available evidence, studies also support beneficial effects of physical exercise for patients with BD, especially with regard to reductions in depressive symptoms [58,59].

Last, the therapeutic effects of dietary interventions in the management of mood disorders have recently been the object of great interest. In addition to their positive effects on reducing metabolic syndrome and decreasing systemic inflammation, dietary strategies have the potential to explore the interesting albeit relatively unexplored link between mood disorder, inflammation, and gut microbiota [58,60,61].

In summary, available evidence does suggest that agents targeting inflammation may have a role in the treatment of mood disorders. However, the heterogeneity of the findings supports the hypothesis that these agents are likely to be of more benefit for specific subgroups of patients, whose mood disorders seem to be more markedly associated with increased inflammatory activity.

Conclusions

The role of inflammation in mood disorders likely corresponds to one of the most relevant advances in the understanding of the pathophysiology of these conditions observed in the past few decades. In addition to its numerous potential therapeutic implications, research on the mood disorders–inflammation association has played a pivotal role in the redefinition of mood disorders as systemic conditions, contributing to a better clarification of the interface between these disorders and comorbid medical conditions. The better characterization of specific mood disorder phenotypes more directly associated with inflammation corresponds to a fertile area for research and will contribute to a better characterization of novel treatment strategies targeting inflammatory processes in mood illnesses.

References

1. Harrison PJ, Geddes JR, Tunbridge EM. The emerging neurobiology of bipolar disorder. *Trends Neurosci*. 2018 Jan;**41**(1):18–30.

2. Sanches M, Keshavan MS, Brambilla P, Soares JC. Neurodevelopmental basis of bipolar disorder: a critical appraisal. *Prog Neuropsychopharmacol Biol Psychiatry*. 2008 Oct 1;**32**(7):1617–27.

3. Kraus C, Castrén E, Kasper S, Lanzenberger R. Serotonin and neuroplasticity – links between molecular, functional and structural pathophysiology in depression. *Neurosci Biobehav Rev*. 2017 Jun;**77**:317–26.

4. Bauer ME, Teixeira AL. Inflammation in psychiatric disorders: what comes first? *Ann N Y Acad Sci*. 2019;**1437**(1):57–67.

5. Beurel E, Toups M, Nemeroff CB. The bidirectional relationship of depression and inflammation: double trouble. *Neuron*. 2020 Jul 22;**107**(2):234–56.

6. Horrobin DF, Lieb J. A biochemical basis for the actions of lithium on behaviour and on immunity: relapsing and remitting disorders of inflammation and immunity such as multiple sclerosis or recurrent herpes as manic-depression of the immune system. *Med Hypotheses*. 1981 Jul;**7**(7):891–905.

7. Rosenblat JD, McIntyre RS. Bipolar disorder and inflammation. *Psychiatr Clin North Am*. 2016 Mar;**39**(1):125–37.

8. Liu CS, Adibfar A, Herrmann N, Gallagher D, Lanctôt KL. Evidence for inflammation-associated depression. In R Dantzer, L Capuron, editors. *Inflammation-Associated Depression: Evidence, Mechanisms and Implications*, Vol. **31**, *Current Topics in Behavioral Neurosciences*. Cham: Springer, 2016; 3–30. Available from: http://link.springer.com/10.1007/7854_2016_2

9. Mohite S, Sanches M, Teixeira AL. Exploring the evidence implicating the renin-angiotensin system (RAS) in the physiopathology of mood disorders. *Protein Pept Lett*. 2020;**27**(6):449–55.

10. Galvez JF, Bauer IE, Sanches M, et al. Shared clinical associations between obesity and impulsivity in rapid cycling bipolar disorder: a systematic review. *J Affect Disord*. 2014 Oct;**168**:306–13.

11. Banks WA, Kastin AJ, Broadwell RD. Passage of cytokines across the blood-brain barrier. *Neuroimmunomodulation*. 1995 Aug;**2**(4):241–8.

12. Singhal G, Baune BT. Inflammatory abnormalities in major depressive disorder. In RS McIntyre, editor. *Major Depressive Disorder*. Elsevier, 2019; 75–89. Available from: https://linkinghub.elsevier.com/retrieve/pii/B9780323581318000069

13. Köhler CA, Freitas TH, Maes M, et al. Peripheral cytokine and chemokine alterations in depression: a meta-analysis of 82 studies. *Acta Psychiatr Scand*. 2017 May;**135**(5):373–87.

14. Haapakoski R, Mathieu J, Ebmeier KP, Alenius H, Kivimäki M. Cumulative meta-analysis of interleukins 6 and 1β, tumour necrosis factor α and C-reactive protein in patients with major depressive disorder. *Brain Behav Immun*. 2015 Oct;**49**:206–15.

15. Fiedorowicz JG, Prossin AR, Johnson CP, et al. Peripheral inflammation during abnormal mood states in bipolar I disorder. *J Affect Disord*. 2015 Nov 15;**187**:172–8.

16. Guloksuz S, Cetin EA, Cetin T, et al. Cytokine levels in euthymic bipolar patients. *J Affect Disord*. 2010 Nov;**126**(3):458–62.

17. van den Ameele S, van Diermen L, Staels W, et al. The effect of mood-stabilizing drugs on cytokine levels in bipolar disorder: a systematic review. *J Affect Disord*. 2016 Oct;**203**:364–73.

18. Duffy A, Goodday SM, Keown-Stoneman C, et al. Epigenetic markers in inflammation-related genes associated with mood disorder: a cross-sectional and longitudinal study in high-risk offspring of bipolar parents. *Int J Bipolar Disord*. 2019 Dec;**7**(1):17.

19. Lima Giacobbo B, Doorduin J, Klein HC, et al. Brain-derived neurotrophic factor in brain disorders: focus on neuroinflammation. *Mol Neurobiol*. 2019 May;**56**(5):3295–312.

20. Baumeister D, Akhtar R, Ciufolini S, Pariante CM, Mondelli V. Childhood trauma and adulthood inflammation: a meta-analysis of peripheral C-reactive protein, interleukin-6 and tumour necrosis factor-α. *Mol Psychiatry*. 2016 May;**21**(5):642–9.

21. Barbosa IG, Machado-Vieira R, Soares JC, Teixeira AL. The immunology of bipolar disorder. *Neuroimmunomodulation*. 2014;**21**(2–3):117–22.

22. Pace TWW, Miller AH. Cytokines and glucocorticoid receptor signaling: relevance to major depression. *Ann N Y Acad Sci*. 2009 Oct;**1179**(1):86–105.

23. Vancampfort D, Vansteelandt K, Correll CU, et al. Metabolic syndrome and metabolic abnormalities in bipolar disorder: a meta-analysis of prevalence rates and moderators. *Am J Psychiatry*. 2013 Mar;**170**(3):265–74.

24. Thom R, Silbersweig DA, Boland RJ. Major depressive disorder in medical illness: a review of assessment, prevalence, and treatment options. *Psychosom Med*. 2019 Apr;**81**(3):246–55.

25. Halaris A. Inflammation-associated co-morbidity between depression and cardiovascular disease. *Curr Top Behav Neurosci*. 2017;**31**:45–70.

26. Izzi B, Tirozzi A, Cerletti C, et al. Beyond haemostasis and thrombosis: platelets in depression and its co-morbidities. *Int J Mol Sci*. 2020 Nov 21;**21**(22):E8817.

27. Limberg JK, Harrell JW, Johansson RE, et al. Microvascular function in younger adults with obesity and metabolic syndrome: role of oxidative stress. *Am J Physiol Heart Circ Physiol*. 2013 Oct 15;**305**(8):H1230-1237.

28. Rosenblat JD, Brietzke E, Mansur RB, et al. Inflammation as a neurobiological substrate of cognitive impairment in bipolar disorder: evidence, pathophysiology and treatment implications. *J Affect Disord*. 2015 Dec 1;**188**:149–59.

29. Derecki NC, Cardani AN, Yang CH, et al. Regulation of learning and memory by meningeal immunity: a key role for IL-4. *J Exp Med*. 2010 May 10;**207** (5):1067–80.

30. Kauer-Sant'Anna M, Kapczinski F, Andreazza AC, et al. Brain-derived neurotrophic factor and inflammatory markers in patients with early- vs. late-stage bipolar disorder. *Int J Neuropsychopharmacol*. 2009 May;**12**(4):447–58.

31. Berk M, Post R, Ratheesh A, et al. Staging in bipolar disorder: from theoretical framework to clinical utility. *World Psychiatry*. 2017;**16**(3):236–44.

32. Worthen RJ, Garzon Zighelboim SS, Torres Jaramillo CS, Beurel E. Anti-inflammatory IL-10 administration rescues depression-associated learning and memory deficits in mice. *J Neuroinflammation*. 2020 Dec;**17**(1):246.

33. Kiecolt-Glaser JK, Wilson SJ. Psychiatric disorders, morbidity, and mortality: tracing mechanistic pathways to accelerated aging. *Psychosom Med*. 2016 Sep;**78**(7):772–5.

34. Lindqvist D, Epel ES, Mellon SH, et al. Psychiatric disorders and leukocyte telomere length: underlying mechanisms linking mental illness with cellular aging. *Neurosci Biobehav Rev*. 2015 Aug;**55**:333–64.

35. Squassina A, Pisanu C, Vanni R. Mood disorders, accelerated aging, and inflammation: is the link hidden in telomeres? *Cells*. 2019 Jan 15;**8**(1):52.

36. Wolkowitz OM, Mellon SH, Epel ES, et al. Leukocyte telomere length in major depression: correlations with chronicity, inflammation and oxidative stress–preliminary findings. *PLoS One*. 2011 Mar 23;**6**(3): e17837.

37. Vasconcelos-Moreno MP, Fries GR, Gubert C, et al. Telomere length, oxidative stress, inflammation and bdnf levels in siblings of patients with bipolar disorder: implications for accelerated cellular aging. *Int J Neuropsychopharmacol*. 2017 Jun 1;**20**(6):445–54.

38. Kramer NE, Cosgrove VE, Dunlap K, et al. A clinical model for identifying an inflammatory phenotype in mood disorders. *J Psychiatr Res*. 2019 Jun;**113**:148–58.

39. Moriarity DP, van Borkulo C, Alloy LB. Inflammatory phenotype of depression symptom structure: a network perspective. *Brain Behav Immun*. 2021 Mar;**93**:35–42.

40. Chamberlain SR, Cavanagh J, de Boer P, et al. Treatment-resistant depression and peripheral C-reactive protein. *Br J Psychiatry J Ment Sci*. 2019 Jan;**214**(1):11–9.

41. Sanches M, Newberg AR, Soares JC. Emerging drugs for bipolar disorder. *Expert Opin Emerg Drugs*. 2010 Sep;**15**(3):453–66.

42. Nery FG, Monkul ES, Hatch JP, et al. Celecoxib as an adjunct in the treatment of depressive or mixed episodes of bipolar disorder: a double-blind, randomized, placebo-controlled study. *Hum Psychopharmacol*. 2008 Mar;**23**(2):87–94.

43. Akhondzadeh S, Jafari S, Raisi F, et al. Clinical trial of adjunctive celecoxib treatment in patients with major depression: a double blind and placebo controlled trial. *Depress Anxiety*. 2009;**26**(7):607–11.

44. Scapagnini G, Davinelli S, Drago F, De Lorenzo A, Oriani G. Antioxidants as antidepressants: fact or fiction? *CNS Drugs*. 2012 Jun 1;**26**(6):477–90.

45. di Michele F, Talamo A, Niolu C, Siracusano A. Vitamin D and N-acetyl cysteine supplementation in treatment-resistant depressive disorder patients: a general review. *Curr Pharm Des*. 2020;**26** (21):2442–59.

46. Yalin N, Young AH. Pharmacological treatment of bipolar depression: what are the current and emerging options? *Neuropsychiatr Dis Treat*. 2020;**16**:1459–72.

47. Fernandes BS, Dean OM, Dodd S, Malhi GS, Berk M. N-Acetylcysteine in depressive symptoms and functionality: a systematic review and meta-analysis. *J Clin Psychiatry*. 2016 Apr;**77**(4):e457-466.

48. Bauer IE, Green C, Colpo GD, et al. A double-blind, randomized, placebo-controlled study of aspirin and N-acetylcysteine as adjunctive treatments for bipolar depression. *J Clin Psychiatry*. 2018 Dec 4;**80**(1).

49. Calder PC. Omega-3 polyunsaturated fatty acids and inflammatory processes: nutrition or pharmacology? *Br J Clin Pharmacol*. 2013 Mar;**75**(3):645–62.

50. Appleton KM, Sallis HM, Perry R, Ness AR, Churchill R. Omega-3 fatty acids for depression in adults. *Cochrane Database Syst Rev*. 2015;**11**:CD004692.

51. Bozzatello P, Rocca P, Mantelli E, Bellino S. Polyunsaturated fatty acids: what is their role in treatment of psychiatric disorders? *Int J Mol Sci*. 2019 Oct 23;**20**(21):E5257.

52. McIntyre RS, Subramaniapillai M, Lee Y, et al. Efficacy of adjunctive infliximab vs placebo in the treatment of adults with bipolar I/II depression: a randomized clinical trial. *JAMA Psychiatry*. 2019 Aug 1;**76**(8):783–90.

53. Ignácio ZM, da Silva RS, Plissari ME, Quevedo J, Réus GZ. Physical exercise and neuroinflammation in major depressive disorder. *Mol Neurobiol*. 2019 Dec;**56**(12):8323–35.

54. Metsios GS, Moe RH, Kitas GD. Exercise and inflammation. *Best Pract Res Clin Rheumatol*. 2020 Apr;**34**(2):101504.

55. Ost M, Coleman V, Kasch J, Klaus S. Regulation of myokine expression: role of exercise and cellular stress. *Free Radic Biol Med*. 2016 Sep;**98**:78–89.

56. Blumenthal JA, Babyak MA, Doraiswamy PM, et al. Exercise and pharmacotherapy in the treatment of major depressive disorder. *Psychosom Med*. 2007 Oct;**69**(7):587–96.

57. Ravindran AV, Balneaves LG, Faulkner G, et al. Canadian Network for Mood and Anxiety Treatments (CANMAT) 2016 Clinical Guidelines for the Management of Adults with Major Depressive Disorder: Section 5. Complementary and Alternative Medicine Treatments. *Can J Psychiatry Rev Can Psychiatr*. 2016 Sep;**61**(9):576–87.

58. Bauer IE, Gálvez JF, Hamilton JE, et al. Lifestyle interventions targeting dietary habits and exercise in bipolar disorder: a systematic review. *J Psychiatr Res*. 2016 Mar;**74**:1–7.

59. Melo MCA, Daher EDF, Albuquerque SGC, de Bruin VMS. Exercise in bipolar patients: a systematic review. *J Affect Disord*. 2016 Jul 1;**198**:32–8.

60. Gondalia S, Parkinson L, Stough C, Scholey A. Gut microbiota and bipolar disorder: a review of mechanisms and potential targets for adjunctive therapy. *Psychopharmacology (Berl)*. 2019 May;**236**(5):1433–43.

61. Null G, Pennesi L. Diet and lifestyle intervention on chronic moderate to severe depression and anxiety and other chronic conditions. *Complement Ther Clin Pract*. 2017 Nov;**29**:189–93.

Genetics of Mood Disorders

Camila Nayane de Carvalho Lima, Christopher Busby, and Gabriel Rodrigo Fries

Introduction

Mood disorders, including bipolar disorder (BD) and major depressive disorder (MDD), are fairly common in the population and are among the most prevalent psychiatric disorders in adults [1,2]. Both disorders are highly heritable, with heritability estimates in BD and MDD [3] ranging as high as 85–93% and 40–50%, respectively [4]. However, their specific genetic underpinnings remain fairly unknown, with recent studies pointing to complex, multifactorial, and highly polygenic architectures. This chapter will provide an overview of the reported genetic landscape of mood disorders, discussing the contributions of earlier genetic epidemiological studies all the way to recent microarray and sequencing findings.

Genetic Basis of BD

Classical Genetic Epidemiology of BD

As mentioned above, genetic studies have suggested very high estimates of heritability for BD, as evidenced by family, twin, and, to a lesser extent, adoption studies [3–6]. The estimated lifetime risk for BD development is approximately 0.5–1.5% for people with no family history of BD; first-degree relatives of patients with BD are seven times more likely to develop BD than the general population. Specifically, the lifetime risk is 5–10% for first-degree relatives and 40–70% for monozygotic co-twins [7], suggesting a significant contribution of genetic factors.

Linkage studies in BD

Genetic linkage studies were among the earliest strategies to identify genetic risk *loci* for neuropsychiatric disorders. Linkage studies are considered more suitable for Mendelian diseases where there are one or few

genetic *loci* exerting a substantial effect on risk [7]. Although several regions have been implicated in BD, the linkage paradigm has been unable to accurately and reproducibly identify the *loci* involved in BD (as for most other common familial diseases).

Candidate Genes and GWAS Studies in BD

To overcome the limitations of linkage methods, many studies have tried to identify genetic markers that were chosen based on their proximity to genes that encoded proteins of known neurobiological importance (i.e., "candidate genes" approach). These studies mainly focused on neurotransmitter systems known to be influenced by medications used in the clinical management of the disorder [8]. These choices were not based on a predicated sophisticated level of hypothesis or understanding of the pathogenesis, which shows that selecting candidate genes with a high-prior probability of involvement in BD has proven to be quite difficult [9]. While at least some meta-analyses support a small contribution from a few well-studied candidates, the most reliable association evidence has come from unbiased screenings in genome-wide association studies (GWAS).

Genome-wide association studies are beginning to illuminate the genetic risk for this complex polygenic disorder and have so far been the most successful strategy for identifying genetic variants associated with BD [10,11]. Since the first BD GWAS was published in 2007 [12], many genetic studies of common variations in BD have detected multiple genome-wide significant associations between disease and single nucleotide polymorphisms (SNPs) [13,14], including a GWAS (~50 K cases) that discovered 30 significant *loci* that encode ion channels, neurotransmitter transporters, and synaptic components and of which 20 were newly identified [15]. The most recent published GWAS compared 41,917 patients and 371,549 controls of European ancestry and identified 64 associated *loci* enriched for synaptic signaling pathways and brain-expressed genes [16]. After integrating GWAS results with gene expression data, the authors identified 15 genes of key relevance for the disorder, including druggable targets for follow-up studies (*HTR6, MCHR1, DCLK3,* and *FURIN*) [16].

A couple of gene associations have been replicated over multiple BD GWAS studies, including *TRANK1, ANK3, CACNA1C,* and *ODZ4* (Table 17.1). *TRANK1*, which was one of the top-ranked associations with BD in the latest GWAS [16], has also been previously associated with schizophrenia [17]. This gene encodes a large, primarily uncharacterized protein, highly expressed in multiple tissues (especially the brain). It may play a role in maintaining the blood–brain barrier, synaptic plasticity, dendritic spine, axon guidance, and circadian rhythm [18]. Of note, the expression of *TRANK1* is increased by treatment with the mood stabilizer valproic acid, and cells

carrying the risk allele show decreased expression of the gene and its protein [19]. *ANK3* was one of the first genes to be implicated in BD's etiology by GWAS [20] and was again identified in the latest GWAS [16]. This gene encodes ankyrin-G, a large protein whose neural-specific isoforms are involved in maintaining ion channels and cell adhesion molecules [21]. *CACNA1C* has also been implicated by genome-wide significant SNP associations in several studies of BD, schizophrenia, and MDD; some of these associated SNPs are also associated with the expression of *CACNA1C* in multiple tissues, including the brain [22]. The *CACNA1C* gene encodes the alpha-1 subunit of the voltage-gated calcium channel with a well-established role in neuronal development and synaptic signaling [23]. Finally, the *ODZ4* gene codes for the teneurin transmembrane protein 4 have been associated with BD since the first BD GWAS iteration from the Psychiatric Genomics Consortium [24]. This protein has been demonstrated to play a role in

Table 17.1 Main genes identified by recent genome-wide association studies in bipolar disorder and major depressive disorder

Condition	Gene	Nomenclature	Location	Significance
MDD	*NEGR1*	Neuronal growth regulator 1	1p31.1	It has been identified in at least 5 GWAS with concordant effect direction for MDD. It has assumed association with the hippocampus.
MDD	*DRD2*	Dopamine receptor D2	11q23.2	Decreased expression of DRD2 has been noted in the nucleus accumbens. Lack of receptors might be linked to depression-like symptom.
MDD	*CELF4*	CUGBP Elav-like family member 4	18q12.2	Deletion has been associated with developmental disorders. Mice studies have shown gene abnormality results in aberrant sodium channel function.
BD	*TRANK1*	Tetratricopeptide repeat and ankyrin repeat containing 1	3p22.2	May play a role in maintaining the blood–brain barrier, synaptic plasticity, dendritic spine, axon guidance, and circadian rhythm. Expression is increased by valproic acid.
BD	*ANK3*	Ankyrin 3	10q21.2	Maintenance of ion channels and cell adhesion molecules.
BD	*CACNA1C*	Calcium voltage-gated channel subunit alpha-1C	12p13.33	*CACNA1C* gene encodes the alpha-1 subunit of the voltage-gated calcium channel with a well-established role in neuronal development and synaptic signaling.
BD	*ODZ4*	Teneurin transmembrane protein 4	11q14.1	This protein has been shown to play a role in neuronal connectivity during development, and the SNP associated with BD has been linked to amygdala activation during reward processing.

Abbreviations: BD: bipolar disorder; GWAS: genome-wide association studies; MDD: major depressive disorder; SNP: single nucleotide polymorphisms.

neuronal connectivity during development, and the SNP associated with BD has been linked to amygdala activation during reward processing [25].

The genetic risk variants in these *loci* show unprecedented statistical support but explain only a minor fraction of BD heritability. However, this is in line with the results of recent studies that provide evidence of a strong polygenic component in BD, suggesting a large number of additional risk *loci*, each mediating a small susceptibility to the disease [26]. In this sense, polygenic risk scores (PRS) that combine the additive effects of many risk alleles can index substantially more genetic risk by including variants that have so far escaped detection of individual genome-wide significance [27]. Recent studies that use the PRS strategy have shown that common variation accounts for about 25% of the total genetic risk for BD (less of the phenotypic variance), that PRS overlap substantially between BD and schizophrenia, and that PRS derived from large schizophrenia samples are associated with increased rates of psychotic symptoms and decreased response to lithium in BD [28].

Data from early GWAS indicated a significant genetic overlap between BD and schizophrenia, but subsequent data have observed significant genetic correlations between BD and MDD [29–31], attention deficit hyperactivity disorder [32], neuroticism [33], and borderline personality disorder [34]. Small but significant genetic correlations have also emerged between BD and educational attainment [15], creativity [35], and leadership [36].

Genetic Basis of MDD

Classical Genetic Epidemiology of MDD

Many studies have reported a significant familial aggregation of MDD [37]. Specifically, offspring of parents with MDD has been shown to present an increased risk for depression with an odds ratio of around 3, with no differences in whether the mother or father was affected [37]. Early twin studies, when analyzed in the aggregate, have estimated the heritability of MDD to be around 30–40% [38,39], which represents a moderate genetic influence with a crucial environmental effect. Overall, these initial reports served as the basis for follow-up investigations of the molecular genetics of MDD.

Linkage Studies in MDD

As MDD is strongly suspected of having polygenic roots, linkage studies have mainly been unfruitful. Between 1998 and 2010, no less than 12 studies with this design were executed without replicable findings [40,41]. Consequently, studies in recent years have largely shifted to GWAS investigations.

Candidate Genes and GWAS Studies in MDD

Initial studies that have tried to identify single candidate genes have failed to pinpoint and replicate individual genes that control the expression of MDD [39,42]. Most research has instead focused on the polygenic nature of MDD through GWAS analyses that simultaneously investigated thousands of single nucleotide variants in large databases of patients and controls. Early GWAS found difficulty reaching the significance threshold in identifying *loci* of interests and SNPs, likely due to their small sample sizes [39]. In particular, the difficulty in identifying the specific genetic factors associated with MDD can be attributed in part to the highly polygenic nature of the disease, meaning that there are multiple contributing genetic factors [43]. Further complicating efforts to identify the genetic regions of interest in MDD is the variability and heterogeneity in phenotypic expression of the disorder, which can vary over the course of an individual's lifetime, as well as vary greatly among identified patients. There is also a strong correlation between MDD and other major psychiatric disorders, including substance abuse disorder, panic disorder, and generalized anxiety [44], which adds an extra layer of complexity to the MDD phenotype and further complicates the efforts to pinpoint its genetic basis.

Across the globe, several major organizations have used increasingly large databases with subjects who have self-reported symptoms of MDD. In 2012, the Major Depressive Working Group of the Psychiatric Genomics Consortium (PGC) published one of the first major GWAS with information from 18,759 individuals by combining several large, previously studied databases. Their analysis discovered 15 *loci* of interest for MDD [45]. In addition, a study published in 2016 by 23andMe included one of the largest databases with 75,607 MDD cases and 231,747 controls, which yielded 17 *loci* of interest [46]. GWAS has gravitated toward increasingly large databases over time, often relying on databases from earlier foundational studies to provide larger pools for meta-analysis.

Consequently, the latest GWAS studies have produced greater numbers of genetic *loci* associated with MDD. In 2018, the PGC published a meta-analysis using 480,359 genetic profiles and found 44 *loci* of significant interest to MDD [47]. A 2018 GWAS with data from 322,580 subjects from the UK Biobank identified 17 independent *loci* of interest to MDD, with 14 of them being novel [48]. Interestingly, a genome-wide by environment interaction study from 2019 identified 2 significant *loci* of relevance in the expression of MDD when exacerbated by a stressful life event, as well as 6 genes associated with depressive symptoms [49]. This same study also revealed shared genetic aetiologies between MDD and schizotypal personality, heart disease, and chronic obstructive pulmonary disorder [49]. Another GWAS published in 2019 by the PGC using data from the UK Biobank drew from a population database of 807,533 individuals to identify 102 independent genetic variants associated with MDD, with 87 being supported as significant in a replicable sample [50]. In an additional analysis of disease and personality traits with genetic roots, 41 of these variants were found to have significant genetic correlations [51]. Finally, a large recent meta-analysis in over 1.2 million subjects identified 178 genomic risk *loci* in MDD [51]. Using a transcriptome-wide association analysis, the authors also found significant associations of MDD with the expression of *NEGR1* in the hypothalamus and *DRD2* in the nucleus accumbens [51] (see Table 17.1). Overall, information provided in these studies and others has allowed researchers to further pursue ideas regarding assessing risk, linking related medical conditions, and providing new information on potential drug therapies for MDD.

Future Directions and Perspectives

The field of psychiatric genetics has seen a dramatic development in the past few years thanks to technical advancements and to a continuing increase in sample sizes under investigation. The ongoing identification of genetic variants underlying BD and MDD has the potential not only to provide a better understanding of their pathophysiology and mechanisms and thereby identify novel and repurposed medications for both conditions but also to lead to the identification of clinically useful genetic markers for early diagnosis, risk assessment, and treatment response. Regarding the latter, the field of pharmacogenetics (and the emerging "pharmacoepigenetics") promises to use genetic variants to aid in the identification of medications with fewer side effects or those with higher probability of response for specific patients, making genetic findings directly applicable to the lives of clinicians and mood disorders patients.

As the field continues to evolve, efforts from research groups worldwide will continue to increase sample sizes through consortia (such as the highly successful PGC) and thereby provide more statistical power for GWAS platforms. In parallel, the field is expected to eventually shift from microarrays to sequencing technologies (whole-exome sequencing and whole-genome sequencing, for instance), as these techniques become more widely available and affordable. This will allow for the interrogation and identification of rare variants thought to significantly contribute to the genetic architecture of mood disorders. In addition, it is expected that more studies incorporate environmental information into their genetic analyses in so-called Genome-Wide Gene-Environment Interaction Analysis so that the contribution of genes by environment interactions can be directly quantified. Overall, although still not fully understood, significant progress has been made in the search for the genetic bases of mood disorders over the past years. The findings hold the potential not only to shed important light in the disorders' pathophysiology, but also to contribute to the clinical care of patients and subjects at high risk.

References

1. M. Bauer, A. Pfennig. Epidemiology of bipolar disorders. *Epilepsia* 2005;**46**:8–13.

2. K. Demyttenaere, R. Bruffaerts, J. Posada-Villa, et al. Prevalence, severity, and unmet need for treatment of mental disorders in the World Health Organization World Mental Health Surveys. *JAMA* 2004;**291**:2581–90.

3. D.F. Levinson. The genetics of depression: a review. *Biol Psychiatry* 2006;**60**:84–92.

4. P. McGuffin, F. Rijsdijk, M. Andrew, et al. The heritability of bipolar affective disorder and the genetic relationship to unipolar depression. *Arch Gen Psychiatry* 2003;**60**:497–502.

5. W.H. Berrettini. Molecular linkage studies of bipolar disorder. *Dialogues Clin Neurosci* 1999;**1**:12–21.

6. F.J. McMahon, P.J Hopkins, J. Xu, et al. Linkage of bipolar affective disorder to chromosome 18 markers

in a new pedigree series. *Am J Hum Genet* 1997;**61**:1397–1404.

7. G. Turecki, P. Grof, P. Cavazzoni, et al. Lithium responsive bipolar disorder, unilineality, and chromosome 18: a linkage study. *Am J Med Genet* 1999;**88**:411–15.

8. N. Craddock, S. Davé, J. Greening. Association studies of bipolar disorder. *Bipolar Disorders* 2001;**3**:284–98.

9. F.J.A. Gordovez, F.J. McMahon. The genetics of bipolar disorder. *Molecular Psychiatry* 2020;**25**:544–59.

10. A.W. Charney, D.M Ruderfer, E.A Stahl, et al. Evidence for genetic heterogeneity between clinical subtypes of bipolar disorder. *Transl Psychiatry* 2017;**7**: e993.

11. K.S. O'Connell, B.J. Coombes. Genetic contributions to bipolar disorder: current status and future directions. *Psycol Med* 2021;**51**:2156–67.

12. P.R. Burton, D.G. Clayton, L.R. Cardon, et al. Genome-wide association study of 14,000 cases of seven common diseases and 3,000 shared controls. *Nature* 2007;**447**:661–78.

13. D.T. Chen, X. Jiang, N. Akula, et al. Genome-wide association study meta-analysis of European and Asian-ancestry samples identifies three novel loci associated with bipolar disorder. *Mol Psychiatry* 2013;**18**:195–205.

14. L. Hou, S.E. Bergen, N. Akula, et al. Genome-wide association study of 40,000 individuals identifies two novel loci associated with bipolar disorder. *Hum Mol Genet* 2016;**25**:3383–94.

15. E.A. Stahl, G. Breen, A.J. Forstner, et al. Genome-wide association study identifies 30 loci associated with bipolar disorder. *Nat Genet* 2019;**51**:793–803.

16. N. Mullins, A.J. Forstner, K.S. O'Connell, et al. Genome-wide association study of more than 40,000 bipolar disorder cases provides new insights into the underlying biology. *Nat Genet.* 2021;**53**(6):817–29.

17. X. Jiang, S.D. Detera-Wadleigh, N. Akula, et al. Sodium valproate rescues expression of TRANK1 in iPSC-derived neural cells that carry a genetic variant associated with serious mental illness. *Mol Psychiatry* 2019;**24**:613–24.

18. J. Lai, J. Jiang, P. Zhang, et al. Impaired blood-brain barrier in the microbiota-gut-brain axis: Potential role of bipolar susceptibility gene *TRANK1*. *J Cell Mol Med* 2021;**00**:jcmm.16611.

19. X. Jiang, S.D. Detera-Wadleigh, N. Akula, et al. Sodium valproate rescues expression of TRANK1 in iPSC-derived neural cells that carry a genetic variant associated with serious mental illness. *Mol Psychiatry* 2019;**24**:613–24.

20. A.E. Baum, N. Akula, M. Cabanero, et al. A genome-wide association study implicates diacylglycerol kinase eta (DGKH) and several other genes in the etiology of bipolar disorder. *Mol Psychiatry* 2008;**13**:197–207.

21. E. Kordeli, S. Lambert, V. Bennett. Ankyrin(G). A new ankyrin gene with neural-specific isoforms localized at the axonal initial segment and node of Ranvier. *J Biol Chem* 1995;**270**:2352–9.

22. M. Maheshwari, J. Shi, J.A. Badner et al. Common and rare variants of DAOA in bipolar disorder. *Am J Med Genet Part B Neuropsychiatr Genet* 2009;**150**:960–966.

23. E.S. Gershon, K. Grennan, J. Busnello, et al. A rare mutation of CACNA1C in a patient with bipolar disorder, and decreased gene expression associated with a bipolar-associated common SNP of CACNA1C in brain. *Mol Psychiatry* 2014;**19**:890–894.

24. P. Sklar, S. Ripke, L.J. Scott, et al. Large-scale genome-wide association analysis of bipolar disorder identifies a new susceptibility locus near ODZ4. *Nat Genet* 2011;**43**:977–85.

25. A. Heinrich, A. Lourdusamy, J. Tzschoppe, et al. The risk variant in ODZ4 for bipolar disorder impacts on amygdala activation during reward processing. *Bipolar Disord* 2013;**15**:440–5.

26. P. Sklar, S. Ripke, L.J. Scott, et al. Large-scale genome-wide association analysis of bipolar disorder identifies a new susceptibility locus near ODZ4. *Nat Genet* 2011;**43**:977–85.

27. S.M. Purcell, N.R. Wray, J.L. Stone, et al. Common polygenic variation contributes to risk of schizophrenia and bipolar disorder. *Nature* 2009;**460**:748–52.

28. D.M. Ruderfer, A.H. Fanous, S. Ripke, et al. Polygenic dissection of diagnosis and clinical dimensions of bipolar disorder and schizophrenia. *Mol Psychiatry* 2014;**19**:1017–24.

29. E.A. Stahl, G. Breen, A.J. Forstner, et al. Genome-wide association study identifies 30 loci associated with bipolar disorder. *Nat Genet* 2019;**51**:793–803.

30. C.M. Middeldorp, M.H.M. De Moor, L.M. McGrath, et al. The genetic association between personality and major depression or bipolar disorder. A polygenic score analysis using genome-wide association data. *Transl Psychiatry* 2011;**1**:e50.

31. J. Huang, R.H. Perlis, P.H. Lee, et al. Cross-disorder genomewide analysis of schizophrenia, bipolar disorder, and depression. *Am J Psychiatry* 2010;**167**:1254–63.

32. H. Weber, S. Kittel-Schneider, A. Gessner, et al. Cross-disorder analysis of bipolar risk genes: further

evidence of dGKH as a risk gene for bipolar disorder, but also unipolar depression and adult ADHD. *Neuropsychopharmacology* 2011;**36**:2076–85.

33. H.E. O'Brien, E. Hannon, M.J. Hill, et al. Expression quantitative trait loci in the developing human brain and their enrichment in neuropsychiatric disorders. *Genome Biol* 2018;**19**:194.

34. S.H. Witt, F. Streit, M. Jungkunz, et al. Genome-wide association study of borderline personality disorder reveals genetic overlap with bipolar disorder, major depression and schizophrenia. *Transl Psychiatry* 2017;**7**:e1155.

35. R.A. Power, S. Steinberg, G. Bjornsdottir, et al. Polygenic risk scores for schizophrenia and bipolar disorder predict creativity. *Nat Neurosci* 2015;**18**:953–5.

36. S. Kyaga, P. Lichtenstein, M. Boman, et al. Bipolar disorder and leadership – a total population study. *Acta Psychiatr Scand* 2015;**131**:111–19.

37. R. Lieb, B. Isensee, M. Höfler, et al. Parental major depression and the risk of depression and other mental disorders in offspring: a prospective-longitudinal community study. *Arch Gen Psychiatry* 2002;**59**:365–74.

38. P.F. Sullivan, M.C. Neale, K.S. Kendler. Genetic epidemiology of major depression: Review and meta-analysis. *Am J Psychiatry* 2000;**157**:1552–62.

39. N. Mullins, C.M. Lewis. Genetics of depression: progress at last. *Curr Psychiatry Rep* 2017;**19**:43.

40. A.M. McIntosh, P.F. Sullivan, C.M. Lewis. Uncovering the genetic architecture of major depression. *Neuron* 2019;**102**:91–103.

41. R. Border, E.C. Johnson, L.M. Evans, et al. No support for historical candidate gene or candidate gene-by-interaction hypotheses for major depression across multiple large samples. *Am J Psychiatry* 2019;**176**:376–87

42. P. Unal-Aydin, O. Aydin, A. Arslan. Genetic architecture of depression: where do we stand now? *Adv Exp Med Biol* 2021;**1305**:203–30.

43. N.R. Wray, S.H. Lee, D. Mehta, et al. Research review: polygenic methods and their application to psychiatric traits. *J Child Psychol Psychiatry* 2014;**55**:1068–87.

44. D.S. Hasin, R.D. Goodwin, F.S. Stinson, et al. Epidemiology of major depressive disorder: results from the National Epidemiologic Survey on Alcoholism and Related Conditions. *Arch Gen Psychiatry* 2005;**62**:1097–1106.

45. P.F. Sullivan, M.J. Daly, S. Ripke, et al. A mega-analysis of genome-wide association studies for major depressive disorder. *Mol Psychiatry* 2013;**18**:497–511.

46. C.L. Hyde, M.W. Nagle, C. Tian, et al. Identification of 15 genetic loci associated with risk of major depression in individuals of European descent. *Nat Genet* 2016;**48**:1031–6.

47. N.R. Wray, S. Ripke, M. Mattheisen, et al. Genome-wide association analyses identify 44 risk variants and refine the genetic architecture of major depression. *Nat Genet* 2018;**50**:668–81.

48. D.M. Howard, M.J. Adams, M. Shirali, et al. Genome-wide association study of depression phenotypes in UK Biobank identifies variants in excitatory synaptic pathways. *Nat Commun* 2018;**9**:1470.

49. A. Arnau-Soler, E. Macdonald-Dunlop, M.J. Adams, et al. Genome-wide by environment interaction studies of depressive symptoms and psychosocial stress in UK Biobank and Generation Scotland. *Transl Psychiatry* 2019;**9**:14.

50. D.M. Howard, M.J. Adams, T.K. Clarke, et al. Genome-wide meta-analysis of depression identifies 102 independent variants and highlights the importance of the prefrontal brain regions. *Nat Neurosci* 2019;**22**:343–52.

51. D.F. Levey, M.B. Stein, F.R. Wendt, et al. Bi-ancestral depression GWAS in the Million Veteran Program and meta-analysis in >1.2 million individuals highlight new therapeutic directions. *Nat Neurosci* 2021;**24**(7):954–63.

Chapter 18

Management of Major Depressive Disorder: Basic Principles

Danilo Arnone, Vaishali Tirumalaraju, and Sudhakar Selvaraj

Initial Workup

Arriving at a Diagnosis

Symptoms of depression consist of a persistent feeling of sadness, called 'dysphoria', which is the cardinal psychological manifestation of this condition. Other psychological manifestations include 'lack of interest in previously enjoyed activities', called 'anhedonia', and a pervasive sense of helplessness and hopelessness for the current situation and often the past and the future. Negative cognitions regarding the self and others are often prevalent. These are not factual beliefs and appear disproportionate to the actual state of affairs. There is frequently an accompanying strong sense of guilt, which encompasses the presentation. More often than not, the affected person feels unjustifiably inadequate and unnecessarily responsible for the lived situation and their inability to exit it. It is not unusual that the individual is unable to consider alternative options so that that thinking can become circular and ruminative. A spiral of negative thinking is a risk factor for suicide. Cognitively, individuals with depression find it difficult to concentrate on tasks, especially if demanding, and make decisions promptly [1].

Somatic manifestations of depression include disturbance of sleep and appetite, decreased energy level, and inability to start and/or complete tasks. The most common sleep disturbance in depression is 'insomnia', or lack of sleep. Difficulties at the beginning of sleep (initial insomnia), in maintaining sleep (middle insomnia), and in waking up early in the morning (late insomnia or early morning wakening) are the commonest documented sleep problems in up to 75% of the cases. The proportion of depressed individuals experiencing 'hypersomnia', or excessive sleep, as sleep disturbance is less frequent overall and commoner in younger individuals (40% under 30) and women of any age. Hypersomnia constitutes a feature of atypical depression [1,2].

Depression may also manifest as decreased interest in food with concomitant weight loss or 'hypophagia'. The opposite presentation, or 'hyperphagia', often accompanied by weight gain, is associated with atypical depression with 15% and 29% at a 1-year prevalence [3]. Most people with depression feel fatigued to the point that they cannot carry out day-to-day activities and look after dependents. Psychomotor disturbance is another feature typically associated with depression and presents as either psychomotor agitation or retardation. Psychomotor agitation is characterized by unintentional, repetitive motor activity resulting in inner restlessness/tension and behaviours such as pacing and fidgeting. Psychomotor retardation instead involves reduced body movements with a concomitant reduction in thinking and speech output, which results in the inability to carry out actions to the point of no motor activity and mutism [4]. Both the *International Classification of Mental and Behavioural Disorders*, 10th edition (ICD-10) and the *Diagnostic and Statistical Manual of Mental Disorders*, 5th edition (DSM-5) allow identification of depressive episodes or major depressive disorder (MDD) [5,6]. The ICD-10 requires the presence of three core symptoms of depression, including low mood, anhedonia, and decreased energy level for a minimum of 2 weeks [5]. The DSM-5/DSM-IV requires the identification of five key symptoms present for 2 weeks, emphasizing significant distress/impairment in social or occupational functioning [6,7].

Differential Diagnosis and Investigations

It is important to ensure that the diagnosis of major depression is a primary mood disorder. The first diagnostic step is to exclude the possibility that symptoms originate from a medical condition or medical treatment. This is generally established by exclusion. Conditions that present with symptoms resembling depression include brain disorders (space-occupying lesions, trauma, cerebrovascular events, multiple sclerosis, Parkinson's disease, normal pressure hydrocephalus, epilepsy, Huntington's disease), cardiovascular disease, cancer and paraneoplastic syndromes, endocrine disorders (hypothyroidism, hyperthyroidism, hypoparathyroidism, hyperparathyroidism), vitamin deficiencies (e.g., D, B3), autoimmune conditions (e.g., rheumatoid arthritis, systemic lupus erythematosus), genetic disorders (e.g., Wilson's disease), sexually transmitted diseases (e.g., HIV/AIDS, syphilis), infectious diseases, and metabolic disorders (e.g., porphyria, diabetes) [1]. Depressive symptoms are, however, commonly comorbid with medical conditions. In outpatient settings, including primary care, the percentage of diagnosed cases reaches 52.8% [8]. However, research suggests that depression can either be overlooked if the focus is centred on the physical presentation or over-diagnosed, so a longitudinal approach is recommended to improve diagnostic specificity [9]. Including case-finding or screening instruments for depression in non-mental health settings can facilitate symptom recognition [10].

Many functional disorders can present with symptoms resembling major depression. Commonly, the duration of the symptoms and course, along with premorbid personality and family history, can help to discriminate [1]. It is challenging to distinguish psychotic depression from schizophrenia / schizoaffective disorder when psychotic symptoms are mood congruent [1]. Another difficult discrimination is depression from cognitive impairment, particularly in older adults. In this situation, aside from important information emerging from the history, resolution of cognitive problems often follows once the depressive syndrome is treated [1]. A range of substances, including prescribed medications, illegal substances, and toxins, can mimic significant depression [1]. In the case of illegal substances, depressive symptoms can become evident due to acute intoxication or during the withdrawal phase. It is essential to allow detoxification prior to establishing evidence of a mood disorder independent from the triggering substance. Known substances of abuse include alcohol, phencyclidine and other hallucinogens, inhalants, opioids, sedative/hypnotic/anxiolytic medications, and amphetamine and other stimulants, including cocaine [1,6]. Different from the DSM-IV, the DSM-5 recognizes that bereavement can trigger a depressive episode [11]. Most bereavement reactions would not meet the criteria for a depressive episode and the intense emotional pain is centred on the preoccupation with the deceased or the circumstances of the death. The DSM-5 recognizes the possibility that a grief reaction might become pathological when there is no resolution of the symptoms beyond 12 months [1,6].

In the absence of diagnostic tests for major depression, all the investigations are conducted to exclude the possibility that biological abnormalities explain depressive symptoms or co-occur with them. Routine blood tests most commonly include full blood count (anaemia, infection, and inflammatory conditions), urine and electrolytes (primary/secondary renal diseases, metabolic disorders, electrolytes imbalances, and others), liver function tests (hepatic disorders), thyroid function tests (hypo/hyperthyroidism), glucose measurements including HbA1c (diabetes), and HIV/VDRL tests (sexually transmitted diseases). Urinalysis is generally carried out to exclude the presence of substances of abuse as part of the differential diagnosis workup [1]. It is also useful to organize a chest X-ray to identify respiratory abnormalities and an electrocardiogram (ECG) to exclude an abnormal heart rhythm while measuring the QTc interval. It is also useful to evaluate weight and height (and calculate the body mass index [BMI]) and a waistline measure. Some of these tests offer important baseline values prior to the commencement of treatment, contribute to profile patients for potential metabolic risk factors, and are routinely monitored as part of medication side effects surveillance (e.g., QTc interval, metabolic parameters). There may be a clinical indication for neuroimaging, including a magnetic resonance imaging (MRI) scan of the brain and electrophysiology [1].

Functional Evaluation

Depression affects several domains of function, including social and family life and occupational and leisurely activities. Symptoms of depression are the source of functional impairment, which can be relatively mild or to a level of complete functional incapacity with an inability to attend to basic self-care needs such as mutism or catatonia [6]. Evidence suggests that functional impairment is present in up to 97% of patients with major depression over a 12-month observational period, with the number of days affected proportionally to the severity of the impairment [12,13]. The level of functional impairment is proportional to the severity of the depressive symptoms [13].

Several rating scales, clinician- or patient-rated, can assess functionality and evaluate a specific domain or global function [13]. A well-known clinician rating scale is the 'Global Assessment of Functioning', which combines symptom severity and functional impairment in a single score [12]. Among the most used self-rated questionnaires are the 'Sheehan Disability Scale', investigating several functional domains [14], and the 'Quality of Life Enjoyment and Satisfaction Questionnaire', assessing satisfaction with daily life [12,15].

Functional outcomes generally improve with depressive symptoms, although the relationship with symptom severity does not appear linear and is negatively affected by partial response. For example, cognitive deficits, consistently described in major depression, do not appear to fully recover with treatment and have a relationship with the number of episodes [16]. Affected cognitive domains include memory, executive function, processing speed, attention, and concentration [16]. Overall, functional improvement appears more favourable for those patients who respond within the first 2 weeks of treatment [13].

Therapeutic Alliance: Discussion, Education, and Collaborative Decision-Making

Shared decisions can improve decision-making quality for patients with major depression and illness self-management with positive health outcomes [17]. Evidence shows that involving patients in making decisions increases patients' participation in their own care and greater treatment satisfaction. Although research remains inconclusive regarding the direct effect of this type of intervention on depression severity [18], there is evidence for improved adherence to treatment [19,20] with no extra consultation time [18].

Risk Management and Safety

Depressed individuals often experience thoughts that 'life is not worth living'. Suicidal thoughts can progress into suicidal ideation and planning. According to a large survey in the United States, up to 26.3% of individuals with depression experienced suicidal ideation in the previous year [21]. Global suicide rates are around 1.4%, equivalent to 10.7 per 100,000 population (male-to-female [M:F] ratio = 1.7) [22,23]. Approximately 50% of the completed suicides are associated with major depression. Although the highest suicide rates are in adolescents and young adults between 15 and 29 years of age, elderly depressed individuals are overall more likely to complete suicide, particularly in cases of severe depression with psychotic symptoms [22]. Suicide risk is best managed longitudinally as fluctuations in risk level are common and influenced by several risk and protective factors. Risk factors positively associated with suicide include young age, widowed/divorced, male sex, low income, low education, unemployment, inequality, low social support, change in individual social or economic circumstances (e.g., level of urbanization, income, housing, and others), inadequate housing, overcrowding, violence, family history of psychiatric disorders, previously attempted suicides, severe depression, hopelessness, comorbid disorders including anxiety, and misuse of alcohol and drugs [22,24]. Some of these factors are influenced by geographical location and ethnicity, which might explain why 78% of suicides globally originate from low- and middle-income countries [22]. Some of the known protective factors against suicide include fear of suicide itself and moral objections, family responsibilities, social disapproval, and effective coping skills [22,25].

Primary prevention strategies include reducing access to lethal suicide methods. Information, education, awareness programmes, helplines, support centres, and support lines can help to reduce stigma and identify predisposing factors and early warning signs, which can encourage help-seeking behaviours, thereby reducing the chance of escalation. It is essential that healthcare professionals screen for suicide risk at any given opportunity, as it is not unusual that individuals who complete suicide consult healthcare professionals prior to attempting suicide [22,26,27]. Secondary prevention applies to patients at high risk of attempting suicide and involves primary healthcare professionals [28]. In this context, a systematic and inclusive approach to risk assessment and minimization is essential and is formulated to offer tailored plans to reduce risk factors and promote protective factors [22]. Escalation in risk of suicide cannot be contained by referring to resources available within the affected individuals, and their proximity requires admission to psychiatric inpatients [29].

Multidisciplinary Framework

Care delivery for patients with major depression is often provided as part of a comprehensive, holistic care plan delivered in a multidisciplinary framework. A typical multidisciplinary team often consists of professionals with complementary skills and knowledge and includes a psychiatrist, psychiatric nurse, psychologist, social worker, and occupational therapist [30]. This approach's described benefits include improved service contact after discharge from the hospital, patients' and carers' agreeability [31], and lower admission rates [32].

Treatment

Treatment strategies for MDD are primarily guided by the severity, risks, and chronicity of presenting symptoms, which can be broadly categorized into the following phases:

- Acute phase
- Continuation phase
- Maintenance phase

Acute Phase

Major depressive disorder (MDD) in the acute phase can be broadly categorized into mild, moderate, and severe types based on the severity of symptoms. Although this categorization is non-encompassing of other variables such as duration and course of illness [33], it continues to be widely used in several guidelines as the approach to treatment [34]. Most mild to moderate depression could be treated in the outpatient setting unless complicated by other factors such as the high risk of suicide, psychosis, and severe impairment of functioning. The estimated lifetime risk of suicide in affective disorders treated in the outpatient setting is about 2.2%, and that in hospitalized patients is about 4% [35]. Furthermore, recent studies with long-term follow-up indicate that the absolute suicide risk in hospitalized MDD patients may be almost 7% in males and about 4% in females [36]. This risk can further increase in the presence of comorbid anxiety [37], cluster B traits [38], psychosis [39], substance use [40], prior suicide attempts, and other demographic factors [40]. Therefore, it is crucial to assess and address various risks factors at every stage to guide the appropriate setting for treatment.

The widely accepted goal of initial treatment in the acute phase is achieving remission, defined as the resolution of depressive symptoms and the return of baseline premorbid functioning [41,42]. There are several validated depression rating scales, but many clinical studies utilize the 17-item Hamilton Rating Scale for Depression (HAMD-17), the Montgomery–Asberg Depression Rating Scale (MDRS), and the Patient Health Questionnaire – Nine Items (PHQ-9), with scores ≤ 7 in the former two and scores ≤ 5 in the latter serving as indicators of remission [43–45]. Furthermore, studies indicate that measurement-based treatment approaches may improve clinical outcomes by improving treatment adherence [46,47]. The most studied treatment modalities in the acute phase are pharmacotherapy and psychotherapy. While practice guidelines from the UK National Institute for Health and Care Excellence (NICE) recommend starting with psychotherapy [48] in the initial treatment of mild depression, those of the American Psychiatric Association (APA) suggest both pharmacotherapy and psychotherapy as acceptable initial interventions for mild to moderate depression [41]. Although there is no evidence of the superiority over the other [49,50], growing evidence from newer meta-analyses suggests that a combination of both pharmacotherapy and psychotherapy may be more effective than stand-alone treatments with either [51–53]. Other therapies such as electroconvulsive therapy (ECT), transcranial magnetic stimulation (TMS), vagus nerve stimulation (VNS), and light therapy can also be considered in the acute phase. However, the ultimate choice of treatment depends on multiple factors such as age, severity of presenting symptoms, adverse effect profiles, comorbid medical and psychiatric illnesses, ease of use, cost, and patient preference [41,54].

Pharmacological Approach

Antidepressants have proven efficacy, at least in the treatment of moderate and severe depression [55]. Commonly used antidepressants can be broadly classified into selective serotonin reuptake inhibitors (SSRIs), serotonin-norepinephrine reuptake inhibitors (SNRIs), serotonin modulators, atypical antidepressants, tricyclic antidepressants (TCAs), and monoamine oxidase inhibitors (MAOIs). SSRIs appear to be first line and are the most prescribed class of antidepressants for initial treatment [56] based upon their efficacy and tolerability in randomized trials [57]. Although SNRIs, atypical antidepressants (bupropion, mirtazapine, and agomelatine), and serotonin modulators (vilazodone, trazodone, vortioxetine, and others) are reasonable alternatives. Meta-analyses of placebo-controlled studies between specific antidepressants, in the same and different antidepressant classes, demonstrate comparable efficacy in inducing remission in patients with MDD regardless of the severity of symptoms [58,59]. Older antidepressants such as TCAs and MAOIs have established efficacies in treating depression but are less widely prescribed due to safety and tolerability concerns and are usually reserved for patients who do not respond to other treatments as second-line and third-line agents, respectively [60,61]. Among the SSRIs, some studies suggest that sertraline and escitalopram appear to be more efficacious, are better tolerated, and lead to less frequent discontinuation than others in their class [55]. However, this was not replicated in another study [58,59]. Mirtazapine was deemed to have a considerably faster onset of antidepressive effects in the same meta-analyses [58,59]. However, it must be noted that all the randomized controlled trials (RCTs) included were funded by the drug manufacturing company and, in a head-to-head comparison, showed similar response rates as other antidepressants after 4 weeks.

Overall, the efficacy of antidepressants is comparable both across and within specific classes of antidepressants [62–65]. Thus, factors such as tolerability profiles, anticipated side effects, drug–drug interactions, medical comorbidities, cost, initial response, and family history play an active role in selecting the appropriate antidepressant for a patient. Regardless of the initial choice of treatment, patients must be closely monitored to assess medication response and the emergence of side effects after the treatment. Most practice guidelines suggest at least 6 to 12 weeks as an adequate trial to gauge the full effects of treatment [41,66,67]. However, studies indicate that patients can start showing a response as early as 1–2 weeks of initiation of antidepressants [68,69], and early improvement seems to be a good prognostic indicator for eventual remission [70–72]. It is, therefore, reasonable to consider a change in treatment (e.g., modifying medication dosage or switching to different antidepressants) for patients who show slight improvement after 4 to 6 weeks and even earlier if emerging side effects are a concern [73–75]. Some of the most typical side effects amongst the newer second-generation antidepressants include gastrointestinal distress, insomnia, sedation, sexual dysfunction, weight changes, and, less commonly, cardiovascular effects, anticholinergic effects, hyponatraemia, and serotonin syndrome [58]. Specific antidepressants have more propensity to induce some of the side effects than others. For example, diarrhoea is

a common side effect with sertraline, and somnolence is more notable with trazodone, weight gain more significant with mirtazapine, sexual dysfunction is more common with paroxetine and least common with bupropion, and nausea and vomiting are more problematic with venlafaxine and other medications [58]. To mitigate the emergence of side effects and improve patient adherence, most guidelines suggest starting the antidepressant at the lowest recommended dose and then titrating upwards to the total therapeutic dose depending on age, psychiatric and medical comorbidities, drug–drug interactions, and patient tolerability [41,48,76]. If side effects do occur, reducing the dose of the antidepressant or switching to a different antidepressant that is not associated with the side effect should be considered.

In severe depression complicated by psychosis or a high risk of suicide, pharmaco-therapeutic augmenting strategies can be utilized. In depressed patients with psychosis, the addition of a second-generation antipsychotic as initial treatment has demonstrable efficacy and is recommended consistently by multiple guidelines [77,78]. No head-to-head trials comparing specific combinations exist, and thus it is reasonable to start any second-generation antipsychotic, keeping in mind side effects, drug interactions, and tolerability profiles. In patients refractory to combination therapy with antipsychotics or ECT [79,80] (discussed further below), lithium augmentation can also be considered [81,82]. In the case of acute suicidality associated with severe depression, ketamine is the only pharmacological agent that appears to demonstrate immediate effects mitigating suicide. The US Food and Drug Administration approved the use of intranasal esketamine and antidepressant combination to treat acute depression with suicidal behaviour [83]. Lithium can also be considered for acute suicidality; however, its benefits seem more apparent with long-term therapy and the prevention of further suicide attempts [84].

Psychotherapeutic Approach

Various forms of depression-focused psychotherapy, particularly cognitive behavioural therapy (CBT) and interpersonal therapy (IPT), have been widely studied in many meta-analyses and deemed an efficacious treatment choice for depression [85–87]. Psychotherapy has been found to have comparable efficacy to pharmacotherapy [88] and appears to have persisting benefits even after discontinuation, potentially prolonging remission times [89]. Thus, a combination of pharmacotherapy and psychotherapy can be a useful intervention strategy in treating depression. Moreover, guidelines from the APA and the UK NICE recommend stand-alone treatment with psychotherapy, particularly in cases of mild to moderate depression and in conjunction with pharmacotherapy in cases of moderate to severe depression, mild cases with major interpersonal and psychosocial problems as well as comorbid Axis 2 diagnoses [48].

Some of the most effective psychotherapy modalities to treat depression include CBT, IPT, problem-solving therapy, supportive psychotherapy, couples and family therapy, and psychodynamic psychotherapy. CBT and IPT are more widely available and hence studied and chosen as treatment options more often. No statistically significant findings suggest any one choice of psychotherapy is better than the other [90,91]. Selecting specific psychotherapy depends on patient preference, cost, availability, initial response, perceived goals of treatment, and others. Like in the case of pharmacotherapy, after the choice of psychological intervention is made, it is important to monitor patients regularly to gauge treatment response and safety. NICE guidelines recommend initial intervention with 16–20 sessions of CBT or IPT over 3–4 months (with two additional sessions per week during the first 2–3 weeks in cases of moderate-severe depression) along with three to four follow-up sessions in the following 3 to 6 months [48].

Psychotherapy can also be considered as an adjunctive treatment for complicated severe depression with associated psychosis [92,93] or increased suicidal and self-harm behaviours [94,95]. Although not first line, specific psychotherapies such as acceptance and commitment therapy have demonstrated added benefit in patients with psychotic depression [92]. CBT and problem-solving psychotherapy have shown some efficacy in reducing suicidal and self-harm behaviours [95].

Other Therapies

Electroconvulsive therapy (ECT) is a reasonable alternative to the interventions mentioned above in treating patients with severe MDD, particularly in patients with suicidal ideations, severe functional impairment, including associated psychosis and catatonia, documented prior response, and treatment-resistant depression [79,80]. Although relatively safe with a faster onset of action, it does have its limitations in terms of availability, patient preference, tolerability

profile, and increased relapse rates on discontinuation [96]. Another emerging alternative treatment option in treating acute depression, specifically after the failure of antidepressant therapy, is repetitive transcranial magnetic stimulation (TMS) with multiple meta-analyses demonstrating its efficacy compared to placebo [97,98]. TMS added as an adjunct or simultaneously with pharmacotherapy might have superior efficacy than antidepressants alone [99]. However, ECT has demonstrably superior efficacy compared to TMS in the treatment of depression [100].

In patients with seasonal affective disorder, artificial light therapy that includes bright light therapy, dawn simulation, or both are first line [101,102]. Invasive surgical approaches for the treatment of depression are generally the very last resort, with vagus nerve stimulation (VNS) [103] and ablative neurosurgery being currently clinically available [104]. Newer approaches such as deep brain stimulation are still in the investigative stage.

Augmentation Strategies

Some guidelines recommend a trial of augmenting interventions, particularly in cases of inadequate response to initial treatment [41,105]. These include add-on therapy with a second antidepressant, second-generation antipsychotics, lithium, thyroid hormone, and psychotherapy modalities such as cognitive behavioural therapy [48,106]. There is limited evidence but growing interest in the use of adjunct stimulants such as modafinil, methylphenidate, and pramipexole [107,108], particularly in the elderly population [109]. Other options with limited evidence include anticonvulsants [106], relaxation techniques [110], physical exercise [111], and nutritional supplementation with omega-3 fatty acids [112] and folate [113]. It may also be beneficial to treat comorbid anxiety and insomnia with selective gamma-aminobutyric acid (GABA) agonists, buspirone, or a short-term course of benzodiazepines [114]. ECT and TMS may also be considered as an add-on to improve response to first- and second-line treatment options.

Special Considerations

Elderly Patients: First-line treatment of depression in this population includes psychotherapy and pharmacotherapy, either singly or in combination [115]. Although antidepressant treatment is efficacious in treating elderly depression, it is not as robust as in the younger population and has comparable efficacy within and across different antidepressant classes [116,117]. Poor tolerability and higher withdrawal rates are seen with TCAs compared to second-generation antidepressants like SSRIs, which remain first line [118]. Some SNRIs such as venlafaxine and duloxetine have shown utility, particularly in patients with concomitant neuropathic pain. Mirtazapine may also be helpful in patients with insomnia, agitation, and anorexia [119]. Some of the main concerns in this population include decreased drug clearance ability, drug–drug interactions, poorer physical health with medical comorbidities, increased propensity for non-adherence, and higher relapse rates. Therefore, it is recommended to start medication at lower doses, stick to monotherapy, closely monitor for side effects, and consider long-term maintenance therapy in this patient population. Psychotherapy appears to be quite beneficial [120], although psychiatric services are grossly underutilized in this population either secondary to lack of insurance coverage, poor availability of services, or logistics. Augmentation strategies such as adding adjunctive lithium [121] or second-generation antipsychotics like aripiprazole [122] or quetiapine [123] can be used but with caution in treatment-resistant patients. ECT is a viable option in elderly patients with treatment-resistant depression.

Pregnancy: The initial treatment choices for mild-moderate cases of antenatal MDD largely depend on patient preference. Antidepressants and psychotherapy are reasonable alternatives, with some evidence that starting antidepressant treatment with SSRIs in mothers with prior history of depression may be more beneficial [124]. In cases of severe depression, most guidelines, including the American Psychiatric Association [41], American College of Obstetricians and Gynecologists [125], and the UK National Institute for Health and Care Excellence [48], recommend that the benefits of antidepressants outweigh the potential risks. However, psychotherapeutic interventions like CBT and IPT can be reasonable alternatives if the patient chooses or has a history of poor prior response to antidepressants. A combination of both treatments may improve clinical outcomes.

It is important to consider potential maternal and fetal adverse effects, plans regarding breastfeeding, prior response to specific interventions, comorbidities, and potential drug interactions when choosing an antidepressant in pregnant women [126]. Patients who have been successfully treated with an antidepressant before pregnancy can continue to receive the same during pregnancy [127]. In anti-depressant naïve patients, sertraline, citalopram, and escitalopram are reasonable choices with little to no risk of teratogenicity amongst the SSRIs [128]. Although fluoxetine is relatively safe, it is not first line owing to its pharmacokinetics, which may cause accumulation in breastfeeding infants. Paroxetine may be associated with a small absolute risk of congenital cardiac defects and thus should be avoided [128,129]. Dosing should be optimized in patients who do not respond adequately to initial treatment before switching to a different SSRI. If a patient fails multiple SSRI trials, it is reasonable to consider an SNRI such as venlafaxine [130]. In treatment-refractory cases, antidepressants such as duloxetine, bupropion, and mirtazapine may be tried, or procedures like TMS and ECT can be considered [131]. Additionally, ECT can supersede multiple medication trials if symptoms include suicidality, functional impairment, and psychosis or catatonia.

Children and Adolescents: Most guidelines recommend avoiding antidepressants and taking the psychotherapy route, such as individual and group CBT and IPT in paediatric cases of mild depression [132]. In the case of moderate-severe depression, psychotherapy continues to remain first line, followed by antidepressant trial if the response is inadequate; however, a reasonable alternative could be combination therapy with antidepressants and psychotherapy. Amongst antidepressants, fluoxetine is the first choice and has the most evidence of efficacy in this population [133]. Patients who do not respond to fluoxetine, sertraline, escitalopram, and citalopram are reasonable options [134]. Antidepressant therapy should be carefully monitored in the paediatric population and should be continued for at least 6 months once remission is achieved with discontinuation over 6–12 weeks to avoid withdrawal syndromes [135]. ECT is reserved for adolescents with intractable severe depression that did not respond to other treatments and otherwise life-threatening behaviours.

Continuation Phase

The main goal of treatment in this phase is to prolong remission and prevent relapse [41]. MDD is a highly recurrent illness, with some meta-analyses estimating that the recurrence rate over 2 years is over 40% and that the risk of recurrence increases by about 16% with each subsequent episode [136]. Studies indicate that a combination of psychotherapy such as CBT or IPT and pharmacotherapy has better outcomes than monotherapy in sustaining remission [137,138]. If remission was achieved with antidepressant treatment alone, the exact dosages used in the acute phase to attain remission are continued in this phase for 4–9 months [139]. It is important to monitor for emerging side effects and signs of relapse carefully. In patients who have remitted on ECT in the acute phase, continuation ECT is administered at an interval of 1–8 weeks for 6 months [140]. Alternatively, ECT plus pharmacotherapy could be considered. Long-term effects might be limited for patients who responded to TMS and would benefit from continuation treatment with pharmacotherapy or pharmacotherapy plus psychotherapy [141]. In the case of MDD complicated by psychosis and requiring antipsychotic medications in addition to antidepressants, studies suggest that it is reasonable to discontinue the antipsychotic after 4 months [142] but imperative to continue antidepressants for long-term maintenance. Continuation and later maintenance treatment with lithium have compelling evidence of utility in preventing suicide associated with depression [143,144]. Studies suggest that physical exercise may help sustain remission for more extended periods, thereby improving prognosis [145].

Maintenance Phase

Patients with recurrent MDD, higher risk of relapse, prior complicated depressive episodes, residual depressive symptoms after remission, persisting psychosocial stressors, and co-occurring disorders are recommended to continue with maintenance therapy for 1–3 years or sometimes indefinitely after the continuation phase [41,42]. As in the case of the continuation phase, the modalities of treatment that helped induce and maintain remission usually continue during the maintenance phase. This includes antidepressant therapy at full therapeutic doses and psychotherapy with reduced frequency of sessions or a combination of both. Maintenance ECT, VNS, and TMS treatments are recommended for patients who responded in the acute and continuation phases. Maintenance treatment should be evaluated periodically with regular follow-ups during this phase, and patients should be educated on the dangers of sudden discontinuation. If a discontinuation decision is made, it is recommended to do so gradually over weeks [41].

References

1. Friedman ES, Anderson IM. *Handbook of Depression*. Tarporley: Springer Healthcare Ltd., 2009. Available from: http://link.springer.com/10.1007/978-1-907673-24-5

2. Nutt D, Wilson S, Paterson L. Sleep disorders as core symptoms of depression. *Dialogues Clin Neurosci*. 2008;**10**(3):329–36.

3. Thase ME. Recognition and diagnosis of atypical depression. *J Clin Psychiatry*. 2007;**68**(Suppl 8):11–16.

4. Sobin C, Sackeim HA. Psychomotor symptoms of depression. *Am J Psychiatry*. 1997 Jan;**154**(1):4–17.

5. *International Statistical Classification of Diseases and Related Health Problems. 3: Alphabetical Index*. 2nd. ed. Geneva: World Health Organization, 2004; 808 p.

6. American Psychiatric Association. *Diagnostic and Statistical Manual of Mental Disorders: DSM-5*. 5th ed. Washington, DC: American Psychiatric Association, 2013.

7. Montgomery S. Are the ICD-10 or DSM-5 diagnostic systems able to define those who will benefit from treatment for depression? *CNS Spectr*. 2016 Aug;**21**(4):283–8.

8. Yates WR, Mitchell J, Rush AJ, et al. Clinical features of depressed outpatients with and without co-occurring general medical conditions in STAR*D. *Gen Hosp Psychiatry*. 2004 Dec;**26**(6):421–9.

9. Mitchell AJ, Vaze A, Rao S. Clinical diagnosis of depression in primary care: a meta-analysis. *Lancet*. 2009 Aug 22;**374**(9690):609–19.

10. Gilbody S, Sheldon T, House A. Screening and case-finding instruments for depression: a meta-analysis. *Can Med Ass J*. 2008 Apr 8;**178**(8):997–1003.

11. Murray Parkes C. Complicated grief in the DSM-5: problems and solutions. *Arch Psychiatr Ment Health*. 2020 Jun 1;**4**(1):048–051.

12. Sheehan DV, Nakagome K, Asami Y, Pappadopulos EA, Boucher M. Restoring function in major depressive disorder: a systematic review. *J Affect Disord*. 2017 Jun;**215**:299–313.

13. Kessler RC, Berglund P, Demler O, et al. The epidemiology of major depressive disorder: results from the National Comorbidity Survey Replication (NCS-R). *JAMA*. 2003 Jun 18;**289**(23):3095.

14. Sheehan KH, Sheehan DV. Assessing treatment effects in clinical trials with the Discan metric of the Sheehan Disability Scale. *Int Clin Psychopharmacol*. 2008 Mar;**23**(2):70–83.

15. Endicott J, Nee J, Harrison W, Blumenthal R. Quality of Life Enjoyment and Satisfaction Questionnaire: a

new measure. *Psychopharmacol Bull.* 1993;**29**(2):321–6.

16. Pan Z, Park C, Brietzke E, et al. Cognitive impairment in major depressive disorder. *CNS Spectr.* 2019 Feb;**24**(1):22–9.

17. Drake RE, Cimpean D, Torrey WC. Shared decision making in mental health: prospects for personalized medicine. *Dialogues Clin Neurosci.* 2009;**11**(4):455–63.

18. Loh A, Simon D, Wills CE, et al. The effects of a shared decision-making intervention in primary care of depression: a cluster-randomized controlled trial. *Patient Educ Couns.* 2007 Aug;**67**(3):324–32.

19. Thompson L, McCabe R. The effect of clinician-patient alliance and communication on treatment adherence in mental health care: a systematic review. *BMC Psychiatry.* 2012 Dec;**12**(1):87.

20. Hopwood M. the shared decision-making process in the pharmacological management of depression. *Patient.* 2020 Feb;**13**(1):23–30.

21. Han B, McKeon R, Gfroerer J. Suicidal ideation among community-dwelling adults in the United States. *Am J Public Health.* 2014 Mar;**104**(3):488–97.

22. Bachmann S. Epidemiology of suicide and the psychiatric perspective. *Int J Environ Res Public Health.* 2018 Jul 6;**15**(7):E1425.

23. Värnik P. Suicide in the World. *IJERPH.* 2012 Mar 2;**9**(3):760–71.

24. Hawton K, Casañas i Comabella C, Haw C, Saunders K. Risk factors for suicide in individuals with depression: a systematic review. *J Affect Disord.* 2013 May;**147**(1–3):17–28.

25. Malone KM, Oquendo MA, Haas GL, et al. Protective factors against suicidal acts in major depression: reasons for living. *AJP.* 2000 Jul;**157**(7):1084–8.

26. Pirkis J, Burgess P. Suicide and recency of health care contacts: a systematic review. *Br J Psychiatry.* 1998 Dec;**173**(6):462–74.

27. Luoma JB, Martin CE, Pearson JL. Contact with mental health and primary care providers before suicide: a review of the evidence. *AJP.* 2002 Jun;**159**(6):909–16.

28. Sher L, Oquendo MA, Mann JJ. Risk of suicide in mood disorders. *Clin Neurosci Res.* 2001 Nov;**1**(5):337–44.

29. Gold LH, Frierson RL, editors. *The American Psychiatric Association Publishing Textbook of Suicide Risk Assessment and Management.* 3rd ed. Washington, DC: American Psychiatric Association, 2020 .

30. Haines A, Perkins E, Evans EA, McCabe R. Multidisciplinary team functioning and decision making within forensic mental health. *MHRJ.* 2018 Aug 15;**23**(3):185–96.

31. Ford R. Providing the safety net: CASE management for people with a serious mental illness. *J Ment Health.* 1995 Jan;**4**(1):91–8.

32. Malone D, Marriott SVL, Newton-Howes G, Simmonds S, Tyrer P. Community mental health teams (CMHTs) for people with severe mental illnesses and disordered personality. *Cochrane Database Syst Rev.* 2007 Jul 18;(3):CD000270.

33. Uher R, Payne JL, Pavlova B, Perlis RH. Major depressive disorder in DSM-5: implications for clinical practice and research of changes from DSM-IV. *Depress Anxiety.* 2014 Jun;**31**(6):459–71. doi: 10.1002/da.22217. PMID: 24272961.

34. American Psychiatric Association. Depressive disorders. In *Diagnostic and Statistical Manual of Mental Disorders: DSM-5.* 5th ed. Washington, DC: American Psychiatric Association, 2013; 155–88.

35. Bostwick JM, Pankratz VS. Affective disorders and suicide risk: a reexamination. *Am J Psychiatry.* 2000 Dec;**157**(12):1925–32. doi: 10.1176/appi.ajp.157.12.1925. PMID: 11097952.

36. Nordentoft M, Mortensen PB, Pedersen CB. Absolute risk of suicide after first hospital contact in mental disorder. *Arch Gen Psychiatry.* 2011;**68**(10):1058–1064. doi:10.1001/archgenpsychiatry.2011.113

37. Sareen J, Cox BJ, Afifi TO, et al. Anxiety disorders and risk for suicidal ideation and suicide attempts: a population-based longitudinal study of adults. *Arch Gen Psychiatry.* 2005 Nov;**62**(11):1249–57. doi: 10.1001/archpsyc.62.11.1249. PMID: 16275812.

38. Dumais A, Lesage AD, Alda M, et al. Risk factors for suicide completion in major depression: a case-control study of impulsive and aggressive behaviors in men. *Am J Psychiatry.* 2005 Nov;**162**(11):2116–24. doi: 10.1176/appi.ajp.162.11.2116. PMID: 16263852.

39. Schaffer A, Flint AJ, Smith E, et al. Correlates of suicidality among patients with psychotic depression. *Suicide Life Threat Behav.* 2008 Aug;**38**(4):403–14. doi: 10.1521/suli.2008.38.4.403. PMID: 18724788.

40. World Health Organization. *Preventing Suicide: A Global Imperative.* Geneva: World Health Organization, 2014.

41. American Psychiatric Association. *Practice Guideline for the Treatment of Patients with Major Depressive Disorder.* 3rd ed. Washington, DC: American Psychiatric Association, 2010. Available at: http://psychiatryonline.org/guidelines.aspx

42. Bauer M, Pfennig A, Severus E, et al. World Federation of Societies of Biological Psychiatry (WFSBP) guidelines for biological treatment of unipolar depressive disorders, part 1: update 2013 on

the acute and continuation treatment of unipolar depressive disorders. *World J Biol Psychiatry*. 2013; **14**:334.

43. Hamilton M. A rating scale for depression. *J Neurol Neurosurg Psychiatry*. 1960 Feb;**23**(1):56–62. doi: 10.1136/jnnp.23.1.56. PMID: 14399272; PMCID: PMC495331.

44. Montgomery SA, Asberg M. A new depression scale designed to be sensitive to change. *Br J Psychiatry*. 1979 Apr;**134**:382–9. doi: 10.1192/bjp.134.4.382. PMID: 444788.

45. Kroenke K, Spitzer RL, Williams JB. The PHQ-9: validity of a brief depression severity measure. *J Gen Intern Med*. 2001;**16**(9):606–13. doi:10.1046/j.1525-1497.2001.016009606.x

46. Knaup C, Koesters M, Schoefer D, Becker T, Puschner B. Effect of feedback of treatment outcome in specialist mental healthcare: meta-analysis. *Br J Psychiatry*. 2009 Jul;**195**(1):15–22. doi: 10.1192/bjp.bp.108.053967. PMID: 19567889.

47. Chang TE, Jing Y, Yeung AS, et al. Depression monitoring and patient behavior in the Clinical Outcomes in MEasurement-Based Treatment (COMET) trial. *Psychiatr Serv*. 2014 Aug 1;**65** (8):1058–61. doi: 10.1176/appi.ps.201300326. PMID: 25082605.

48. National Collaborating Centre for Mental Health (UK). *Depression: The Treatment and Management of Depression in Adults* (updated edition). Leicester: British Psychological Society, 2010. PMID: 22132433.

49. Cuijpers P, Sijbrandij M, Koole SL, et al. The efficacy of psychotherapy and pharmacotherapy in treating depressive and anxiety disorders: a meta-analysis of direct comparisons. *World Psychiatry*. 2013 Jun;**12** (2):137–48. doi: 10.1002/wps.20038. PMID: 23737423; PMCID: PMC3683266.

50. Spielmans GI, Berman MI, Usitalo AN. Psychotherapy versus second-generation antidepressants in the treatment of depression: a meta-analysis. *J Nerv Ment Dis*. 2011 Mar;**199**(3):142–9. doi: 10.1097/NMD.0b013e31820caefb. PMID: 21346483.

51. Amick HR, Gartlehner G, Gaynes BN, et al. Comparative benefits and harms of second generation antidepressants and cognitive behavioral therapies in initial treatment of major depressive disorder: systematic review and meta-analysis. *BMJ*. 2015 Dec 8;**351**:h6019. doi: 10.1136/bmj.h6019. PMID: 26645251; PMCID: PMC4673103.

52. Cuijpers P, Dekker J, Hollon SD, Andersson G. Adding psychotherapy to pharmacotherapy in the treatment of depressive disorders in adults: a meta-analysis. *J Clin Psychiatry*. 2009 Sep;**70**(9):1219–29. doi: 10.4088/JCP.09r05021. PMID: 19818243.

53. Cuijpers P, van Straten A, Warmerdam L, Andersson G. Psychotherapy versus the combination of psychotherapy and pharmacotherapy in the treatment of depression: a meta-analysis. *Depress Anxiety*. 2009;**26**(3):279–88. doi: 10.1002/da.20519. PMID: 19031487.

54. Gartlehner G, Thaler K, Hill S, Hansen RA. How should primary care doctors select which antidepressants to administer? *Curr Psychiatry Rep*. 2012 Aug;**14**(4):360–9. doi: 10.1007/s11920-012-0283-x. PMID: 22648236.

55. Cipriani A, Furukawa TA, Salanti G, et al. Comparative efficacy and acceptability of 21 antidepressant drugs for the acute treatment of adults with major depressive disorder: a systematic review and network meta-analysis. *Lancet*. 2018 Apr 7;**391** (10128):1357–66. doi: 10.1016/S0140-6736(17)32802-7. PMID: 29477251; PMCID: PMC5889788.

56. Mojtabai R, Olfson M. National patterns in antidepressant treatment by psychiatrists and general medical providers: results from the national co-morbidity survey replication. *J Clin Psychiatry*. 2008 Jul;**69**(7):1064–74. doi: 10.4088/jcp.v69n0704. PMID: 18399725.

57. Geddes JR, Freemantle N, Mason J, Eccles MP, Boynton J. SSRIs versus other antidepressants for depressive disorder. *Cochrane Database Syst Rev*. 2000;(2):CD001851. doi: 10.1002/14651858. CD001851. Update in *Cochrane Database Syst Rev*. 2006;(3):CD001851. PMID: 10796826.

58. Gartlehner G, Hansen RA, Morgan LC, et al. Comparative benefits and harms of second-generation antidepressants for treating major depressive disorder: an updated meta-analysis. *Ann Intern Med*. 2011 Dec 6;**155**(11):772–85. doi: 10.7326/0003-4819-155-11-201112060-00009. PMID: 22147715.

59. Gartlehner G, Hansen RA, Morgan LC, et al. *Second-Generation Antidepressants in the Pharmacologic Treatment of Adult Depression: An Update of the 2007 Comparative Effectiveness Review* [Internet]. Report No.: 12-EHC012-EF. Rockville, MD: Agency for Healthcare Research and Quality (US); 2011 Dec.

60. Anderson IM. Selective serotonin reuptake inhibitors versus tricyclic antidepressants: a meta-analysis of efficacy and tolerability. *J Affect Disord*. 2000 Apr;**58** (1):19–36. doi: 10.1016/s0165-0327(99)00092-0. PMID: 10760555.

61. Suchting R, Tirumalajaru V, Gareeb R, et al. Revisiting monoamine oxidase inhibitors for the treatment of depressive disorders: a systematic review and network meta-analysis. *J Affect Disord*. 2021 Mar 1;**282**:1153–60. doi: 10.1016/j.jad.2021.01.021. PMID: 33601690.

62. Machado M, Iskedjian M, Ruiz I, Einarson TR. Remission, dropouts, and adverse drug reaction rates in major depressive disorder: a meta-analysis of head-to-head trials. *Curr Med Res and Opinions.* 2006;**22**:10825–37.

63. Anderson IM. Meta analysis of antidepressant drugs: selectivity versus multiplicity. In JA den Boer, MGM Westenberg, editors. *Antidepressants: Selectivity versus Multiplicity.* Amsterdam: Benecke NI, 2001; 85–99.

64. Williams JW, Mulrow CD, Chiquette E et al. A systematic review of newer pharmacotherapies for depression in adults: evidence report summary. *Ann Intern Med.* 2000;**132**:749–56.

65. Gibbons RD, Hur K, Brown CH, Davis JM, Mann JJ. Benefits from antidepressants: synthesis of 6-week patient-level outcomes from double-blind placebo-controlled randomized trials of fluoxetine and venlafaxine. *Arch Gen Psychiatry.* 2012;**69**(6):572–9. doi:10.1001/archgenpsychiatry.2011.2044

66. Lam RW, Kennedy SH, Grigoriadis S, et al.; Canadian Network for Mood and Anxiety Treatments (CANMAT). Canadian Network for Mood and Anxiety Treatments (CANMAT) clinical guidelines for the management of major depressive disorder in adults. III. Pharmacotherapy. *J Affect Disord.* 2009 Oct;**117**(Suppl 1):S26–43. doi: 10.1016/j.jad.2009.06.041. PMID: 19674794.

67. Bauer M, Pfennig A, Severus E, et al.; World Federation of Societies of Biological Psychiatry. Task Force on Unipolar Depressive Disorders. World Federation of Societies of Biological Psychiatry (WFSBP) guidelines for biological treatment of unipolar depressive disorders, part 1: update 2013 on the acute and continuation treatment of unipolar depressive disorders. *World J Biol Psychiatry.* 2013 Jul;**14**(5):334–85. doi: 10.3109/15622975.2013.804195. PMID: 23879318.

68. Uher R, Mors O, Rietschel M, et al. Early and delayed onset of response to antidepressants in individual trajectories of change during treatment of major depression: a secondary analysis of data from the Genome-Based Therapeutic Drugs for Depression (GENDEP) study. *J Clin Psychiatry.* 2011 Nov;**72**(11):1478–84. doi: 10.4088/JCP.10m06419. PMID: 22127194.

69. Posternak MA, Zimmerman M. Is there a delay in the antidepressant effect? A meta-analysis. *J Clin Psychiatry.* 2005 Feb;**66**(2):148–58. doi: 10.4088/jcp.v66n0201. PMID: 15704999.

70. Katz MM, Meyers AL, Prakash A, Gaynor PJ, Houston JP. Early symptom change prediction of remission in depression treatment. *Psychopharmacol Bull.* 2009;**42**(1):94–107. PMID: 19204654.

71. Ciudad A, Álvarez E, Roca M, et al. Early response and remission as predictors of a good outcome of a major depressive episode at 12-month follow-up: a prospective, longitudinal, observational study. *J Clin Psychiatry.* 2012 Feb;**73**(2):185–91. doi: 10.4088/JCP.10m06314. PMID: 22053897.

72. Szegedi A, Jansen WT, van Willigenburg AP, et al. Early improvement in the first 2 weeks as a predictor of treatment outcome in patients with major depressive disorder: a meta-analysis including 6562 patients. J Clin Psychiatry. 2009 Mar;**70**(3):344–53. doi: 10.4088/jcp.07m03780. PMID: 19254516.

73. Fava M. Diagnosis and definition of treatment-resistant depression. *Biol Psychiatry.* 2003 Apr 15;**53**(8):649–59. doi: 10.1016/s0006-3223(03)00231-2. PMID: 12706951.

74. Papakostas GI. Managing partial response or nonresponse: switching, augmentation, and combination strategies for major depressive disorder. *J Clin Psychiatry.* 2009;**70**(suppl 6):16–25. doi: 10.4088/JCP.8133su1 c.03. PMID: 19922740.

75. McIntyre RS. When should you move beyond first-line therapy for depression? *J Clin Psychiatry.* 2010;**71**(suppl 1):16–20. doi: 10.4088/JCP.9104su1 c.03. PMID: 20977871.

76. Wu CH, Farley JF, Gaynes BN. The association between antidepressant dosage titration and medication adherence among patients with depression. *Depress Anxiety.* 2012 Jun;**29**(6):506–14. doi: 10.1002/da.21952. PMID: 22553149.

77. Wijkstra J, Lijmer J, Balk FJ, Geddes JR, Nolen WA. Pharmacological treatment for unipolar psychotic depression: systematic review and meta-analysis. *Br J Psychiatry.* 2006 May;**188**:410–5. doi: 10.1192/bjp.bp.105.010470. PMID: 16648526.

78. Farahani A, Correll CU. Are antipsychotics or antidepressants needed for psychotic depression? A systematic review and meta-analysis of trials comparing antidepressant or antipsychotic monotherapy with combination treatment. *J Clin Psychiatry.* 2012 Apr;**73**(4):486–96. doi: 10.4088/JCP.11r07324. PMID: 22579147; PMCID: PMC4537657.

79. Pagnin D, de Queiroz V, Pini S, Cassano GB. Efficacy of ECT in depression: a meta-analytic review. *J ECT.* 2004 Mar;**20**(1):13–20. doi: 10.1097/00124509-200403000-00004. PMID: 15087991.

80. UK ECT Review Group. Efficacy and safety of electroconvulsive therapy in depressive disorders: a systematic review and meta-analysis. *Lancet.* 2003 Mar 8;**361**(9360):799–808. doi: 10.1016/S0140-6736(03)12705-5. PMID: 12642045.

81. Price LH, Conwell Y, Nelson JC. Lithium augmentation of combined neuroleptic-tricyclic

treatment in delusional depression. *Am J Psychiatry.* 1983 Mar;**140**(3):318–22. doi: 10.1176/ajp.140.3.318. PMID: 6131612.

82. Birkenhäger TK, van den Broek WW, Wijkstra J, et al. Treatment of unipolar psychotic depression: an open study of lithium addition in refractory psychotic depression. *J Clin Psychopharmacol.* 2009 Oct;**29**(5):513–15. doi: 10.1097/JCP.0b013e3181b6744e. PMID: 19745662.

83. US Food and Drug Administration. Label for esketamine nasal spray. www.accessdata.fda.gov/drugsatfda_docs/label/2020/211243s004lbl.pdf

84. Cipriani A, Hawton K, Stockton S, Geddes JR. Lithium in the prevention of suicide in mood disorders: updated systematic review and meta-analysis. *BMJ.* 2013 Jun 27;**346**:f3646. doi: 10.1136/bmj.f3646. PMID: 23814104.

85. Driessen E, Cuijpers P, Hollon SD, Dekker JJ. Does pretreatment severity moderate the efficacy of psychological treatment of adult outpatient depression? A meta-analysis. *J Consult Clin Psychol.* 2010 Oct;**78**(5):668–80. doi: 10.1037/a0020570. PMID: 20873902.

86. Bai Z, Luo S, Zhang L, Wu S, Chi I. Acceptance and Commitment Therapy (ACT) to reduce depression: a systematic review and meta-analysis. *J Affect Disord.* 2020 Jan 1;**260**:728–37. doi: 10.1016/j.jad.2019.09.040PMID: 31563072.

87. Cuijpers P, Karyotaki E, Weitz E, et al. The effects of psychotherapies for major depression in adults on remission, recovery and improvement: a meta-analysis. *J Affect Disord.* 2014 Apr;**159**:118–26. doi: 10.1016/j.jad.2014.02.026. PMID: 24679399.

88. Cuijpers P, van Straten A, van Oppen P, Andersson G. Are psychological and pharmacologic interventions equally effective in the treatment of adult depressive disorders? A meta-analysis of comparative studies. *J Clin Psychiatry.* 2008 Nov;**69**(11):1675–85; quiz 1839–41. doi: 10.4088/jcp.v69n1102. PMID: 18945396.

89. Imel ZE, Malterer MB, McKay KM, Wampold BE. A meta-analysis of psychotherapy and medication in unipolar depression and dysthymia. *J Affect Disord.* 2008 Oct;**110**(3):197–206. doi: 10.1016/j.jad.2008.03.018. PMID: 18456340.

90. Shinohara K, Honyashiki M, Imai H, et al. Behavioural therapies versus other psychological therapies for depression. *Cochrane Database Syst Rev.* 2013 Oct 16;**2013**(10):CD008696. doi: 10.1002/14651858.CD008696.pub2. PMID: 24129886; PMCID: PMC7433301.

91. Cuijpers P, van Straten A, Andersson G, van Oppen P. Psychotherapy for depression in adults: a meta-analysis of comparative outcome studies. *J Consult Clin Psychol.* 2008 Dec;**76**(6):909–22. doi: 10.1037/a0013075. PMID: 19045960.

92. Gaudiano BA, Miller IW, Herbert JD. The treatment of psychotic major depression: is there a role for adjunctive psychotherapy? *Psychother Psychosom.* 2007;**76**(5):271–7. doi: 10.1159/000104703. PMID: 17700047.

93. Bach PA, Gaudiano B, Pankey J, Herbert J., Hayes SC. Acceptance, mindfulness, values, and psychosis: applying Acceptance and Commitment Therapy (ACT) to the chronically mentally ill. In RA Baer, editor. *Mindfulness-Based Treatment Approaches: Clinician's Guide to Evidence Base and Applications.* Elsevier Academic Press, 2006; 93–116. https://doi.org/10.1016/B978-012088519-0/50006-X

94. Erlangsen A, Lind BD, Stuart EA, et al. Short-term and long-term effects of psychosocial therapy for people after deliberate self-harm: a register-based, nationwide multicentre study using propensity score matching. *Lancet Psychiatry.* 2015 Jan;**2**(1):49–58. doi: 10.1016/S2215-0366(14)00083-2. PMID: 26359612.

95. Hawton K, Witt KG, Salisbury TLT, et al. Psychosocial interventions following self-harm in adults: a systematic review and meta-analysis. *Lancet Psychiatry.* 2016 Aug;**3**(8):740–50. doi: 10.1016/S2215-0366(16)30070-0. PMID: 27422028.

96. Sackeim HA, Haskett RF, Mulsant BH, et al. Continuation pharmacotherapy in the prevention of relapse following electroconvulsive therapy: a randomized controlled trial. *JAMA.* 2001 Mar 14;**285**(10):1299–307. doi: 10.1001/jama.285.10.1299. PMID: 11255384.

97. Slotema CW, Blom JD, Hoek HW, Sommer IE. Should we expand the toolbox of psychiatric treatment methods to include repetitive transcranial magnetic stimulation (rTMS)? A meta-analysis of the efficacy of rTMS in psychiatric disorders. *J Clin Psychiatry.* 2010 Jul;**71**(7):873–84. doi: 10.4088/JCP.08m04872gre. PMID: 20361902.

98. Brunoni AR, Chaimani A, Moffa AH, et al. Repetitive transcranial magnetic stimulation for the acute treatment of major depressive episodes: a systematic review with network meta-analysis. *JAMA Psychiatry.* 2017 Feb 1;**74**(2):143–52. doi: 10.1001/jamapsychiatry.2016.3644. Erratum in: *JAMA Psychiatry.* 2017 Apr 1;**74**(4):424. PMID: 28030740.

99. Health Quality Ontario. Repetitive transcranial magnetic stimulation for treatment-resistant depression: a systematic review and meta-analysis of randomized controlled trials. *Ont Health Technol Assess Ser.* 2016 Mar 1;**16**(5):1–66. PMID: 27099642; PMCID: PMC4808719.

189

100. Berlim MT, Van den Eynde F, Daskalakis ZJ. Efficacy and acceptability of high frequency repetitive transcranial magnetic stimulation (rTMS) versus electroconvulsive therapy (ECT) for major depression: a systematic review and meta-analysis of randomized trials. *Depress Anxiety*. 2013 Jul;**30**(7):614–23. doi: 10.1002/da.22060. PMID: 23349112.

101. Mårtensson B, Pettersson A, Berglund L, Ekselius L. Bright white light therapy in depression: a critical review of the evidence. *J Affect Disord*. 2015 Aug 15;**182**:1–7. doi: 10.1016/j.jad.2015.04.013. PMID: 25942575.

102. Golden RN, Gaynes BN, Ekstrom RD, et al. The efficacy of light therapy in the treatment of mood disorders: a review and meta-analysis of the evidence. *Am J Psychiatry*. 2005 Apr;**162**(4):656–62. doi: 10.1176/appi.ajp.162.4.656. PMID: 15800134.

103. Bottomley JM, LeReun C, Diamantopoulos A, Mitchell S, Gaynes BN. Vagus nerve stimulation (VNS) therapy in patients with treatment resistant depression: a systematic review and meta-analysis. *Compr Psychiatry*. 2019 Dec 12;**98**:152156. doi: 10.1016/j.comppsych.2019.152156. PMID: 31978785.

104. Volpini M, Giacobbe P, Cosgrove GR, et al. The history and future of ablative neurosurgery for major depressive disorder. *Stereotact Funct Neurosurg*. 2017;**95**(4):216–28. doi: 10.1159/000478025. PMID: 28723697.

105. Lam RW, Kennedy SH, Grigoriadis S, et al.; Canadian Network for Mood and Anxiety Treatments (CANMAT). Canadian Network for Mood and Anxiety Treatments (CANMAT) clinical guidelines for the management of major depressive disorder in adults. III. *Pharmacotherapy. J Affect Disord*. 2009 Oct;**117**(Suppl 1):S26–43. doi: 10.1016/j.jad.2009.06.041. PMID: 19674794.

106. Taylor RW, Marwood L, Oprea E, et al. Pharmacological augmentation in unipolar depression: a guide to the guidelines. *Int J Neuropsychopharmacology*. 2020;**23**(9):587–625. https://doi.org/10.1093/ijnp/pyaa033

107. Corp SA, Gitlin MJ, Altshuler LL. A review of the use of stimulants and stimulant alternatives in treating bipolar depression and major depressive disorder. *J Clin Psychiatry*. 2014 Sep;**75**(9):1010–18. doi: 10.4088/JCP.13r08851. PMID: 25295426.

108. Cusin C, Iovieno N, Iosifescu DV, et al. A randomized, double-blind, placebo-controlled trial of pramipexole augmentation in treatment-resistant major depressive disorder. *J Clin Psychiatry*. 2013 Jul;**74**(7):e636–41. doi: 10.4088/JCP.12m08093. PMID: 23945458.

109. Lavretsky H, Reinlieb M, St Cyr N, et al. Citalopram, methylphenidate, or their combination in geriatric depression: a randomized, double-blind, placebo-controlled trial. *Am J Psychiatry*. 2015 Jun;**172**(6):561–9. doi: 10.1176/appi.ajp.2014.14070889. PMID: 25677354; PMCID: PMC4451432.

110. Jorm AF, Morgan AJ, Hetrick SE. Relaxation for depression. *Cochrane Database Syst Rev*. 2008 Oct 8;(4):CD007142. doi: 10.1002/14651858.CD007142.pub2. PMID: 18843744.

111. Cooney GM, Dwan K, Greig CA, et al. Exercise for depression. *Cochrane Database Syst Rev*. 2013 Sep 12;(9):CD004366. doi: 10.1002/14651858.CD004366.pub6. PMID: 24026850.

112. Osher Y, Belmaker RH. Omega-3 fatty acids in depression: a review of three studies. *CNS Neurosci Ther*. 2009 Summer;**15**(2):128–33. doi: 10.1111/j.1755-5949.2008.00061.x. PMID: 19499625; PMCID: PMC6494070.

113. Morris DW, Trivedi MH, Rush AJ. Folate and unipolar depression. *J Altern Complement Med*. 2008 Apr;**14**(3):277–85. doi: 10.1089/acm.2007.0663. PMID: 18370582.

114. Ballenger JC. Anxiety and depression: optimizing treatments. *Prim Care Companion J Clin Psychiatry*. 2000;**2**(3):71–79. doi:10.4088/pcc.v02n0301

115. Areán PA, Cook BL. Psychotherapy and combined psychotherapy/pharmacotherapy for late life depression. *Biol Psychiatry*. 2002 Aug 1;**52**(3):293–303. doi: 10.1016/s0006-3223(02)01371-9. PMID: 12182934.

116. Tedeschini E, Levkovitz Y, Iovieno N, et al. Efficacy of antidepressants for late-life depression: a meta-analysis and meta-regression of placebo-controlled randomized trials. *J Clin Psychiatry*. 2011 Dec;**72**(12):1660–8. doi: 10.4088/JCP.10r06531. PMID: 22244025.

117. Gibbons RD, Hur K, Brown CH, Davis JM, Mann JJ. Benefits from antidepressants: synthesis of 6-week patient-level outcomes from double-blind placebo-controlled randomized trials of fluoxetine and venlafaxine. *Arch Gen Psychiatry*. 2012 Jun;**69**(6):572–9. doi: 10.1001/archgenpsychiatry.2011.2044. PMID: 22393205; PMCID: PMC3371295.

118. Wilson K, Mottram P. A comparison of side effects of selective serotonin reuptake inhibitors and tricyclic antidepressants in older depressed patients: a meta-analysis. *Int J Geriatr Psychiatry*. 2004 Aug;**19**(8):754–62. doi: 10.1002/gps.1156. PMID: 15290699

119. Mottram P, Wilson K, Strobl J. Antidepressants for depressed elderly. *Cochrane Database Syst Rev*. 2006 Jan 25;**2006**(1):CD003491. doi: 10.1002/14651858.

CD003491.pub2. PMID: 16437456; PMCID: PMC8406818.

120. Huang AX, Delucchi K, Dunn LB, Nelson JC. A systematic review and meta-analysis of psychotherapy for late-life depression. *Am J Geriatr Psychiatry*. 2015 Mar;**23**(3):261–73. doi: 10.1016/j.jagp.2014.04.003. PMID: 24856580.

121. Dew MA, Whyte EM, Lenze EJ, et al. Recovery from major depression in older adults receiving augmentation of antidepressant pharmacotherapy. *Am J Psychiatry*. 2007 Jun;**164**(6):892–9. doi: 10.1176/ajp.2007.164.6.892. PMID: 17541048.

122. Lenze EJ, Mulsant BH, Blumberger DM, et al. Efficacy, safety, and tolerability of augmentation pharmacotherapy with aripiprazole for treatment-resistant depression in late life: a randomised, double-blind, placebo-controlled trial. *Lancet*. 2015 Dec 12;**386**(10011):2404–12. doi: 10.1016/S0140-6736(15)00308-6. Erratum in: *Lancet*. 2015 Dec 12;**386**(10011):2394. PMID: 26423182; PMCID: PMC4690746.

123. Katila H, Mezhebovsky I, Mulroy A, et al. Randomized, double-blind study of the efficacy and tolerability of extended release quetiapine fumarate (quetiapine XR) monotherapy in elderly patients with major depressive disorder. *Am J Geriatr Psychiatry*. 2013 Aug;**21**(8):769–84. doi: 10.1016/j.jagp.2013.01.010. PMID: 23567397.

124. Nillni YI, Mehralizade A, Mayer L, Milanovic S. Treatment of depression, anxiety, and trauma-related disorders during the perinatal period: a systematic review. *Clin Psychol Rev*. 2018 Dec;**66**:136–48. doi: 10.1016/j.cpr.2018.06.004. PMID: 29935979; PMCID: PMC6637409.

125. Yonkers KA, Wisner KL, Stewart DE, et al. The management of depression during pregnancy: a report from the American Psychiatric Association and the American College of Obstetricians and Gynecologists. *Gen Hosp Psychiatry*. 2009 Sep-Oct;**31**(5):403–13. doi: 10.1016/j.genhosppsych.2009.04.003. PMID: 19703633; PMCID: PMC3094693.

126. Chaudron LH. Complex challenges in treating depression during pregnancy. *Am J Psychiatry*. 2013 Jan;**170**(1):12–20. doi: 10.1176/appi.ajp.2012.12040440. PMID: 23288385.

127. McAllister-Williams RH, Baldwin DS, Cantwell R, et al.; endorsed by the British Association for Psychopharmacology. British Association for Psychopharmacology consensus guidance on the use of psychotropic medication preconception, in pregnancy and postpartum 2017. *J Psychopharmacol*. 2017 May;**31**(5):519–52. doi: 10.1177/0269881117699361. PMID: 28440103.

128. Larsen ER, Damkier P, Pedersen LH, et al.; Danish Psychiatric Society; Danish Society of Obstetrics and Gynecology; Danish Paediatric Society; Danish Society of Clinical Pharmacology. Use of psychotropic drugs during pregnancy and breast-feeding. *Acta Psychiatr Scand*. 2015;**445**:1–28. doi: 10.1111/acps.12479. PMID: 26344706.

129. Byatt N, Deligiannidis KM, Freeman MP. Antidepressant use in pregnancy: a critical review focused on risks and controversies. *Acta Psychiatr Scand*. 2013 Feb;**127**(2):94–114. doi: 10.1111/acps.12042. PMID: 23240634; PMCID: PMC4006272.

130. Malhi GS, Bassett D, Boyce P, et al. Royal Australian and New Zealand College of Psychiatrists clinical practice guidelines for mood disorders. *Aust N Z J Psychiatry*. 2015 Dec;**49**(12):1087–206. doi: 10.1177/0004867415617657. PMID: 26643054.

131. Yonkers KA, Vigod S, Ross LE. Diagnosis, pathophysiology, and management of mood disorders in pregnant and postpartum women. *Obstet Gynecol*. 2011 Apr;**117**(4):961–77. doi: 10.1097/AOG.0b013e31821187a7. PMID: 21422871.

132. NICE guideline [NG134]. Depression in children and young people: identification and management. Published 25 June 2019

133. Hetrick SE, McKenzie JE, Bailey AP, et al. New generation antidepressants for depression in children and adolescents: a network meta-analysis. *Cochrane Database Syst Rev*. 2021 May 24;**5**(5):CD013674. doi: 10.1002/14651858.CD013674.pub2. PMID: 34029378; PMCID: PMC8143444.

134. Brent DA, Gibbons RD, Wilkinson P, Dubicka B. Antidepressants in paediatric depression: do not look back in anger but around in awareness. *BJPsych Bull*. 2018 Feb;**42**(1):1–4. doi: 10.1192/bjb.2017.2. PMID: 29388523; PMCID: PMC6001874.

135. Emslie GJ, Rush AJ, Weinberg WA, et al. Fluoxetine in child and adolescent depression: acute and maintenance treatment. *Depress Anxiety*. 1998;**7**(1):32–9. doi: 10.1002/(sici)1520-6394(1998)7:1<32::aid-da4>3.0.co;2-7. PMID: 959263

136. Solomon DA, Keller MB, Leon AC, et al. Multiple recurrences of major depressive disorder. *Am J Psychiatry*. 2000 Feb;**157**(2):229–33. doi: 10.1176/appi.ajp.157.2.229. PMID: 10671391.

137. Karyotaki E, Smit Y, Holdt Henningsen K, et al. Combining pharmacotherapy and psychotherapy or monotherapy for major depression? A meta-analysis on the long-term effects. *J Affect Disord*. 2016 Apr;**194**:144–52. doi: 10.1016/j.jad.2016.01.036. PMID: 26826534.

138. Oestergaard S, Møldrup C. Optimal duration of combined psychotherapy and pharmacotherapy for patients with moderate and severe depression: a

meta-analysis. *J Affect Disord*. 2011 Jun;**131**(1–3):24–36. doi: 10.1016/j.jad.2010.08.014. PMID: 20950863.

139. Hansen R, Gaynes B, Thieda P, et al. Meta-analysis of major depressive disorder relapse and recurrence with second-generation antidepressants. *Psychiatr Serv*. 2008 Oct;**59**(10):1121–30. doi: 10.1176/appi.ps.59.10.1121. PMID: 18832497; PMCID: PMC2840386.

140. Jelovac A, Kolshus E, McLoughlin DM. Relapse following successful electroconvulsive therapy for major depression: a meta-analysis. *Neuropsychopharmacology*. 2013 Nov;**38**(12):2467–74. doi: 10.1038/npp.2013.149. PMID: 23774532; PMCID: PMC3799066.

141. Kedzior KK, Reitz SK, Azorina V, Loo C. Durability of the antidepressant effect of the high-frequency repetitive transcranial magnetic stimulation (rTMS) in the absence of maintenance treatment in major depression: a systematic review and meta-analysis of 16 double-blind, randomized, sham-controlled trials. *Depress Anxiety*. 2015 Mar;**32**(3):193–203. doi: 10.1002/da.22339. PMID: 25683231.

142. Rothschild AJ, Duval SE. How long should patients with psychotic depression stay on the antipsychotic medication? *J Clin Psychiatry*. 2003 Apr;**64**(4):390–6. doi: 10.4088/jcp.v64n0405. PMID: 12716238.

143. Cipriani A, Hawton K, Stockton S, Geddes JR. Lithium in the prevention of suicide in mood disorders: updated systematic review and meta-analysis. *BMJ*. 2013 Jun 27;**346**:f3646. doi: 10.1136/bmj.f3646. PMID: 23814104.

144. Cipriani A, Pretty H, Hawton K, Geddes JR. Lithium in the prevention of suicidal behavior and all-cause mortality in patients with mood disorders: a systematic review of randomized trials. *Am J Psychiatry*. 2005 Oct;**162**(10):1805–19. doi: 10.1176/appi.ajp.162.10.1805. PMID: 16199826.

145. Hoffman BM, Babyak MA, Craighead WE, et al. Exercise and pharmacotherapy in patients with major depression: one-year follow-up of the SMILE study. *Psychosom Med*. 2011 Feb-Mar;**73**(2):127–33. doi: 10.1097/PSY.0b013e31820433a5. PMID: 21148807; PMCID: PMC3671874

Chapter 19

Treatment-Resistant Depression: Pharmacological Approach

Alexandre Paim Diaz, Joao Quevedo, Marsal Sanches, and Jair C. Soares

Concept of Treatment-Resistant Depression

There is no consensus for the concept of treatment-resistant depression (TRD). How TRD has been defined in each study also varies according to the investigators' concept of depression over the years. For instance, Haskovec and Rysanek (1967) investigated clinical and biochemical effects of reserpine in "imipramine-resistant depressive" patients. The criteria for "imipramine-resistant" included no improvement of depression after three weeks of imipramine administration for patients with "at least one previous depressive illness". The diagnosis criteria of depression encompassed "prolonged pathological depressive emotional disposition, loss of interest and energy, psychomotor inhibition, sleep disturbances, anorexia with loss of weight, feeling of hopelessness, self-reproach, morning depression and an indication of suicidal tendencies" [1]. In a randomized controlled trial (RCT) for pharmacological treatment of TRD, Drago et al. (1983) investigated the efficacy of maprotiline 100 mg daily and clomipramine 100 mg daily by the intravenous route. TRD was considered if the participant had not responded to three different antidepressants in the previous six months of the study [2]. The diagnosis of depression was made according to the Feighner criteria, which, together with the Research Diagnostic Criteria, influenced the third version of the *Diagnostic and Statistical Manual of Mental Disorders* (DSM-III) [2,3]. Hardy defined resistant depression as "those depressions in which the spontaneous course is not influenced by therapeutic measures". The author points out the need for clear criteria for the characterization of the clinical condition; otherwise, the definition of TRD would vary significantly [4].

Given the difficulty to reflect the complexity of treatment response, the persistence of symptoms even among those patients considered remitted, and the

questionable validity of the TRD concept, Malhi and Byrow argue whether TRD is a useful definition [5]. Despite the criticisms, the authors recognize some benefits of research with TRD patients – for instance, the identification of "therapy-defined depressive subtypes", which can provide more homogeneous samples, probably in terms of clinical and biological characteristics, to investigate new therapies [5]. An expert consensus for the definition and assessment of TRD states that an operational conceptualization of TRD might help improve the identification of predictors and interventions for depression nonresponsive to different trials. In this consensus, most of the experts agreed that TRD is a meaningful concept in clinical practice and that it should be defined by "the failure of two adequately dosed and evidence supported trials of antidepressant medications". However, although the categorical approach would be helpful to identify patients with treatment resistance initially, a continuous approach would better delineate the progression or severity of TRD [6]. Nevertheless, other authors argue that to consider TRD as a subtype of depression is not supported by evidence, as only part of the resistance can be explained through pharmacodynamics or pharmacokinetic mechanisms [7]. Dodd et al. critically reviewed treatment resistance in patients with depression, providing a thorough discussion on the topic. The authors agree that pharmacokinetics or pharmacodynamic mechanisms can explain only part of TRD; that is, most TRD are related to psychosocial variables, personality disorders, substance use, or nonadherence. Thus, they suggest the evaluation of treatment resistance should be personalized, which also contributes to the individualization of the further treatment strategies [7].

Despite no consensus regarding TRD, most commonly, it is considered when the patient does not present remission after two or more treatments in adequate duration and dosage. However, as this definition can accommodate different criteria, as a response rather than remission, minimum severity of symptoms, or type of interventions, we will describe how TRD was determined in the studies cited in this chapter.

Epidemiology and Impact of Treatment-Resistant Depression

The 12-month prevalence of major depressive disorder (MDD) in the US adult population is 7.1%. Among them, around 50% use medication to treat the depression [8]. In a register-based cohort study, the authors identified all adult patients registered first time with MDD and classified those with TRD according to the following criteria: "two shifts in treatment for MDD, which was assessed by patients' use of antidepressants or electroconvulsive therapy (ECT) 12 months before and after first hospital contact with MDD" [9]. According to this definition, 15% of the 197,615 individuals with depression met the criteria for TRD, most of them female (64.5%), mean age of 51 years, with mild to moderate depression (78.4%). Among the pharmacological treatments used by these patients, the most common ever-use medications were serotonin and noradrenaline reuptake inhibitors (SNRIs) (92.3%), followed by selective serotonin reuptake inhibitors (SSRIs) (91.6%), antipsychotic agents (44.6%), tricyclic antidepressants (TCA) (31.9%), lithium (3.9%), and monoamine oxidase inhibitor (MAOI) (1.1%) [9].

The Sequenced Treatment Alternatives to Relieve Depression (STAR*D) study, funded by the National Institutes of Health (NIH), is the largest prospective clinical trial to investigate the sequenced treatment of major depression. The design included four levels of treatment: level 1 – citalopram; level 2 – switch to bupropion, or venlafaxine, or sertraline, or cognitive therapy; or augment with bupropion, or buspirone, or cognitive therapy; level 3 – switch to mirtazapine or nortriptyline, or augment with lithium or T3 thyroid hormone; level 4 – switch to tranylcypromine or mirtazapine plus venlafaxine. The study also includes a level 2a for participants receiving cognitive therapy in level 2: switch to bupropion or venlafaxine [10]. The study included 4,041 participants between 18 and 75 years old. The researchers found that approximately 30% achieved remission at level 1, 25% at level 2, 13–16% at level 3, and 7–16% at level 4. The cumulative remission showed that after the four levels, one-third of patients do not

reach remission [11]. Mojtabai reported that greater severity, poorer physical health, poor adherence, unemployment, not having higher education, and longer duration of current episode were associated with nonremission [12]. The prevalence of TRD among patients in UK primary care was even higher in a cross-sectional study by Thomas et al., although their criteria for TRD were less restricted. In this study, TRD was defined as scores ≥ 14 on the Beck Depression Inventory (BDI) in patients taking antidepressant medication at an adequate dose for at least six weeks [13]. Among 2,129 patients, 55.3% met the study's criteria for TRD. SSRIs were the antidepressants most prescribed (79%), the majority of the sample was female (70.3%) and approximately 50 years old on average [13].

Zhdavana et al. estimated the 12-month prevalence and burden of TRD in the US population. The definition of TRD for this study was the initiation of a third antidepressant treatment course after changing two antidepressant trials of adequate dose and duration. The prevalence of TRD among adults with medication-treated MDD varied from 21.4% (data from Medicare) to 44.2% (data from Medicaid), 30.9% overall (about 1.1% of the US adult population) [14]. The incremental annual healthcare cost of adults with TRD was $9,323 compared to individuals without MDD. This amount is more than $6,000 higher than the incremental annual cost for non-TRD MDD individuals, which was $3,197. Despite only 30.9% of adult medication-treated MDD presented TRD, the proportions of healthcare costs and unemployment costs attributable to TRD were 56.6% and 47.7%, respectively [14]. Results from a Danish nationwide register-based cohort study found that individuals with TRD had significantly higher mortality than those without TRD, with an adjusted mortality rate ratio of 1.39 (95% confidence interval [CI]: 1.19–1.63) for women and 1.34 (95% CI: 1.18–1.52) for men. In addition, women and men presented 1.24 and 1.21 shorter years of life expectancy, respectively, than non-TRD patients, mostly accounted by suicide [15]. In fact, results from the same nationwide register-based cohort reported significantly higher rates of suicide and self-harming behavior in one year (adjusted hazard ratio [HR] of 2.2 and 1.5, respectively) in individuals with TRD compared to non-TRD patients [16]. In terms of absolute number of excess deaths, a Swedish national register study reported 7 to 16 excess deaths per 1,000 patients during 5 years among individuals with TRD (defined as patients who initiated a third consecutive treatment trial) compared to non-TRD patients [17]. Considering the sizable prevalence and the significant impact of TRD on the individual and society, novel efficacious and safe treatments are necessary. Understanding the neurobiology of depression, and TRD in particular, can help identify novel targets for interventions. As already discussed, despite the heterogeneity of TRD and its limitations to be considered a valid subtype of depression, several studies explored the neurobiology of TRD, elucidating at least part of its pathophysiology.

Neurobiology of Treatment-Resistant Depression

Understanding the neurobiology associated with TRD may provide insights for novel targets and interventions [18]. One of the potential neurobiological mechanisms underlying depression is the hyperactivity of the hypothalamic–pituitary–adrenal (HPA) axis, which is also highly related to early life stress, a risk factor for depression [19,20]. Juruena et al. found significantly lower salivary cortisol levels in individuals with TRD (no remission after at least two different classes of antidepressants) compared to placebo at baseline and after dexamethasone and prednisolone administration. The authors also reported a distinct response of dexamethasone and prednisolone administration on HPA axis activity (impaired suppression and normal suppression, respectively) in the TRD individuals [21]. Allen et al. investigated the influence of ketamine, an N-methyl-D-aspartate (NMDA) receptor antagonist, on kynurenine pathway metabolism in patients with TRD compared to healthy controls (HC), as well as before and after ECT, an intervention usually indicated for patients with more severe and treatment-resistant disease. For this study, TRD was considered as failure to respond to at least two adequate trials of antidepressants [22]. The authors found greater salivary cortisol at baseline in the ECT group than in the ketamine and HC groups. On the other hand, plasma kynurenine concentrations were significantly higher in the ketamine group compared to the other two groups. Both ketamine and ECT groups presented lower kynurenic acid and kynurenic acid / kynurenine ratios compared to HC. However, treatment with ketamine or ECT did not significantly change kynurenine pathway metabolism [22].

Caraci et al. reviewed the neurobiology of TRD, including genetics, the role of glutamatergic systems, and neurotrophic mechanisms. The authors reported that despite the fact that genetic variants can explain about 42% of the variance in antidepressant response, genome-wide association studies (GWAS) did not find common genetic variants related to TRD [18]. However, Fabbri et al. reported that *FKBP5* polymorphisms, which are associated with glucocorticoid signaling, may be related to antidepressant efficacy [23], as well as the *PPP3CC* gene, which is involved in the regulation of immune system and synaptic plasticity [24]. In 2006, Zarate et al. published positive results from an RCT study that investigated the efficacy of ketamine in treating TRD [25]. Since then, several studies have shown the efficacy of ketamine in treating patients with TRD, suggesting a role of the glutamatergic system in the neurobiology of depression resistant to treatment [26]. The rapid antidepressant response to ketamine is associated with decreased metabolism in the right habenula and the medial and orbital prefrontal networks in patients with TRD [27]. This finding has stimulated the investigation of novel glutamatergic agents for TRD [28,29].

Considering the clinical heterogeneity of depression, some studies explored the neurobiology of transdiagnostic symptoms of depression and its association with TRD. For example, anhedonia, a core component of depression [30], is related to the limbic–cortical–striatal–pallidal–thalamic pathway and may be useful in predicting TRD [31]. Anhedonia was the only depressive symptom that predicted a longer time until remission after adjustment for several covariates in a randomized clinical trial with TRD adolescents [32]. In the same way, the HPA axis hyperactivity may be associated with a different profile of depressive symptoms. For instance, Iob et al. found higher cortisol and C-reactive protein (CRP) levels more strongly related to somatic rather than cognitive-affective symptoms [33].

Pharmacological Interventions for Patients with Treatment-Resistant Depression

The pharmacological management of depression may involve administering drugs in monotherapy, in association, or augmented by another agent. This section will present data from several systematic reviews of RCTs that assessed the efficacy of pharmacological interventions for TRD and RCTs of medications published in the past five years not yet covered by these reviews.

In the Edwards et al. study, the authors estimated the clinical effectiveness of augmentation with either lithium or atypical antipsychotics in the treatment with selective serotonin reuptake inhibitors (SSRIs). The results showed a statistically significant benefit for fluoxetine plus olanzapine over fluoxetine in monotherapy for both response and remission, with no significant differences regarding treatment discontinuation. One RCT from this review compared fluoxetine plus lithium to fluoxetine alone, and the results did not show statistically significant differences between the groups regarding both response and changes in depressive symptoms scores [34]. However, in the systematic review of Nelson et al., augmentation of tricyclic antidepressants (TCA) or second-generation antidepressants with lithium was superior to placebo (combined odds ratio [OR] 2.89, CI: 1.65–5.05) for patients with non-response to at least 21 days of treatment with one antidepressant [35]. Zhou et al. reported a higher efficacy (mean change scores in depressive symptoms) for atypical antipsychotics augmentation at standard doses compared to placebo (the results were not significant for low-dose atypical antipsychotics) to treat TRD ("inadequate response to at least one course of conventional antidepressant treatment"). A network meta-analysis of this study did not find differences between the atypical antipsychotics [36]. A systematic review that included 11 augmentation agents in TRD did not find statistically significant differences between the agents (including comparisons among them) and placebo regarding discontinuation rates (percentage of patients who terminated the study for any reason). However, quetiapine, olanzapine, aripiprazole, and lithium were significantly less well tolerated than placebo. TRD was considered as a history of failure to at least one treatment and nonresponse to at least one first-line antidepressant during the current depressive episode. Quetiapine (OR = 1.92), aripiprazole (OR = 1.85), thyroid hormone (OR = 1.84), and lithium (OR = 1.56) were superior to placebo in terms of clinical response. Thyroid hormone, risperidone, quetiapine, buspirone, olanzapine, and aripiprazole were superior to placebo in terms of remission [37]. Adjunctive aripiprazole was also found to provide therapeutic benefits for TRD in a systematic review that included 8 RCTs totalizing 2,260 patients [38]. The results showed that aripiprazole was associated with statistically significant higher remission and response than placebo (risk ratio [RR] = 1.64, 95% CI: 1.43–1.90 and RR = 1.50, 95% CI: 1.14–1.98, respectively). However, adjunctive aripiprazole was associated with significantly higher adverse events discontinuation rates than placebo (RR = 2.21, 95% CI: 1.23–3.67) and significantly higher incidence of adverse events, mainly constipation, fatigue, akathisia, insomnia, restlessness, and blurred vision [38]. Brexpiprazole is a serotonin-dopamine activity modulator that has lower intrinsic activity at the D2 receptor than aripiprazole, potentially inducing fewer D2 agonist-mediated adverse events, including akathisia [39]. Despite its apparent more favorable profile, adjunctive brexpiprazole was associated with a higher discontinuation rate, akathisia, and restlessness than placebo for individuals with a history of treatment failure, as aripiprazole and brexpiprazole were associated with significantly higher response and remission rates with data from nine RCTs. Doses lower than 2 mg/day presented a better risk/benefit relationship [40]. Pindolol, a β-adrenoceptor and 5-HT1A/1B receptor ligand that has been associated with an increase of 5-HT synthesis in animal models [41,42], was investigated as adjunctive treatment in five RCTs involving 154 patients who had failed to respond to at least one SSRI [43]. The results showed that adjunctive pindolol was not more effective than placebo plus SSRI or SSRI alone (standardized mean difference [SMD] in depressive symptoms scores of –0.43, 95% CI: –1.14 to 0.29) [43]. Olanzapine/fluoxetine combination was associated with a significant reduction of depressive symptoms in individuals with TRD compared with olanzapine or fluoxetine monotherapy, according to a meta-analysis of five RCTs [44]. The combination treatment was also associated with a significantly higher response rate (RR = 1.35, 95% CI: 1.12–1.63) and remission rate (RR = 1.71, 95% CI: 1.31–2.23), with no significant differences regarding the incidence of adverse events [44]. A meta-analysis of four RCTs with infliximab, a tumor necrosis factor inhibitor, to treat TRD did not find a therapeutic benefit of the intervention compared to placebo. Studies' duration varied from 8 to 12 weeks and all of them used 5 mg/day of infliximab compared to placebo [45]. Ketamine has been extensively investigated for TRD. A meta-analysis of RCTs of ketamine for unipolar or bipolar depression included 20 studies, most of them with TRD patients and compared to placebo. TRD was defined as a lack of response to at least two different antidepressant drugs at an adequate dose and duration of administration [46]. For patients with TRD, single-dose ketamine was associated with a significantly greater reduction of depressive symptoms at 24 hours, 3–4 days, and 7 days of administration [46]. Similar results were found in a network meta-analysis in which ketamine was superior to other pharmacological interventions in terms of response rates and velocity for reducing depression severity [47].

A Cochrane systematic review with pharmacological interventions for TRD included 10 RCTs totalizing 2,731 participants [48]. The results showed that despite no benefit being found for switching to mianserin, augmenting the antidepressant treatment with this medication was associated with a significant decrease in depressive symptoms (mean difference [MD] = –4.8, 95% CI: –8.18 to –1.42). The authors also reported that augmentation with buspirone did not show therapeutic benefits but was associated with a significant decrease in depressive symptoms with cariprazine, olanzapine, quetiapine, or ziprasidone compared to monotherapy [48]. Table 19.1 summarizes RCTs published in the past five years for pharmacological interventions not covered by the systematic reviews and meta-analyses already discussed.

Guidelines Recommendations for Pharmacological Treatment of Treatment-Resistant Depression

Guidelines to treat depression try to summarize the best evidence available systematically and translate it to clinicians to implement the evidence in clinical practice. This helps to provide the most effective and safe treatment in the real world [49]. Several guidelines are available to help clinicians in the pharmacological management of depression [49–53], and some are specific for TRD [54–56]. Malhi et al. recommend that, for partial and nonresponse, clinicians should first reevaluate the diagnosis and consider discussing with a colleague. The authors also suggest approaching the clinical situation by assessing predisposing, precipitating, perpetuating, and protective factors, psychological interventions, and lifestyle management [51]. Clinicians should also consider longer evaluation periods until response [52,57], and maybe direct more emphasis on functioning and quality of life rather than symptoms remission [52]. The Canadian Network for Mood and Anxiety Treatments (CANMAT)

publishes one of the most prestigious guidelines for treating depression. In the 2016 CANMAT for pharmacological treatments, the authors provide an algorithm for managing the inadequate response to an antidepressant, including switching to a second-line or third-line antidepressant, switching to an antidepressant with superior efficacy or adding an adjunctive medication. Among the options of adjunctive medication, the authors include aripiprazole, quetiapine, and risperidone as first-line and level I evidence. This guideline recommends considering an adjunctive medication when there have been two or more antidepressant trials, and there is less time to wait for a response (for instance, in the presence of more severe symptoms and more functional impairment) [52]. Specifically regarding TRD, Bennabi et al. published the French Association for Biological Psychiatry and Neuropsychopharmacology and the foundation Fonda Mental clinical guidelines, with detailed information about adjuvant treatments, minimal duration of the antidepressant trial, switching, combination, and add-on strategies. For instance, for treatment potentiation, the authors suggest as first intention lithium and quetiapine, and as a second intention, aripiprazole, lamotrigine, and tri-iodothyronine [54]. Caraci et al. describe strategies usually applied in the clinical practice of treating patients with TRD as increasing the dose, switching to another new antidepressant, a combination of two or more antidepressants, augmentation of the current medication, and finally the use of "innovative psychopharmacotherapy" as ketamine [18].

However, despite the usefulness and importance of guidelines in treating depression in clinical practice, their implementation is inadequately planned, reported, and measured, according to Lee et al. [49]. The authors reviewed the development and implementation of guidelines to treat depression and compared those from low-, middle-, and high-income countries to characterize their differences [49]. The authors found that many low- and lower-middle-income countries do not have clinical guidelines to treat depression, a multidisciplinary team authored the minority, and only 10% of low- and middle-income countries and 19% of high-income countries' guidelines provided plans to evaluate quality indicators or recommendation implementation. The authors suggest that narrowing the gap between guideline development and implementation should be a priority [49].

Table 19.1 Summary of randomized controlled trials for treatment-resistant depression published in the past five years (access date 5/12/2021)

Authors and year	Sample size	TRD criteria	Intervention	Mechanism of action	Comparison	Primary outcome	Main results
Dichtel et al., 2020 [84]	101 women	MADRS score ≥12, and current treatment with an antidepressant at an adequate dosage for at least 8 weeks	Adjunctive low-dose testosterone	Hormone's metabolite 5α-androstane-3α,17β-diol has GABAergic-related effects	Placebo	Changes in MADRS score at weeks 2 through 8	No statistical difference between the groups
Umbricht et al., 2020 [85]	357	MADRS scores ≥ 25 and CGI-Severity of Illness scale score ≥ 4, despite up to two adequate trials	Decoglurant	Selective metabotropic glutamate receptor type 2/3 (mGlu2/3) negative allosteric modulator	Placebo	Changes in the MADRS total score in six weeks	No significant differences between decoglurant and placebo
Popova et al, 2019 [86]	227	Nonresponse to one to five antidepressants in the current depressive episode	Intranasal esketamine combined with a newly initiated oral antidepressant	NMDA receptor antagonist	Placebo	Changes in the MADRS scores from baseline to day 28	Changes in MADRS scores with esketamine plus antidepressant were significantly greater than with antidepressant plus placebo
Palhano-Fontes et al., 2019 [87]	29	Inadequate responses to at least two antidepressant medications from different classes	Ayahuasca	Psychedelic with serotonin and sigma–1 receptors agonism and reversible monoamine oxidase inhibition properties	Placebo	Changes in the HAM-D scores from baseline to day seven	MADRS scores were significantly lower in the ayahuasca group and associated with significantly higher response rates
Daly et al, 2018 [88]	67	Inadequate response to two or more antidepressants with at least ne inadequate response in the current depression episode.	Intranasal esketamine	NMDA receptor antagonist	Placebo	Changes from baseline in MADRS total score from baseline to day eight	Superior efficacy of esketamine for all three twice-weekly doses (28 mg, 56 mg, and 84 mg)

Study	N	Inclusion criteria	Intervention	Mechanism	Control	Outcome	Results
Miyaoka et al., 2018 [89]	40	Inadequate or nonresponse to two or more 8-week trials with two different classes of antidepressants	Clostridium butyricum MIYAIRI 588 (CBM588)	It produces short-chain fatty acids that may have potential anti-inflammatory effects	Control	Mean change in HAMD–17 at the end of the 8-week trial	CBM588 was associated with significant decrease in median HAMD–17 scores. No serious adverse events were reported.
Mathew et al., 2017 [90]	104	Inadequate response to at least one but no greater than four adequate trials of an antidepressant	Riluzole	Inhibition of presynaptic release of glutamate	Placebo	Changes in the MADRS score during each 4-week phase of the trial	Differences between riluzole and placebo was not statistically significant
Husain et al., 2017 [91]	41	Failed to respond to at least two antidepressant treatments	Minocycline	Tetracycline antibiotic with anti-inflammatory, anti-oxidant, anti-apoptotic, and modulation of glutamate and monoamine neurotransmission properties	Minocycline added to TAU vs. TAU	Mean change in HAMD–17 scores from baseline to week 12	Large reduction in HAM-D scores and CGI scores in the minocycline group
Mehdi et al., 2017 [92]	12	Failure of clinical improvement after 6 weeks with an approved, clinically adequate dose of an antidepressant	Intravenous infusion of magnesium sulfate	Ca antagonist and a voltage-dependent blocker of the NMDA channel	Placebo (5% dextrose)	Changes were noted on the HAM-D scores 24 h post-treatment	No statistically significant differences between the groups
Sanacora et al., 2017 [93]	302	Inadequate response to three or more antidepressants	Adjunctive lanicemine (AZD6765) 50 mg or 100 mg	NMDA channel blocker	Placebo (saline)	Changes in MADRS total score from baseline to week 6	No differences compared to placebo

Abbreviations: Ca: calcium; CGI: Clinical Global Impressions; HAMD–17: Hamilton Depression Rating Scale; MADRS: Montgomery–Asberg Depression Rating Scale; NMDA: N-methyl-D-aspartate19.1; TAU: treatment as usual; TRD: treatment-resistant depression.

Pharmacological Interventions under Investigation for Treatment-Resistant Depression

Among the neurobiological targets that have been investigated for drug discovery in TRD, Caraci et al. include the glutamatergic system, inflammatory system, opioid system, cholinergic system, dopaminergic system, and neurotrophin signaling [18]. We searched for registered clinical trials with pharmacological interventions for TRD on clinicaltrials.gov to find ongoing studies active/not recruiting, not yet recruiting, or recruiting as accessed on May 17, 2021 [58]. Among the 83 studies found, 30 were interventional studies related to pharmacological interventions to TRD, including: aripiprazole, AXS-05 (dextromethorphan in combination with bupropion), dextromethorphan, esketamine, ethosuximide, fecal microbiota, 5-methoxy-N,N-dimethyltryptamine (5-MeO-DMT), ketamine, lithium, minocycline, propofol, quetiapine, salicylic acid, simvastatin, tianeptine, TS-161, and psilocybin.

Regarding the pharmacological properties of these drugs under investigation for TRD, TS-161 is a metabotropic glutamate receptor modulator [59], and dextromethorphan is a weak antagonist of the NMDA receptor [60]. The combination of dextromethorphan with bupropion (AXS-05) is associated with a synergistic therapeutic effect [60,61]. In addition to acting through the norepinephrine transporter (NET) and dopamine transporter (DAT), bupropion inhibits cytochrome P450 2D6 (CYP450 2D6), which rapidly metabolizes dextromethorphan [61]. Ethosuximide is an anticonvulsant used in the management of absence epilepsy, which mechanism of action consists of blocking low-voltage-sensitive T-type calcium channels [62], a property that may have rapid antidepressant effects [63]. Gut microbiota transplantation from mice submitted to unpredictable chronic mild stress is associated with a reduction in adult hippocampal neurogenesis and induction of depressive-like behaviors, effects mediated by the endocannabinoid system [64]. In the opposite direction, the restoration of gut microbiota by the transplantation of fecal microbiota from a healthy donor can improve depressive symptoms, which the regulation of astrocyte dysfunction via circular RNA HIPK2 may be one of the mechanisms involved [65,66]. The 5-MeO-DMT is a serotoninergic psychedelic with anti-inflammatory activity, for instance, inhibiting the secretion of IL-1β, IL-6, and TNFα and increasing IL-10 levels [67]. The administration of 5-MeO-DMT has also been associated with increased dentate gyrus cell proliferation in a preclinical study, which may be related to its antidepressant properties [68]. Psilocybin (phosphoryloxy-N,N-dimethyltryptamine) is another psychedelic that affects serotoninergic signaling and increases striatal dopamine concentration via 5-HT1A receptor activation and in the amygdala reduces neural response to negative stimuli [69]. Propofol is an intravenous anesthetic agent with GABA-A agonism activity and affinity at the NMDA receptor, with demonstrated antidepressant-like effects in preclinical studies [70,71]. The use of salicylic acid, an inhibitor of the activity of the enzyme cyclooxygenase (COX) [72], was associated with a lower rate of depression in a cohort study with 316,904 individuals [73]. In an animal model of depression, salicylic acid was associated with depressive-like behavior improvement alongside decreased serum cortisol and increased brain serotonin levels [74]. Simvastatin is an HMG-CoA reductase inhibitor with antidepressant effects demonstrated in preclinical studies. For instance, Wu et al. showed that simvastatin administered to mice was able to attenuate depressive-like behavior and to reduce the overexpression of pro-inflammatory cytokines in the hippocampus, neuronal injury, and serotoninergic system dysfunction induced by the model of depression [75]. Tianeptine is associated with pre-synaptic serotonin uptake and affects NMDA and AMPA receptors, which has been related to its antidepressant properties [76,77].

Predictors of Treatment Response

One of the biggest challenges in clinical practice is identifying which treatment would best fit an individual patient. The trial-and-error treatment approach can be frustrating for both clinicians and patients, compromising adherence and exposing the patients to more prolonged periods with disabling symptoms. Another critical issue is the ideal period of time clinicians should wait for symptoms remission until they opt to change the therapeutic strategy. Henssler et al. addressed this question by investigating trajectories of acute antidepressant efficacy through a systematic review of randomized, double-blind placebo-controlled trials [57]. The authors found that despite no further increase in response rates expected after 12 weeks, compared to placebo, after 12 weeks the response rates for the active treatment were significantly higher (OR = 2.25, CI 95%: 1.58–3.19). However, between 9 and 12 weeks, the probability of achieving response and remission among nonresponders and nonremitters with the active treatment is 10% (response) and 14% (remission) [57]. Thus, it is reasonable to state that if the patient does not present a remission in up to 12 weeks of the initiation of the trial, most probably the clinician should consider another strategy.

Although applicable to predict adverse effects, pharmacogenetic tests are still not helpful in predicting treatment outcomes as response or remission [78,79]. However, it is possible that pharmacogenomic information could help to improve the predictive power of treatment outcomes that some studies have demonstrated, for instance, with neurobiological data and with machine learning techniques. For example, with a combination of machine learning with a Personalized Advantage Index, Webb et al. investigated whether it is possible to identify the most appropriate treatment for patients with depression. The authors found that individuals with older age, employed, with less cognitive control impairment, higher neuroticism, and depressive symptoms would present better outcomes with sertraline than placebo [80]. Another study with machine learning evaluated the predictive power of electroencephalographic data (EEG) for treatment outcomes with escitalopram. The results showed that baseline data had an accuracy for treatment response (50% decreased Montgomery–Asberg Depression Rating Scale [MADRS] scores in week 8 of the treatment) of 79.2% (67.3% sensitivity and 91% specificity). This accuracy was optimized to 82.4% (79.2% sensitivity and 85.5% specificity) when data of week 2 were added to the model [81]. Electroencephalographic data and a machine learning algorithm were also able to predict treatment response to sertraline in another study, findings that were validated in three independent samples of individuals with depression [82]. The authors also showed that the EEG predictive signature was different between sertraline and transcranial magnetic stimulation treatments, suggesting that EEG data could help in the identification of which treatment is more appropriate for specific individuals [82,83].

Conclusion

Pharmacological interventions are the mainstream of TRD. Considering the most common classification of TRD, individuals with treatment resistance to two or more trials in adequate dose and duration are at higher risk of worse outcomes, including mortality. Several guidelines provide algorithms that can help clinicians to manage TRD. However, more research is necessary to evaluate how these guidelines have been implemented and their effectiveness in the "real world". Numerous pharmacological interventions are under investigation for TRD, especially targeting the immune, serotoninergic, and glutamatergic systems. At the same time, findings from studies using advanced computational analyses combining clinical and neurobiological data to predict treatment response give hope that the trial-and-error approach will one day be replaced by a more effective and personalized procedure to identify the proper treatment for an individual patient.

References

1. Haskovec L, Rysanek K. The action of reserpine in imipramine-resistant depressive patients. Clinical and biochemical study. *Psychopharmacologia*. 1967;**11**(1):18–30.

2. Drago F, Motta A, Grossi E. Intravenous maprotiline in severe and resistant primary depression: a double-blind comparison with clomipramine. *J Int Med Res*. 1983;**11**(2):78–84.

3. Decker HS. *The Making of DSM-III: A Diagnostic Manual's Conquest of American Psychiatry*. New York: Oxford University Press, 2013.

4. Hardy P. [Concept of resistant depression]. *Encephale*. 1986;**12**:Spec No:191–6.

5. Malhi GS, Byrow Y. Is treatment-resistant depression a useful concept? *Evid Based Ment Health*. 2016;**19**(1):1–3.

6. Rybak YE, Lai KSP, Ramasubbu R, et al. et al. Treatment-resistant major depressive disorder: Canadian expert consensus on definition and assessment. *Depress Anxiety*. 2021;**38**(4):456–67.

7. Dodd S, Bauer M, Carvalho AF, et al. A clinical approach to treatment resistance in depressed patients: what to do when the usual treatments don't work well enough? *World J Biol Psychiatry*. 2021;**22**(7):483–94.

8. National Institute of Mental Health. Major depression. 2017. Available from: www.nimh.nih.gov/health/statistics/major-depression.

9. Gronemann FH, Petersen J, Alulis S, et al. Treatment patterns in patients with treatment-resistant depression in Danish patients with major depressive disorder. *J Affect Disord*. 2021;**287**:204–13.

10. Gaynes BN, Warden D, Trivedi MH, et al. What did STAR*D teach us? Results from a large-scale, practical, clinical trial for patients with depression. *Psychiatr Serv*. 2009;**60**(11):1439–45.

11. Gaynes BN, Rush AJ, Trivedi MH, et al. The STAR*D study: treating depression in the real world. *Cleve Clin J Med*. 2008;**75**(1):57–66.

12. Mojtabai R. Nonremission and time to remission among remitters in major depressive disorder: revisiting STAR*D. *Depress Anxiety*. 2017;**34**(12):1123–33.

13. Thomas L, Kessler D, Campbell J, et al. Prevalence of treatment-resistant depression in primary care: cross-sectional data. *Br J Gen Pract*. 2013;**63**(617):e852-8.

14. Zhdanava M, Pilon D, Ghelerter I, et al. The prevalence and national burden of treatment-resistant depression and major depressive disorder in the United States. *J Clin Psychiatry*. 2021;**82**(2).

15. Madsen KB, Plana-Ripoll O, Musliner KL, et al. Cause-specific life years lost in individuals with treatment-resistant depression: a Danish nationwide register-based cohort study. *J Affect Disord*. 2021;**280**(Pt A):250–7.

16. Gronemann FH, Jorgensen MB, Nordentoft M, Andersen PK, Osler M. Treatment-resistant depression and risk of all-cause mortality and suicidality in Danish patients with major depression. *J Psychiatr Res*. 2021;**135**:197–202.

17. Brenner P, Reutfors J, Nijs M, Andersson TM. Excess deaths in treatment-resistant depression. *Ther Adv Psychopharmacol*. 2021;**11**:20451253211006508.

18. Caraci F, Calabrese F, Molteni R, et al. International Union of Basic and Clinical Pharmacology CIV: the neurobiology of treatment-resistant depression: from antidepressant classifications to novel pharmacological targets. *Pharmacol Rev*. 2018;**70**(3):475–504.

19. Ceruso A, Martinez-Cengotitabengoa M, Peters-Corbett A, Diaz-Gutierrez MJ, Martinez-Cengotitabengoa M. Alterations of the HPA axis observed in patients with major depressive disorder and their relation to early life stress: a systematic review. *Neuropsychobiology*. 2020;**79**(6):417–27.

20. LeMoult J, Humphreys KL, Tracy A, et al. Meta-analysis: exposure to early life stress and risk for depression in childhood and adolescence. *J Am Acad Child Adolesc Psychiatry*. 2020;**59**(7):842–55.

21. Juruena MF, Cleare AJ, Papadopoulos AS, et al. Different responses to dexamethasone and prednisolone in the same depressed patients. *Psychopharmacology (Berl)*. 2006;**189**(2):225–35.

22. Allen AP, Naughton M, Dowling J, et al. Kynurenine pathway metabolism and the neurobiology of treatment-resistant depression: comparison of multiple ketamine infusions and electroconvulsive therapy. *J Psychiatr Res*. 2018;**100**:24–32.

23. Fabbri C, Corponi F, Albani D, et al. Pleiotropic genes in psychiatry: calcium channels and the stress-related FKBP5 gene in antidepressant resistance. *Prog Neuropsychopharmacol Biol Psychiatry*. 2018;**81**:203–10.

24. Fabbri C, Marsano A, Albani D, et al. PPP3CC gene: a putative modulator of antidepressant response through the B-cell receptor signaling pathway. *Pharmacogenomics J*. 2014;**14**(5):463–72.

25. Zarate CA Jr, Singh JB, Carlson PJ, et al. A randomized trial of an N-methyl-D-aspartate antagonist in treatment-resistant major depression. *Arch Gen Psychiatry*. 2006;**63**(8):856–64.

26. Marcantoni WS, Akoumba BS, Wassef M, et al. A systematic review and meta-analysis of the efficacy of intravenous ketamine infusion for treatment resistant depression: January 2009–January 2019. *J Affect Disord*. 2020;**277**:831–41.

27. Carlson PJ, Diazgranados N, Nugent AC, et al. Neural correlates of rapid antidepressant response to ketamine in treatment-resistant unipolar depression: a preliminary positron emission tomography study. *Biol Psychiatry*. 2013;**73**(12):1213–21.

28. Kadriu B, Musazzi L, Henter ID, et al. Glutamatergic neurotransmission: pathway to developing novel rapid-acting antidepressant treatments. *Int J Neuropsychopharmacol*. 2019;**22**(2):119–35.

29. Du J, Machado-Vieira R, Maeng S, et al. Enhancing AMPA to NMDA throughput as a convergent mechanism for antidepressant action. *Drug Discov Today Ther Strateg*. 2006;**3**(4):519–26.

30. Pizzagalli DA. Depression, stress, and anhedonia: toward a synthesis and integrated model. *Annu Rev Clin Psychol*. 2014;**10**:393–423.

31. Sternat T, Katzman MA. Neurobiology of hedonic tone: the relationship between treatment-resistant depression, attention-deficit hyperactivity disorder, and substance abuse. *Neuropsychiatr Dis Treat*. 2016;**12**:2149–64.

32. McMakin DL, Olino TM, Porta G, et al. Anhedonia predicts poorer recovery among youth with selective serotonin reuptake inhibitor treatment-resistant depression. *J Am Acad Child Adolesc Psychiatry*. 2012;**51**(4):404–11.

33. Iob E, Kirschbaum C, Steptoe A. Persistent depressive symptoms, HPA-axis hyperactivity, and inflammation: the role of cognitive-affective and somatic symptoms. *Mol Psychiatry*. 2020;**25**(5):1130–40.

34. Edwards SJ, Hamilton V, Nherera L, Trevor N. Lithium or an atypical antipsychotic drug in the

management of treatment-resistant depression: a systematic review and economic evaluation. *Health Technol Assess*. 2013;**17**(54):1–190.

35. Nelson JC, Baumann P, Delucchi K, Joffe R, Katona C. A systematic review and meta-analysis of lithium augmentation of tricyclic and second generation antidepressants in major depression. *J Affect Disord*. 2014;**168**:269–75.

36. Zhou X, Keitner GI, Qin B, et al. Atypical antipsychotic augmentation for treatment-resistant depression: a systematic review and network meta-analysis. *Int J Neuropsychopharmacol*. 2015;**18**(11): pyv060.

37. Zhou X, Ravindran AV, Qin B, et al. Comparative efficacy, acceptability, and tolerability of augmentation agents in treatment-resistant depression: systematic review and network meta-analysis. *J Clin Psychiatry*. 2015;**76**(4):e487-98.

38. Luan S, Wan H, Zhang L, Zhao H. Efficacy, acceptability, and safety of adjunctive aripiprazole in treatment-resistant depression: a meta-analysis of randomized controlled trials. *Neuropsychiatr Dis Treat*. 2018;**14**:467–77.

39. Citrome L, Ota A, Nagamizu K, et al. The effect of brexpiprazole (OPC-34712) and aripiprazole in adult patients with acute schizophrenia: results from a randomized, exploratory study. *Int Clin Psychopharmacol*. 2016;**31**(4):192–201.

40. Kishi T, Sakuma K, Nomura I, et al. Brexpiprazole as adjunctive treatment for major depressive disorder following treatment failure with at least one antidepressant in the current episode: a systematic review and meta-analysis. *Int J Neuropsychopharmacol*. 2019;**22**(11):698–709.

41. Skelin I, Fikre-Merid M, Diksic M. Both acute and subchronic treatments with pindolol, a 5-HT(1A) and beta(1) and beta(2) adrenoceptor antagonist, elevate regional serotonin synthesis in the rat brain: an autoradiographic study. *Neurochem Int*. 2012;**61**(8):1417–23.

42. Artigas F, Celada P, Laruelle M, Adell A. How does pindolol improve antidepressant action? *Trends Pharmacol Sci*. 2001;**22**(5):224–8.

43. Liu Y, Zhou X, Zhu D, et al. Is pindolol augmentation effective in depressed patients resistant to selective serotonin reuptake inhibitors? A systematic review and meta-analysis. *Hum Psychopharmacol*. 2015;**30**(3):132–42.

44. Luan S, Wan H, Wang S, Li H, Zhang B. Efficacy and safety of olanzapine/fluoxetine combination in the treatment of treatment-resistant depression: a meta-analysis of randomized controlled trials. *Neuropsychiatr Dis Treat*. 2017;**13**:609–20.

45. Bavaresco DV, Uggioni MLR, Ferraz SD, et al. Efficacy of infliximab in treatment-resistant depression: a systematic review and meta-analysis. *Pharmacol Biochem Behav*. 2020;**188**:172838.

46. Kryst J, Kawalec P, Mitoraj AM, et al. Efficacy of single and repeated administration of ketamine in unipolar and bipolar depression: a meta-analysis of randomized clinical trials. *Pharmacol Rep*. 2020;**72**(3):543–62.

47. Papadimitropoulou K, Vossen C, Karabis A, Donatti C, Kubitz N. Comparative efficacy and tolerability of pharmacological and somatic interventions in adult patients with treatment-resistant depression: a systematic review and network meta-analysis. *Curr Med Res Opin*. 2017;**33**(4):701–11.

48. Davies P, Ijaz S, Williams CJ, et al. Pharmacological interventions for treatment-resistant depression in adults. *Cochrane Database Syst Rev*. 2019;**12**: CD010557.

49. Lee Y, Brietzke E, Cao B, et al. Development and implementation of guidelines for the management of depression: a systematic review. *Bull World Health Organ*. 2020;**98**(10):683-97 H.

50. Simons P, Cosgrove L, Shaughnessy AF, Bursztajn H. Antipsychotic augmentation for major depressive disorder: a review of clinical practice guidelines. Int J Law Psychiatry. 2017;**55**:64–71.

51. Malhi GS, Hitching R, Berk M, et al. Pharmacological management of unipolar depression. *Acta Psychiatr Scand Suppl*. 2013(443):6–23.

52. Kennedy SH, Lam RW, McIntyre RS, et al. Canadian Network for Mood and Anxiety Treatments (CANMAT) 2016 Clinical Guidelines for the Management of Adults with Major Depressive Disorder: Section 3. *Pharmacological Treatments*. *Can J Psychiatry*. 2016;**61**(9):540–60.

53. Bauer M, Severus E, Moller HJ, Young AH, Disorders WTFoUD. Pharmacological treatment of unipolar depressive disorders: summary of WFSBP guidelines. *Int J Psychiatry Clin Pract*. 2017;**21**(3):166–76.

54. Bennabi D, Charpeaud T, Yrondi A, et al. Clinical guidelines for the management of treatment-resistant depression: French recommendations from experts, the French Association for Biological Psychiatry and Neuropsychopharmacology and the Foundation FondaMental. *BMC Psychiatry*. 2019;**19**(1):262.

55. Dold M, Kasper S. Evidence-based pharmacotherapy of treatment-resistant unipolar depression. *Int J Psychiatry Clin Pract*. 2017;**21**(1):13–23.

56. MacQueen G, Santaguida P, Keshavarz H, et al. Systematic review of clinical practice guidelines for failed antidepressant treatment response in major depressive disorder, dysthymia, and subthreshold

depression in adults. *Can J Psychiatry*. 2017;**62**(1):11–23.

57. Henssler J, Kurschus M, Franklin J, Bschor T, Baethge C. Trajectories of acute antidepressant efficacy: how long to wait for response? A systematic review and meta-analysis of long-term, placebo-controlled acute treatment trials. *J Clin Psychiatry*. 2018;**79**(3).

58. National institutes of Health. Recruiting studies | treatment resistant depression. 2021. Available from: https://clinicaltrials.gov/ct2/results?cond=Treatment+Resistant+Depression&Search=Apply&recrs=a&age_v=&gndr=&type=&rslt=.

59. Henter ID, Park LT, Zarate CA Jr. Novel glutamatergic modulators for the treatment of mood disorders: current status. *CNS Drugs*. 2021;**35**(5):527–43.

60. Wilkinson ST, Sanacora G. A new generation of antidepressants: an update on the pharmaceutical pipeline for novel and rapid-acting therapeutics in mood disorders based on glutamate/GABA neurotransmitter systems. *Drug Discov Today*. 2019;**24**(2):606–15.

61. Stahl SM. Dextromethorphan/bupropion: a novel oral NMDA (N-methyl-d-aspartate) receptor antagonist with multimodal activity. *CNS Spectr*. 2019;**24**(5):461–6.

62. Hanrahan B, Carson RP. *Ethosuximide*. Treasure Island, FL: StatPearls Publishing, 2021.

63. Yang Y, Cui Y, Sang K, et al. Ketamine blocks bursting in the lateral habenula to rapidly relieve depression. *Nature*. 2018;**554**(7692):317–22.

64. Chevalier G, Siopi E, Guenin-Mace L, et al. Effect of gut microbiota on depressive-like behaviors in mice is mediated by the endocannabinoid system. *Nat Commun*. 2020;**11**(1):6363.

65. Chinna Meyyappan A, Forth E, Wallace CJK, Milev R. Effect of fecal microbiota transplant on symptoms of psychiatric disorders: a systematic review. *BMC Psychiatry*. 2020;**20**(1):299.

66. Zhang Y, Huang R, Cheng M, et al. Gut microbiota from NLRP3-deficient mice ameliorates depressive-like behaviors by regulating astrocyte dysfunction via circHIPK2. *Microbiome*. 2019;**7**(1):116.

67. Szabo A. Psychedelics and immunomodulation: novel approaches and therapeutic opportunities. *Front Immunol*. 2015;**6**:358.

68. Lima da Cruz RV, Moulin TC, Petiz LL, Leao RN. A single dose of 5-MeO-DMT stimulates cell proliferation, neuronal survivability, morphological and functional changes in adult mice ventral dentate gyrus. *Front Mol Neurosci*. 2018;**11**:312.

69. Vollenweider FX, Preller KH. Psychedelic drugs: neurobiology and potential for treatment of psychiatric disorders. *Nat Rev Neurosci*. 2020;**21**(11):611–24.

70. Daniel DG, Daniel NG, Daniel DT, Flynn LC, Allen MH. The effect of propofol on a forced swim test in mice at 24 hours. *Curr Ther Res Clin Exp*. 2020;**92**:100590.

71. Daniel DG, Daniel NG, Daniel DT, Flynn LC, Allen MH. The effect of acutely administered propofol on forced swim test outcomes in mice. *Innov Clin Neurosci*. 2019;**16**(9–10):22–6.

72. Vane JR, Botting RM. The mechanism of action of aspirin. *Thromb Res*. 2003;**110**(5–6):255–8.

73. Hu K, Sjolander A, Lu D, et al. Aspirin and other non-steroidal anti-inflammatory drugs and depression, anxiety, and stress-related disorders following a cancer diagnosis: a nationwide register-based cohort study. *BMC Med*. 2020;**18**(1):238.

74. Bhatt S, Pundarikakshudu K, Patel P, et al. Beneficial effect of aspirin against interferon-alpha-2b-induced depressive behavior in Sprague Dawley rats. *Clin Exp Pharmacol Physiol*. 2016;**43**(12):1208–15.

75. Wu H, Lv W, Pan Q, et al. Simvastatin therapy in adolescent mice attenuates HFD-induced depression-like behavior by reducing hippocampal neuroinflammation. *J Affect Disord*. 2019;**243**:83–95.

76. Wilde MI, Benfield P. Tianeptine. A review of its pharmacodynamic and pharmacokinetic properties, and therapeutic efficacy in depression and coexisting anxiety and depression. *Drugs*. 1995;**49**(3):411–39.

77. Wlaz P, Kasperek R, Wlaz A, et al. NMDA and AMPA receptors are involved in the antidepressant-like activity of tianeptine in the forced swim test in mice. *Pharmacol Rep*. 2011;**63**(6):1526–32.

78. Zeier Z, Carpenter LL, Kalin NH, et al. Clinical implementation of pharmacogenetic decision support tools for antidepressant drug prescribing. *Am J Psychiatry*. 2018;**175**(9):873–86.

79. Zubenko GS, Sommer BR, Cohen BM. On the marketing and use of pharmacogenetic tests for psychiatric treatment. *JAMA Psychiatry*. 2018;**75**(8):769–70.

80. Webb CA, Trivedi MH, Cohen ZD, et al. Personalized prediction of antidepressant v. placebo response: evidence from the EMBARC study. *Psychol Med*. 2019;**49**(7):1118–27.

81. Zhdanov A, Atluri S, Wong W, et al. Use of machine learning for predicting escitalopram treatment outcome from electroencephalography recordings in adult patients with depression. *JAMA Netw Open*. 2020;**3**(1):e1918377.

82. Wu W, Zhang Y, Jiang J, et al. An electroencephalographic signature predicts

antidepressant response in major depression. *Nat Biotechnol.* 2020;**38**(4):439–47.

83. Michel CM, Pascual-Leone A. Predicting antidepressant response by electroencephalography. *Nat Biotechnol.* 2020;**38**(4):417–9.

84. Dichtel LE, Carpenter LL, Nyer M, et al. Low-dose testosterone augmentation for antidepressant-resistant major depressive disorder in women: an 8-week randomized placebo-controlled study. *Am J Psychiatry.* 2020;**177**(10):965–73.

85. Umbricht D, Niggli M, Sanwald-Ducray P, et al. randomized, double-blind, placebo-controlled trial of the mGlu2/3 negative allosteric modulator decoglurant in partially refractory major depressive disorder. *J Clin Psychiatry.* 2020;**81**(4).

86. Popova V, Daly DJ, Trivedi M, et al. Efficacy and safety of flexibly dosed esketamine nasal spray combined with a newly initiated oral antidepressant in treatment-resistant depression: a randomized double-blind active-controlled study. *Am J Psychiatry.* 2019;**176**(6):428–38.

87. Palhano-Fontes F, Barreto D, Onias H, et al. Rapid antidepressant effects of the psychedelic ayahuasca in treatment-resistant depression: a randomized placebo-controlled trial. *Psychol Med.* 2019;**49**(4):655–63.

88. Daly EJ, Singh JB, Fedgchin M, et al. Efficacy and safety of intranasal esketamine adjunctive to oral antidepressant therapy in treatment-resistant depression: a randomized clinical trial. *JAMA Psychiatry.* 2018;**75**(2):139–48.

89. Miyaoka T, Kanayama M, Wake R, et al. Clostridium butyricum MIYAIRI 588 as adjunctive therapy for treatment-resistant major depressive disorder: a prospective open-label trial. *Clin Neuropharmacol.* 2018;**41**(5):151–5.

90. Mathew SJ, Gueorguieva R, Brandt C, Fava M, Sanacora G. A randomized, double-blind, placebo-controlled, sequential parallel comparison design trial of adjunctive riluzole for treatment-resistant major depressive disorder. *Neuropsychopharmacology.* 2017;**42**(13):2567–74.

91. Husain MI, Chaudhry IB, Husain N, et al. Minocycline as an adjunct for treatment-resistant depressive symptoms: a pilot randomised placebo-controlled trial. *J Psychopharmacol.* 2017;**31**(9):1166–75.

92. Mehdi SM, Atlas SE, Qadir S, et al. Double-blind, randomized crossover study of intravenous infusion of magnesium sulfate versus 5% dextrose on depressive symptoms in adults with treatment-resistant depression. *Psychiatry Clin Neurosci.* 2017;**71**(3):204–11.

93. Sanacora G, Johnson MR, Khan A, et al. Adjunctive lanicemine (AZD6765) in patients with major depressive disorder and history of inadequate response to antidepressants: a randomized, placebo-controlled study. *Neuropsychopharmacology.* 2017;**42**(4):844–53.

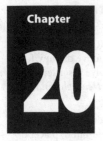

Chapter 20

An Update on the Treatment of Manic and Hypomanic States

Sameer Jauhar and Sui Liem Alexandre Wong

Introduction

Bipolar disorder is a relapsing/remitting illness with a degree of symptomatic and functional recovery between episodes [1]. As defined by both the *International Classification of Disorders 11th Revision* (ICD-11), and the *Diagnostic and Statistical Manual of Mental Disorders*, 5th edition (DSM-5), a diagnosis of bipolar disorder type I requires at least one episode of mania, whilst a diagnosis of bipolar disorder type II requires at least one hypomanic episode and at least one depressive episode [2,3].

With an estimated global lifetime prevalence between 0.6 to 1.0% for bipolar type I and between 0.4 to 1.1% for bipolar type II [4], bipolar disorder is a leading cause of disability amongst young people with wide-reaching effects across personal, social, and occupational functioning [5]. Not only does it carry significant economic burden – total annual cost of bipolar type I in the United States alone has been estimated to be in excess of US$200 billion [6] when direct costs (e.g., medical and pharmacy) and indirect costs (e.g., loss of occupational productivity) are combined – it carries significant mortality, with up to 12 years of life expectancy lost for those diagnosed between 25 and 45 years old [7].

In the ICD-11 and DSM-5, the definitions of mania and hypomania are nearly identical. Mania without psychosis is defined as, at its core, an abnormally elevated mood state, irritability, and a subjective sense of increased energy or overactivity, lasting at least one week or to the extent that a hospital admission is required. In addition, there must be several (ICD-11) or at least three (DSM-5) of the following classical symptoms: rapid or pressured speech, flight of ideas, a decreased need for sleep, an inflated self-esteem or grandiosity, impulsive or reckless behaviour, an increase in sexual drive or sociability, and marked distractibility resulting in poorly sustained attention [5]. There should also be an accompanied marked impairment in one's level of social and occupational functioning.

In mania with psychosis, symptoms as listed above are more pronounced. Common psychotic symptoms include delusions of grandeur; delusions of persecution; rapid speech and flight of ideas may present in the context of formal thought disorder; there may be evidence of abnormal perceptions, in particular mood-congruent auditory hallucinations; and there will invariably be lack of insight. It should be noted that, although psychotic symptoms in affective disorder can be differentiated from those in nonaffective disorder [8], people with mania can present with first rank symptoms.

Considered a less severe form of mania, hypomania is defined as a persistently elevated mood state lasting several days (ICD-11) or at least four days (DSM-5) together with irritability, increased activity, and a subjective sense of increased energy, accompanied by other classical symptoms such as racing thoughts, rapid speech, decreased need for sleep, elevated self-esteem, increased sociability or overfamiliarity, distractibility, or impulsive behaviours. Importantly, these symptoms must not be severe enough to warrant a hospital admission or cause marked disruption to normal social and occupational functioning, and psychotic symptoms must not be present; otherwise, a diagnosis of mania should be considered.

General Treatment Principles

Assessment

When assessing an acutely unwell patient, the identification and management of risks will likely be at the forefront of most clinicians' minds. In the case of those experiencing a manic episode, the associated risks are often difficult to fully and adequately contain, even in a hospital environment, let alone the community. Impulsive and reckless behaviours can be prominent and pose significant risk both to the patient and to those around them. Reckless behaviours may include driving dangerously or making potentially life-altering financial decisions without due diligence. Uncharacteristic sexual promiscuity leaves the patient vulnerable to exploitation and engaging in sexual encounters they may not ordinarily agree to; it would also put them at risk of sexually transmitted infections. Irritability and persecutory ideas may merge and manifest as aggression towards others, which in turn may put them at risk of retaliatory violence. Delusions of grandeur, impulsivity, and overactivity in combination may lead the patient to accidental harm or even death by misadventure, if, for example, they believed themselves to be immortal or to possess the power of flight. A significantly reduced need for sleep is often accompanied by reduced appetite and when persistent are likely to pose a risk to physical health by means of exhaustion and dehydration. A lack of insight significantly increases risk of poor engagement with services and poor adherence with treatment. These are some of the risks associated with a manic episode and whilst not an exhaustive list, they demonstrate the wide variety of sources that risks can arise from and the difficulty faced by clinicians attempting to treat acute mania in the community. The first consideration when assessing acute mania, therefore, should be whether an admission into hospital is necessary for the person's own health, for their own safety, or for the safety of others.

It should be considered early on whether the patient's acute presentation may have an organic or iatrogenic component, or whether concurrent medical problems may complicate treatment. A physical examination with laboratory testing should be offered, but in many cases they are not tolerated and may be postponed. An electrocardiogram should be offered, particularly if it is foreseeable that pharmacological therapy will be imminently required. A pregnancy test should be considered in women of childbearing age. Abrupt onset mania with neurological signs should prompt further investigations such as brain imaging and a lumbar puncture under the care of a physician.

Substance misuse should be explored, in particular the use of stimulants, and any physiological withdrawal symptoms should be managed. Systemic steroids for inflammatory disorders may have to be discontinued with guidance from the prescribing physician. Endocrine disorders, such as hyperthyroidism, should be tested for and treated if present, and those with a history of cardiovascular, hepatic, or renal diseases may not be suitable for certain pharmacological treatments, or may require closer monitoring. Existing antidepressant therapy should be discontinued.

Treatment

The treatment of mania in modern practice is predominantly pharmacological, with the aim of rapidly controlling any agitation, distress, aggression, and impulsivity, which are the driving force behind much of mania's associated risks.

Nonpharmacological

Consideration should be given to lower environmental stimulation, which may ease any agitation or distress. Though it may be challenging in the case of severe mania, a strong therapeutic alliance should be established early on, as this helps maintain adherence to treatment [9]. Attempts should be made to explain the current situation at hand and the patient should be involved as much as feasibly possible with regard to treatment decisions which should be tailored to each individual according to their specific clinical presentation, past history, and needs. Any advanced treatment plan whilst they were well and capacious should be respected, except in extraordinary circumstances. In most cases, the patient's family should be involved and kept updated, unless there is good reason not to, such as suspicion of abuse or exploitation, or the person had previously stated certain family members were not to be contacted. Psychoeducation, both during and following the acute episode, should focus on addressing the different experiences and expectations that each party brings in, whilst making use of the available evidence to highlight the nature of bipolar disorder, the risks and benefits of treatment, and reducing the likelihood of future relapses.

Treatment of Acute Mania and Hypomania

In the absence of adequate evidence, hypomania should be treated similarly to mania; in general, hypomania is likely to require relatively lower doses of psychotropic medication. Whilst the neurobiological pathophysiology of mania is not fully understood, it is generally accepted to be a hyper-dopaminergic state [10]; it follows that the mainstay of pharmacological treatment revolves around blockade of D_2 and D_3 receptors. Mood stabilisers, namely lithium, sodium valproate, and carbamazepine, also have an important role [11,12]. This is reflected by their recommendations as first-line agents found in multiple international guidelines such as the International College of Neuropsychopharmacology (CINP [13], which suggest valproate as a first-line option) and the Canadian Network for Mood and Anxiety Treatments (CANMAT [14], which suggest both lithium and valproate as first-line options). Notably, network meta-analysis ranks their efficacy below that of dopamine antagonists / partial agonists [15], which may have contributed to them being slightly less favoured in other guidelines, such as the British Association for Psychopharmacology (BAP) [16]. In addition to anti-manic agents, sedatives and anxiolytics are also utilised as aids to restore sleep and calm episodes of acute behavioural disturbance or agitation.

There is currently no evidence to support the efficacy of psychotherapy in the treatment of acute mania [16,17]. This is unsurprising given the inherently chaotic and distractible mental state invariably seen in acute mania, making any sustained and focused conversation required for effective psychotherapy near impossible.

For those presenting to psychiatric services with mania and who are psychotropic-naïve, there is generally good consensus amongst international and national guidelines [13,14,16,18,19,20] for trials with one of the following agents as first-line treatment:

First-line agents Ranges of typical effective daily dose

- Aripiprazole 15–30 mg
- Asenapine 10–20 mg
- Cariprazine 3–12 mg
- Haloperidol 5 – 20 mg
- Olanzapine 10–20 mg
- Paliperidone 3–12 mg
- Quetiapine 400–800 mg
- Risperidone 2–6 mg
- Lithium 600–1,200 mg (will depend on serum lithium levels)
- Divalproex 1,000–2,000 mg

The general efficacy of the above treatments is broadly similar (Cohen's d = 0.32–0.66; effect size between small and medium) [21]; the decision of which of these first-line agents to prescribe will therefore be guided by other aspects that ought to be considered, such as tolerability, teratogenicity, need for monitoring, and the patient's clinical presentation. A response should generally be expected within one to two weeks.

Of the list of first-line agents above, cariprazine is the latest addition, having been approved by the US Food and Drug Administration (FDA) for treatment of acute mania and mixed mania in September 2015. In May 2019, cariprazine was also approved by the FDA for treatment of bipolar depression, becoming the third agent to be approved for treatment of bipolar disorder across illness poles from depression to mania [22]. It is a dopamine-serotonin partial agonist which binds to D_3 dopamine, D_2 dopamine, and $5HT_{2B}$ serotonin receptors with high potency. Meta-analysis indicates cariprazine is comparable to other more established second-generation antipsychotics (SGAs) in treatment of mania, and that it was not associated with treatment discontinuation due to adverse effects, suggesting it may be better tolerated than aripiprazole [23], whilst producing statistically significant improvements across all 11 items in the Young Mania Rating Scale [24].

Olanzapine has recently had its status as a first-line agent downgraded to second-line in a number of international guidelines [13,14,16] despite evidence for its efficacy in acute mania. This is predominantly a result of concerns over its long-term tolerability and effects on metabolism. Whilst these concerns are well-founded, its potent anxiolytic effect remains very valuable in the acute phase of mania; it can be argued that olanzapine could remain a first-line treatment with the singular aim of achieving euthymia, after which it can be switched to a better tolerated option for long-term maintenance therapy.

Monotherapy with one of the above listed agents is a viable option which can be effective for some patients [22]. First-line combination options primarily include a mood stabiliser (either lithium or sodium valproate) combined with one of the second-generation antipsychotics listed above (aripiprazole, asenapine, olanzapine, quetiapine, or risperidone). There is good evidence to support the superior efficacy of combination therapy over monotherapy, with 20% more people showing response, particularly in those with more severe illness [25,26]. This is with the exception of paliperidone, which at the time of writing lacks evidence supporting its efficacy in combination therapy [14].

In the event of inadequate response with a first-line treatment, dosing should be reviewed and, if tolerated, gradually increased to the maximum licenced dose. Adherence to medication should be reviewed, as should contributing factors such as substance misuse. In the absence of any such factors, those with inadequate clinical response should have their treatment switched to another first-line agent. Treatment with second- and third-line agents, listed below, should only be considered following unsuccessful trials of multiple first-line agents.

Second-line agents

- Carbamezapine
- Ziprasidone
- Electroconvulsive therapy

These agents are recommended as second-line despite their proven efficacy, due to concerns over safety and tolerability [12,27]. In addition to pharmacological treatments, electroconvulsive therapy (ECT) should also be considered as a second-line option, particularly in the most severe forms of illness where there is an imminent and serious risk to life. ECT's efficacy is well established, but has been relegated from a first-line treatment for mania due to stigma, logistics, and ethical considerations [28].

Third-line agents

- Chlorpromazine
- Clozapine
- Tamoxifen

Tamoxifen has promising results from several small, randomised controlled trials from 2007 onwards, and has demonstrated efficacy both when added to lithium and as monotherapy [29]. There is evidence to support clozapine as being effective in treatment-resistant mania [28], but its monitoring requirements and significant adverse effect profile limit it to a third-line agent in most international guidelines [13,14,16,18].

Not recommended

- Allopurinol
- Gabapentin
- Lamotrigine
- Phenytoin
- Topiramate
- Memantine
- Verapamil

Other psychotropic medications have been mentioned as potential options should all of the above strategies fail in acute mania, but the following agents cannot be recommended at the time of writing due to either a lack of convincing evidence or evidence disproving their efficacy: allopurinol [30], gabapentin [31], lamotrigine, phenytoin, topiramate, memantine [32], and verapamil [33].

For those presenting with a relapse of mania, having had pharmacological treatment in the past or currently on treatment, more information will be required to make an informed decision. Firstly, antidepressant agents should be tapered and discontinued. If the relapse occurred whilst on a pharmacological regimen, it would be imperative to first assess the level of adherence; if adherence has been poor, the reason behind this should be explored and any concerns or adverse effects should be addressed, either through psychoeducation, dose reduction, or switching to another agent with a more tolerable adverse effect profile. If adherence is not an issue, the dosage (and possibly blood levels) should be optimised, and increased to the highest tolerated dose. For those already on lithium, serum levels should be checked, and optimised to the higher end of normal therapeutic range, namely, 0.8–1.0 mmol/L. In those with a history of a manic episode that responded to treatment but are no longer on treatment, consideration should be given to resuming the same regimen; any agent that had in the past been trialled (for an adequate duration and at an adequate dose) without success should be avoided.

Agitation is common in acute mania and, when present, should be managed appropriately. Its severity can range from fidgeting and pacing to outright aggression and physical violence. Nonpharmacological approaches should be attempted, such as reducing the level of stimulation in the person's environment, or verbal de-escalation when their agitation increases. Iatrogenic causes, namely, akathisia secondary to an antipsychotic medication, should be ruled out. Should their acute behavioural disturbance require pharmacological treatment to ensure their safety and those around them, agents with inherent antimanic properties are preferred seeing as their agitation is secondary to their underlying mania. Table 20.1 includes those agents recommended for use in severe behavioural disturbances in the context of acute mania, based on available evidence and current guidelines [12,16,33–38].

It should be kept in mind that a lack of evidence does not necessarily constitute lack of efficacy, and

Table 20.1 Agents recommended for use in acute mania

Adjunctive agent for agitation	Recommended single dose	Recommended daily maximum [18]
First-line		
Olanzapine (IM)	2.5–5 mg	10 mg
Aripiprazole (IM)	9.75 mg	15 mg
Loxapine (Inhaled)	5 mg	10 mg
Second-line		
Haloperidol (IM)	5 mg	15 mg
Asenapine (SL)	10 mg	20 mg
Risperidone (ODT)	2 mg	4 mg
Lorazepam (IM)	1–2 mg	4 mg
Third-line		
Haloperidol (PO)	5 mg	15 mg
Quetiapine (PO)	-	Around 300 mg

Abbreviations: IM = intramuscular; SL = sublingual; ODT = orally disintegrating tablet; PO = per oral.

there will be limits on the available evidence in light of understandable issues with informed consent in this population. Clinical experience also suggests oral preparations of antipsychotics (such as haloperidol and olanzapine), benzodiazepines (such as lorazepam and clonazepam), and antihistamines (such as promethazine) to be effective and should be preferred if the oral route is readily accepted; intramuscular administration (with or without physical restraint) should only be used as a last resort, if oral administration has been ineffective or has been declined.

Maintenance Treatment Following Mania or Hypomania

Given the relapsing-remitting nature of bipolar disorder, those who have been diagnosed are often advised to remain on long-term maintenance treatment, in some cases indefinitely. One-off episodes of mania or hypomania are rare, and without treatment, relapses can be expected, on average, every one to two years [34].

Unfortunately, there is a considerable lack of concrete evidence to guide clinical practices when it comes to determining which agents should be discontinued, or which agents should be introduced, if any at all, during maintenance treatment [1]. Generally, the antimanic regimen which was effective at treating the acute manic or hypomanic episode should be continued for 6 to 12 months to minimise the risk of an early relapse [13]. Adherence to maintenance treatment is generally poor [35], and can severely impact prognosis. This necessitates good quality care, at times through specialist services, providing interventions such as psychoeducation.

The choice of agent in maintenance treatment should be a joint decision made with the patient and tailored to their clinical presentation and needs. Lithium is one of the most established maintenance treatments in bipolar disorders and is considered the current gold standard of treatment. Its efficacy in preventing mania and anti-suicidal effects has been clearly demonstrated [36]. There is a general consensus that as maintenance therapy, a serum level between 0.4 and 0.6 mmol/L should be aimed for, which provides adequate cover against further affective episodes but also reduces the burden of potential adverse effects. Most guidelines continue to advocate for lithium as first-line monotherapy in maintenance treatment [13,14,18], but despite this, lithium prescription appears to be falling [37]. Increasingly, second-generation antipsychotics are used either as monotherapy or as adjunct with a mood stabiliser; whilst there is some evidence for this practice [38], this is not without its controversies and limitations [39]. A heavier reliance on second-generation antipsychotics by clinicians will likely lead to more prominent metabolic side effects and weight gain, which will negatively impact adherence, a major predictive factor in future relapse.

In summary, there are a variety of options for people and their clinicians in acute mania, well supported by available evidence. Following the acute episode, people will require assiduous care in making decisions about maintenance treatment to ensure adequate relapse prevention and maintain high levels of functioning.

References

1. McIntyre RS, Berk M, Brietzke E, et al. Bipolar disorders. *Lancet* 2020;**396**:1841–56.

2. *International Classification of Diseases 11th Revision.* Geneva: World Health Organization, 2019. https://icd.who.int/en (accessed May 8, 2022).

3. American Psychiatric Association. *Diagnostic and Statistical Manual of Mental Disorders: DSM-5.* 5th ed. Washington, DC: American Psychiatric Association, 2013.

4. Merikangas KR, Jin R, He J-P, et al. Prevalence and correlates of bipolar spectrum disorder in the world mental health survey initiative. *Arch Gen Psychiatry* 2011;**68**:241–51.

5. Bessonova L, Ogden K, Doane MJ, O'Sullivan AK, Tohen M. the economic burden of bipolar disorder in the United States: a systematic literature review. *Clinicoecon Outcomes Res* 2020;**12**:481–97.

6. Cloutier M, Greene M, Guerin A, Touya M, Wu E. The economic burden of bipolar I disorder in the United States in 2015. *J Affect Disord* 2018;**226**: 45–51.

7. Kessing LV, Vradi E, Andersen PK. Life expectancy in bipolar disorder. *Bipolar Disord* 2015;**17**:543–8.

8. Jauhar S, Krishnadas R, Nour MM, et al. Is there a symptomatic distinction between the affective psychoses and schizophrenia? A machine learning approach. *Schizophr Res* 2018;**202**:241–7.

9. García S, Martínez-Cengotitabengoa M, López-Zurbano S, et al. Adherence to antipsychotic medication in bipolar disorder and schizophrenic patients. *J Clin Psychopharmacol* 2016;**36**:355–71.

10. Jauhar S, Nour MM, Veronese M, et al. A test of the transdiagnostic dopamine hypothesis of psychosis using positron emission tomographic imaging in bipolar affective disorder and schizophrenia. *JAMA Psychiatry* 2017;**74**:1206–13.

11. Yildiz A, Vieta E, Leucht S, Baldessarini RJ. Efficacy of antimanic treatments: meta-analysis of randomized, controlled trials. *Neuropsychopharmacology* 2011;**36**: 375–89.

12. Yildiz A, Nikodem M, Vieta E, Correll CU, Baldessarini RJ. A network meta-analysis on comparative efficacy and all-cause discontinuation of antimanic treatments in acute bipolar mania. *Psychol Med* 2015;**45**:299–317.

13. Fountoulakis KN, Grunze H, Vieta E, et al. The International College of Neuro-Psychopharmacology (CINP) Treatment Guidelines for Bipolar Disorder in Adults (CINP-BD-2017), part 3: the clinical guidelines. *Int J Neuropsychopharmacol* 2016;**20**:180–95.

14. Yatham LN, Kennedy SH, Parikh SV, et al. Canadian Network for Mood and Anxiety Treatments (CANMAT) and International Society for Bipolar Disorders (ISBD) 2018 guidelines for the management of patients with bipolar disorder. *Bipolar Disord* 2018;**20**:97–170.

15. Cipriani A, Barbui C, Salanti G, et al. Comparative efficacy and acceptability of antimanic drugs in acute mania: a multiple-treatments meta-analysis. *Lancet* 2011;**378**:1306–15.

16. Goodwin GM, Haddad PM, Ferrier IN, et al. Evidence-based guidelines for treating bipolar disorder: revised third edition recommendations from the British Association for Psychopharmacology. *J Psychopharmacol (Oxford)* 2016;**30**:495–553.

17. Geddes JR, Miklowitz DJ. Treatment of bipolar disorder. *Lancet* 2013;**381**:1672–82.

18. Malhi GS, Bassett D, Boyce P, et al. Royal Australian and New Zealand College of Psychiatrists clinical practice guidelines for mood disorders. *Aust N Z J Psychiatry* 2015;**49**:1087–206.

19. Morriss R. Mandatory implementation of NICE Guidelines for the care of bipolar disorder and other conditions in England and Wales. *BMC Medicine* 2015;**13**:246.

20. Taylor DM, Barnes TRE, Young AH. *The Maudsley Prescribing Guidelines in Psychiatry.* 13th ed. New York: Wiley-Blackwell, 2018.

21. Pacchiarotti I, Anmella G, Colomer L, Vieta E. How to treat mania. *Acta Psychiatr Scand* 2020;**142**(3):173–92.

22. Stahl SM, Laredo S, Morrissette DA. Cariprazine as a treatment across the bipolar I spectrum from depression to mania: mechanism of action and review of clinical data. *Ther Adv Psychopharmacol* 2020;**10**. doi:10.1177/2045125320905752.

23. Pinto JV, Saraf G, Vigo D et al. Cariprazine in the treatment of bipolar disorder: a systematic review and meta-analysis. *Bipolar Disord* 2020;**22**:360–71.

24. Vieta E, Durgam S, Lu K et al. Effect of cariprazine across the symptoms of mania in bipolar I disorder: analyses of pooled data from phase II/III trials. *Eur Neuropsychopharmacol* 2015;**25**:1882–91.

25. Ogawa Y, Tajika A, Takeshima N, Hayasaka Y, Furukawa TA. Mood stabilizers and antipsychotics for acute mania: a systematic review and

meta-analysis of combination/augmentation therapy versus monotherapy. *CNS Drugs* 2014;**28**:989–1003.

26. Glue P, Herbison P. Comparative efficacy and acceptability of combined antipsychotics and mood stabilizers versus individual drug classes for acute mania: network meta-analysis. *Aust N Z J Psychiatry* 2015;**49**:1215–20.

27. Vieta E, Ramey T, Keller D et al. in the treatment of acute mania: a 12-week, placebo-controlled, haloperidol-referenced study. *J Psychopharmacol* 2010;**24**:547–58.

28. Elias A, Thomas N, Sackeim HA. Electroconvulsive therapy in mania: a review of 80 years of clinical experience. *Am J Psychiatry* 2021;**178**:229–39.

29. Yildiz A, Guleryuz S, Ankerst DP, Ongür D, Renshaw PF. Protein kinase C inhibition in the treatment of mania: a double-blind, placebo-controlled trial of tamoxifen. *Arch Gen Psychiatry* 2008;**65**:255–63.

30. Weiser M, Burshtein S, Gershon AA, et al. Allopurinol for mania: a randomized trial of allopurinol versus placebo as add-on treatment to mood stabilizers and/or antipsychotic agents in manic patients with bipolar disorder. *Bipolar Disord* 2014;**16**:441–7.

31. Rosa AR, Fountoulakis K, Siamouli M, Gonda X, Vieta E. Is anticonvulsant treatment of mania a class effect? Data from randomized clinical trials. *CNS Neurosci Ther* 2011;**17**:167–77.

32. Veronese N, Solmi M, Luchini C, et al. Acetylcholinesterase inhibitors and memantine in bipolar disorder: a systematic review and best evidence synthesis of the efficacy and safety for multiple disease dimensions. *J Affect Disord* 2016; **197**:268–80.

33. Fountoulakis KN, Yatham LN, Grunze H, et al. The CINP guidelines on the definition and evidence-based interventions for treatment-resistant bipolar disorder. *Int J Neuropsychopharmacol* 2020;**23**: 230–56.

34. Baldessarini RJ, Tondo L, Vázquez GH. Pharmacological treatment of adult bipolar disorder. *Mol Psychiatry* 2019;**24**:198–217.

35. Kessing LV, Søndergård L, Kvist K, Andersen PK. Adherence to lithium in naturalistic settings: results from a nationwide pharmacoepidemiological study. *Bipolar Disord* 2007;**9**:730–6.

36. Severus E, Taylor MJ, Sauer C, et al. Lithium for prevention of mood episodes in bipolar disorders: systematic review and meta-analysis. *Int J Bipolar Disord* 2014;**2**:15.

37. Winstanley J, Young AH, Jauhar S. Back to basics – a UK perspective on 'Make lithium great again' Malhi et al. *Bipolar Disord* 2021;**23**:97–8.

38. Lindström L, Lindström E, Nilsson M, Höistad M. Maintenance therapy with second generation antipsychotics for bipolar disorder – a systematic review and meta-analysis. *J Affect Disord* 2017;**213**: 138–50.

39. Jauhar S, Young AH. Controversies in bipolar disorder; role of second-generation antipsychotic for maintenance therapy. *Int J Bipolar Disord* 2019;**7**:10.

Chapter 21

The Burden of Bipolar Depression

Allan Young and Dominic Cottrell

Bipolar affective disorder is a severe and enduring mental illness, estimated to affect 1–3% of people. It has an enormous impact on the individual, those who care for them, and the wider systems in which they live over the course of decades [1].

Manic or hypomanic episodes are the cardinal features of bipolar I and bipolar II, respectively, and have a significant impact on patients in terms of rates of hospitalisation, disruption to their lives, and the consequences of impulsive or reckless behaviour. However, it is increasingly apparent that it is the *depressive* period of the illness that accounts for most of the illness burden for many individuals with bipolar disorder [2,3]. A series of long-term follow-up studies revealed that in bipolar I disorder, patients would spend 31.9% of the total follow-up time in a depressive phase, as opposed to 8.9% in a manic or hypomanic phase [4]; this is even more pronounced in bipolar II, with patients reporting depressive symptoms 50% of the time [5]. Depressive symptoms in bipolar disorder appear harder to treat than manic, hypomanic, or mixed symptoms, with poorer rates of recovery from depressive episodes and a less pronounced response to treatment noted [6,7].

Attempts to distinguish bipolar depression from unipolar depression according to symptomatic features have suggested a greater degree of diurnal variation, psychomotor abnormalities, and psychosis, though whether these have utility in terms of prognostic diagnosis (i.e., predicting 'converters' to bipolar disorder) is unclear [6]. More recently, affective lability has been mooted as a predictor of patients with depressive symptoms who will 'convert' to a bipolar illness [8], though this requires further investigation.

The BRIDGE study (a multi-centre, multinational, cross-sectional diagnostic study of over 5,000 patients with a major depressive episode [9]) indicated that a family history of mania, multiple mood episodes, and an onset prior to the age of 30 were suggestive of a 'bipolar-signifier' – people who would not strictly meet criteria for bipolar disorder but show a degree of 'bipolarity'. This group of patients are far more likely to report emerging manic or hypomanic symptoms during antidepressant therapy, findings which have since been replicated [10].

Alongside the lifetime morbidity of bipolar disorder is the risk of elevated mortality. The risk of attempted suicide in bipolar disorder is high (one study put the rate of attempted suicide as high as 4% [11]). Furthermore, people with bipolar disorder who attempt to take their own life are more likely to complete suicide than the general population [12]. This is important for this clinical topic, as it is the depressive phase (as opposed to mixed or purely manic periods) that is particularly associated with suicidal thoughts [13]. Comparisons with unipolar depression show that though the risk of attempted suicide is higher in those with bipolar depression, this appears to be related to the amount of time spent in bipolar depression, as opposed to a quality of the depressive state itself [14].

Diagnosis and Delays

The clinical features of unipolar and bipolar depression are similar, but not identical. In bipolar depression, symptom onset tends to be earlier [9], mood episodes are more frequent, and patients experiencing a bipolar depressive episode report a worse quality of life than their unipolar counterparts [15].

Despite the importance of early recognition of bipolar illness, delays to diagnosis are common. Only 20% of those affected receive their diagnosis within a year and a treatment latency of 5–10 years appears common [16].

Perhaps most importantly, the two disorders differ greatly in terms of clinical response, especially to standard antidepressant therapy. Evidence regarding unipolar depression does not translate simply to bipolar depression. This means that the period whereby a patient with a bipolar illness is misdiagnosed as suffering from unipolar depression is time spent receiving, at best, suboptimal care. Furthermore, in those patients with a bipolar illness, standard antidepressant treatment can carry risks – emergence of hypomanic and manic symptoms is common [2,9] and antidepressants are harmful in those showing both manic and depressive features simultaneously (i.e., those in a 'mixed-affective' state) as they worsen manic features without ameliorating the depressive [17]. Encouragingly, delayed diagnosis does not appear to contribute to the emergence of treatment resistance, however [16].

The Challenge of Pharmacotherapy

Pharmacotherapy remains the mainstay for treating and preventing depressive episodes in bipolar disorder. However, in contrast to the manic phase of the illness, there remains limited consensus concerning which treatment options are first line or second line and which are to be used only cautiously. A brief summary of clinical guidance gives a sense of the breadth of opinion (see Table 21.1). Aside from quetiapine (which is the most consistently advocated treatment for bipolar depression), the role of lithium and mood stabilisers in contrast to second generation antipsychotics remains uncertain.

Antidepressants

The use of antidepressants in bipolar depression remains widespread, often on a long-term basis. One international sample of 186 bipolar patients showed over 80% had been prescribed an antidepressant over the course of their illness [20]. Studies typically show high rates (50–58%) of current antidepressant prescription in patients diagnosed with bipolar disorder [21,22] and high rates of antidepressant monotherapy [23]. However, the use of antidepressants in patients with confirmed bipolar disorder remains highly controversial. This is reflected in international guidelines, which recommend only fluoxetine in bipolar depression (in conjunction with olanzapine) and counsel against the use of antidepressant monotherapy, citing risk of 'manic switching' [24].

The evidence base for antidepressant efficacy in acute bipolar depression is equivocal. In a large ($N = 740$), multi-centre, randomised controlled trial (EMBOLDEN-II), paroxetine was significantly inferior in reducing depressive symptoms in bipolar patients, compared to those given even modest (i.e., 300 mg) doses of quetiapine. In fact, paroxetine offered no improvement beyond that seen in placebo for depression (though an improvement in anxiety was seen). Even in patients already being treated with a mood stabiliser, the evidence for incremental improvement with the addition of an antidepressant is sparse. A further double-blind study (STEP-BD)

Table 21.1 Pharmacotherapy: a brief summary

Agent	NICE	BAP [18]	Royal Australian and New Zealand College of Psychiatrists Guidelines [19]	CANMAT [12]
Fluoxetine + olanzapine	✓	✓	Not specifically, but endorsed as part of a broader 2nd line strategy	2nd line
Quetiapine	✓	✓	✓	✓
Lamotrigine	2nd line	✓	✓	✓
Lithium	Optimise if taking	✓	✓	✓
Valproate	Optimise if taking	✗	✓	2nd line
Lurasidone	✗	✓	✓	✓
Cariprazine	✗	✓	✓	2nd line
Olanzapine	✗	✓	2nd line	✗
Electroconvulsive therapy	✗	✓	2nd line	✓

Broad summary of guidelines, where a tick (✓) indicates status as a first-line or recommended treatment strategy. N.B.: This is a simplification of detailed information for clarity and brevity. The reader is advised to review the guidelines individually, which differ in their approach to recommendations and given evidence base.

found that in those patients already taking a mood stabiliser, adding in an antidepressant offered minimal benefit over mood stabiliser alone [25]. Follow-ups to this study further noted that antidepressant discontinuation had no impact in terms of more frequent or severe depressive relapse and rates of self-reported manic switching were high [26], further underlining that adjunctive antidepressant use be confined to the depressive period itself, if at all, and not in the maintenance phase.

A recent meta-analysis (summarising the treatment of 1,383 patients) updated the above findings, noting that adjunctive antidepressant treatment offered only modest improvement in depressive symptoms and had no impact on clinical remission [27]. Further, similar analyses have suggested some role for monoamine oxidase inhibitors and tricyclic antidepressants [28], though these are limited by the relatively few trials exploring these agents, as well as short trial time.

Of further concern, treatment with adjunctive antidepressants in the longer term (i.e., over 12 months) was associated with a higher rate of emerging manic symptoms (though other studies have argued the risk of manic switching in the longer term is limited to patients not receiving a mood stabiliser [23]).

A final note of caution in the use of antidepressants for bipolar depression: there is evidence that, at least in some patients, longer-term use of antidepressants (even those receiving a mood stabiliser) predisposes to more frequent mood episodes (i.e., rapid cycling) [29]. Considering this risk, the evidence for modest clinical benefit and the side effect burden of polypharmacy, the role of antidepressants in bipolar disorder is, at best, limited.

Antipsychotics

In contrast to antidepressants, the evidence base for atypical antipsychotics is much more favourable (as reflected in clinical guidelines). Large-scale syntheses of available data reflect these recommendations, finding good efficacy for lurasidone, olanzapine, and quetiapine [28,30,31,32]. The size of the clinical response for these treatments is robust (with number needed to treat [NNT] ranging from 5, for lurasidone, to 10, for olanzapine) [32]. Of note, aripiprazole (a commonly prescribed antipsychotic on account of its favourable metabolic profile) and ziprasidone have consistently fared poorly in large-scale meta-analyses described

above. More novel atypical antipsychotics such as cariprazine (a D3 and 5-HT1A partial agonist) also show promise, several randomised controlled trials showing a good degree of efficacy with a minimal impact on metabolic parameters (though the risk of akathisia remains) [33,34].

Given the broadly consistent efficacy of a relatively small number of antipsychotics, the choice between them is largely driven by side effect burden. Both quetiapine and olanzapine are associated with metabolic complications (most especially obesity and dyslipidaemia) [35], with significant weight gain (2.9 kg for olanzapine; 1.2 kg for quetiapine) noted even over relatively short trial periods [32]. The metabolic burden of treatment is especially important, as patients with bipolar disorder show a greater rate of cardiovascular disease and associated mortality than the general population [36,37]. This said, lurasidone is not without risks, most especially of akathisia – which has a strong association with suicidality – though the risks of benefit versus harm seem favourable [38].

Mood Stabilisers

The term 'mood stabiliser' is in common usage and is typically used to refer to lithium and anticonvulsant agents used in affective disorders (valproate, carbamazepine, and lamotrigine, chiefly). The term would imply efficacy in the acute treatment, and maintenance, of both manic and depressive episodes, as well as in mixed and rapid cycling states. The question of whether these agents have earned this title is not new [39] and is particularly important in bipolar depression (where the majority of the burden of affective illness is arguably found).

Lithium was the earliest agent identified in the treatment of bipolar disorder and has proven efficacy in the treatment of both acute mania and the prevention of manic episodes, with an estimated NNT of about 5 or 6 [40]. However, its role in the acute treatment of a bipolar depressive episode is less clear. The EMBOLDEN-I study compared lithium with quetiapine as monotherapies in a large ($N = 802$) randomised placebo-controlled trial and found lithium no better than placebo by 8 weeks of treatment [41]. A study looking at the efficacy of lithium in preventing depressive episodes over a substantial follow-up period (up to 18 months), which compared lithium with lamotrigine at therapeutic doses (0.8–1.1 mmol/L), found that lithium served to reduce the number of manic, but not depressive, episodes [42].

Recent reviews and meta-analyses have equally struggled to find as clear a benefit for lithium in the depressive phase as seen in the manic phase [28,40,43]. Given the importance of close concordance with lithium in preventing early relapse [44], the risk of renal and thyroid impairment and the dangers of lithium in overdose – with a narrow gap between the minimum effective serum level and toxicity [45] – the use of lithium in those with a predominately depressive presentation needs to be pursued cautiously.

Valproate is the most widely prescribed anticonvulsant, though its usage is increasingly limited by teratogenicity, multiple interactions with other medications, and numerous side effects. It has established efficacy in treating acute mania and preventing manic relapses. It is harder to evaluate its antidepressant qualities in bipolar disorder compared to lithium, as there have been fewer large studies looking at its efficacy. A Cochrane review found evidence to suggest that valproate was effective in preventing a depressive episode compared to placebo (as has been confirmed by other systematic reviews [28,46,47]) but was no different to lithium in this regard [48]).

Lamotrigine is another anticonvulsant that has become increasingly favoured in the depressive phase of bipolar disorder. It appears to have a degree of efficacy in terms of preventing depressive episodes [49,50], though its efficacy in treating acute depressive episodes is equivocal [51]. This prophylactic effect is phase-specific, with limited evidence that it prevents the emergence of manic episodes [52]. The use of lamotrigine is somewhat limited by the risk of significant dermatological side effects, including Stevens–Johnson syndrome / toxic epidermolytic necrosis which, while rare, has a high mortality rate [53].

Nonpharmacological and Emerging Treatment Options

Aside from established pharmacotherapy, a range of treatment modalities exists with a robust or growing evidence base.

Psychotherapy

Alongside pharmacological interventions, there is good evidence that psychosocial interventions have a key role in managing the impact of bipolar depression. Several interventions have been developed, with aims ranging from early recognition of affective switching, avoiding factors likely to cause relapse, through to direct treatment of mood episodes [12].

The evidence base for such interventions is encouraging. Much of the research conducted to date explores the role of psychotherapies as adjuncts to pharmacotherapy. In this context, psychotherapy seems to improve depressive symptoms, reduce the proportion of patients who relapse, and boost overall functioning [54]. Encouragingly, given the frequency of relapse in bipolar disorder, the protective effect of psychotherapy appears to persist up to at least a year, across a range of modalities [55]. Finally, psychotherapy does not carry the side effect burden associated with pharmacotherapies and so represents an opportunity to bolster existing treatment avenues, without the typical costs incurred by polypharmacy.

Electroconvulsive Therapy

In unipolar and treatment-resistant depression, electroconvulsive therapy (ECT) has a strong evidence base as an effective and rapid treatment option in the acute setting [56]. Its use is limited by uncertainty around the persistence of its effects, an adverse perception in the public domain, and concerns regarding longer-term cognitive impairment, especially relating to memory. Given the propensity for bipolar depressive episodes to be severe, protracted, and treatment resistant, a quick-onset and robust treatment option is especially attractive. However, the evidence base for antidepressants argues against assuming ECT will be as effective in bipolar depression, or that the side effects will be similar.

Earlier, shorter-term observational studies have been promising. One such study found that approximately two-thirds of a cohort of depressed, treatment-non-responsive bipolar patients responded to a course of ECT (with a pronounced response in those with a bipolar II diagnosis). Of note, no instances of affective switching were noted over the course of the treatment [57]. There are relatively few randomised controlled trials (RCTs) on ECT which focus exclusively on bipolar depression. One such study compared the response rate to either ECT or pharmacotherapy over 6 weeks; the ECT group showed a greater rate of response and a more rapid antidepressant effect. Encouragingly, the remission rate between ECT and pharmacotherapy was similar (albeit over a relatively short time frame). From a longer-term, retrospective cohort study, it may also be the case that rates of suicide are reduced in patients receiving ECT as opposed to pharmacotherapy alone, an effect also seen in just bipolar depressed patients [58].

Larger, pooled analyses (involving both prospective and retrospective studies) are suggestive that ECT is just as effective [59,60], if not more so [61], in bipolar patients as in those with unipolar depression. These results are encouraging, though there remains few if any longer-term studies to ascertain the long-term efficacy of ECT. The evidence for the cognitive impact of unilateral ECT (the predominant method used in the studies cited above) on patients with bipolar depression is mixed. One study found no worsening in cognitive function found in those treated with ECT at 6 months compared with those receiving pharmacotherapy alone [62].

Adjunctive and Novel Treatments

Ketamine

Over the past decade, ketamine (an N-methyl-D-aspartate [NMDA] receptor antagonist, otherwise used as an anaesthetic agent and as an illicit recreational substance) has, along with its racemic enantiomer esketamine, emerged as an effective antidepressant agent with a novel mechanism of action, a robust antidepressant effect (with an estimated NNT of 6 to 7), and, perhaps most excitingly, an unusually rapid onset of effect [63,64].

The evidence base for ketamine in bipolar depression is, however, less well developed. The pool of studies assessing ketamine in bipolar depression is smaller (meta-analyses published within the past few years have drawn on aggregate treatment groups which are typically less than a fifth the size of those seen in the meta-analyses of treatment-resistant depression, with roughly a quarter the number of studies to collate) [65]. Estimates of clinical efficacy are therefore tentative. There appears to be evidence for a prompt antidepressant effect with a single dose of intravenous ketamine, though the effect does not seem to persist more than a week or so [66]. However, one-off, intravenous ketamine is rarely used in routine clinical practice for depression and there is a paucity of studies looking at other routes of administration or dosing regimens; how best to maximise the effect of ketamine in routine clinical practice remains unanswered and ripe for further research.

Light Therapy and Circadian Rhythms

There is ample evidence that the biological mechanisms underlying sleep and wakefulness have a bearing on affective disorders. Sleep disturbances are common in depression and many individuals experience alterations in their mood relating to the ambient light (most classically in seasonal affective disorder, or SAD).

Sleep is especially important in bipolar disorder. Insomnia is well described as both a trigger and a manifestation of an emerging mood episode. Even in recovered bipolar patients, residual sleep disturbances are common [67], those with bipolar disorder tend to have a delayed chronotype (i.e., be 'night-owls') [68], and sleep dysfunction predicts earlier relapse [69]. Changes in sleep patterns seem to herald developing mood episodes, leading to development of a theory that there is a close interaction between internal circadian rhythms, external time cues (such as environmental light exposure, externally enforced sleep patterns), and mood regulation [70,71]. The most well established of these is Bright Light Therapy (BLT), whereby a fluorescent lamp is targeted towards the patient during waking hours to mimic the effect of environmental light-givers, especially sunlight. The evidence for this treatment in both seasonal and non-seasonal depression is robust, both as a monotherapy and an adjunctive therapy, though preliminary data raise concerns regarding emerging hypomania [72,73].

Given the evidence for sleep having a role in bipolar disorder and the potential value of nonpharmacological adjunctive therapies, there have been increasing attempts to target disrupted sleep patterns in bipolar disorder. However, to date there have been relatively few studies of high quality assessing the efficacy of BLT on bipolar depression specifically. However, systematic reviews of the role of BLT as an adjunctive suggest a marked antidepressant effect in bipolar depression when used as adjunctive therapy, with minimal risk of side effects (most especially manic switching) [74,75].

Other Treatment Modalities

Bright Light Therapy and ketamine are far from the only promising emerging treatments for bipolar depression. Possible options under assessment include the novel antipsychotics brexpiprazole and pramipexole, modafinil, and triiodothyronine (T3) (for a detailed overview of emerging treatment options, see Yalin and Young [51]). Furthermore, there is a developing literature on a range of adjunctive treatment options, which, while unlikely to be efficacious in isolation, may boost the efficacy of more established treatments [43].

Conclusions

Bipolar depression imposes a significant challenge to those working to care for people with bipolar disorder. It is far more than just unipolar depression in those who happen to have had manic or hypomanic episodes. It tends to appear earlier; absorb more of a person's time they would otherwise expect to be well; and represents much of the reduced quality of life and increased risk of completed suicide seen in bipolar disorder.

Furthermore, the principles for treating unipolar depression or mania do not necessarily translate to the depressive phase of bipolar disorder. Any professional looking to treat it adequately needs to understand it *sui generis* and cultivate an awareness of the specific treatment options required. Encouragingly, a range of novel treatments is emerging that will, it is hoped, herald a broader armamentarium for the clinician and a better outlook for their patient.

References

1. Ferrari AJ, Stockings E, Khoo JP, et al. The prevalence and burden of bipolar disorder: findings from the Global Burden of Disease Study 2013. *Bipolar Disord* 2016 Aug;**18**(5):440–50.

2. Manning JS. Burden of illness in bipolar depression. *Prim Care Companion J Clin Psychiatry* 2005;**7**(6):259–67.

3. Vojta C, Kinosian B, Glick H, Altshuler L, Bauer MS. Self-reported quality of life across mood states in bipolar disorder. *Compr Psychiatry* 2001 May–Jun;**42**(3):190–5.

4. Judd LL, Akiskal HS, Schettler PJ, et al. The long-term natural history of the weekly symptomatic status of bipolar I disorder. *Arch Gen Psychiatry* 2002 Jun;**59**(6):530–7.

5. Judd LL, Akiskal HS, Schettler PJ, et al. A prospective investigation of the natural history of the long-term weekly symptomatic status of bipolar II disorder. *Arch Gen Psychiatry* 2003 Mar;**60**(3):261–9.

6. Mitchell PB, Malhi GS. Bipolar depression: phenomenological overview and clinical characteristics. *Bipolar Disord* 2004 Dec;**6**(6):530–9.

7. Keller MB, Lavori PW, Coryell W, et al. Differential outcome of pure manic, mixed/cycling, and pure depressive episodes in patients with bipolar illness. *JAMA* 1986 Jun 13;**255**(22):3138–42.

8. Taylor RH, Ulrichsen A, Young AH, Strawbridge R. Affective lability as a prospective predictor of subsequent bipolar disorder diagnosis: a systematic review. *Int J Bipolar Disord* 2021 Nov 1;**9**(1):33-021–00237–1.

9. Angst J, Azorin JM, Bowden CL, et al. Prevalence and characteristics of undiagnosed bipolar disorders in patients with a major depressive episode: the BRIDGE study. *Arch Gen Psychiatry* 2011 Aug;**68**(8):791–7.

10. Valentí M, Pacchiarotti I, Bonnín CM, et al. Risk factors for antidepressant-related switch to mania. *J Clin Psychiatry* 2012 Feb;**73**(2):e271–6.

11. Tondo L, Pompili M, Forte A, Baldessarini RJ. Suicide attempts in bipolar disorders: comprehensive review of 101 reports. *Acta Psychiatr Scand* 2016 Mar;**133**(3):174–86.

12. Yatham LN, Kennedy SH, Parikh SV, et al. Canadian Network for Mood and Anxiety Treatments (CANMAT) and International Society for Bipolar Disorders (ISBD) 2018 guidelines for the management of patients with bipolar disorder. *Bipolar Disord* 2018 Mar;**20**(2):97–170.

13. Dilsaver SC, Chen YW, Swann AC, et al. Suicidality, panic disorder and psychosis in bipolar depression, depressive-mania and pure-mania. *Psychiatry Res* 1997 Nov 14;**73**(1–2):47–56.

14. Holma KM, Haukka J, Suominen K, et al. Differences in incidence of suicide attempts between bipolar I and II disorders and major depressive disorder. *Bipolar Disord* 2014 Sep;**16**(6):652–61.

15. Berlim MT, Pargendler J, Caldieraro MA, et al. Quality of life in unipolar and bipolar depression: are there significant differences? *J Nerv Ment Dis* 2004 Nov;**192**(11):792–5.

16. Baldessarini RJ, Tondo L, Baethge CJ, Lepri B, Bratti IM. Effects of treatment latency on response to maintenance treatment in manic-depressive disorders. *Bipolar Disord* 2007 Jun;**9**(4):386–93.

17. Fagiolini A, Coluccia A, Maina G, et al. Diagnosis, epidemiology and management of mixed states in bipolar disorder. *CNS Drugs* 2015 Sep;**29**(9):725–40.

18. Goodwin GM, Haddad PM, Ferrier IN, et al. Evidence-based guidelines for treating bipolar disorder: revised third edition recommendations from the British Association for Psychopharmacology. *J Psychopharmacol* 2016 Jun;**30**(6):495–553.

19. Malhi GS, Bell E, Boyce P, et al. The 2020 Royal Australian and New Zealand College of psychiatrists clinical practice guidelines for mood disorders:

bipolar disorder summary. *Bipolar Disord* 2020 Dec;**22**(8):805–21.

20. Mauer S, Alahmari R, Vöhringer PA, et al. International prescribing patterns for mood illness: the International Mood Network (IMN). *J Affect Disord* 2014;**167**:136–9.

21. Baldessarini RJ, Leahy L, Arcona S, et al. Patterns of psychotropic drug prescription for U.S. patients with diagnoses of bipolar disorders. *Psychiatr Serv* 2007 Jan;**58**(1):85–91.

22. Serafini G, Vazquez G, Monacelli F, et al. The use of antidepressant medications for bipolar I and II disorders. *Psychiatry Res* 2021 Feb;**296**:113273.

23. Viktorin A, Lichtenstein P, Thase ME, et al. The risk of switch to mania in patients with bipolar disorder during treatment with an antidepressant alone and in combination with a mood stabilizer. *Am J Psychiatry* 2014 Oct;**171**(10):1067–73.

24. Pacchiarotti I, Bond DJ, Baldessarini RJ, et al. The International Society for Bipolar Disorders (ISBD) task force report on antidepressant use in bipolar disorders. *Am J Psychiatry* 2013 Nov;**170**(11):1249–62.

25. Sachs GS, Nierenberg AA, Calabrese JR, et al. Effectiveness of adjunctive antidepressant treatment for bipolar depression. *N Engl J Med* 2007 Apr 26;**356**(17):1711–22.

26. Truman CJ, Goldberg JF, Ghaemi SN, et al. Self-reported history of manic/hypomanic switch associated with antidepressant use: data from the Systematic Treatment Enhancement Program for Bipolar Disorder (STEP-BD). *J Clin Psychiatry* 2007 Oct;**68**(10):1472–9.

27. McGirr A, Vöhringer PA, Ghaemi SN, Lam RW, Yatham LN. Safety and efficacy of adjunctive second-generation antidepressant therapy with a mood stabiliser or an atypical antipsychotic in acute bipolar depression: a systematic review and meta-analysis of randomised placebo-controlled trials. *Lancet Psychiatry* 2016 Dec;**3**(12):1138–46.

28. Bahji A, Ermacora D, Stephenson C, Hawken ER, Vazquez G. Comparative efficacy and tolerability of pharmacological treatments for the treatment of acute bipolar depression: a systematic review and network meta-analysis. *J Affect Disord* 2020 May 15;**269**:154–84.

29. El-Mallakh RS, Vöhringer PA, Ostacher MM, et al. Antidepressants worsen rapid-cycling course in bipolar depression: a STEP-BD randomized clinical trial. *J Affect Disord* 2015 Sep 15;**184**:318–21.

30. Taylor DM, Cornelius V, Smith L, Young AH. Comparative efficacy and acceptability of drug treatments for bipolar depression: a

multiple-treatments meta-analysis. *Acta Psychiatr Scand* 2014 Dec;**130**(6):452–69.

31. Ostacher M, Ng-Mak D, Patel P, et al. Lurasidone compared to other atypical antipsychotic monotherapies for bipolar depression: a systematic review and network meta-analysis. *World J Biol Psychiatry* 2018 Dec;**19**(8):586–601.

32. Kadakia A, Dembek C, Heller V, et al. Efficacy and tolerability of atypical antipsychotics for acute bipolar depression: a network meta-analysis. *BMC Psychiatry* 2021 May 11;**21**(1):249-021–03220-3.

33. Earley W, Burgess MV, Rekeda L, et al. Cariprazine treatment of bipolar depression: a randomized double-blind placebo-controlled phase 3 study. *Am J Psychiatry* 2019 Jun 1;**176**(6):439–48.

34. Earley WR, Burgess MV, Khan B, et al. Efficacy and safety of cariprazine in bipolar I depression: a double-blind, placebo-controlled phase 3 study. *Bipolar Disord* 2020 Jun;**22**(4):372–84.

35. Kishi T, Yoshimura R, Sakuma K, Okuya M, Iwata N. Lurasidone, olanzapine, and quetiapine extended-release for bipolar depression: a systematic review and network meta-analysis of phase 3 trials in Japan. *Neuropsychopharmacol Rep* 2020 Dec;**40**(4):417–22.

36. Weiner M, Warren L, Fiedorowicz JG. Cardiovascular morbidity and mortality in bipolar disorder. *Ann Clin Psychiatry* 2011 Feb;**23**(1):40–4.

37. Penninx BWJH, Lange SMM. Metabolic syndrome in psychiatric patients: overview, mechanisms, and implications. *Dialogues Clin Neurosci* 2018 Mar;**20**(1):63–73.

38. Citrome L, Ketter TA, Cucchiaro J, Loebel A. Clinical assessment of lurasidone benefit and risk in the treatment of bipolar I depression using number needed to treat, number needed to harm, and likelihood to be helped or harmed. J Affect Disord 2014 Feb;**155**:20–7.

39. Goodwin GM, Malhi GS. What is a mood stabilizer? *Psychol Med* 2007 May;**37**(5):609–14.

40. Fountoulakis KN, Tohen M, Zarate CA Jr. Lithium treatment of bipolar disorder in adults: a systematic review of randomized trials and meta-analyses. *Eur Neuropsychopharmacol* 2022 Jan;**54**:100–15.

41. Young AH, McElroy SL, Bauer M, et al. A double-blind, placebo-controlled study of quetiapine and lithium monotherapy in adults in the acute phase of bipolar depression (EMBOLDEN I). *J Clin Psychiatry* 2010 Feb;**71**(2):150–62.

42. Bowden CL, Calabrese JR, Sachs G, et al. A placebo-controlled 18-month trial of lamotrigine and lithium maintenance treatment in recently manic or

hypomanic patients with bipolar I disorder. *Arch Gen Psychiatry* 2003 Apr;**60**(4):392–400.

43. Bahji A, Ermacora D, Stephenson C, Hawken ER, Vazquez G. Comparative efficacy and tolerability of adjunctive pharmacotherapies for acute bipolar depression: a systematic review and network meta-analysis. *Can J Psychiatry* 2021 Mar;**66**(3):274–88.

44. Goodwin GM. Recurrence of mania after lithium withdrawal. Implications for the use of lithium in the treatment of bipolar affective disorder. *Br J Psychiatry* 1994 Feb;**164**(2):149–52.

45. Nolen WA, Licht RW, Young AH, et al. What is the optimal serum level for lithium in the maintenance treatment of bipolar disorder? A systematic review and recommendations from the ISBD/IGSLI Task Force on treatment with lithium. *Bipolar Disord* 2019 Aug;**21**(5):394–409.

46. Bond DJ, Lam RW, Yatham LN. Divalproex sodium versus placebo in the treatment of acute bipolar depression: a systematic review and meta-analysis. *J Affect Disord* 2010 Aug;**124**(3):228–34.

47. Smith LA, Cornelius VR, Azorin JM, et al. Valproate for the treatment of acute bipolar depression: systematic review and meta-analysis. *J Affect Disord* 2010 Apr;**122**(1–2):1–9.

48. Jochim J, Rifkin-Zybutz RP, Geddes J, Cipriani A. Valproate for acute mania. *Cochrane Database Syst Rev* 2019 Oct 7;**10**(10):CD004052.

49. Hashimoto Y, Kotake K, Watanabe N, Fujiwara T, Sakamoto S. Lamotrigine in the maintenance treatment of bipolar disorder. *Cochrane Database Syst Rev* 2021 Sep 15;**9**(9):CD013575.

50. Besag FMC, Vasey MJ, Sharma AN, Lam ICH. Efficacy and safety of lamotrigine in the treatment of bipolar disorder across the lifespan: a systematic review. *Ther Adv Psychopharmacol* 2021 Oct 8;**11**:20451253211045870.

51. Yalin N, Young AH. Pharmacological treatment of bipolar depression: what are the current and emerging options? *Neuropsychiatr Dis Treat* 2020 Jun 9;**16**:1459–72.

52. Cipriani A, Barbui C, Salanti G, et al. Comparative efficacy and acceptability of antimanic drugs in acute mania: a multiple-treatments meta-analysis. *Lancet* 2011 Oct 8;**378**(9799):1306–15.

53. Edinoff AN, Nguyen LH, Fitz-Gerald MJ, et al. Lamotrigine and Stevens-Johnson syndrome prevention. *Psychopharmacol Bull* 2021 Mar 16;**51**(2):96–114.

54. Chiang KJ, Tsai JC, Liu D, et al. Efficacy of cognitive-behavioral therapy in patients with bipolar disorder: a meta-analysis of randomized controlled trials. *PLoS One* 2017 May 4;**12**(5):e0176849.

55. Miklowitz DJ, Efthimiou O, Furukawa TA, et al. Adjunctive psychotherapy for bipolar disorder: a systematic review and component network meta-analysis. *JAMA Psychiatry* 2021 Feb 1;**78**(2):141–50.

56. UK ECT Review Group. Efficacy and safety of electroconvulsive therapy in depressive disorders: a systematic review and meta-analysis. *Lancet* 2003 Mar 8;**361**(9360):799–808.

57. Perugi G, Medda P, Toni C, et al. Role of electroconvulsive therapy (ECT) in bipolar disorder: effectiveness in 522 patients with bipolar depression, mixed-state, mania and catatonic features. *Curr Neuropharmacol* 2017 Apr;**15**(3):359–71.

58. Liang CS, Chung CH, Ho PS, Tsai CK, Chien WC. Superior anti-suicidal effects of electroconvulsive therapy in unipolar disorder and bipolar depression. *Bipolar Disord* 2018 Sep;**20**(6):539–46.

59. Loo C, Katalinic N, Mitchell PB, Greenberg B. Physical treatments for bipolar disorder: a review of electroconvulsive therapy, stereotactic surgery and other brain stimulation techniques. *J Affect Disord* 2011 Jul;**132**(1–2):1–13.

60. Dierckx B, Heijnen WT, van den Broek WW, Birkenhäger TK. Efficacy of electroconvulsive therapy in bipolar versus unipolar major depression: a meta-analysis. *Bipolar Disord* 2012 Mar;**14**(2):146–50.

61. Bahji A, Hawken ER, Sepehry AA, Cabrera CA, Vazquez G. ECT beyond unipolar major depression: systematic review and meta-analysis of electroconvulsive therapy in bipolar depression. *Acta Psychiatr Scand* 2019 Mar;**139**(3):214–26.

62. Bjoerke-Bertheussen J, Schoeyen H, Andreassen OA, et al. Right unilateral electroconvulsive therapy does not cause more cognitive impairment than pharmacologic treatment in treatment-resistant bipolar depression: a 6-month randomized controlled trial follow-up study. *Bipolar Disord* 2018 Sep;**20**(6):531–8.

63. McIntyre RS, Carvalho IP, Lui LMW, et al. The effect of intravenous, intranasal, and oral ketamine in mood disorders: a meta-analysis. *J Affect Disord* 2020 Nov 1;**276**:576–84.

64. McIntyre RS, Rosenblat JD, Nemeroff CB, et al. Synthesizing the evidence for ketamine and esketamine in treatment-resistant depression: an international expert opinion on the available evidence and implementation. *Am J Psychiatry* 2021 May 1;**178**(5):383–99.

65. Bahji A, Zarate CA, Vazquez GH. Ketamine for bipolar depression: a systematic review. *Int J Neuropsycho pharmacol* 2021 Jul 23;**24**(7):535–41.

66. Dean RL, Marquardt T, Hurducas C, et al. Ketamine and other glutamate receptor modulators for

depression in adults with bipolar disorder. *Cochrane Database Syst Rev* 2021 Oct 8;**10**(10):CD011611.

67. Ng TH, Chung KF, Ho FY, et al. Sleep-wake disturbance in interepisode bipolar disorder and high-risk individuals: a systematic review and meta-analysis. *Sleep Med Rev* 2015 Apr;**20**:46–58.

68. Melo MCA, Abreu RLC, Linhares Neto VB, de Bruin PFC, de Bruin VMS. Chronotype and circadian rhythm in bipolar disorder: a systematic review. *Sleep Med Rev* 2017 Aug;**34**:46–58.

69. Cretu JB, Culver JL, Goffin KC, Shah S, Ketter TA. Sleep, residual mood symptoms, and time to relapse in recovered patients with bipolar disorder. *J Affect Disord* 2016 Jan 15;**190**:162–6.

70. Takaesu Y. Circadian rhythm in bipolar disorder: a review of the literature. *Psychiatry Clin Neurosci* 2018 Sep;**72**(9):673–82.

71. Gold AK, Kinrys G. Treating circadian rhythm disruption in bipolar disorder. *Curr Psychiatry Rep* 2019 Mar 2;**21**(3):14–019–1001–8.

72. Maruani J, Geoffroy PA. Bright light as a personalized precision treatment of mood disorders. *Front Psychiatry* 2019 Mar 1;**10**:85.

73. Tuunainen A, Kripke DF, Endo T. Light therapy for non-seasonal depression. *Cochrane Database Syst Rev* 2004;**2004**(2):CD004050.

74. Hirakawa H, Terao T, Muronaga M, Ishii N. Adjunctive bright light therapy for treating bipolar depression: a systematic review and meta-analysis of randomized controlled trials. *Brain Behav* 2020 Dec;**10**(12):e01876.

75. Dallaspezia S, Benedetti F. Antidepressant light therapy for bipolar patients: a meta-analyses. *J Affect Disord* 2020 Sep 1;**274**:943–8.

Chapter 22

The Management of Neurocognitive Impairment in Mood Disorders

Peter Gallagher and Allan Young

Neurocognitive Dysfunction in Mood Disorders: An Overview

Mood disorders – major depressive disorder (MDD) and bipolar disorder (BD) – are associated with dysfunction* in a range of neurocognitive domains and processes [1–5]. These deficits are of greater magnitude during symptomatic episodes, although there is some evidence of their persistence during remission [6–8], particularly in euthymic BD [9–11]. It has been recognised that such deficits are associated with, and may contribute to, reduced psychological wellbeing, and social and occupational functioning [12–17]. Therefore, neurocognitive dysfunction represents a specific target for potential therapeutic intervention in both MDD and BD [18–21].

When assessing potential treatment avenues, it is necessary to consider the aetiological and pathophysiological underpinnings of neurocognitive deficits in mood disorders. An understanding of these mechanisms has direct relevance to, and will likely dictate, the approach to potential intervention. For example, we could broadly conceptualise treatments or interventions acting mechanistically in the following different ways:

(i) General symptomatic improvement: where neurocognitive deficits are one of a cluster of co-occurring symptoms of a mood disorder, which are amenable to improvement with successful treatment. In this circumstance, neurocognition would improve concurrently with other psychological, somatic, and physical symptoms.

(ii) Secondary symptomatic improvement: where neurocognitive deficits are the result – either wholly or in part – of other symptoms of mood disorders which, when targeted, lead to a downstream improvement. Here, examples may include the psychological (such as motivation) where a treatment/intervention targets an amotivational state, or physical (such as sleep), where a resolution of sleep problems or circadian dysregulation results in neurocognitive improvement.

(iii) Procognitive: where treatments or interventions directly stimulate/activate neuronal or neuroendocrine function, or neurotransmission, leading to improved neurocognitive function.

(iv) Restorative: where a treatment/intervention is specifically targeting neuronal or neuroendocrine functions, or neurotransmission, which has been reduced or affected by the mood disorder.†

In the current chapter, we review the current evidence base of treatments for improving and managing neurocognitive impairment in mood disorders. Given that reviews have already synthesised existing work [18,20,21,23,24], our purpose here is to discuss the evidence in the context of their general mechanism (or mechanisms) outlined above, to better understand the most promising approaches. To increase the scope

---

* Within the literature on neurocognitive performance in mood disorders, the terms *dysfunction*, *deficit*, and *impairment* are used interchangeably. In most cases this simply refers to statistically poorer performance in the patient group compared to healthy controls or other normative reference. A smaller proportion of studies specify *clinically significant impairment*, often defined as the proportion of clinical cases falling below a specific healthy control-derived cut-off, such as < 5th percentile or < 1.5 standard deviations in one or more domains. As such, we will adopt the same position here, where these terms simply reflect significantly poorer performance, unless otherwise specified (i.e., where a defined cut-off has been referenced).

---

† We distinguish this from the point above in that, in (iii), an intervention would potentially improve neurocognitive function in any individual. In (iv), an intervention is restoring function in a deficient system and therefore, while improving function in mood disorders, it may have no effect or even be detrimental to neurocognition in a non-affected individual (if we consider optimal performance in the context of the Yerkes–Dodson [22] curve).

of the chapter we will consider experimental candidate interventions along with clinical trials.

Pharmacological Interventions

As we have introduced above, one of the primary questions to understanding the utility for interventions to improve neurocognitive function in mood disorders is the core mechanism of action: Are neurocognitive improvements a consequence of general symptomatic improvement or a more specific effect? This question is of direct relevance to the neurocognitive effects of conventional treatments – antidepressants, antipsychotics, and mood stabilisers.

Despite clear evidence for the efficacy of antidepressants in the acute treatment of MDD [25], until recently there has been relatively little focus on their neurocognitive effects. Two meta-analyses [26,27] have suggested that overall, antidepressants do have significant positive effects on some cognitive processes such psychomotor speed (Digit Symbol Substitution Test [DSST] pooled standardised mean difference [SMD] 0.16) and delayed recall (SMD 0.24). Although it is of note that the significance of these effects were entirely consequent on two drugs – duloxetine [28–30] and vortioxetine [28,31,32]. One of these studies used path analysis to dissociate the direct effect of vortioxetine on cognition (from general mood improvement, with depression used as a mediator) and found that around two-thirds of the treatment effect was direct on neurocognition [31].

Further studies of vortioxetine in MDD have now examined neurocognitive function as a primary endpoint with generally negative results, although this may be a consequence of the trial design and principal study aims. For example, no significant difference in DSST improvement was observed following a treatment switch to either vortioxetine or escitalopram in MDD patients who had not adequately responded to SSRI or SNRI treatment [33]. In a study of 8 weeks of treatment with vortioxetine, paroxetine or placebo in working adults with MDD, no significant difference in DSST performance was observed between treatment arms, despite a significant improvement from baseline in all [34]. However, on a subsequent analysis of an overall cognitive z-score composite, vortioxetine (not paroxetine) did separate significantly from placebo (standardised effect size 0.49) with a path analysis demonstrating that 72% of the effect was direct on neurocognition and not mediated by mood improvement [34]. Similarly, in one recent trial in remitted MDD patients with only residual depressive symptoms, despite an improvement in cognition from baseline in all arms of the study, vortioxetine did not separate from a selective serotonin reuptake inhibitor (SSRI) comparator (either alone or in combination with the SSRI) [35].

In BD, there has been a greater focus on the role of mood stabilisers [36] and antipsychotic [37] – rather than antidepressant – medications on neurocognitive outcomes, but evidence of direct effects is difficult to establish. In a recent review of the topic [38], it was noted that it is broadly inconclusive due to the cross-sectional nature of most studies and a general failure to consider residual symptoms, illness severity, and comorbidities. It was also concluded that, as is the case in MDD, it is difficult to disambiguate observed neurocognitive effects of 'standard' treatments from general symptom reduction following remission of acute episodes.

Overall, the evidence of neurocognitive improvement from clinically indicated pharmacological treatments is mixed. Although there is some evidence of positive effects with specific antidepressant medications in MDD, evidence of a direct effect – rather than following general symptomatic remission – comes from statistical modelling and not through study design. This reflects the difficulty in establishing the most promising mechanistic approaches to facilitate neurocognitive improvement. Within cross-sectional or short-term studies, a finding of cognitive improvement in the absence of significant mood change may indicate a primary effect of the intervention, but it could equally be a consequence of differences in sensitivity of the two outcomes or even a temporal dissociation of mood from neurocognitive change. And although it is feasible to recruit patients outside of acute episodes, in full or partial remission, this creates its own difficulties due to the fact that while neurocognitive dysfunction can be evident, deficits are less pronounced than in symptomatic episodes [3,39], leading to potential floor effects (and the need for samples to be much larger to detect small effect size changes).

Direct Biological Targets for Neurocognitive Improvement

Glucocorticoid Dysregulation

An alternative approach to the treatment of neurocognitive dysfunction has been to target specific biological processes that are dysfunctional in mood disorders and known to be involved in cognition.

Hypothalamic–pituitary–adrenal (HPA) axis dysregulation and consequent hypercortisolaemia have been observed in mood disorders [40–48] and have been a treatment target for multiple studies. Given the role of corticosteroids and their receptors (the mineralocorticoid receptor [MR] and glucocorticoid receptor [GR]) in human cognition, a focus for many studies has been the potential amelioration of neurocognitive deficits [43,49–54].

The cortisol synthesis inhibitor metyrapone has been shown to have adjunctive antidepressant effects in MDD [55,56]. However, a large-scale randomised controlled trial (RCT) in treatment-resistant MDD did not find any significant effects on either mood symptoms or neurocognitive function across a range of domains, including spatial working memory, attention, memory, and affective processing [57,58]. The use of the GR-antagonist mifepristone (RU-486) has also been suggested in the treatment of cognitive deficits and depression in alcohol dependence [59]; however, the trial fell short of its recruitment target and conclusions were not possible from the limited sample.

In BD, significant neurocognitive improvement has been observed following 7-day adjunctive treatment with the GR-antagonist mifepristone (RU-486). In a small, randomised crossover study in 19 BD patients with depressive symptoms, spatial working memory performance was improved 19.8% over placebo when assessed 2 weeks after cessation of treatment; depressive symptoms also significantly improved from baseline [60]. In a larger follow-up study, a randomised, double-blind, parallel-group trial in 60 patients with BD depression, the same spatial working memory measure was found to have improved significantly over placebo 7 weeks after cessation of treatment (although the week 2 difference was not significant, nor was mood change) [61]. Interestingly, the magnitude of the spatial working memory improvement was directly related to the magnitude of the cortisol response to mifepristone. And although this is correlational, considered along with evidence of a sustained cortisol response to the GR-antagonist [62] in the absence of mood change, this may suggest a direct mechanism of action for the neurocognitive effects. However, it is not possible to say definitively if this is specific to mood disorders, as the effect of GR-antagonism on this cognitive process in unaffected individuals is not known.

Dopamine Dysregulation

Although the precise neurobiology of neurocognitive impairment is not known, and is likely to involve multiple interacting systems, improving dopamine function has been suggested as a potential target for treatment [63,64]. Early single-case investigations of drugs such as apomorphine on cognitive processes showed no significant response [65]. Other treatments such as lisdexamfetamine dimesylate similarly showed no objective neurocognitive improvements, although self-report measures did improve [66]. However, several studies have now demonstrated positive symptom change [67–70] as well as some suggestion of neurocognitive effects [71] of the D_2/D_3 agonist pramipexole. One recent RCT in 45 BD patients, with neurocognitive function as the primary outcome measure, found no significant treatment effect in the overall sample, but a subsequent analysis of the subgroup of 35 euthymic patients indicated significant improvement in working memory (reverse digit span) and executive function (Stroop) following pramipexole compared to placebo [72].

Glutamate Dysregulation

Glutamate is the most abundant excitatory neurotransmitter in the human brain and has been implicated in the pathogenesis of mood disorders [73,74]. There is growing interest in the clinical utility of drugs that target excess glutamate release for their potential to treat mood disorders, including neurocognitive symptoms. Ketamine, a potent glutamatergic N-methyl-D-aspartate (NMDA) receptor antagonist has been found to have antidepressant effects in both MDD and BD [75,76]. Repeated ketamine infusion has been found to improve speed of cognitive processing in treatment-resistant depression, but only in those patients with anxiety [77]. Similarly, memantine, a non-competitive NMDA receptor antagonist, has been reported to have positive effects on neurocognitive function in single case studies in BD depression [78,79].

Overall, there is mixed evidence supporting the targeting of dysregulation in specific neurobiological systems to improve neurocognitive function. Some of these approaches are promising, but further trials are needed before more definitive conclusions are possible. Focussing on individuals in clinical remission or euthymia seems particularly warranted. However, one potential note of caution in adopting this approach is that targeting one system may be of limited use unless that system is the primary underpinning of the neurocognitive deficit under investigation. This highlights the need to use outcome measures that are sensitive and specific to the action of the intervention, rather than general neurocognition. Some studies have adopted this approach, for example, the use of spatial working memory as the primary outcome in studies of GR antagonists was a direct result of evidence in animals and healthy humans, demonstrating that this measure was sensitive to cortisol/HPA axis manipulations [80–82]. A similar approach – such as a focus on reward processing [83,84] in relation to dopaminergic treatments – may be warranted.

Procognitive Interventions

Direct Effect or Multiple Mechanisms?

One of the mechanisms outlined above is that of agents that enhance cognition directly, without being specifically related to mood disorder. Several interventions have been trialled that follow this principle.

Non-invasive brain stimulation methods (transcranial direct current stimulation [tDCS], repetitive transcranial magnetic stimulation [rTMS]) have been used extensively to explore the links between the brain and behaviour, including facilitating functional improvements in neurocognitive processes in both healthy and clinical populations [85,86]. Several studies have examined these methods in mood disorders. One study in older remitted MDD patients examined the effects of a 10-day course of bilateral anodal tDCS of the dorsolateral prefrontal cortex (DLPFC) reported no significant improvement in working memory or global cognition [87]. Other studies of rTMS to the left DLPFC in MDD have been mixed, with some negative [88], and others positive [89,90] in terms of neurocognitive improvement. With tDCS, some positive effects have been noted, including in cognitive control following a single administration in a crossover trial [91], and in working memory, in a small proof-of-concept study [92]. In BD, findings with rTMS have again been mixed, with some studies in BD depression showing no specific improvement over sham [93], while others in remitted BD patients have reported significant neurocognitive improvements in visuospatial memory and fluency [94]. Prefronto-cerebellar tDCS has also been found to

enhance neurocognition in euthymic bipolar patients [95,96].

Pharmacological options have similarly been explored. Modafinil is a wakefulness-enhancing agent that is indicated for narcolepsy, daytime somnolence, and fatigue associated with shift work disorder. Modafinil has been demonstrated to selectively improve neurocognitive function in healthy, non-sleep-deprived individuals [97–99] and has been explored as a procognitive treatment in mood disorders. It has been shown that augmentation with modafinil/armodafinil is associated with significantly greater rates of treatment response in BD depression [100]. In one prospective open-label study in MDD partial responders, augmenting antidepressant treatment with modafinil was found to improve symptoms of fatigue and depression as well as selectively improving neurocognitive performance (executive inhibition, but not set-shifting or working memory) [101].

The use of modafinil to improve cognitive function is an interesting illustration of an intervention that could be of utility through multiple mechanisms of action. It is discussed here in terms of its procognitive effects (having been found to improve performance in healthy subjects). However, attributing effects to one system is difficult given that neurobiological systems often interact [102] and drugs such as modafinil may exert their effects through a pro-dopaminergic / dopamine-reregulating mechanism [103]. Modafinil has also been demonstrated to improve neurocognitive functioning in subjects with primary sleep disorders such as obstructive sleep apnoea (OSA) [104,105]. Given the well-documented evidence of sleep disturbance (including OSA) in mood disorders [106,107], this provides yet another potential mechanism through which to improve neurocognitive function – specifically, if its efficacy is greater in those patients with sleep disorders when several mechanisms of action work synergistically.

This principle may also apply to other physical comorbidities in mood disorders. Cardiovascular and metabolic dysfunction, diabetes, and physical health problems have been found to be increased in severe mood disorders [108–110], and are possibly exacerbated by some treatments [111–114]. These physical health problems are also known to cause neurocognitive impairment [115–118] and therefore represent a potential treatment target in patients whose neurocognitive impairment is secondary to – or exacerbated by – such problems. Metformin, a widely used treatment for type 2 diabetes mellitus (T2DM), has been shown to significantly improve a range of neurocognitive functions (verbal, general and delayed memory, attention, and concentration) and mood in MDD patients with T2DM [119]. However, a recent RCT found that intranasal insulin improved one test of executive function in euthymic BD, although no other effects were observed in the wider neurocognitive battery, and patients were specifically screened to be free from cardiovascular and metabolic problems [120]. So, while such interventions may not be primarily 'procognitive', they may still hold potential to alleviate neurocognitive problems in a subset of patients.

Repurposing Procognitive Treatments from Other Conditions

Methylene blue, a derivative of phenothiazine used for the treatment of methemoglobinemia, has actions that may be neuroprotective and cognitive enhancing [121,122]. The use of methylene blue to treat mood disorders was first suggested 40 years ago [123–126], and it has been examined as a prophylactic treatment in BD [127] and severe depression [128]. In a recent randomised crossover study in 37 BD patients, methylene blue (195 mg) or placebo (a subtherapeutic dose of methylene blue, 15 mg) was administered over 6 months with neurocognitive assessments at baseline, week 13 and week 26. Although there were improvements in mood (Hamilton Depression Rating Scale [HAM-D], $d = 0.71$; Montgomery–Asberg Depression Rating Scale [MADRS], $d = 0.80$), there were no significant effects on the battery of neurocognitive tests assessing verbal learning and memory, executive set shifting, process dissociation, visual backward masking, and reaction time priming [129].

Erythropoietin (EPO), used for treatment of anaemia in individuals with cancer, has been found to exhibit neuroprotective and neurotrophic effects [130]. Several trials have explored its utility as a procognitive intervention [131]. Verbal memory improvement has been observed in treatment-resistant MDD [132] and improvements in attention and executive function in BD [133] after 8 weekly EPO infusions versus saline. These effects were associated with changes in functional and volumetric brain correlates [134,135].

Drugs that target the cholinergic system have been studied extensively for the treatment or slowing of neurocognitive decline in mild cognitive impairment (MCI)

and dementia [136,137]. Donepezil, a cholinesterase inhibitor, has been found to improve verbal memory in healthy volunteers [138], and early case reports have suggested it may also improve neurocognition in BD [139]. Positive neurocognitive effects have also been demonstrated in older MDD patients in whom improved neurocognitive function has been reported with adjunctive administration [140,141], although not in older BD patients [142]. The cholinesterase inhibitor and nicotinic receptor agonist galantamine has similarly been found to have beneficial cognitive effects independent of mood in several case series and one small trial in BD [143,144]. One further RCT demonstrated significant neurocognitive improvement from baseline, but not over placebo [145]. A study of donepezil in healthy older adults has highlighted an important consideration in the application of such treatments, suggesting evidence of a Yerkes–Dodson effect, where reduced cognitive function was induced in some subjects, potentially through perturbation of an already optimised cholinergic system [146]. This further suggests that patient stratification is an important consideration in relation to study design.

Dietary Supplements and Herbal Remedies

There has been interest several supplements for their potential in improving neurocognitive function in mood disorders. At present these trials are small and await replication. The medication N-acetyl cysteine has been proposed [147], given its neurobiological actions, although in a trial in BD no improvements were observed [148]. Omega-3 polyunsaturated fatty acids have well-demonstrated antioxidant properties [149,150], although studies in MDD have shown no neurocognitive effects [151]. *Withania somnifera* extract (WSE; ashwagandha) also known as 'Indian winter cherry' or 'Indian ginseng', is a widely used herb in traditional medicine with a number of biochemical properties that suggest it may have procognitive actions [152]. In a randomised placebo-controlled trial in 53 BD patients on standard maintenance treatment, adjunctive WSE was found to significantly improve working memory (reverse digit span; $d = 0.51$), and specific aspects of attention (Flanker test, neutral RT; $d = 0.62$) and emotion processing (Penn Emotional Acuity Test RT; $d = 0.26$) compared to the placebo arm of the study, in the absence of any changes in mood [153].

Behavioural and Psychological Interventions

Two approaches that are receiving growing interest for their potential to improve neurocognitive function in mood disorders are cognitive remediation and functional remediation [154–156]. There is a degree of overlap between these interventions: Cognitive remediation tends to employ focussed 'drill and practice' on neurocognitive tasks (either pen-and-paper or computerised) sometimes with metacognitive reflection or methods of strategic application. Functional remediation includes neurocognitive training, but this is alongside broader aspects of psychoeducation for contextualising and understanding the effect of these on daily life, psychosocial functioning, and sometimes with input from an individual's wider supporting/family network [157–159]. Here we focus particularly on those studies assessing neurocognitive improvement (rather than symptomatic or general functional recovery).

In MDD, cognitive remediation has been found to significantly improve attention/processing speed and verbal memory [160]. Improvements in memory have also been observed with cognitive training [161]. However, an open-label study in a mixed MDD and BD sample in partial remission observed no changes in verbal memory, although working memory was significantly improved [162]. A pilot study has examined the efficacy of computerised neurocognitive remediation therapy in community-living remitted MDD patients and found significant improvements in neurocognitive function [163], which is in line with meta-analytic findings, particularly in the case of working memory (mean effect size estimate, $g = 0.72$) and attention (mean effect size estimate, $g = 0.67$) [164]. One further recent study screened for the presence of cognitive impairment in MDD (< 16th percentile in two tests) and found significant improvements in attention following cognitive remediation therapy ($d = 0.763$; and after controlling for medication use, $d = 0.582$), which had been administered either as a group or individualised based on specific neurocognitive impairment [165].

In BD, following positive neurocognitive outcomes in preliminary studies [166], several trials have been completed using these interventions [167]. One trial of a short-term cognitive remediation intervention did not show any neurocognitive or psychosocial improvements [168]. However, a study of group-based cognitive remediation found positive effects on neurocognition, but similarly, no effect on psychosocial outcomes [169]. A 70-hour computerised cognitive remediation programme has been shown to improve processing speed and visual learning and memory [170], while a recent trial of action-based cognitive rehabilitation (which combines computer training, use of strategies, and practical activities with the aim to facilitate transfer to daily life) found improvements in executive function (planning) and subjective cognition [171].

In a comparison of functional remediation to psychoeducation or 'treatment as usual', one trial selected BD patients based on the presence of neurocognitive impairment at baseline ($n = 188/239$ who scored < 2 standard deviations [SD] below normative average) and found that functional remediation significantly improved verbal memory [172,173]. A previous study had not found any specific intervention-related neurocognitive improvement, as all groups improved significantly from baseline [174,175]. However, longitudinal follow-up revealed that patients with better cognitive performance at baseline, especially verbal memory, and executive function had better functional outcome [176]. This is in line with longitudinal observational causal modelling studies that have suggested that baseline neurocognitive function can predict and is causally primary to 1-year functional outcome [177].

There have also been attempts to combine several elements of these different interventions. A recent randomised controlled trial of an *integrative approach* (combining psychoeducation, mindfulness training, and functional remediation) observed significant improvements in psychosocial/functional outcome measures, including in the cognitive domain, although there were no changes in general neurocognitive function [178]. Combining neurostimulation with cognitive remediation has also been examined. Based on the hypothesis that MDD is associated with reduced dorsolateral prefrontal cortical activity, adding tDCS or sham to a trial of cognitive control therapy (CCT; a cognitive intervention of computer-based working memory exercises) resulted in greater efficacy of CCT under the active intervention [179]. Combining interventions across modalities selected for their association with underlying neurobiological deficits holds important therapeutic potential.

Numerous studies have shown a link between neurocognitive function and psychosocial function in mood disorders [15,177,180–182]. It is therefore of interest to note that behavioural interventions that target cognition such as those discussed in this chapter consistently have positive effects on function and outcome. Although there is the caveat that cognitive rehabilitation and remediation interventions do not solely train neurocognition but do so along with other psychosocial and reflective techniques, it may be that part of their efficacy derives from this approach.

Discussion and Recommendations

In this chapter we presented an overview of studies of interventions to improve neurocognitive functioning in major depressive and bipolar disorders. We have focussed specifically on the conceptual and broader methodological approaches underlying these studies to better consider the most promising directions for further research. While there are several directions that hold promise, it is of note that numerous trials have found no neurocognitive effects following intervention, sometimes despite seeing positive effects on mood or functional outcomes. There are a number of potential methodological and conceptual reasons why this may have occurred.

There is increasing recognition of the heterogeneity in neurocognition within mood disorders. While deficits are most frequently explored at cohort or group level, within any given study a proportion of cases will be indistinguishable from healthy controls, with statistical significance being driven by more substantive deficits in a subset of individuals, often meeting criteria for clinically significant impairment [10,183–186]. This is an often overlooked but important factor when considering potential management or treatment interventions for neurocognitive dysfunction. Using targeted treatment, after patient stratification based on defined neurocognitive impairment, may increase efficacy.

As we have seen in the studies presented, it is also crucial to consider the variety of mechanisms through which interventions may be acting. Successful approaches to neurocognitive improvement can be found in some treatments that lead to broad symptomatic improvement, of which one symptom may be neurocognitive dysfunction. Most commonly this has been in symptomatic patients, or those with evident residual symptoms. This may well be *pseudospecific* in terms of a mechanism but is still clinically important if we are looking to expand the available armamentarium. Similarly, the targeting of specific physical symptoms in affected subgroups, for example, those with metabolic or sleep dysregulation, could be a fruitful direction for

further research as much as focussing on direct *procognitive* treatments. Taking sleep as an example, there is strong evidence for the use of cognitive behavioural therapy for insomnia (CBT-I) in those with primary sleep disorders, which also improves depressive symptoms and cognition [187–191]. Along with other pharmacological approaches that target fatigue (reviewed above) or psychoeducation/functional remediation with 'sleep hygiene' components, using these interventions in stratified patient samples[‡] with both neurocognitive and sleep disturbance would be of great interest.

Finally, it should be acknowledged that in many cases the approaches we have reviewed could involve more than one mode of action. In some cases, neurocognitive improvement may come with general symptomatic response, for others, from specific targeting of a circumscribed neurobiological dysfunction. For some, it may come by addressing other symptoms such as metabolic or sleep disorders, or perhaps by using direct 'cognitive enhancing' treatments. This is crucial as, given the heterogeneity in both the overall presence of neurocognitive deficits and the underlying neurobiology for a given individual, it is unlikely we are seeking a 'one-size-fits-all' solution. Work on neurocognitive treatments needs to coincide with work on developing a deeper understanding of such deficits in mood disorders, reliable patient stratification, and biomarkers. These would provide the field with much clearer avenues to further progress clinical research into methods of ameliorating and managing neurocognitive dysfunction in mood disorders.

References

1. Rock PL, Roiser JP, Riedel WJ, Blackwell AD. Cognitive impairment in depression: a systematic review and meta-analysis. *Psychol Med* 2014;44:2029–40.

2. Zakzanis KK, Leach L, Kaplan E. On the nature and pattern of neurocognitive function in major depressive disorder. *Neuropsychiatry Neuropsychol Behav Neurol* 1998;11:111–19.

[‡] It is important to note that, as we have reviewed in this chapter, dysregulated neurobiological systems and physical symptoms such as those discussed have been observed in individuals whose primary mood symptoms have partially or fully remitted (especially in euthymic BD). Therefore, in such samples, treatments working via these mechanisms that lead to neurocognitive improvement cannot be doing so as a secondary consequence of primary mood change.

3. Kurtz MM, Gerraty RT. A meta-analytic investigation of neurocognitive deficits in bipolar illness: profile and effects of clinical state. *Neuropsychol Rev* 2009;**23**:551–62.

4. Goodall J, Fisher C, Hetrick S, et al. Neurocognitive functioning in depressed young people: a systematic review and meta-analysis. *Neuropsychol Rev* 2018;**28**:216–31.

5. Lee RSC, Hermens DF, Porter MA, Redoblado-Hodge MA. A meta-analysis of cognitive deficits in first-episode major depressive disorder. *J Affect Disord* 2012;**140**:113–24.

6. Hasselbalch BJ, Knorr U, Kessing LV. Cognitive impairment in the remitted state of unipolar depressive disorder: a systematic review. *J Affect Disord* 2011;**134**:20–31.

7. Preiss M, Kucerova H, Lukavsky J, et al. Cognitive deficits in the euthymic phase of unipolar depression. *Psychiatry Res* 2009;**169**:235–9.

8. Gallagher P, Robinson LJ, Gray JM, Porter RJ, Young AH. Neurocognitive function following remission in major depressive disorder: potential objective marker of response? *Aust N Z J Psychiatry* 2007;**41**:54–61.

9. Robinson LJ, Thompson JM, Gallagher P, et al. A meta-analysis of cognitive deficits in euthymic bipolar subjects. *J Affect Disord* 2006;**93**:105–15.

10. Cullen B, Ward J, Graham NA, et al. Prevalence and correlates of cognitive impairment in euthymic adults with bipolar disorder: a systematic review. *J Affect Disord* 2016;**205**:165–81.

11. Thompson JM, Gallagher P, Hughes JH, et al. Neurocognitive impairment in euthymic bipolar disorder. *Br J Psychiatry* 2005;**186**:32–40.

12. Withall A, Harris LM, Cumming SR. The relationship between cognitive function and clinical and functional outcomes in major depressive disorder. *Psychol Med* 2009;**39**:393–402.

13. Zubieta JK, Huguelet P, O'Neil RL, Giordani BJ. Cognitive function in euthymic bipolar I disorder. *Psychiatry Res* 2001;**102**:9–20.

14. Tabarés-Seisdedos R, Balanzá-Martínez V, Sánchez-Moreno J, et al. Neurocognitive and clinical predictors of functional outcome in patients with schizophrenia and bipolar I disorder at one-year follow-up. *J Affect Disord* 2008;**109**:286–99.

15. Mur M, Portella MJ, Martinez-Aran A, Pifarre J, Vieta E. Influence of clinical and neuropsychological variables on the psychosocial and occupational outcome of remitted bipolar patients. *Psychopathology* 2009;**42**:148–56.

16. Duarte W, Becerra R, Cruise K. The relationship between neurocognitive functioning and occupational functioning in bipolar disorder: a literature review. *Eur J Psychol* 2016;**12**:659–78.

17. Drakopoulos J, Sparding T, Clements C, Pålsson E, Landén M. Executive functioning but not IQ or illness severity predicts occupational status in bipolar disorder. *Int J Bipolar Disord* 2020;**8**:7.

18. Bortolato B, Miskowiak KW, Köhler CA, et al. Cognitive remission: a novel objective for the treatment of major depression? *BMC Med* 2016;**14**.

19. Sanches M, Bauer IE, Galvez JF, Zunta-Soares GB, Soares JC. The management of cognitive impairment in bipolar disorder: current status and perspectives. *Am J Ther* 2015;**22**:477–86.

20. Miskowiak KW, Carvalho AF, Vieta E, Kessing LV. Cognitive enhancement treatments for bipolar disorder: a systematic review and methodological recommendations. *Eur Neuropsychopharmacol* 2016;**26**:1541–61.

21. Miskowiak KW, Ott CV, Petersen JZ, Kessing LV. Systematic review of randomized controlled trials of candidate treatments for cognitive impairment in depression and methodological challenges in the field. *Eur Neuropsychopharmacol* 2016;**26**:1845–67.

22. Yerkes RM, Dodson JD. The relation of strength of stimulus to rapidity of habit-formation. *J Comp Neurol Psychol* 1908;**18**:459–82.

23. Tamura JK, Carvalho IP, Leanna LMW, et al. Management of cognitive impairment in bipolar disorder: a systematic review of randomized controlled trials. *CNS Spectr* 2021;**28**:1–22.

24. Solé B, Jiménez E, Torrent C, et al. Cognitive impairment in bipolar disorder: treatment and prevention strategies. *Int J Neuropsychopharmacol* 2017;**20**:670–80.

25. Cipriani A, Furukawa TA, Salanti G, et al. Comparative efficacy and acceptability of 21 antidepressant drugs for the acute treatment of adults with major depressive disorder: a systematic review and network meta-analysis. *Lancet* 2018;**391**:1357–66.

26. Rosenblat JD, Kakar R, McIntyre RS. The cognitive effects of antidepressants in major depressive disorder: a systematic review and meta-analysis of randomized clinical trials. *Int J Neuropsychopharmacol* 2015;**19**.

27. Baune BT, Brignone M, Larsen KG. a network meta-analysis comparing effects of various antidepressant classes on the Digit Symbol Substitution Test (DSST) as a measure of cognitive dysfunction in patients with major depressive disorder. *Int J Neuropsychopharmacol* 2018;**21**:97–107.

28. Katona C, Hansen T, Olsen CK. A randomized, double-blind, placebo-controlled,

duloxetine-referenced, fixed-dose study comparing the efficacy and safety of Lu AA21004 in elderly patients with major depressive disorder. *Int Clin Psychopharmacol* 2012;**27**:215–23.

29. Raskin J, Wiltse CG, Siegal A, et al. Efficacy of duloxetine on cognition, depression, and pain in elderly patients with major depressive disorder: an 8-week, double-blind, placebo-controlled trial. *Am J Psychiatry* 2007;**164**:900–9.

30. Robinson M, Oakes TM, Raskin J, et al. Acute and long-term treatment of late-life major depressive disorder: duloxetine versus placebo. *Am J Geriatr Psychiatry* 2014;**22**:34–45.

31. McIntyre RS, Lophaven S, Olsen CK. A randomized, double-blind, placebo-controlled study of vortioxetine on cognitive function in depressed adults. *Int J Neuropsychopharmacol* 2014;**17**:1557–67.

32. Mahableshwarkar AR, Zajecka J, Jacobson W, Chen Y, Keefe RS. A randomized, placebo-controlled, active-reference, double-blind, flexible-dose study of the efficacy of vortioxetine on cognitive function in major depressive disorder. *Neuropsychopharmacology* 2015;**40**:2025–37.

33. Vieta E, Sluth LB, Olsen CK. The effects of vortioxetine on cognitive dysfunction in patients with inadequate response to current antidepressants in major depressive disorder: a short-term, randomized, double-blind, exploratory study versus escitalopram. *J Affect Disord* 2018;**227**:803–9.

34. Baune BT, Sluth LB, Olsen CK. The effects of vortioxetine on cognitive performance in working patients with major depressive disorder: a short-term, randomized, double-blind, exploratory study. *J Affect Disord* 2018;**229**:421–8.

35. Nierenberg AA, Loft H, Olsen CK. Treatment effects on residual cognitive symptoms among partially or fully remitted patients with major depressive disorder: a randomized, double-blinded, exploratory study with vortioxetine. *J Affect Disord* 2019;**250**:35–42.

36. Mur M, Portella MJ, Martínez-Arán A, Pifarré J, Vieta E. Neuropsychological profile in bipolar disorder: a preliminary study of monotherapy lithium-treated euthymic bipolar patients evaluated at a 2-year interval. *Acta Psychiatr Scand* 2008;**118**:373–81.

37. Yatham LN, Mackala S, Basivireddy J, et al. Lurasidone versus treatment as usual for cognitive impairment in euthymic patients with bipolar I disorder: a randomised, open-label, pilot study. *Lancet Psychiatry* 2017;**4**:208–17.

38. Xu N, Huggon B, Saunders KEA. Cognitive impairment in patients with bipolar disorder: impact of pharmacological treatment. *CNS Drugs* 2020;**34**:29–46.

39. Porter RJ, Robinson LJ, Mahli GS, Gallagher P. The neurocognitive profile of mood disorders – a review of the evidence and methodological issues. *Bipolar Disord* 2015;**17**:21–40.

40. Gallagher P, Watson S, Smith MS, Young AH, Ferrier IN. Plasma cortisol-dehydroepiandrosterone (DHEA) ratios in schizophrenia and bipolar disorder. *Schizophr Res* 2007;**90**:258–65.

41. Maes M, Calabrese J, Meltzer HY. The relevance of the inpatient versus the outpatient status for studies on HPA-axis in depression – spontaneous hypercortisolism is a feature of major depressed inpatients and not of major depression per se. *Prog Neuropsychopharmacol Biol Psychiatry* 1994;**18**:503–17.

42. Arborelius L, Owens MJ, Plotsky PM, Nemeroff CB. The role of corticotropin-releasing factor in depression and anxiety disorders. *J Endocrinol* 1999;**160**:1–12.

43. Gallagher P, Reid KS, Ferrier IN. Neuropsychological functioning in health and mood disorder: modulation by glucocorticoids and their receptors. *Psychoneuroendocrinology* 2009;**34** 196–207.

44. Girshkin L, Matheson SL, Shepherd AM, Green MJ. Morning cortisol levels in schizophrenia and bipolar disorder: a meta-analysis. *Psychoneuroendocrinology* 2014;**49**:187–206.

45. Fries GR, Vasconcelos-Moreno MP, Gubert C, et al. Hypothalamic-pituitary-adrenal axis dysfunction and illness progression in bipolar disorder. *Int J Neuropsychopharmacol* 2015;**18**:pyu043-pyu. Erratum in: *Int J Neuropsychopharmacol*. 2016 Apr 27: PMID: 25522387; PMCID: PMC4368875.

46. Watson S, Gallagher P, Del-Estal D, et al. Hypothalamic-pituitary-adrenal axis function in patients with chronic depression. *Psychol Med* 2002;**32**:1021–8.

47. Watson S, Gallagher P, Ritchie JC, Ferrier IN, Young AH. Hypothalamic-pituitary-adrenal axis function in patients with bipolar disorder. *Br J Psychiatry* 2004;**184**:496–502.

48. Young AH, Gallagher P, Porter RJ. Elevation of the cortisol-dehydroepiandrosterone ratio in drug-free depressed patients. *Am J Psychiatry* 2002;**159**:1237–9.

49. Wolkowitz OM, Reus VI, Weingartner H, et al. Cognitive effects of corticosteroids. *Am J Psychiatry* 1990;**147**:1297–303.

50. Heffelfinger AK, Newcomer JW. Glucocorticoid effects on memory function over the human life span. *Dev Psychopathol* 2001;**13**:491–513.

51. Jameison K, Dinan TG. Glucocorticoids and cognitive function: from physiology to pathophysiology. *Hum Psychopharmacol* 2001;**16**:293–302.

52. McAllister-Williams RH, Rugg MD. Effects of repeated cortisol administration on brain potential correlates of episodic memory retrieval. *Psychopharmacology (Berl)* 2002;**160**:74–83.

53. Lupien SJ, Wilkinson CW, Briere S, et al. The modulatory effects of corticosteroids on cognition: studies in young human populations. *Psychoneuroendocrinology* 2002;**27**:401–16.

54. McQuade R, Young AH. Future therapeutic targets in mood disorders: the glucocorticoid receptor. *Br J Psychiatry* 2000;**177**:390–5.

55. Jahn H, Schick M, Kiefer F, et al. Metyrapone as additive treatment in major depression: a double-blind and placebo-controlled trial. *Arch Gen Psychiatry* 2004;**61**:1235–44.

56. O'Dwyer A-M, Lightman SL, Marks MN, Checkley SA. Treatment of major depression with metyrapone and hydrocortisone. *J Affect Disord* 1995;**33**:123–8.

57. McAllister-Williams RH, Anderson IM, Finkelmeyer A, et al. Antidepressant augmentation with metyrapone for treatment-resistant depression (the ADD study): a double-blind, randomised, placebo-controlled trial. *Lancet Psychiatry* 2016;**3**:117–27.

58. Ferrier IN, Anderson IM, Barnes J, et al. Randomised controlled trial of Antiglucocorticoid augmentation (metyrapone) of antiDepressants in Depression (ADD Study). *Efficacy Mech Eval* 2015;**2**.

59. Donoghue K, Rose A, Coulton S, et al. Double-blind, placebo-controlled trial of mifepristone on cognition and depression in alcohol dependence. *Trials* 2020;**21**:796.

60. Young AH, Gallagher P, Watson S, et al. Improvements in neurocognitive function and mood following adjunctive treatment with mifepristone (RU-486) in bipolar disorder. *Neuropsychopharmacology* 2004;**29**:1538–45.

61. Watson S, Gallagher P, Porter RJ, et al. A randomized trial to examine the effect of mifepristone on neuropsychological performance and mood in patients with bipolar depression. *Biol Psychiatry* 2012;**72**:943–9.

62. Gallagher P, Watson S, Dye CE, Young AH, Ferrier IN. Persistent effects of mifepristone (RU-486) on cortisol levels in bipolar disorder and schizophrenia. *J Psychiatr Res* 2008;**42**:1037–41.

63. Harrison PJ. Molecular neurobiological clues to the pathogenesis of bipolar disorder. *Curr Opin Neurobiol* 2015;**36**:1–6.

64. Kalia M. Neurobiological basis of depression: an update. *Metabolism* 2005;**54**:24–7.

65. Austin MP, Mitchell P, Hadzi-Pavlovic D, et al. Effect of apomorphine on motor and cognitive function in melancholic patients: a preliminary report. *Psychiatry Res* 2000;**97**:207–15.

66. Madhoo M, Keefe RSE, Roth RM, et al. Lisdexamfetamine dimesylate augmentation in adults with persistent executive dysfunction after partial or full remission of major depressive disorder. *Neuropsychopharmacology* 2014;**39**:1388–98.

67. Goldberg JF, Burdick KE, Endick CJ. Preliminary randomized, double-blind, placebo-controlled trial of pramipexole added to mood stabilizers for treatment-resistant bipolar depression. *Am J Psychiatry* 2004;**161**:564–6.

68. Cusin C, Iovieno N, Iosifescu DV, et al. A randomized, double-blind, placebo-controlled trial of pramipexole augmentation in treatment-resistant major depressive disorder. *J Clin Psychiatry* 2013;**74**: e636-41.

69. Zarate J, Carlos A., Payne JL, et al. Pramipexole for bipolar II depression: a placebo-controlled proof of concept study. *Biol Psychiatry* 2004;**56**:54–60.

70. Hori H, Kunugi H. The efficacy of pramipexole, a dopamine receptor agonist, as an adjunctive treatment in treatment-resistant depression: an open-label trial. *ScientificWorldJournal* 2012;**2012**:372474.

71. Burdick KE, Braga RJ, Goldberg JF, Malhotra AK. Cognitive dysfunction in bipolar disorder: future place of pharmacotherapy. *CNS Drugs* 2007;**21**:971–81.

72. Burdick KE, Braga RJ, Nnadi CU, et al. Placebo-controlled adjunctive trial of pramipexole in patients with bipolar disorder: targeting cognitive dysfunction. *J Clin Psychiatry* 2012;**73**:103–12.

73. Li C-T, Yang K-C, Lin W-C. Glutamatergic dysfunction and glutamatergic compounds for major psychiatric disorders: evidence from clinical neuroimaging studies. *Front Psychiatry* 2019;**9**:767.

74. Gigante AD, Bond DJ, Lafer B, et al. Brain glutamate levels measured by magnetic resonance spectroscopy in patients with bipolar disorder: a meta-analysis. *Bipolar Disord* 2012;**14**:478–87.

75. Berman RM, Cappiello A, Anand A, et al. Antidepressant effects of ketamine in depressed patients. *Biol Psychiatry* 2000;**47**:351–4.

76. Joseph B, Parsaik AK, Ahmed AT, Erwin PJ, Singh B. A systematic review on the efficacy of intravenous racemic ketamine for bipolar depression. *J Clin Psychopharmacol* 2021;**41**:71–5.

77. Liu W, Zhou Y, Zheng W, et al. Repeated intravenous infusions of ketamine: Neurocognition in patients

with anxious and nonanxious treatment-resistant depression. *J Affect Disord* 2019;**259**:1–6.

78. Chei TT, Demetrio FN. Memantine may acutely improve cognition and have a mood stabilizing effect in treatment-resistant bipolar disorder. *Braz J Psychiatry* 2006;**28**:252–4.

79. Strzelecki D, Tabaszewska A, Barszcz Z, et al. A 10-week memantine treatment in bipolar depression: a case report. Focus on depressive symptomatology, cognitive parameters and quality of life. *Psychiatry Investig* 2013;**10**:421–4.

80. Young AH, Sahakian BJ, Robbins TW, Cowen PJ. The effects of chronic administration of hydrocortisone on cognitive function in normal male volunteers. *Psychopharmacology (Berl)* 1999;**145**:260–6.

81. Oitzl MS, Fluttert M, de Kloet ER. Acute blockade of hippocampal glucocorticoid receptors facilitates spatial learning in rats. *Brain Res* 1998;**797**:159–62.

82. Oitzl MS, Fluttert M, Sutanto W, de Kloet ER. Continuous blockade of brain glucocorticoid receptors facilitates spatial learning and memory in rats. *Eur J Neurosci* 1998;**10**:3759–66.

83. Ashok AH, Marques TR, Jauhar S, et al. The dopamine hypothesis of bipolar affective disorder: the state of the art and implications for treatment. *Mol Psychiatry* 2017;**22**(5):666–79.

84. Whitton AE, Treadway MT, Pizzagalli DA. Reward processing dysfunction in major depression, bipolar disorder and schizophrenia. *Curr Opin Psychiatr* 2015;**28**:7–12.

85. Valero-Cabré A, Amengual JL, Stengel C, Pascual-Leone A, Coubard OA. Transcranial magnetic stimulation in basic and clinical neuroscience: a comprehensive review of fundamental principles and novel insights. *Neurosci Biobehav Rev* 2017;**83**:381–404. Erratum in Corrigendum to 'Transcranial magnetic stimulation in basic and clinical neuroscience: a comprehensive review of fundamental principles and novel insights' [Neurosci. Biobehav. Rev. 83 (2017) 381–404].

86. Moreno ML, Vanderhasselt MA, Carvalho AF, et al. Effects of acute transcranial direct current stimulation in hot and cold working memory tasks in healthy and depressed subjects. *Neurosci Lett* 2015;**591**:126–31.

87. Kumar S, Batist J, Ghazala Z, et al. Effects of bilateral transcranial direct current stimulation on working memory and global cognition in older patients with remitted major depression: a pilot randomized clinical trial. *Int J Geriatr Psychiatry* 2020;**35**:1233–42.

88. Mogg A, Pluck G, Eranti SV, et al. A randomized controlled trial with 4-month follow-up of adjunctive repetitive transcranial magnetic stimulation of the left prefrontal cortex for depression. *Psychol Med* 2008;**38**:323–33.

89. O'Connor MG, Jerskey BA, Robertson EM, et al. The effects of repetitive transcranial magnetic stimulation (rTMS) on procedural memory and dysphoric mood in patients with major depressive disorder. *Cogn Behav Neurol* 2005;**18**.

90. Schulze-Rauschenbach SC, Harms U, Schlaepfer TE, et al. Distinctive neurocognitive effects of repetitive transcranial magnetic stimulation and electroconvulsive therapy in major depression. *Br J Psychiatry* 2005;**186**:410–6.

91. Wolkenstein L, Plewnia C. Amelioration of cognitive control in depression by transcranial direct current stimulation. *Biol Psychiatry* 2013;**73**:646–51.

92. Fregni F, Boggio PS, Nitsche MA, Rigonatti SP, Pascual-Leone A. Cognitive effects of repeated sessions of transcranial direct current stimulation in patients with depression. *Depress Anxiety* 2006;**23**:482–4.

93. Myczkowski ML, Fernandes A, Moreno M, et al. Cognitive outcomes of TMS treatment in bipolar depression: safety data from a randomized controlled trial. *J Affect Disord* 2018;**235**:20–6.

94. Yang LL, Zhao D, Kong LL, et al. High-frequency repetitive transcranial magnetic stimulation (rTMS) improves neurocognitive function in bipolar disorder. *J Affect Disord* 2019;**246**:851–6.

95. Bersani FS, Minichino A, Bernabei L, et al. Prefronto-cerebellar tDCS enhances neurocognition in euthymic bipolar patients. Findings from a placebo-controlled neuropsychological and psychophysiological investigation. *J Affect Disord* 2017;**209**:262–9.

96. Minichino A, Bersani FS, Bernabei L, et al. Prefronto-cerebellar transcranial direct current stimulation improves visuospatial memory, executive functions, and neurological soft signs in patients with euthymic bipolar disorder. *Neuropsychiatr Dis Treat* 2015;**11**:2265–70.

97. Turner DC, Robbins TW, Clark L, et al. Cognitive enhancing effects of modafinil in healthy volunteers. *Psychopharmacology (Berl)* 2003;**165**:260–9.

98. Battleday RM, Brem AK. Modafinil for cognitive neuroenhancement in healthy non-sleep-deprived subjects: a systematic review. *Eur Neuropsychopharmacol* 2015;**25**:1865–81.

99. Cope ZA, Minassian A, Kreitner D, et al. Modafinil improves attentional performance in healthy, non-sleep deprived humans at doses not inducing hyperarousal across species. *Neuropharmacology* 2017;**125**:254–62.

100. Nunez NA, Singh B, Romo-Nava F et al. Efficacy and tolerability of adjunctive modafinil/armodafinil in bipolar depression: a meta-analysis of randomized controlled trials. *Bipolar Disord* 2020;**22**:109–20.

101. DeBattista C, Lembke A, Solvason HB, Ghebremichael R, Poirier J. A prospective trial of modafinil as an adjunctive treatment of major depression. *J Clin Psychopharmacol* 2004;**24**:87–90.

102. Peters KZ, Cheer JF, Tonini R. Modulating the neuromodulators: dopamine, serotonin, and the endocannabinoid system. *Trends Neurosci* 2021;**44**:464–77.

103. Federici M, Latagliata EC, Rizzo FR, et al. Electrophysiological and amperometric evidence that modafinil blocks the dopamine uptake transporter to induce behavioral activation. *Neuroscience* 2013;**252**:118–24.

104. Dinges DF, Weaver TE. Effects of modafinil on sustained attention performance and quality of life in OSA patients with residual sleepiness while being treated with nCPAP. *Sleep Med* 2003;**4**:393–402.

105. Wang D, Bai XX, Williams SC, et al. Modafinil increases awake EEG activation and improves performance in obstructive sleep apnea during continuous positive airway pressure withdrawal. *Sleep* 2015;**38**:1297–303.

106. Bradley AJ, Anderson KN, Gallagher P, McAllister-Williams RH. The association between sleep and cognitive abnormalities in bipolar disorder. *Psychol Med* 2020;**50**:125–32.

107. Bradley AJ, Webb-Mitchell R, Hazu A, et al. Sleep and circadian rhythm disturbance in bipolar disorder. *Psychol Med* 2017;**47**:1678–89.

108. Garcia-Portilla MP, Saiz PA, Bascaran MT, et al. Cardiovascular risk in patients with bipolar disorder. *J Affect Disord* 2009;**115**:302–8.

109. Murray DP, Weiner M, Prabhakar M, Fiedorowicz JG. Mania and mortality: why the excess cardiovascular risk in bipolar disorder? *Curr Psychiatry Rep* 2009;**11**:475.

110. Vargas HO, Nunes SOV, Barbosa DS, et al. Castelli risk indexes 1 and 2 are higher in major depression but other characteristics of the metabolic syndrome are not specific to mood disorders. *Life Sci* 2014;**102**:65–71.

111. Carli M, Kolachalam S, Longoni B, et al. Atypical antipsychotics and metabolic syndrome: from molecular mechanisms to clinical differences. *Pharmaceuticals (Basel)* 2021;**14**.

112. Mackin P, Bishop D, Watkinson H, Gallagher P, Ferrier IN. Metabolic disease and cardiovascular risk in people treated with antipsychotics in the community. *Br J Psychiatry* 2007;**191**:23–9.

113. Mackin P, Waton T, Watkinson HM, Gallagher P. A four-year naturalistic prospective study of cardiometabolic disease in antipsychotic-treated patients. *Eur Psychiatry* 2012;**27**:50–5.

114. Wang Y, Liu D, Li X, Liu Y, Wu Y. Antidepressants use and the risk of type 2 diabetes mellitus: a systematic review and meta-analysis. *J Affect Disord* 2021;**287**:41–53.

115. Panza F, Frisardi V, Capurso C, et al. Metabolic syndrome and cognitive impairment: current epidemiology and possible underlying mechanisms. *J Alzheimers Dis* 2010;**21**:691–724.

116. Yaffe K, Kanaya A, Lindquist K, et al. The metabolic syndrome, inflammation, and risk of cognitive decline. *JAMA* 2004;**292**:2237–42.

117. Brands AMA, Biessels GJ, de Haan EHF, Kappelle LJ, Kessels RPC. The effects of type 1 diabetes on cognitive performance: a meta-analysis. *Diabetes Care* 2005;**28**:726–35.

118. Awad N, Gagnon M, Messier C. The relationship between impaired glucose tolerance, type 2 diabetes, and cognitive function. *J Clin Exp Neuropsychol* 2004;**26**:1044–80.

119. Guo M, Mi J, Jiang QM, et al. Metformin may produce antidepressant effects through improvement of cognitive function among depressed patients with diabetes mellitus. *Clin Exp Pharmacol Physiol* 2014;**41**:650–6.

120. McIntyre RS, Soczynska JK, Woldeyohannes HO, et al. A randomized, double-blind, controlled trial evaluating the effect of intranasal insulin on neurocognitive function in euthymic patients with bipolar disorder. *Bipolar Disord* 2012;**14**:697–706.

121. Sikka P, Bindra VK, Kapoor S, Jain V, Saxena KK. Blue cures blue but be cautious. *J Pharm Bioallied Sci* 2011;**3**:543–5.

122. Poteet E, Winters A, Yan LJ, et al. Neuroprotective actions of methylene blue and its derivatives. *PLoS One* 2012;**7**.

123. Naylor GJ, Dick DAT, Johnston BB, et al. Possible explanation for the therapeutic actions of lithium, and a possible substitute (methylene blue). *Lancet* 1981;**318**:1175–6.

124. Narsapur SL, Naylor GJ. Methylene blue: a possible treatment for manic depressive psychosis. *J Affect Disord* 1983;**5**:155–61.

125. Thomas RD, Callender K. Methylene blue in treatment of bipolar illness. *Biol Psychiatry* 1985;**20**:120–1.

126. Naylor GJ, Smith AH, Connelly P. Methylene blue in mania. *Biol Psychiatry* 1988;**24**:941–2.

127. Naylor GJ, Martin B, Hopwood SE, Watson Y. A two-year double-blind crossover trial of the prophylactic effect of methylene blue in manic-depressive psychosis. *Biol Psychiatry* 1986;**21**:915–20.

128. Naylor GJ, Smith AH, Connelly P. A controlled trial of methylene blue in severe depressive illness. *Biol Psychiatry* 1987;**22**:657–9.

129. Alda M, McKinnon M, Blagdon R, et al. Methylene blue treatment for residual symptoms of bipolar disorder: randomised crossover study. *Br J Psychiatry* 2017;**210**:54–60.

130. Sargin D, Friedrichs H, El-Kordi A, Ehrenreich H. Erythropoietin as neuroprotective and neuroregenerative treatment strategy: comprehensive overview of 12 years of preclinical and clinical research. *Best Pract Res Clin Anaesthesiol* 2010;**24**:573–94.

131. Ott CV, Vinberg M, Kessing LV, Miskowiak KW. The effect of erythropoietin on cognition in affective disorders – associations with baseline deficits and change in subjective cognitive complaints. *Eur Neuropsychopharmacol* 2016;**26**:1264–73.

132. Miskowiak KW, Vinberg M, Christensen EM, et al. Recombinant human erythropoietin for treating treatment-resistant depression: a double-blind, randomized, placebo-controlled phase 2 trial. *Neuropsychopharmacology* 2014;**39**:1399–408.

133. Miskowiak KW, Ehrenreich H, Christensen EM, Kessing LV, Vinberg M. Recombinant human erythropoietin to target cognitive dysfunction in bipolar disorder: a double-blind, randomized, placebo-controlled phase 2 trial. *J Clin Psychiatry* 2014;**75**:1347–55.

134. Miskowiak KW, Macoveanu J, Vinberg M, et al. Effects of erythropoietin on memory-relevant neurocircuitry activity and recall in mood disorders. *Acta Psychiatr Scand* 2016;**134**:249–59.

135. Miskowiak KW, Vinberg M, Macoveanu J, et al. Effects of erythropoietin on hippocampal volume and memory in mood disorders. *Biol Psychiatry* 2015;**78**:270–7.

136. Freo U, Pizzolato G, Dam M, Ori C, Battistin L. A short review of cognitive and functional neuroimaging studies of cholinergic drugs: implications for therapeutic potentials. *J Neural Transm (Vienna)* 2002;**109**:857–70.

137. Hampel H, Mesulam MM, Cuello AC, et al. The cholinergic system in the pathophysiology and treatment of Alzheimer's disease. *Brain* 2018;**141**:1917–33.

138. Zaninotto AL, Bueno OF, Pradella-Hallinan M, et al. Acute cognitive effects of donepezil in young, healthy volunteers. *Hum Psychopharmacol* 2009;**24**:453–64.

139. Kelly T. Is donepezil useful for improving cognitive dysfunction in bipolar disorder? *J Affect Disord* 2008;**107**:237–40.

140. Pelton GH, Harper OL, Tabert MH, et al. Randomized double-blind placebo-controlled donepezil augmentation in antidepressant-treated elderly patients with depression and cognitive impairment: a pilot study. *Int J Geriatr Psychiatry* 2008;**23**:670–6.

141. Reynolds CF III, Butters MA, Lopez O, et al. Maintenance treatment of depression in old age: a randomized, double-blind, placebo-controlled evaluation of the efficacy and safety of donepezil combined with antidepressant pharmacotherapy. *Arch Gen Psychiatry* 2011;**68**:51–60.

142. Gildengers AG, Butters MA, Chisholm D, Reynolds CF III, Mulsant BH. A 12-week open-label pilot study of donepezil for cognitive functioning and instrumental activities of daily living in late-life bipolar disorder. *Int J Geriatr Psychiatry* 2008;**23**:693–8.

143. Schrauwen E, Ghaemi SN. Galantamine treatment of cognitive impairment in bipolar disorder: four cases. *Bipolar Disord* 2006;**8**:196–9.

144. Iosifescu DV, Moore CM, Deckersbach T, et al. Galantamine-ER for cognitive dysfunction in bipolar disorder and correlation with hippocampal neuronal viability: a proof-of-concept study. *CNS Neurosci Ther* 2009;**15**:309–19.

145. Ghaemi SN, Gilmer WS, Dunn RT, et al. A double-blind, placebo-controlled pilot study of galantamine to improve cognitive dysfunction in minimally symptomatic bipolar disorder. *J Clin Psychopharmacol* 2009;**29**:291–5.

146. Beglinger LJ, Tangphao-Daniels O, Kareken DA, et al. Neuropsychological test performance in healthy elderly volunteers before and after donepezil administration: a randomized, controlled study. *J Clin Psychopharmacol* 2005;**25**.

147. Dean O, Giorlando F, Berk M. N-acetylcysteine in psychiatry: current therapeutic evidence and potential mechanisms of action. *J Psychiatry Neurosci* 2011;**36**:78–86.

148. Dean OM, Bush AI, Copolov DL, et al. Effects of N-acetyl cysteine on cognitive function in bipolar disorder. *Psychiatry Clin Neurosci* 2012;**66**:514–7.

149. Ciappolino V, DelVecchio G, Prunas C, et al. The effect of DHA supplementation on cognition in patients with bipolar disorder: an exploratory randomized control trial. *Nutrients* 2020;**12**.

150. McNamara RK, Carlson SE. Role of omega-3 fatty acids in brain development and function: potential

implications for the pathogenesis and prevention of psychopathology. *Prostaglandins Leukot Essent Fatty Acids* 2006;75:329–49.

151. Antypa N, Smelt AHM, Strengholt A, Van der Does AJW. Effects of omega-3 fatty acid supplementation on mood and emotional information processing in recovered depressed individuals. *J Psychopharmacol (Oxf)* 2011;26:738–43.

152. Singh N, Bhalla M, de Jager P, Gilca M. An overview on ashwagandha: a Rasayana (rejuvenator) of Ayurveda. *Afr J Tradit Complement Altern Med* 2011;8:208–13.

153. Chengappa KNR, Bowie CR, Schlicht PJ, et al. Randomized placebo-controlled adjunctive study of an extract of *Withania somnifera* for cognitive dysfunction in bipolar disorder. *J Clin Psychiatry* 2013;74:1076–83.

154. Douglas KM, Peckham A, Porter R, Hammar A. Cognitive enhancement therapy for mood disorders: a new paradigm? *Aust N Z J Psychiatry* 2019;53:1148–50.

155. Burdick KE, Lewandowski KE, Van Rheenen TE. Entering the debate: cognitive enhancement therapy for mood disorders: a new paradigm? *Bipolar Disord* 2020;22:305–6.

156. Porter RJ, Bowie CR, Jordan J, Malhi GS. Cognitive remediation as a treatment for major depression: a rationale, review of evidence and recommendations for future research. *Aust N Z J Psychiatry* 2013;47:1165–75.

157. Listunova L, Roth C, Bartolovic M, et al. Cognitive impairment along the course of depression: non-pharmacological treatment options. *Psychopathology* 2018;51:295–305.

158. Bowie CR, Gupta M, Holshausen K. Cognitive remediation therapy for mood disorders: rationale, early evidence, and future directions. *Can J Psychiatry* 2013;58:319–25.

159. Martínez-Arán A, Torrent C, Solé B, et al. Functional remediation for bipolar disorder. *Clin Pract Epidemiol Ment Health* 2011;7:112–16.

160. Bowie CR, Gupta M, Holshausen K, et al. Cognitive remediation for treatment-resistant depression: effects on cognition and functioning and the role of online homework. *J Nerv Ment Dis* 2013;201.

161. Naismith SL, Redoblado-Hodge MA, Lewis SJ, Scott EM, Hickie IB. Cognitive training in affective disorders improves memory: a preliminary study using the NEAR approach. *J Affect Disord* 2010;121:258–62.

162. Meusel L-AC, Hall GBC, Fougere P, McKinnon MC, MacQueen GM. Neural correlates of cognitive remediation in patients with mood disorders. *Psychiatry Res* 2013;214:142–52.

163. Semkovska M, Ahern E. Online neurocognitive remediation therapy to improve cognition in community-living individuals with a history of depression: a pilot study. *Internet Interv* 2017;9:7–14.

164. Motter JN, Pimontel MA, Rindskopf D, et al. Computerized cognitive training and functional recovery in major depressive disorder: a meta-analysis. *J Affect Disord* 2016;189:184–91.

165. Listunova L, Kienzle J, Bartolovic M, et al. Cognitive remediation therapy for partially remitted unipolar depression: a single-blind randomized controlled trial. *J Affect Disord* 2020;276:316–26.

166. Deckersbach T, Nierenberg AA, Kessler R, et al. Cognitive rehabilitation for bipolar disorder: an open trial for employed patients with residual depressive symptoms. *CNS Neurosci Ther* 2010;16:298–307.

167. Strawbridge R, Tsapekos D, Hodsoll J, et al. Cognitive remediation therapy for patients with bipolar disorder: a randomised proof-of-concept trial. *Bipolar Disord* 2021;23:196–208.

168. Demant KM, Vinberg M, Kessing LV, Miskowiak KW. Effects of short-term cognitive remediation on cognitive dysfunction in partially or fully remitted individuals with bipolar disorder: results of a randomised controlled trial. *PLoS One* 2015;10:e0127955.

169. Gomes BC, Rocca CC, Belizario GO, et al. Cognitive behavioral rehabilitation for bipolar disorder patients: a randomized controlled trial. *Bipolar Disord* 2019;21:621–33.

170. Lewandowski KE, Sperry SH, Cohen BM, et al. Treatment to Enhance Cognition in Bipolar Disorder (TREC-BD): efficacy of a randomized controlled trial of cognitive remediation versus active control. *J Clin Psychiatry* 2017;78:e1242-e9.

171. Ott CV, Vinberg M, Kessing LV, et al. Effect of action-based cognitive remediation on cognitive impairment in patients with remitted bipolar disorder: a randomized controlled trial. *Bipolar Disord* 2020;23(5):487–99.

172. Bonnin CM, Reinares M, Martínez-Arán A, et al. Effects of functional remediation on neurocognitively impaired bipolar patients: enhancement of verbal memory. *Psychol Med* 2016;46:291–301.

173. Bonnin CM, Torrent C, Arango C, et al. Functional remediation in bipolar disorder: 1-year follow-up of neurocognitive and functional outcome. *Br J Psychiatry* 2016;208:87–93.

174. Torrent C, del Mar Bonnin C, Martínez-Arán A, et al. Efficacy of functional remediation in bipolar disorder: a multicenter randomized controlled study. *Am J Psychiatry* 2013;**170**:852–9.

175. Solé B, Bonnin CM, Mayoral M, et al. Functional remediation for patients with bipolar II disorder: improvement of functioning and subsyndromal symptoms. *Eur Neuropsychopharmacol* 2015;**25**:257–64.

176. Solé B, Bonnín CM, Radua J, et al. Long-term outcome predictors after functional remediation in patients with bipolar disorder. *Psychol Med* 2022;**52** (2):314–922.

177. Ehrminger M, Brunet-Gouet E, Cannavo A-S, et al. Longitudinal relationships between cognition and functioning over 2 years in euthymic patients with bipolar disorder: a cross-lagged panel model approach with the FACE-BD cohort. *Br J Psychiatry* 2021;**218**:80–7.

178. Valls È, Bonnín CM, Torres I, et al. Efficacy of an integrative approach for bipolar disorder: preliminary results from a randomized controlled trial. *Psychol Med* 2021;**52**(16):1–12.

179. Brunoni AR, Boggio PS, De Raedt R, et al. Cognitive control therapy and transcranial direct current stimulation for depression: a randomized, double-blinded, controlled trial. *J Affect Disord* 2014;**162**:43–9.

180. Martinez-Aran A, Vieta E, Colom F, et al. Neuropsychological performance in depressed and euthymic bipolar patients. *Neuropsychobiology* 2002;**46**:16–21.

181. Martinez-Aran A, Penades R, Vieta E, et al. Executive function in patients with remitted bipolar disorder and schizophrenia and its relationship with functional outcome. *Psychother Psychosom* 2002;**71**:39–46.

182. Silverstein ML, Harrow M, Mavrolefteros G, Close D. Neuropsychological dysfunction and clinical outcome in psychiatric disorders: a two-year follow-up study. *J Nerv Ment Dis* 1997;**185**:722–9.

183. Douglas KM, Gallagher P, Robinson LJ, et al. Prevalence of cognitive impairment in major depression and bipolar disorder. *Bipolar Disord* 2018;**20**:260–74.

184. Van Rheenen TE, Lewandowski KE, Tan EJ, et al. Characterizing cognitive heterogeneity on the schizophrenia-bipolar disorder spectrum. *Psychol Med* 2017;**47**:1848–64.

185. Burdick KE, Russo M, Frangou S, et al. Empirical evidence for discrete neurocognitive subgroups in bipolar disorder: clinical implications. *Psychol Med* 2014;**44**:3083–96.

186. Iverson GL, Brooks BL, Langenecker SA, Young AH. Identifying a cognitive impairment subgroup in adults with mood disorders. *J Affect Disord* 2011;**132**:360–7.

187. Cunningham JEA, Shapiro CM. Cognitive behavioural therapy for insomnia (CBT-I) to treat depression: a systematic review. *J Psychosom Res* 2018;**106**:1–12.

188. Lancee J, van Straten A, Morina N, Kaldo V, Kamphuis JH. Guided online or face-to-face cognitive behavioral treatment for insomnia: a randomized wait-list controlled trial. *Sleep* 2016;**39**:183–91.

189. Sweetman A, Lovato N, Micic G, et al. Do symptoms of depression, anxiety or stress impair the effectiveness of cognitive behavioural therapy for insomnia? A chart-review of 455 patients with chronic insomnia. *Sleep Med* 2020;**75**:401–10.

190. Manber R, Edinger JD, Gress JL, et al. Cognitive behavioral therapy for insomnia enhances depression outcome in patients with comorbid major depressive disorder and insomnia. *Sleep* 2008;**31**:489–95.

191. Cheng P, Luik AI, Fellman-Couture C, et al. Efficacy of digital CBT for insomnia to reduce depression across demographic groups: a randomized trial. *Psychol Med* 2019;**49**:491–500.

Progress in Biomarkers to Improve Treatment Outcomes in Major Depressive Disorder

Sophie R. Vaccarino, Amanda K. Ceniti, Susan Rotzinger, and Sidney H. Kennedy

Introduction

Precision medicine is often considered the 'next frontier' of medical research and treatment, taking into account an individual's variability in several domains, including genes, neurobiology, environment, and lifestyle [1]. Precision medicine offers the promise of earlier disease diagnosis, identification of prognosis, and development of a personalized treatment plan based on a patient's unique characteristics. The application of precision medicine relies on the identification and use of biomarkers: 'characteristics that are objectively measured and evaluated as indicators of normal biological processes, [or] pathogenic processes' [2].

The treatment of major depressive disorder (MDD) would be greatly improved with the application of a precision medicine approach. MDD is a heterogeneous disorder that likely represents a group of disorders with multiple causes and phenotypic presentations. Based on the *Diagnostic and Statistical Manual of Mental Disorders*, 5th edition (DSM-5) diagnostic criteria, there are over 200 possible combinations of symptoms to meet criteria for a major depressive episode (MDE) [3,4]. Given this immense variability, it is unrealistic to think that a single treatment would work for all individuals with MDD. Instead, precision psychiatry aims to provide a biosignature by profiling genetics, neurobiology, environment, symptom presentation, and more that can identify which treatment approach would work best on an individual level.

While biomarkers have been evaluated in a range of contexts, including diagnosis, prognosis, and monitoring of disease progression [5,6], the current chapter will focus on predictive biomarkers to identify individuals who are more or less likely to experience a therapeutic benefit from a particular treatment [5].

These biomarkers are typically measured at baseline, but may also be reassessed at different phases of treatment to identify early clinical or biological changes that may predict treatment response or nonresponse. In particular, this chapter will focus on clinical, molecular, and neuroimaging indices of treatment outcome. We will also discuss the future of biomarker research, including integration of large databases through data-sharing platforms and the application of machine-learning methodologies.

Clinical Phenotypes

Clinical biomarkers include measures of demographic data, personal history, symptom severity, and behavioural dimensions (Figure 23.1). They are typically derived from clinical interviews, behavioural assessments, or self-reports; while they do not measure biological processes directly, they may reflect underlying biology. Clinical measures that are predictive of poor outcome include greater illness duration, number of previous episodes, quality of remission, and number of previous failed treatments [7–9]. Psychiatric or physical comorbidities are also associated with poor outcomes [8,10,11], as are life experiences such as childhood maltreatment and major life stressors [12–15].

Reward processing, personality, and cognitive factors have received considerable attention as potential clinical markers of underlying biological processes that can predict treatment outcome. Anhedonia, or loss of interest or pleasure in things that used to bring enjoyment, is a central characteristic of MDD with neuroimaging correlates, and therefore has frequently been studied as a potential biomarker. Early changes in reward sensitivity during the first 2 weeks of treatment with escitalopram are predictive of positive outcomes in MDD [16]. Findings from the first Canadian Biomarker

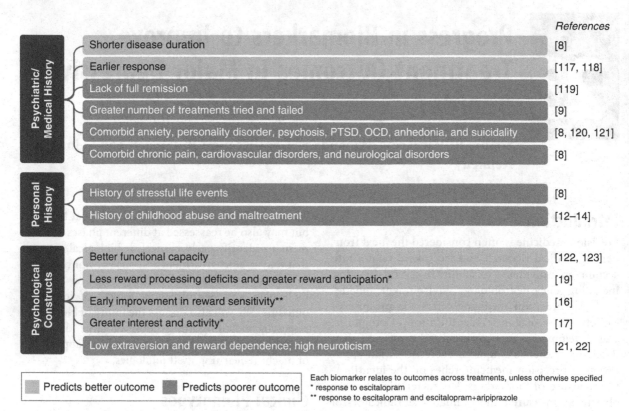

References

Psychiatric/Medical History	Shorter disease duration	[8]
	Earlier response	[117, 118]
	Lack of full remission	[119]
	Greater number of treatments tried and failed	[9]
	Comorbid anxiety, personality disorder, psychosis, PTSD, OCD, anhedonia, and suicidality	[8, 120, 121]
	Comorbid chronic pain, cardiovascular disorders, and neurological disorders	[8]
Personal History	History of stressful life events	[8]
	History of childhood abuse and maltreatment	[12–14]
Psychological Constructs	Better functional capacity	[122, 123]
	Less reward processing deficits and greater reward anticipation*	[19]
	Early improvement in reward sensitivity**	[16]
	Greater interest and activity*	[17]
	Low extraversion and reward dependence; high neuroticism	[21, 22]

■ Predicts better outcome ■ Predicts poorer outcome

Each biomarker relates to outcomes across treatments, unless otherwise specified
* response to escitalopram
** response to escitalopram and escitalopram+aripiprazole

Figure 23.1 Clinical biomarkers of treatment outcome.
Abbreviations: OCD: obsessive-compulsive disorder; PTSD: post-traumatic stress disorder.

Integration Network in Depression (CAN-BIND-1) dataset indicate that individuals with prominent loss of interest and reduced activity have worse treatment outcomes during treatment with escitalopram monotherapy, but show a favourable response to adjunctive aripiprazole [17], supporting previous findings suggesting that pro-dopaminergic medications are indicated in individuals with loss of interest and activity [17,18]. Consistent with this finding, individuals in the same trial who displayed less severe reward deficits at baseline during a reward task captured with functional magnetic resonance imaging (MRI) showed a better response to escitalopram at 8 weeks, while those individuals with greater reward deficits had poorer response to escitalopram [19].

Dimensions of personality also are associated with outcome. High neuroticism, low extraversion, and low conscientiousness are associated prospectively with the development of depressive symptoms [20], but in most cases are associated with poor outcome [21,22] and poor response to selective serotonin reuptake inhibitors (SSRIs)

[21–23]. However, a study comparing cognitive behavioural therapy (CBT) to pharmacotherapy found that individuals with high neuroticism respond better to pharmacotherapy than to CBT [24].

Functional impairment in cognition is frequently seen in MDD and has been evaluated as a potential marker for treatment selection. Participants with MDD in the CAN-BIND-1 trial had poorer baseline global cognition compared with non-depressed participants [25]. Neither escitalopram monotherapy nor adjunctive aripiprazole resulted in improvements in cognition. In another study, a subgroup of depressed patients was identified who had impaired cognitive performance, and this general cognitive impairment predicted non-remission to escitalopram with 72% accuracy based on the 16-item Quick Inventory of Depressive Symptomatology (QIDS-SR16) scores [26]. Finally, a report from the Establishing Moderators and Biosignatures of Antidepressant Response for Clinical Care for Depression (EMBARC) study noted that better baseline cognitive performance and early improvements in cognition were associated with higher likelihood of response to placebo [27].

Molecular Biomarkers

In many areas of medicine such as surgery, molecular biomarkers are derived from solid tissue biopsies, although there is increasing recognition of the value of 'liquid biomarkers'. In contrast, the majority of biomarkers examined in mental disorders are derived from plasma, serum, cerebrospinal fluid, saliva, or biopsy and act as objective physiological indicators of molecular properties [28,29]. Unlike biomarkers derived from source tissue, as is possible in other fields, there is debate about how well peripheral blood profiles correlate with those derived directly from organ-based tissue – in this case, the brain [30]. The most frequently studied molecular biomarkers of antidepressant response are cytochrome P450 genotypes [31], hypothalamic–pituitary–adrenal (HPA) axis markers [32–35], inflammatory cytokines [36–41], and functional genomic markers (Figure 23.2); however, larger controlled trials and meta-analyses must be completed.

'Omics' technologies, including transcriptomics, proteomics, genomics, metabolomics, and epigenomics, are sources of molecular biomarkers in psychiatry [42,43], and provide a window into biological systems. They may ultimately facilitate the development of omics-based tests to determine diagnosis, prognosis, and likelihood of treatment response [44].

Only two biomarkers have been approved by the US Food and Drug Administration (FDA) for use in psychiatry: CYP2D6 and CYP2C19, two enzymes of the cytochrome P450 (CYP) class, and these are safety biomarkers [45]. Underexpression of these enzymes can increase the risk of adverse drug effects related to elevated drug serum levels, while overexpression may decrease drug efficacy [46]. However, CYP2D6 and CYP2C19 enzymes metabolize a wide variety of drugs, including many non-psychiatric medications such as analgesics and oral contraceptives [45]. Genome-wide association studies (GWAS) are a common way in which molecular biomarkers are studied to identify genetic variations associated with illness or treatment response. Through GWAS, biomarker 'panels' may be identified, in which patterns across multiple genetic loci are combined to predict treatment response, rather than relying on a single polymorphism.

GWAS typically employs machine-learning approaches to identify biomarker panels [47,48]. Further, biomarker panels may combine clinical and physiological markers (e.g., clinical, molecular, and neuroimaging) to develop a biosignature to increase predictive specificity and sensitivity [49].

The use of biomarker panels aims to increase statistical power and accuracy [50]. However, in practice, results from GWAS are typically limited by relatively small effect sizes and the need for extremely high significance levels (typically a p-value $< 5 \times 10^{-8}$) to correct for multiple testing [51]. Further, GWAS are not hypothesis driven, and often biomarkers identified using this approach have no apparent functional relationship to the disease of interest [29]. Some argue that by taking this completely data-driven approach, GWAS will implicate too many genetic loci, all with small effect sizes, and the loci with actual clinical relevance will be missed [52,53]. However, others contend that since GWAS is a mathematical technique based on probability, there is no need for GWAS findings to be understood in terms of their relationship to the disease pathology [54]. One of the largest cohorts ever evaluated for GWAS of antidepressant response employed the 23andMe database of >50,000 research participants [55]. After analysing for treatment resistance versus non-treatment resistance, SSRI and serotonin and norepinephrine reuptake inhibitor (SNRI) response, three loci associated with immune process were identified [55]. Given the large number of samples required, and the low success rate with GWAS studies in depression, other molecular markers may be more promising.

Messenger RNAs (mRNA) have also been studied as potential antidepressant treatment biomarkers; expression of mRNA provides important information about protein expression and polymorphisms in key proteins involved in MDD pathophysiology [43]. Small non-coding microRNAs (miRNAs) play an important role in regulating gene expression [43,56], and have been linked to MDD aetiology [57]. Changes in various miRNA have also been associated with treatment response [56] and side effects [58], and have been found to change with treatment [59]. Exosomes are a class of extracellular vesicles that contain a variety of biological materials and are rich in miRNA. They can be measured in plasma, urine, or saliva, but since they can cross the blood–brain barrier, they may be very useful markers of brain processes in depression [60].

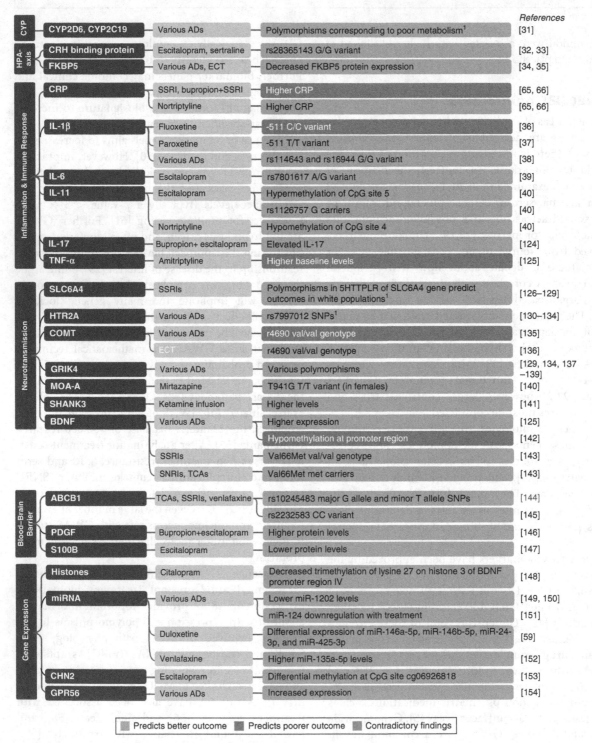

Figure 23.2 Molecular biomarkers of treatment outcome.

[1] Findings not replicated across studies

Abbreviations: 5-HTTLPR: serotonin-transporter-linked polymorphic region; ABCB1: ATP-binding cassette subfamily B member 1; AD: antidepressant; BDNF: blood-derived neurotrophic factor; COMT: catechol-O-methyltransferase; CRH: corticotropin-releasing hormone; CRP: C-reactive protein; CYP: cytochrome P450; ECT: electroconvulsive therapy; FKBP5: FK506 binding protein 5; GRIK4: glutamate ionotropic receptor kainate type subunit 4; HTR2A: 5-hydroxytryptamine receptor 2A (serotonin receptor gene); IL: interleukin; miRNA: micro-ribonucleic acid; MOA-A: monoamine oxidase A gene; PDGF: platelet-derived growth factor; S100B: S100 calcium binding protein B; SHANK3: SH3 and multiple ankyrin repeat; SNP: single nucleotide polymorphism; SNRI: serotonin and norepinephrine reuptake inhibitor; SSRI: selective serotonin reuptake inhibitor; TCA: tricyclic antidepressant; TNF-α: tumour necrosis factor alpha.

There is a large literature implicating inflammatory processes in depression and showing changes in inflammatory markers with antidepressant treatment (reviewed in [61]). C-reactive protein (CRP) is a plasma protein that increases markedly in response to infection or inflammation [62], and levels are heightened among some, but not all, individuals with MDD [63,64]. There are some reports that CRP levels predict treatment response to antidepressants, representing a potential tool for personalized treatment: participants with lower CRP levels experienced a greater improvement in depressive severity with escitalopram, while those with higher CRP levels improved more with nortriptyline [65]. Multiple studies have produced similar findings, showing significant associations between CRP levels and response to various antidepressants [66–69]. More recently, genetic polymorphisms associated with CRP levels have been discovered as potential biomarkers of antidepressant response [70,71]. Many inflammatory cytokines including interleukin-6 (IL-6) and tumour necrosis factor alpha (TNF-α) were found to be elevated in depressed patients compared with controls in a meta-analysis of the literature [72,73], whereas antidepressant treatments tend to reduce inflammatory cytokines [74]. Specific combinations of medications and individual interleukin markers are being investigated for potential in guiding treatment selection [41].

Neuroimaging Biomarkers

Neuroimaging biomarkers are generally derived from structural and functional imaging techniques. Structural biomarkers may be derived from structural MRI, diffusion tensor imaging (DTI), and computerized tomography (CT), while functional neuroimaging markers may be obtained from functional MRI (fMRI), positron emission tomography (PET), electroencephalogram (EEG), and near-infrared spectroscopy (NIRS).

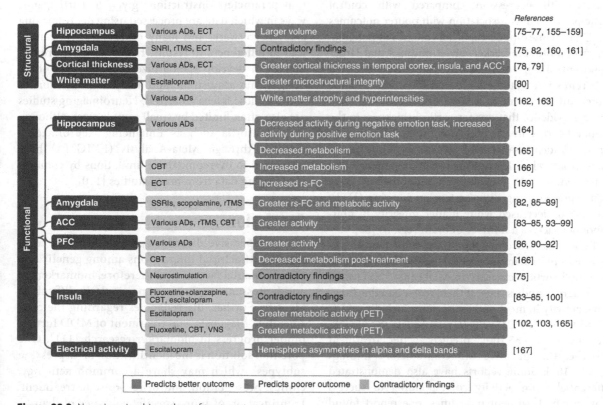

Figure 23.3 Neuroimaging biomarkers of treatment outcome.

[1] Findings not replicated across studies.

Abbreviations: ACC: anterior cingulate cortex; AD: antidepressant; CBT: cognitive behavioural therapy; ECT: electroconvulsive therapy; PET: positron emission tomography; PFC: prefrontal cortex; rs-FC: resting-state functional connectivity; rTMS: repetitive transcranial magnetic stimulation; VNS: vagal nerve stimulation.

The range of neuroimaging modalities presents both pros and cons in the advancement of biomarker research. Each modality has its strengths and weaknesses, but results from multiple neuroimaging modalities may be combined to achieve more accurate results and account for the limitations of each. For example, EEG is a direct measure of brain activity in real time, but has relatively low spatial resolution. Functional MRI, on the other hand, is an indirect measure of brain activity (measuring changes in brain tissue oxygenation after neural activity) but has high spatial resolution. Results from these two modalities may be interpreted together to obtain results that can more reliably identify patterns in activity within specific brain structures.

The most frequently identified structural brain regions associated with treatment outcome are fronto-limbic regions including the prefrontal cortex (PFC), anterior cingulate cortex (ACC), amygdala, insula, and hippocampus [75] (Figure 23.3). A consistent structural finding is reduced hippocampal volume in participants with depression compared with control participants, and its association with poorer outcomes [76,77]. Baseline hippocampal tail volume has potential as a prognostic biomarker, given findings that larger hippocampal tail volumes were positively associated with remission status after 8 and 16 weeks of antidepressant treatment in a large open-label trial [76]. There is evidence that greater cortical thickness in the temporal cortex, insula, and ACC predicts response to various antidepressants and ECT [78,79]. White matter microstructural differences between responders and non-responders to escitalopram monotherapy have been reported using diffusor tension imaging (DTI), implicating decreased white matter integrity in non-responders across a number of brain regions [80].

Functional neuroimaging studies consistently highlight disruptions in subcortical limbic network and prefrontal cortical circuitry in MDD [81–92]. Overall trends across studies suggest that greater baseline functional activity in most of these regions, including ACC [83–85,93–99], PFC [86,90–92], amygdala [82 85–89], and insula [83–85,100], predicts better treatment response, though there are contradictory findings [75,101–103]. Some reports have also demonstrated differential brain activity corresponding to success with specific treatment modalities: one report found insula hypometabolism was associated with remission with pharmacotherapy, whereas hypermetabolism in the same region was associated with remission to cognitive behavioural therapy [103].

Although a meta-analysis published in 2019 did not find support for the use of EEG as a biomarker for treatment response prediction [104], several more recent studies report positive findings for EEG signatures that predict antidepressant response using machine-learning algorithms [105,106]. The CAN-BIND network has also reported that baseline and early changes in EEG activity predict treatment response with high accuracy [107]. This study used a machine-learning feature selection process to identify features predicting antidepressant response that included parietal alpha, ACC activity, and frontal theta activity, as well as asymmetry in complexity of neural activity between hemispheres. Further studies are currently underway to validate this finding.

One of the limiting issues surrounding neuroimaging biomarker research is the lack of standardization across centres in data collection and analytic methods. Differences in imaging machines, acquisition parameters, instructions given to participants, ways in which data are processed using neuroimaging analysis software, and many other variables can all lead to differences in results. However, there are initiatives to develop standardized pipelines for study design, data acquisition, and analysis in an effort to address these issues [108,109]. Neuroimaging studies are also often limited by small sample sizes, although large consortia such as Enhancing NeuroImaging Genetics through Meta-Analysis (ENIGMA) have attempted to overcome these limitations by combining imaging data from many studies [110].

Conclusion

Major depressive disorder appears to reflect complex, multifactorial interactions among genetic and environmental factors, and therefore, biomarkers of antidepressant response are particularly difficult to identify. Further, discrepancies regarding the classification, diagnosis, and treatment of MDD further hinder progress in biomarker research [111]. One potential solution is the identification of 'depression subtypes', which may share a common aetiology, clinical presentation, and/or response to treatment. Identification of more specific subtypes of depression may allow for more targeted biomarker research [112].

Other ways to improve the discovery of psychiatric biomarkers include studies with large sample sizes and replication across different cohorts and study sites. Further, data-sharing platforms should be developed so that many data can be combined in meta-analyses. This will ultimately increase the statistical power of biomarker findings. Importantly, as data sharing and large data platforms become more common, quality control will become increasingly important. When combining data across multiple sites, clear protocols surrounding recruitment, data collection, and data management must be developed, and protocols across sites should be as similar as possible to allow for reliable data amalgamation [109]. For instance, technical guidelines have been developed for the collection of blood biomarkers, including standardized clinical protocols and pre-analysis methods, in an effort to reduce variability across studies [113].

Concerns about data sharing still exist. Researchers may be concerned that others will not understand the exact methodology of their study and therefore use their data inappropriately [114]. Further, many researchers worry about so-called research parasites, that is, those who did not contribute to data collection but may use another's data for their own benefit [114]. To overcome these obstacles, full transparency throughout the data-collection process and active collaboration among research groups is required. Transition from a competitive research towards 'open science' has begun, and while this change may take time, the benefits of data sharing are monumental. Data sharing will allow for very large samples of diverse populations to be obtained, thus providing reliable and statistically powerful results. An example of an effective data-sharing platform is CAN-BIND, which integrates data collected from 28 sites across Canada using an informatics platform [115,116] in order to study biomarkers of depression [116,117].

In the past several years, there has been progress in the development of biomarker technology and in identifying potential clinical, molecular, and neuroimaging treatment biomarkers. However, the heterogeneity of MDD and inconsistent biomarker measures limit progress in biomarker research. Consortia with large datasets, data sharing, and common methodologies are one way to advance biomarker research. Further, in order to identify reliable and generalizable biomarkers, large-scale replication studies and meta-analyses are required. This may be achieved through data-sharing platforms.

Acknowledgements

We would like to thank Rachel Laframboise of the Canadian Biomarker Integration Network in Depression for her assistance with the literature review. This research was conducted as part of CAN-BIND, an Integrated Discovery Program supported by the Ontario Brain Institute, which is an independent non-profit corporation, funded partially by the Ontario government. The opinions, results, and conclusions are those of the authors and no endorsement by the Ontario Brain Institute is intended or should be inferred.

Dr Kennedy has received research funding or honoraria from the following sources: Abbott, Abbvie, Alkermes, Brain Canada, Canadian Institutes for Health Research (CIHR), Janssen, Lundbeck, Lundbeck Institute, Ontario Brain Institute, Ontario Research Fund (ORF), Otsuka, Pfizer, Servier, and Sunovion. Dr Kennedy holds stock in Field Trip Health.

References

1. Committee on a Framework for Developing a New Taxonomy of Disease. *Toward Precision Medicine: Building a Knowledge Network for Biomedical Research and a New Taxonomy Of Disease*. Washington, DC: National Academies Press, 2011. doi: 10.17226/13284.

2. Biomarkers Definitions Working Group. Biomarkers and surrogate endpoints: preferred definitions and conceptual framework. *Clin Pharmacol Ther* 2001;**69**:89–95.

3. American Psychiatric Association. *Diagnostic and Statistical Manual of Mental Disorders: DSM-5*. 5th ed. Washington, DC: American Psychiatric Association, 2013.

4. Zimmerman M, Ellison W, Young D, et al. How many different ways do patients meet the diagnostic criteria for major depressive disorder? *Compr Psychiatry* 2015;**56**:29–34.

5. Califf RM. Biomarker definitions and their applications. *Exp Biol Med* 2018;**243**:213–21.

6. Mayeux R. Biomarkers: potential uses and limitations. *NeuroRX* 2004;**1**:182–8.

7. McAllister-Williams RH, Arango C, Blier P, et al. The identification, assessment and management of difficult-to-treat depression: an international consensus statement. *J Affect Disord* 2020;**267**:264–82.

8. Kraus C, Kadriu B, Lanzenberger R, et al. Prognosis and improved outcomes in major depression: a review. *Transl Psychiatry* 2019;**9**:127.

9. Rush AJ, Trivedi MH, Wisniewski SR, et al. Acute and longer-term outcomes in depressed outpatients requiring one or several treatment steps: a STAR*D report. *Am J Psychiatry* 2006;**163**:1905–17.

10. Souery D, Oswald P, Massat I, et al. Clinical factors associated with treatment resistance in major depressive disorder: results from a European multicenter study. *J Clin Psychiatry* 2007;**68**:1062–70.

11. Spijker J, Bijl R V, de Graaf R, et al. Determinants of poor 1-year outcome of DSM-III-R major depression in the general population: results of the Netherlands Mental Health Survey and Incidence Study (NEMESIS). *Acta Psychiatr Scand* 2001;**103**:122–30.

12. Nanni V, Uher R, Danese A. Childhood maltreatment predicts unfavorable course of illness and treatment outcome in depression: a meta-analysis. *Am J Psychiatry* 2012;**169**:141–51.

13. Harkness KL, Bagby RM, Kennedy SH. Childhood maltreatment and differential treatment response and recurrence in adult major depressive disorder. *J Consult Clin Psychol* 2012;**80**:342–53.

14. Nelson J, Klumparendt A, Doebler P, et al. Childhood maltreatment and characteristics of adult depression: meta-analysis. *Br J Psychiatry* 2017;**210**:96–104.

15. Quilty LC, Marshe V, Lobo DSS, et al. Childhood abuse history in depression predicts better response to antidepressants with higher serotonin transporter affinity: a pilot investigation. *Neuropsychobiology* 2016;**74**:78–83.

16. Allen TA, Lam RW, Milev R, et al. Early change in reward and punishment sensitivity as a predictor of response to antidepressant treatment for major depressive disorder: a CAN-BIND-1 report. *Psychol Med* 2019;**49**:1629–38.

17. Uher R, Frey BN, Quilty LC, et al. Symptom dimension of interest-activity indicates need for aripiprazole augmentation of escitalopram in major depressive disorder. *J Clin Psychiatry* 2020;**81**:20m13229.

18. Uher R, Perlis RH, Henigsberg N, et al. Depression symptom dimensions as predictors of antidepressant treatment outcome: replicable evidence for interest-activity symptoms. *Psychol Med* 2012;**42**:967–80.

19. Dunlop K, Rizvi SJ, Kennedy SH, et al. Clinical, behavioral, and neural measures of reward processing correlate with escitalopram response in depression: a Canadian Biomarker Integration Network in Depression (CAN-BIND-1) Report. *Neuropsychopharmacology* 2020;**45**:1390–7.

20. Hakulinen C, Elovainio M, Pulkki-Råback L, et al. Personality and depressive symptoms: individual participant meta-analysis of 10 cohort studies. *Depress Anxiety* 2015;**32**:461–70.

21. Takahashi M, Shirayama Y, Muneoka K, et al. Low openness on the revised NEO personality inventory as a risk factor for treatment-resistant depression. *PLoS One* 2013;**8**:e71964.

22. Takahashi M, Shirayama Y, Muneoka K, et al. Personality traits as risk factors for treatment-resistant depression. *PLoS One* 2013;**8**:e63756.

23. Allen TA, Harkness KL, Lam RW, et al. Interactions between neuroticism and stressful life events predict response to pharmacotherapy for major depression: a CAN-BIND 1 report. *Personal Ment Health* 2021;**15** (4):273–82.

24. Bagby RM, Quilty LC, Segal ZV, et al. Personality and differential treatment response in major depression: a randomized controlled trial comparing cognitive-behavioural therapy and pharmacotherapy. *Can J Psychiatry* 2008;**53**:361–370.

25. Chakrabarty T, McInerney SJ, Torres IJ, et al. Cognitive outcomes with sequential escitalopram monotherapy and adjunctive aripiprazole treatment in major depressive disorder: a Canadian Biomarker Integration Network in Depression (CAN-BIND-1) report. *CNS Drugs* 2021;**35**(3):291–304.

26. Etkin A, Patenaude B, Song YJC, et al. A cognitive-emotional biomarker for predicting remission with antidepressant medications: a report from the iSPOT-D trial. *Neuropsychopharmacology* 2015;**40**:1332–42.

27. Ang YS, Bruder GE, Keilp JG, et al. Exploration of baseline and early changes in neurocognitive characteristics as predictors of treatment response to bupropion, sertraline, and placebo in the EMBARC clinical trial. *Psychol Med* 2022;**52**(12):2441–9.

28. Gururajan A, Clarke G, Dinan TG, et al. Molecular biomarkers of depression. *Neurosci Biobehav Rev* 2016;**64**:101–33.

29. Gururajan A, Cryan JF, Dinan TG. Molecular biomarkers in depression: toward personalized psychiatric treatment. In BT Baune, editor. *Personalized Psychiatry*. Cambridge, MA: Academic Press, 2020;319–38.

30. Hayashi-Takagi A, Vawter MP, Iwamoto K. Peripheral biomarkers revisited: integrative profiling of peripheral samples for psychiatric research. *Biol Psychiatry* 2014;**75**:920–8.

31. Solomon H V., Cates KW, Li KJ. Does obtaining CYP2D6 and CYP2C19 pharmacogenetic testing predict antidepressant response or adverse drug reactions? *Psychiatry Res* 2019;**271**:604–13.

32. O'Connell CP, Goldstein-Piekarski AN, Nemeroff CB, et al. Antidepressant outcomes

predicted by genetic variation in corticotropin-releasing hormone binding protein. *Am J Psychiatry* 2018;**175**:251–61.

33. Fabbri C, Tansey KE, Perlis RH, et al. Effect of cytochrome CYP2C19 metabolizing activity on antidepressant response and side effects: meta-analysis of data from genome-wide association studies. *Eur Neuropsychopharmacol* 2018;**28**:945–54.

34. Ising M, Maccarrone G, Brückl T, et al. FKBP5 gene expression predicts antidepressant treatment outcome in depression. *Int J Mol Sci* 2019;**20**:485.

35. Sarginson JE, Lazzeroni LC, Ryan HS, et al. FKBP5 polymorphisms and antidepressant response in geriatric depression. *Am J Med Genet Part B Neuropsychiatr Genet* 2010;**153B**:554–60.

36. Yu YW-Y, Chen T-J, Hong C-J, et al. Association study of the interleukin-1beta (C-511T) genetic polymorphism with major depressive disorder, associated symptomatology, and antidepressant response. *Neuropsychopharmacology* 2003;**28**:1182–5.

37. Tadic A. Association analysis between variants of the interleukin-1beta and the interleukin-1 receptor antagonist gene and antidepressant treatment response in major depression. *Neuropsychiatr Dis Treat* 2008;**4**(1):269–76.

38. Baune BT, Dannlowski U, Domschke K, et al. The Interleukin 1 beta (IL1B) gene is associated with failure to achieve remission and impaired emotion processing in major depression. *Biol Psychiatry* 2010;**67**:543–9.

39. Uher R, Perroud N, Ng MYM, et al. Genome-wide pharmacogenetics of antidepressant response in the GENDEP project. *Am J Psychiatry* 2010;**167**:555–64.

40. Powell TR, Smith RG, Hackinger S, et al. DNA methylation in interleukin-11 predicts clinical response to antidepressants in GENDEP. *Transl Psychiatry* 2013;**3**:e300.

41. Jha MK, Minhajuddin A, Gadad BS, et al. Interleukin 17 selectively predicts better outcomes with bupropion-SSRI combination: novel T cell biomarker for antidepressant medication selection. *Brain Behav Immun* 2017;**66**:103–10.

42. Laterza OF, Hendrickson RC, Wagner JA. Molecular biomarkers. *Drug Inf J* 2007;**41**:573–85.

43. Belzeaux R, Lin R, Ju C, et al. Transcriptomic and epigenomic biomarkers of antidepressant response. *J Affect Disord* 2018;**233**:36–44.

44. Committee on the Review of Omics-Based Tests for Predicting Patient Outcomes in Clinical Trials, Board on Health Care Services, Board on Health Sciences Policy, et al. Omics-based clinical discovery: science, technology, and applications. In CM Micheel, SJ Nass, GS Omenn, editors. *Evolution of Translational Omics: Lessons Learned and the Path Forward*. Washington, DC: National Academies Press, 2012; chapter 2.

45. U.S. Food and Drug Administration. Table of Pharmacogenomic Biomarkers in Drug Labeling. www.fda.gov/drugs/science-and-research-drugs/table-pharmacogenomic-biomarkers-drug-labeling.

46. Meyer UA. Pharmacogenetics and adverse drug reactions. *Lancet* 2000;**356**:1667–71.

47. Maciukiewicz M, Marshe VS, Hauschild A-C, et al. GWAS-based machine learning approach to predict duloxetine response in major depressive disorder. *J Psychiatr Res* 2018;**99**:62–8.

48. Lin E, Kuo P-H, Liu Y-L, et al. A deep learning approach for predicting antidepressant response in major depression using clinical and genetic biomarkers. *Front Psychiatry* 2018;**9**:290.

49. Chekroud AM, Zotti RJ, Shehzad Z, et al. Cross-trial prediction of treatment outcome in depression: a machine learning approach. *Lancet Psychiatry* 2016;**3**:243–50.

50. Heinzel A, Mühlberger I, Fechete R, et al. Functional molecular units for guiding biomarker panel design. In VD Kumar, HJ Tipney editors. *Biomedical Literature Mining: Methods in Molecular Biology (Methods and Protocols)*. New York: Humana Press, 2014;109–33.

51. Tam V, Patel N, Turcotte M, et al. Benefits and limitations of genome-wide association studies. *Nat Rev Genet* 2019;**20**:467–84.

52. Goldstein JM, Seidman LJ, Makris N, et al. Hypothalamic abnormalities in schizophrenia: sex effects and genetic vulnerability. *Biol Psychiatry* 2007;**61**:935–45.

53. Boyle EA, Li YI, Pritchard JK. An expanded view of complex traits: from polygenic to omnigenic. *Cell* 2017;**169**:1177–86.

54. Paulus MP. Pragmatism instead of mechanism. *JAMA Psychiatry* 2015;**72**:631–2.

55. Li QS, Tian C, Hinds D, et al. Genome-wide association studies of antidepressant class response and treatment-resistant depression. *Transl Psychiatry* 2020;**10**:360.

56. Lopez JP, Kos A, Turecki G. Major depression and its treatment: microRNAs as peripheral biomarkers of diagnosis and treatment response. *Curr Opin Psychiatry* 2018;**31**:7–16.

57. Belzeaux R, Lin R, Turecki G. Potential use of microRNA for monitoring therapeutic response to antidepressants. *CNS Drugs* 2017;**31**:253–62.

58. Yrondi A, Fiori LM, Frey BN, et al. Association between side effects and blood microRNA expression

levels and their targeted pathways in patients with major depressive disorder treated by a selective serotonin reuptake inhibitor, escitalopram: a CAN-BIND-1 Report. *Int J Neuropsychopharmacol* 2021;**23**:88–95.

59. Lopez JP, Fiori LM, Cruceanu C, et al. MicroRNAs 146a/b-5 and 425-3p and 24-3p are markers of antidepressant response and regulate MAPK/Wnt-system genes. *Nat Commun* 2017;**8**:15497.

60. Saeedi S, Israel S, Nagy C, et al. The emerging role of exosomes in mental disorders. *Transl Psychiatry* 2019;**9**:1–11.

61. Jha M, Trivedi M. Personalized antidepressant selection and pathway to novel treatments: clinical utility of targeting inflammation. *Int J Mol Sci* 2018;**19**:233.

62. Sproston NR, Ashworth JJ. Role of C-reactive protein at sites of inflammation and infection. *Front Immunol* 2018;**9**:754.

63. Haapakoski R, Mathieu J, Ebmeier KP, et al. Cumulative meta-analysis of interleukins 6 and 1β, tumour necrosis factor α and C-reactive protein in patients with major depressive disorder. *Brain Behav Immun* 2015;**49**:206–15.

64. Miller AH, Raison CL. The role of inflammation in depression: from evolutionary imperative to modern treatment target. *Nat Rev Immunol* 2016;**16**:22–34.

65. Uher R, Tansey KE, Dew T, et al. An inflammatory biomarker as a differential predictor of outcome of depression treatment with escitalopram and nortriptyline. *Am J Psychiatry* 2014;**171**:1278–86.

66. Jha MK, Minhajuddin A, Gadad BS, et al. Can C-reactive protein inform antidepressant medication selection in depressed outpatients? Findings from the CO-MED trial. *Psychoneuroendocrinology* 2017;**78**:105–13.

67. Vogelzangs N, Duivis HE, Beekman ATF, et al. Association of depressive disorders, depression characteristics and antidepressant medication with inflammation. *Transl Psychiatry* 2012;**2**:e79.

68. Mocking RJT, Nap TS, Westerink AM, et al. Biological profiling of prospective antidepressant response in major depressive disorder: associations with (neuro)inflammation, fatty acid metabolism, and amygdala-reactivity. *Psychoneuroendocrinology* 2017;**79**:84–92.

69. Zhang J, Yue Y, Thapa A, et al. Baseline serum C-reactive protein levels may predict antidepressant treatment responses in patients with major depressive disorder. *J Affect Disord* 2019;**250**:432–8.

70. Li X, Sun N, Yang C, et al. C-Reactive protein gene variants in depressive symptoms & antidepressants efficacy. *Psychiatry Investig* 2019;**16**:940–7.

71. Zwicker A, Fabbri C, Rietschel M, et al. Genetic disposition to inflammation and response to antidepressants in major depressive disorder. *J Psychiatr Res* 2018;**105**:17–22.

72. Köhler CA, Freitas TH, Maes M, et al. Peripheral cytokine and chemokine alterations in depression: a meta-analysis of 82 studies. *Acta Psychiatr Scand* 2017;**135**:373–87.

73. Osimo EF, Pillinger T, Rodriguez IM, et al. Inflammatory markers in depression: a meta-analysis of mean differences and variability in 5,166 patients and 5,083 controls. *Brain Behav Immun* 2020;**87**:901–9.

74. Köhler CA, Freitas TH, Stubbs B, et al. Peripheral alterations in cytokine and chemokine levels after antidepressant drug treatment for major depressive disorder: systematic review and meta-analysis. *Mol Neurobiol* 2018;**55**:4195–4206.

75. Fonseka TM, MacQueen GM, Kennedy SH. Neuroimaging biomarkers as predictors of treatment outcome in major depressive disorder. *J Affect Disord* 2018;**233**:21–35.

76. Nogovitsyn N, Muller M, Souza R, et al. Hippocampal tail volume as a predictive biomarker of antidepressant treatment outcomes in patients with major depressive disorder: a CAN-BIND report. *Neuropsychopharmacology* 2020;**45**:283–91.

77. MacQueen GM, Yucel K, Taylor VH, et al. Posterior hippocampal volumes are associated with remission rates in patients with major depressive disorder. *Biol Psychiatry* 2008;**64**:880–3.

78. Suh JS, Schneider MA, Minuzzi L, et al. Cortical thickness in major depressive disorder: a systematic review and meta-analysis. *Prog Neuro-Psychopharmacology Biol Psychiatry* 2019;**88**:287–302.

79. Suh JS, Minuzzi L, Raamana PR, et al. An investigation of cortical thickness and antidepressant response in major depressive disorder: a CAN-BIND study report. *NeuroImage Clin* 2020;**25**:102178.

80. Davis AD, Hassel S, Arnott SR, et al. White matter indices of medication response in major depression: a diffusion tensor imaging study. *Biol Psychiatry Cogn Neurosci Neuroimaging* 2019;**4**:913–24.

81. Seminowicz DA, Mayberg HS, McIntosh AR, et al. Limbic-frontal circuitry in major depression: a path modeling metanalysis. *Neuroimage* 2004;**22**:409–18.

82. Furtado CP, Hoy KE, Maller JJ, et al. An investigation of medial temporal lobe changes and cognition following antidepressant response: a prospective rTMS study. *Brain Stimul* 2013;**6**:346–54.

83. Straub J, Metzger CD, Plener PL, et al. Successful group psychotherapy of depression in adolescents

alters fronto-limbic resting-state connectivity. *J Affect Disord* 2017;**209**:135–9.

84. Fu CHY, Williams SCR, Cleare AJ, et al. Neural responses to sad facial expressions in major depression following cognitive behavioral therapy. *Biol Psychiatry* 2008;**64**:505–12.

85. Langenecker SA, Kennedy SE, Guidotti LM, et al. Frontal and limbic activation during inhibitory control predicts treatment response in major depressive disorder. *Biol Psychiatry* 2007;**62**: 1272–80.

86. Ruhé HG, Booij J, Veltman DJ, et al. Successful pharmacologic treatment of major depressive disorder attenuates amygdala activation to negative facial expressions: a functional magnetic resonance imaging study. *J Clin Psychiatry* 2012;**73**:451–9.

87. Szczepanik J, Nugent AC, Drevets WC, et al. Amygdala response to explicit sad face stimuli at baseline predicts antidepressant treatment response to scopolamine in major depressive disorder. *Psychiatry Res Neuroimaging* 2016;**254**:67–73.

88. Cullen KR, Klimes-Dougan B, Vu DP, et al. Neural correlates of antidepressant treatment response in adolescents with major depressive disorder. *J Child Adolesc Psychopharmacol* 2016;**26**:705–12.

89. Drysdale AT, Grosenick L, Downar J, et al. Resting-state connectivity biomarkers define neurophysiological subtypes of depression. *Nat Med* 2017;**23**:28–38.

90. Wang L, Xia M, Li K, et al. The effects of antidepressant treatment on resting-state functional brain networks in patients with major depressive disorder. *Hum Brain Mapp* 2015;**36**:768–78.

91. Miller JM, Schneck N, Siegle GJ, et al. fMRI response to negative words and SSRI treatment outcome in major depressive disorder: a preliminary study. *Psychiatry Res Neuroimaging* 2013;**214**:296–305.

92. Gyurak A, Patenaude B, Korgaonkar MS, et al. Frontoparietal activation during response inhibition predicts remission to antidepressants in patients with major depression. *Biol Psychiatry* 2016;**79**:274–81.

93. Guo W, Liu F, Xue Z, et al. Alterations of the amplitude of low-frequency fluctuations in treatment-resistant and treatment-response depression: a resting-state fMRI study. *Prog Neuro-Psychopharmacology Biol Psychiatry* 2012;**37**:153–60.

94. Keedwell PA, Drapier D, Surguladze S, et al. Subgenual cingulate and visual cortex responses to sad faces predict clinical outcome during antidepressant treatment for depression. *J Affect Disord* 2010;**120**:120–5.

95. Furey ML, Drevets WC, Szczepanik J, et al. Pretreatment differences in BOLD response to emotional faces correlate with antidepressant response to scopolamine. *Int J Neuropsychopharmacol* 2015;**18**:pyv028.

96. Costafreda SG, Chu C, Ashburner J, et al. Prognostic and diagnostic potential of the structural neuroanatomy of depression. *PLoS One* 2009;**4**: e6353.

97. Baeken C, De Raedt R, Van Hove C, et al. HF-rTMS treatment in medication-resistant melancholic depression: results from 18 FDG-PET brain imaging. *CNS Spectr* 2009;**14**:439–48.

98. Li C-T, Wang S-J, Hirvonen J, et al. Antidepressant mechanism of add-on repetitive transcranial magnetic stimulation in medication-resistant depression using cerebral glucose metabolism. *J Affect Disord* 2010;**127**:219–29.

99. Baeken C, Marinazzo D, Everaert H, et al. The impact of accelerated HF-rTMS on the subgenual anterior cingulate cortex in refractory unipolar major depression: insights from 18FDG PET brain imaging. *Brain Stimul* 2015;**8**:808–15.

100. Rizvi SJ, Salomons TV, Konarski JZ, et al. Neural response to emotional stimuli associated with successful antidepressant treatment and behavioral activation. *J Affect Disord* 2013;**151**:573–81.

101. Mayberg HS, Brannan SK, Tekell JL, et al. Regional metabolic effects of fluoxetine in major depression: serial changes and relationship to clinical response. *Biol Psychiatry* 2000;**48**:830–43.

102. Conway CR, Chibnall JT, Gebara MA, et al. Association of cerebral metabolic activity changes with vagus nerve stimulation antidepressant response in treatment-resistant depression. *Brain Stimul* 2013;**6**:788–97.

103. McGrath CL, Kelley ME, Holtzheimer PE III, et al. Toward a neuroimaging treatment selection biomarker for major depressive disorder. *JAMA Psychiatry* 2013;**70**:821–9.

104. Widge AS, Taha Bilge M, Montana R, et al. electroencephalographic biomarkers for treatment response prediction in major depressive illness: a meta-analysis. *Am J Psychiatry* 2019;**176**:44–56.

105. Wu W, Zhang Y, Jiang J, et al. An electroencephalographic signature predicts antidepressant response in major depression. *Nat Biotechnol* 2020;**38**:439–47.

106. Rolle CE, Fonzo GA, Wu W, et al. Cortical connectivity moderators of antidepressant vs placebo treatment response in major depressive disorder: secondary analysis of a randomized clinical trial. *JAMA Psychiatry* 2020;**77**:397–408.

107. Zhdanov A, Atluri S, Wong W, et al. Use of machine learning for predicting escitalopram treatment

outcome from electroencephalography recordings in adult patients with depression. *JAMA Netw Open* 2020;3:e1918377.

108. Farzan F, Atluri S, Frehlich M, et al. Standardization of electroencephalography for multi-site, multi-platform and multi-investigator studies: insights from the Canadian Biomarker Integration Network in Depression. *Sci Rep* 2017;7:1–11.

109. MacQueen GM, Hassel S, Arnott SR, et al. The Canadian Biomarker Integration Network in Depression (CAN-BIND): magnetic resonance imaging protocols. *J Psychiatry Neurosci* 2019;44:223–36.

110. Thompson PM, Stein JL, Medland SE, et al. The ENIGMA Consortium: large-scale collaborative analyses of neuroimaging and genetic data. *Brain Imaging Behav* 2014;8:153–82.

111. Strawbridge R, Young AH, Cleare AJ. Biomarkers for depression: recent insights, current challenges and future prospects. *Neuropsychiatr Dis Treat* 2017;13:1245–62.

112. Lenze EJ, Nicol GE, Barbour DL, et al. Precision clinical trials: a framework for getting to precision medicine for neurobehavioural disorders. *J Psychiatry Neurosci* 2021;46:E97–E110.

113. Andreazza AC, Laksono I, Fernandes BS, et al. Guidelines for the standardized collection of blood-based biomarkers in psychiatry: steps for laboratory validity – a consensus of the Biomarkers Task Force from the WFSBP. *World J Biol Psychiatry* 2019;20:340–51.

114. Longo DL, Drazen JM. Data sharing. *N Engl J Med* 2016;374:276–7.

115. Lefaivre S, Behan B, Vaccarino A, et al. Big data needs big governance: best practices from Brain-CODE, the Ontario-Brain Institute's neuroinformatics platform. *Front Genet* 2019;10:191.

116. Lam RW, Milev R, Rotzinger S, et al. Discovering biomarkers for antidepressant response: protocol from the Canadian biomarker integration network in depression (CAN-BIND) and clinical characteristics of the first patient cohort. *BMC Psychiatry* 2016;16:105.

117. Kennedy SH, Lam RW, Rotzinger S, et al. Symptomatic and functional outcomes and early prediction of response to escitalopram monotherapy and sequential adjunctive aripiprazole therapy in patients with major depressive disorder: a CAN-BIND-1 report. *J Clin Psychiatry* 2019;80:18m12202.

118. Habert J, Katzman MA, Oluboka OJ, et al. Functional recovery in major depressive disorder.

Prim Care Companion CNS Disord 2016;18(5). doi: 10.4088/PCC.15r01926.

119. Dudek D, Rybakowski JK, Siwek M, et al. Risk factors of treatment resistance in major depression: association with bipolarity. *J Affect Disord* 2010;126:268–71.

120. Souery D, Oswald P, Massat I, et al. Clinical factors associated with treatment resistance in major depressive disorder. *J Clin Psychiatry* 2007;68:1062–70.

121. Spijker J, Bijl R V., de Graaf R, et al. Determinants of poor 1-year outcome of DSM-III-R major depression in the general population: results of the Netherlands Mental Health Survey and Incidence Study (NEMESIS). *Acta Psychiatr Scand* 2001;103:122–30.

122. Trivedi MH, Rush AJ, Wisniewski SR, et al. Evaluation of outcomes with citalopram for depression using measurement-based care in STAR*D: implications for clinical practice. *Am J Psychiatry* 2006;163:28–40.

123. Katon W, Üntzer J, Russo J. Major depression: The importance of clinical characteristics and treatment response to prognosis. *Depress Anxiety* 2010;27:19–26.

124. Jha MK, Minhajuddin A, Gadad BS, et al. Interleukin 17 selectively predicts better outcomes with bupropion-SSRI combination: novel T cell biomarker for antidepressant medication selection. *Brain Behav Immun* 2017;66:103–10.

125. Cattaneo A, Gennarelli M, Uher R, et al. Candidate genes expression profile associated with antidepressants response in the GENDEP study: differentiating between baseline 'predictors' and longitudinal 'targets'. *Neuropsychopharmacology* 2013;38:377–85.

126. Mrazek DA, Rush AJ, Biernacka JM, et al. SLC6A4 variation and citalopram response. *Am J Med Genet Part B Neuropsychiatr Genet* 2009;150B:341–51.

127. Porcelli S, Fabbri C, Serretti A. Meta-analysis of serotonin transporter gene promoter polymorphism (5-HTTLPR) association with antidepressant efficacy. *Eur Neuropsychopharmacol* 2012;22:239–58.

128. Maron E, Tammiste A, Kallassalu K, et al. Serotonin transporter promoter region polymorphisms do not influence treatment response to escitalopram in patients with major depression. *Eur Neuropsychopharmacol* 2009;19:451–6.

129. Perlis RH, Fijal B, Dharia S, et al. Failure to replicate genetic associations with antidepressant treatment response in duloxetine-treated patients. *Biol Psychiatry* 2010;67:1110–13.

130. McMahon FJ, Buervenich S, Charney D, et al. Variation in the gene encoding the serotonin 2A receptor is associated with outcome of antidepressant treatment. *Am J Hum Genet* 2006;**78**:804–14.

131. Peters EJ, Slager SL, Jenkins GD, et al. Resequencing of serotonin-related genes and association of tagging SNPs to citalopram response. *Pharmacogenet Genomics* 2009;**19**:1–10.

132. Lucae S, Ising M, Horstmann S, et al. HTR2A gene variation is involved in antidepressant treatment response. *Eur Neuropsychopharmacol* 2010;**20**:65–8.

133. Uher R, Huezo-Diaz P, Perroud N, et al. Genetic predictors of response to antidepressants in the GENDEP project. *Pharmacogenomics J* 2009;**9**:225–33.

134. Horstmann S, Lucae S, Menke A, et al. Polymorphisms in GRIK4, HTR2A, and FKBP5 show interactive effects in predicting remission to antidepressant treatment. *Neuropsychopharmacology* 2010;**35**:727–40.

135. Baune BT, Hohoff C, Berger K, et al. Association of the COMT val158 met variant with antidepressant treatment response in major depression. *Neuropsychopharmacology* 2008;**33**:924–32.

136. Anttila S, Huuhka K, Huuhka M, et al. Catechol-O-methyltransferase (COMT) polymorphisms predict treatment response in electroconvulsive therapy. *Pharmacogenomics J* 2008;**8**:113–16.

137. Paddock S, Laje G, Charney D, et al. Association of GRIK4 with outcome of antidepressant treatment in the STAR*D cohort. *Am J Psychiatry* 2007;**164**:1181–8.

138. Pu M, Zhang Z, Xu Z, et al. Influence of genetic polymorphisms in the glutamatergic and GABAergic systems and their interactions with environmental stressors on antidepressant response. *Pharmacogenomics* 2013;**14**:277–88.

139. Serretti A, Chiesa A, Crisafulli C, et al. Failure to replicate influence of GRIK4 and GNB3 polymorphisms on treatment outcome in major depression. *Neuropsychobiology* 2012;**65**:70–5.

140. Tadić A, Müller MJ, Rujescu D, et al. The MAOA T941G polymorphism and short-term treatment response to mirtazapine and paroxetine in major depression. *Am J Med Genet Part B Neuropsychiatr Genet* 2007;**144B**:325–31.

141. Ortiz R, Niciu MJ, Lukkahati N, et al. Shank3 as a potential biomarker of antidepressant response to ketamine and its neural correlates in bipolar depression. *J Affect Disord* 2015;**172**:307–11.

142. Tadić A, Müller-Engling L, Schlicht KF, et al. Methylation of the promoter of brain-derived neurotrophic factor exon IV and antidepressant response in major depression. *Mol Psychiatry* 2014;**19**:281–3.

143. Colle R, Deflesselle E, Martin S, et al. BDNF/TRKB/P75NTR polymorphisms and their consequences on antidepressant efficacy in depressed patients. *Pharmacogenomics* 2015;**16**:997–1013.

144. Schatzberg AF, DeBattista C, Lazzeroni LC, et al. ABCB1 genetic effects on antidepressant outcomes: a report from the iSPOT-D trial. *Am J Psychiatry* 2015;**172**(8);751–9.

145. Uhr M, Tontsch A, Namendorf C, et al. Polymorphisms in the drug transporter gene ABCB1 predict antidepressant treatment response in depression. *Neuron* 2008;**57**:203–9.

146. Jha MK, Minhajuddin A, Gadad BS, et al. Platelet-derived growth factor as an antidepressant treatment selection biomarker: higher levels selectively predict better outcomes with bupropion-SSRI combination. *Int J Neuropsychopharmacol* 2017;**20**:919–27.

147. Jha M, Minhajuddin A, Gadad B, et al. Blood brain barrier dysfunction selectively predicts poorer outcomes with SSRI monotherapy vs. antidepressant combinations: clinical utility of novel astrocytic marker. *Biol Psychiatry* 2018;**83**:S28.

148. Lopez JP, Mamdani F, Labonte B, et al. Epigenetic regulation of BDNF expression according to antidepressant response. *Mol Psychiatry* 2013;**18**:398–9.

149. Lopez JP, Lim R, Cruceanu C, et al. miR-1202 is a primate-specific and brain-enriched microRNA involved in major depression and antidepressant treatment. *Nat Med* 2014;**20**:764–8.

150. Fiori LM, Lopez JP, Richard-Devantoy S, et al. Investigation of miR-1202, miR-135a, and miR-16 in major depressive disorder and antidepressant response. *Int J Neuropsychopharmacol* 2017;**20**:619–23.

151. He S, Liu X, Jiang K, et al. Alterations of microRNA-124 expression in peripheral blood mononuclear cells in pre- and post-treatment patients with major depressive disorder. *J Psychiatr Res* 2016;**78**:65–71.

152. Marshe VS, Islam F, Maciukiewicz M, et al. Validation study of microRNAs previously associated with antidepressant response in older adults treated for late-life depression with venlafaxine. *Prog Neuro-Psychopharmacology Biol Psychiatry* 2020;**100**:109867.

153. Ju C, Fiori LM, Belzeaux R, et al. Integrated genome-wide methylation and expression analyses reveal functional predictors of response to antidepressants. *Trsansl Psychiatry* 2019;**9**:254.

154. Belzeaux R, Gorgievski V, Fiori LM, et al. GPR56/ADGRG1 is associated with response to antidepressant treatment. *Nat Commun* 2020;**11**:1635.

155. Vakili K, Pillay SS, Lafer B, et al. Hippocampal volume in primary unipolar major depression: a magnetic resonance imaging study. *Biol Psychiatry* 2000;**47**:1087–90.

156. Hsieh M-H, McQuoid DR, Levy RM, et al. Hippocampal volume and antidepressant response in geriatric depression. *Int J Geriatr Psychiatry* 2002;**17**:519–525.

157. Frodl T, Meisenzahl EM, Zetzsche T, et al. Hippocampal and amygdala changes in patients with major depressive disorder and healthy controls during a 1-year follow-up. *J Clin Psychiatry* 2004;**65**:492–9.

158. Frodl T, Jäger M, Smajstrlova I, et al. Effect of hippocampal and amygdala volumes on clinical outcomes in major depression: a 3-year prospective magnetic resonance imaging study. *J Psychiatry Neurosci* 2008;**33**:423–30.

159. Abbott CC, Jones T, Lemke NT, et al. Hippocampal structural and functional changes associated with electroconvulsive therapy response. *Transl Psychiatry* 2014;**4**:e483.

160. Li C-T, Li n C-P, Chou K-H, et al. Structural and cognitive deficits in remitting and non-remitting recurrent depression: a voxel-based morphometric study. *Neuroimage* 2010;**50**:347–56.

161. ten Doesschate F, van Eijndhoven P, Tendolkar I, et al. Pre-treatment amygdala volume predicts electroconvulsive therapy response. *Front Psychiatry* 2014;**5**:169.

162. Baldwin R, Jeffiries S, Jackson A, et al. Treatment response in late-onset depression: Relationship to neuropsychological, neuroradiological and vascular risk factors. *Psychol Med* 2004;**34**:125–36.

163. Iosifescu D V., Renshaw PF, Lyoo IK, et al. Brain white-matter hyperintensities and treatment outcome in major depressive disorder. *Br J Psychiatry* 2006;**188**:180–5.

164. Toki S, Okamoto Y, Onoda K, et al. Hippocampal activation during associative encoding of word pairs and its relation to symptomatic improvement in depression: a functional and volumetric MRI study. *J Affect Disord* 2014;**152–154**:462–7.

165. Mayberg HS, Brannan SK, Tekell JL, et al. Regional metabolic effects of fluoxetine in major depression: serial changes and relationship to clinical response. *Biol Psychiatry* 2000;**48**:830–43.

166. Goldapple K, Segal Z, Garson C, et al. Modulation of cortical-limbic pathways in major depression. *Arch Gen Psychiatry* 2004;**61**:34.

167. Baskaran A, Farzan F, Milev R, et al. The comparative effectiveness of electroencephalographic indices in predicting response to escitalopram therapy in depression: a pilot study. *J Affect Disord* 2018;**227**:542–9.

Chapter 24

Pharmacogenomics and the Management of Mood Disorders

Roos van Westrhenen

Pharmacogenetics (PGx) is a discipline that investigates genetic factors affecting the absorption, metabolism, and transport of drugs, thereby influencing therapy outcome. These genetic factors can, among other things, lead to differences in the activity of enzymes that metabolize drugs. Recent studies in depressed patients show that genotyping of drug-metabolizing enzymes can increase the effectiveness of treatment, which could benefit millions of patients worldwide.

Introduction

Treatment-resistant depression (TRD) is typically described as the occurrence of an inadequate response after an adequate treatment with antidepressant agents (in terms of dose, duration, and compliance), among patients suffering from a depressive disorder [1]. The European Union's Committee for Human Proprietary Medicinal Products (CHMP) defines TRD as follows: "A patient is considered therapy-resistant when consecutive treatments with two products of different classes, used for a sufficient length of time at an adequate dose, fail to induce an acceptable effect" [1].

Effective treatments for mental disorders are available, but their effect is limited because of patients' (genetic) heterogeneity and poor treatment compliance due to frequent adverse events. Only one-third of the patients respond to treatment and experience remission [2,3]. Studies have shown that psychiatry relies on a trial-and-error approach that combines physicians' experience with clinical indicators [4,5]. Pharmacogenetic testing can help in this process by determining the person-specific genetic factors that may predict clinical response and side effects associated with genetic variants that impact drug-metabolizing enzymes, drug transporters, or drug targets [4–6].

Pharmacogenetics is a discipline that investigates genetic factors that affect the absorption, metabolism, and transport of drugs, thereby affecting therapy outcome. These genetic factors can, among other things, lead to differences in the activity of enzymes that metabolize drugs.

Genetic variants that are less than 1% present in the population are referred to as a mutation and those that are more than 1% present as genetic polymorphism. For several polymorphisms in genes encoding for metabolizing enzymes, the effect on the activity of the enzyme has been established. Besides genetic polymorphisms, also other (non-genetic) factors can influence enzyme activity, such as co-medication, smoking, diet, and diseases [5]. The genetic composition of the genes, referred to as the "genotype", is translated into a predicted "phenotype" [6].

Phenotypes

Traditional classification usually divides patients into four groups: (1) Poor metabolizers are homozygous carriers of two loss-of-function alleles (CYP2C19Null/Null or CYP2D6Null/Null, also sometimes referred to as CYP2C19PM/PM or CYP2D6PM/PM); they do not possess active enzyme, and therefore, their specific enzymatic capacity is completely abolished. (2) Intermediate metabolizers carry genotypes that cause substantially reduced, but not absent, enzyme capacity. (3) Normal metabolizers homozygously carry wild type (Wt) alleles and are associated with reference or expected enzymatic capacity. Normal metabolizers may also carry other genotypes as long as the enzymatic capacity is not significantly different compared with Wt/Wt carriers. (4) Ultrarapid metabolizers carry genotypes connected with significantly increased enzymatic capacity compared with Wt/Wt carriers [6].

Variants in cytochrome enzyme CYP2D6 are known to have the poor metabolizer (PM) phenotype in 5 to 10% of the population with a northwestern European background [7]. These individuals have little or no CYP2D6 enzyme activity. They have an increased risk of side effects of medication that is metabolized by this particular enzyme, due to a slower degradation of certain drugs (e.g., with nortriptyline), and therefore higher blood drug concentrations. There also may be undertreatment if the drug has to be converted by CYP2D6 to the active metabolite, as is the case with some opioids (e.g., tramadol). Genetic polymorphisms influencing drug metabolism are common. Besides PM status, intermediate metabolizer status (IM: decreased enzyme activity) and ultrarapid metabolizer status (UM: increased enzyme activity) may predispose patients for an increased risk on both side effects and therapeutic ineffectiveness. For example, in the Caucasian population, 3% are CYP2C19 PM, 8% are CYP2D6 PM. Also, 17% are CYP2C19 IM and 30% CYP2D6 IM [6,7].

Potential Benefit of Pharmacogenetics in Treatment-Resistant Depression

Antidepressants in general aim to increase monoaminergic neurotransmission by blocking monoamine reuptake. However, these effects are neither necessary nor sufficient for treatment response, and the effectiveness of therapy is therefore less than optimal [6]. Despite intensive effort in neuroscience research, very few new psychopharmacological agents have entered the market in recent decades. Therefore, since molecular targets for psychiatric drugs are not yet fully elucidated, and many of the currently available drugs will likely remain the cornerstone of pharmacotherapy in psychiatry for the foreseeable future, it is of paramount value to maximize their effectiveness [6]. Current selection of an appropriate antidepressant drug to a great extent still relies on psychiatrists' clinical experience as well as on a potentially long trial-and-error approach, with potential serious adverse consequences that may include, for example, untreated suicidal ideation and behaviors [6–9].

Clinical Pharmacogenomic Studies in Psychiatry

To date, 14 prospective clinical studies have been published on the effect of genotyping compared to standard care (not further specified) in mood disorder patients [10–16] (Table 24.1).

Eleven studies describe the results of randomized studies [12–18,20–23]. The studies by Hall-Flavin [10,11] describe the results of prospective observational cohort studies and the study by Oslin and colleagues describes the result of an open-label controlled trial [19]. All 14 studies were targeted at depressed patients, only the study by Bradly et al. also included patients with anxiety disorder [15]. One study was found investigating the use of genotyping in psychotic patients in comparison with standard care.

Six studies used the Genesight test [10–12,16,18,19], two studies used NeuroPharmagen [14,17], another two studies used TaqMan probe–PCR and mass array [20,21], one study used the CNSDose [13], another used Genecept [22], one used the NeuroIDgenetix test [15], and one study did not report on the used test [23].

The Genesight test used was a combination test for allele variations in five genes: *CYP1A2*, *CYP2D6*, *CYP2C19*, the serotonin transporter gene (*SLC6A4*), and serotonin receptor 2A (*HTR2A*).

Hall-Flavin was the first to examine whether the use of pharmacogenetic information (Genesight test) yielded gains in the clinical outcome of depressed patients (MDD; major depressive disorder) in a prospective pilot study (Genesight-I study) [10]. Adults aged 25–75 years with psychiatrist-diagnosed MDD and a minimum score of 14 on the Hamilton Depression Scale (HAMD-17) were included. The study was sponsored by the industry (AssureRx Inc.) and two authors were still employed by the Mayo Clinic at the time of design of the study but joined AssureRx during the course of the study. After 8 weeks, the decrease in severity of depressive disorder was greater in the group of patients treated based on pharmacogenetic advice (30.8% decrease in HAMD-17 score) compared to the group of patients receiving standard care (18.2% decrease in HAMD-17 score, $p = 0.04$) [10].

Hall-Flavin conducted a second prospective cohort study with 227 depressed patients (Genesight-II study [11]). As in the previous study by this group [10], the diagnosis was supported by a HAMD-17 score of at least 14. This time, the study involved patients between the ages of 18 and 72 with a depressive disorder. It was reported that after 8 weeks there was a greater reduction in depressive symptoms when pharmacotherapy was prescribed using genotyping (intervention group: 46.9% decrease in score on the HAMD-17 vs. 29.9% decrease in score on this questionnaire in the standard care group, $p < 0.01$). The response rate, defined as > 50% decrease in score, was also higher in the intervention group than in the standard care group, 44.4% versus 23.7%, respectively (odds ratio [OR] = 2.58,

Table 24.1 Prospective RCTs comparing PGx-guided versus non-guided pharmacotherapy (TAU)

Study design	Genotyping method	Number of patients	Outcome
Open-label, prospective cohort [10]	CYP1A2, CYP2D6, CYP2C19 (Genesight)	n =25 Genotyping guided vs. n = 26 TAU	Genotyping leads to more reduction in depression scores
Open-label, prospective cohort [11]	CYP1A2, CYP2D6 CYP2C19 (Genesight)	n = 114 Genotyping guided vs. n = 113 TAU	Genotyping leads to more reduction in depression symptoms
RCT, double-blind [12]	CYP1A2, 2C9, 2C19, 2D6, SCL6A4, 5HTR2A (Genesight)	n = 26 guided vs. n =2 5 TAU	Genotyping results in higher response and remission rates
RCT, double-blind [13]	CYP2D6, CYP2C19, ABCB1, not otherwise specified	n = 74 Genotyping guided vs. n =74 TAU	Genotyping 2.52 times more likely to remit
RCT, double-blind [14]	CYP2D6 and others, not specified (NeuroPharmagen)	n = 155 guided vs n = 161 TAU	Genotyping results in higher response rate and better tolerability
RCT, double-blind, both depressed and anxiety patients [15]	CYP1A2, 2C9, 2C19, 2D6, 3A4, 3A5, SCL6A4, COMT, HTR2A, MHFR (NeurolDgenetix)	n = 352 Genotyping guided vs. n = 3 33 TAU	Genotyping leads to higher response rates and remission rates in patients with depression or anxiety
RCT, double-blind [16]	CYP1A2, 2C9, 2C19, 2B6, 2D6, HTR2A, SCL6A4	n = 1,167 in total	Genotyping leads to higher response and remission rates in depressed patients
RCT, double blind [17]	CYP2D6 and others, not specified (NeuroPharmagen)	n = 52 genotyping guided vs. n = 48 TAU	Genotyping leads to more reduction in depression scores and higher response rates
RCT, double-blind [18]	CYP1A2, CYP2B6, CYP2C9, CYP2C19, CYP2D6, CYP3A4, HTR2A, and SLC6A4 (Genesight) and MC4 R, CNR1, NPY, GCG, HCRTR2, NDUFS1 (in enhanced Genesight)	n = 90 genotyping guided, n = 93 enhanced genotyping guided vs. n = 93 TAU	Genotyping did not lead to a higher decrease in depressive symptoms or higher response or remission
Open-label, prospective cohort [19]	CYP1A2, CYP2B6, CYP2C9, CYP2C19, CYP2D6, CYP3A4, UGT1A4, UGT2B15, SLC6A4, HTR2A, HLA-B*1502 and HLA-B*1502 (Genesight)	n = 966 Genotyping guided vs. n = 978 TAU	Genotyping-based medication advice reduced the number of prescribed drugs with a drug–gene interaction compared to usual care
RCT, double-blind [20]	CYP2C19, CYP2D6, CYP1A2, SLC6A4, and 5-HTR2A (TaqMan probe–PCR and mass array)	n =.31 Genotyping guided vs. n = 40 TAU	Genotyping might not considerably improve the clinical efficiency and safety.
RCT, single-blind [21]	CYP1A2, CYP2B6, CYP2C9, CYP2C19, CYP2D6, CYP3A4, HLA, 5HTTLPR, HTR2A HTR2C, POLG, SLC6A4 and UGT1A4 (TaqMan probe–PCR and mass array)	n = 55 Genotyping guided vs. n = 47 TAU	Genotyping did not lead to significant group differences although a trend was shown
RCT, double-blind [22]	Genecept (7 CYP enzymes genes with 45 variants, 11 pharmacodynamic or other genes)	n =151 Genotyping guided vs. n = 153 TAU	Pharmacogenomic testing was not associated with an improvement of symptoms
RCT, double-blind [23]	CYP2D6 and CYP2C19 (not otherwise specified)	n = 56 Genotyping guided vs. n = 55 TAU	Pharmacogenomic testing was associated with a faster achievement of therapeutic drug concentrations and a decrease in adverse reactions, but not with a decrease in depressive symptoms

Abbreviations: PGx: pharmacogenetics; RCT: randomized controlled trial; TAU: treatment as usual.

95% confidence interval [CI]: 1.33–5.03). Similar results were found for the percentage of patients with remission (defined as a score of < 8 on the HAMD-17), intervention group: 26.4%, standard care group: 12.9%; OR = 2.42, 95% CI: 1.09–5.39, p = 0.03 [11].

The third study using the Genesight panel in depressed patients was a double-blind randomized trial [12]. The clinical effect was measured with the HAMD-17 and the Quick Inventory of Depressive symptoms (QIDS-SR and QIDS-CR) for 10 weeks. All authors were employed by industry (AssureRx Health, Inc.). The mean improvement in HAMD-17 scores at week 10 was higher in the group with a dosing recommendation based on genotyping (30.8% vs. 20.7%; p = 0.28). Response, which was defined as a 50% reduction in HAMD-17 scores, was higher in the Genesight arm compared to the usual treatment arm (36,0% and 20.8%, respectively, OR = 2.14; 95% CI: 0.59–7.69). As well, remission at 10 weeks, a HAMD-17 score < 7, was 20.0% in the Genesight arm compared to 8.3% in the treatment as usual (TAU) arm (OR = 2.14; 95% CI: 0.59–7.69). Together this means that both remission and response improved greatly in the genotyped group. Next to this, reduction in depressive symptoms was greater in the Genesight group compared to TAU (30.8% vs. 20.7%; p = 0.28). Lastly, TAU patients who started a contraindicated medication based on their genotype had very little improvement (only 0.8%) in depressive symptoms. This was a great contrast compared to the Genesight group who started on a contraindicated medication but had a 33.1% improvement (p = 0.06).

The fourth study, using the Genesight

Panel included n = 1,167 outpatients with depressive disorder with a score > 14 on the HAMD-17 [16] and with a patient- or clinician-reported inadequate response to at least one antidepressant. Clinical effect was measured at 0 (baseline), 4, 8, 12, and 24 weeks by a blinded central rater with HAMD-17 (primary), as well as with QIDS and Patient Health Questionnaire (PHQ). In this study there was no significant difference in symptom improvement at 8 weeks between the two treatment groups (27.2% guided vs. 24.4% standard care, p = 0.107), but this was the case for response (≥ 50% decrease in HAMD-17) at week 8 (26.0% vs. 19.9%, p = 0.013) and remission defined as HAMD-17 < 7 (15.3% vs. 10.1%, p = 0.007) [16].

In another study, a test for polymorphisms of CYP2D6, CYP2C19, and ABCB1 (CNSDose) was used [13]. This 12-week, double-blind randomized study was industry sponsored (n = 152). In half of the patients, the prescriber received dosage recommendations (intervention group). The HAMD-17 was measured after 12 weeks. There was a greater improvement in depressive symptoms after 10 weeks: in the intervention group there was 30.8% improvement in HAMD-17 compared to 20.7% improvement in the standard care group, but this difference was not statistically significant (p = 0.28). No statistically significant differences in response rate and percentage of patients with remission were found either: response rate OR = 2.14; 95% CI: 0.59–7.69. With the reported data (9 of 25 cases in the intervention group and 5 of 24 cases in the control group, 1 dropout in both groups), there was a relative risk of 1.73 (95% CI: 0.68–4.42). For the percentage of patients with remission, an OR of 2.75 (95% CI: 0.48–15.80) was reported. With the reported data (5 of 25 cases in the intervention group and 2 of 24 cases in the control group), the relative risk can again be calculated: 2.4 (95% CI: 0.51–11.21). Remission is defined here as a final score on HAMD-17 of less than or equal to 7. The authors further reported that the intervention group had progressed on average 27.6% on the QIDSC-16 and the standard care group 22.1%; this difference was not statistically significant [13].

The next study used the Neuropharmagen panel, which contained CYP2D6 and others (not clearly specified). Patients treated with genotype-guided medication, n = 155, were compared to n = 161 patients in the standard care group in a double-blind set-up [14]. The PGx-guided treatment group had a higher responder rate compared to standard care at 12 weeks (47.8% vs. 36.1%, p = 0.0476; OR = 1.62 [95% CI: 1.00–2.61]), and this difference increased after removing subjects in the PGx-guided group when clinicians explicitly reported not to follow the test recommendations (51.3% vs. 36.1%, p = 0.0135; OR = 1.86 [95% CI: 1.13–3.05]). Effects were more consistent in patients with 1–3 failed drug trials [14].

Bradley et al. investigated a total of n = 685 patients with depression and/or anxiety, of which n = 246 were diagnosed with depression, and n = 204 with both depression and anxiety (n = 450 with depression) in a prospective, randomized, subject- and rater-blinded approach [15]. They assessed HAMD-17 and HAM-A scores at 0, 4, 8, and 12 weeks using the NeuroIDgenetix panel, investigating 10 genes including *CYP1A2, 2C9, 2C19, 2D6, 3A4, 3A5, SCL6A4, COMT, HTR2A,* and *MHFR* [15]. It was described that in patients diagnosed with severe depression, response rates at 8 weeks were 55% in the experimental group versus 28% in the control group, and response rates ($p = 0.001$; OR: 4.72 [1.93–11.52]) and remission rates ($p = 0.02$; OR: 3.54 [1.27–9.88]) were significantly higher in the pharmacogenetics-guided group as compared to the control group at 12 weeks. Also, when both moderate and severe patients were included in the analysis at 8 weeks comparing the experimental and control group, the response rates were 49% and 41%, respectively. At 12 weeks the response rates were significantly higher in the experimental group ($p = 0.01$, OR: 2.03, 1.23–3.33). However, for mild depression patients, no significant effect of pharmacogenomic guided treatment was found. In addition, patients in the experimental group diagnosed with anxiety showed a meaningful improvement in HAM-A scores at both 8 and 12 weeks ($p = 0.02$ and 0.02, respectively), along with higher response rates ($p = 0.04$; OR: 1.76 [1.03–2.99]). From these results, they concluded that pharmacogenetic-guided medication selection significantly improves outcomes of patients diagnosed with severe depression or anxiety, in a variety of healthcare settings [15].

Han et al. conducted an 8-week randomized, rater- and participant-blinded clinical trial [17]. Participants with MDD, $N = 100$, were included and divided into either the PGx or a TAU treatment arm. Treatment was based on either pharmacogenetic analysis using the Neuropharmagen testing panel or treatment left to the assessment of their own healthcare provider. Treatments were compared at 8 weeks using HAM D-17 questionnaire. There was a significant mean change in HAMD score in favor of the PGx group with a –4.1-point difference at the end of the 8th week (-16.1 ± 6.8 -12.1 ± 8.2, $p = 0.010$). Similarly, response rates based on HAMD score, were also significantly higher in the PGx group with a 28.1% difference ($p = 0.014$). Remission rates were higher in the PGx group, although not significant ($p = 0.071$). Additionally, adverse reactions as reason for dropout was higher in the TAU group compared to the PGx group ($n = 9$ in TAU compared to $n = 4$ in PGx). With these results they concluded that PGx may be a better option for treatment of MDD with respect to tolerability and effectiveness.

A 52-week study was launched by Tiwari et al. In this participant- and rater-blinded three-arm randomized controlled trial (RCT) [18], patients were randomized into one of three groups. The first group consisted of patients where the medication prescribers received a standard pharmacogenomic test report (GEN) and could provide medication advice based on these results. In the second group, medication prescribers received an enhanced pharmacogenomic test report (EGEN) or received advice to give the usual treatment (TAU). The pharmacogenomic test reports were based on the Genesight panel. The enhanced report consisted of additional genes, which could give insight into antipsychotic-induced weight gain. The primary endpoint was symptom recovery (change in HAMD-17 score) at week 8, and secondary endpoints were remission and response rates at week 8. A total of $n = 570$ patients were planned for enrolment, of which 276 were finally included in the per protocol analysis. There was no significant difference in the primary endpoints between the GEN and TAU arms (GEN 24.4 vs. TAU 22.6, $p = 0.738$) nor was there a significant difference in EGEN and GEN arms ($p = 0.244$). The guided treatment also did not prove significantly more effective in response (30.3% vs. 22.7%), and remission rates (15.7% vs. 8.3%) compared to TAU. However, the trial was underpowered to detect statistically significant differences.

Oslin and colleagues also utilized the Genesight panel [19]. They initiated a 24-week non-commercially sponsored open-label trial. In this study they investigated remission rates and the risks for receiving an antidepressant with drug–gene interactions as measured by the Patient Health Questionnaire-9 (PHQ-9), comparing a PGx guided group versus a TAU group. A total of $n = 1,944$ patients between 18 and 80 years of age with an MDD diagnosis were included in the final analysis. The results indicated that the risk of a predicted drug–gene interaction was lower in the PGx-guided group compared to the TAU group ($p < 0.001$, no gene interaction vs. moderate/substantial interaction). At 24 weeks there was no significant effect of treatment on remission observed in the PGx versus TAU groups ($p = 0.45$). Oslin et al. concluded that providing PGx test results reduced the number of prescribed drugs with a drug–gene interaction compared to usual care.

Another non-commercially funded study was performed by Shan and colleagues [20]. They investigated $n = 71$ participants between the ages of 18 and 51 with MDD as described by the American Psychiatric Association's *Diagnostic and Statistical Manual of Mental Disorders* (DSM-5) with an HAMD-17 score of ≥ 17. Pharmacogenomic testing was done by a non-commercial laboratory. Genomic DNA was isolated and analyzed using TaqMan probe–PCR and mass array, which detects genetic polymorphisms including *CYP2C19*, *CYP2D6*, *CYP1A2*, *SLC6A4*, and *5-HTR2A*. Participants received either PGx-based treatment or TAU. Analysis revealed no statistically significant difference ($p > 0.05$) in HAMD-17 reduction rates (60.68% guided vs. 52.38% in unguided) as well as response rates, and remission rates between the PGx-guided and unguided groups. There were also no significant differences in adverse effects incidence (55.56% guided and 57.89% unguided). Based on these findings, Shan et al. suggested that pharmacogenomic testing might not considerably improve the clinical efficiency and safety for the PGx-guided group [20].

Another study utilizing the TaqMan probe–PCR and mass array was done by McCarthy et al. In that study, $n = 102$ patients with MDD were subjected to PGx-guided treatment or TAU for 8 weeks [21]. Endpoints were measured using the Clinical Global Impressions (CGI) scale. Remission was also measured using CGI and was defined as any patient ending the trial with a CGI score of either 1 or 2. Subjects significantly improved over the course of the trial ($p = 0.01$); however, between the treatment arms there was no significant effect, although it favored PGx-guided treatment ($p = 0.08$). Correction for diagnosis revealed that patients with MDD ($n = 49$), recovered similarly over time independent of treatment arm ($p = 0.55$). The authors concluded that there were no significant group differences, although a trend was shown.

An 8-week multicenter, participant- and rater-blinded RCT, conducted by Perlis and colleagues, examined PGx-guided treatment versus TAU using a Genecept assay kit [22]. The Genecept assay included 7 CYP enzyme genes with a total of 45 variants and 11 pharmacodynamic or other genes (no further specifications). Included participants had to be diagnosed with MDD with a minimum Structured Interview Guide for the Hamilton Depression Scale (SIGH-D) score of 18 and had a failure of treatment with at least one antidepressant. A total of $n = 296$ participants yielded valuable outcomes. The primary outcome of interest was change in SIGH-D score. No significant difference was observed between the PGx and TAU groups at week 8 ($p = 0.53$). Likewise, no significant effect of guided treatment was detected on response rates (39.7% PGx

vs. 48.0% TAU; −7.8% difference, $p = 0.17$) and remission rates (24.0% PGx vs. 30.7% TAU; −6.1% difference, $p = 0.23$). Based on these results, it was concluded that pharmacogenomic testing was not associated with an improvement of symptoms.

Lastly, one study looked at the effect of pharmacogenetics-informed treatment on the use of tricyclic antidepressants (TCA) [23]. Vos and colleagues investigated and analyzed $n = 111$ patients from whom CYP2D6 and CYP2C19 genotypes were assessed. The primary outcome was days until attainment of a therapeutic TCA plasma concentration. They found that treatment based on pharmacogenetics led to a faster achievement of therapeutic concentrations as assessed by therapeutic drug monitoring (mean [standard deviation, SD], 17.3 [11.2] vs. 22.0 [10.2] days; $p = .04$). Next to this, ($p = .001$), severity ($p = 0.008$), and burden ($p = 0.02$) also decreased.

Side Effects

One study examined the effectiveness of genotyping versus standard care with respect to adverse events measured by the prespecified relevant outcome measures [17]. Adverse reactions as reason for dropout was higher in the TAU group compared to the PGx group ($n = 9$ in TAU compared to $n = 4$ in PGx) in the trial conducted by Han and colleagues.

Therapeutic Drug Monitoring (TDM)

Only one study was found comparing the effect of treatment based on pharmacogenetics with standard care in psychiatric patients taking antidepressants while analyzing therapeutic plasma concentrations [23]. With the use of therapeutic drug monitoring (TDM), Vos and colleagues found out that genotyping led to a faster achievement of therapeutic TCA plasma concentrations compared to TAU.

For certain drugs, such as TCAs, lithium, and clozapine, as well as haloperidol, the German Laborgemeinschaft für Neuropsychopharmakologie und Pharmacopsychiatrie (AGNP) recommends TDM in their guidelines. However, TDM is not required by default for all psychopharmaceuticals. According to the latest update of the German guideline, TDM is not necessary for all selective serotonin reuptake inhibitors (SSRIs) and serotonin and norepinephrine reuptake inhibitors (SNRIs) since large interindividual differences in drug concentrations in the blood result in the absence of a reliable therapeutic window [24]. Monographs are also available at www.tdm-monografie.org. However, it should be realized that the recommendations regarding TDM for psychopharmaceuticals are mostly based on pharmacokinetic (PK) data. RCTs have rarely been conducted in which the added value of TDM in clinical practice has been demonstrated in terms of clinical outcomes measured with correct measurement scales. In patient care, it is more common to make recommendations based on available theoretical knowledge without information from good RCTs and thus clinically relevant scientific evidence.

After starting treatment with TCAs, lithium, and clozapine, TDM can be used to further adjust the dosage [24]. TDM is of added value when using these drugs, because here the risk of relapse is higher at low exposures to the drug, or to prevent toxicity at higher levels (especially for TCAs). For lithium, clozapine, and TCAs such as nortriptyline, imipramine, and amitriptyline, target concentrations are well defined. If TCAs are prescribed for an indication other than depressive or anxiety disorder, such as for pain in general practice, this is at a lower dose and TDM makes little sense [25].

It therefore seems useful to consider genotyping if there are adverse events or abnormal kinetics during treatment with a TCA based on TDM (e.g., strikingly high levels at low doses or low levels at high doses). Genotyping is a way to explain these discrepancies with regard to the levels found, so that this can be taken into account in the future when adjusting dosages or starting other drugs [25]. Lithium is excreted by the kidneys and therefore no CYP enzymes are involved [25].

Although the AGNP Consensus Guideline also recommends TDM for haloperidol, it is currently not the case that TDM for haloperidol is widely used and usually it is only determined on indication. For antipsychotics, TDM is not considered necessary by default, except for clozapine for which a reliable therapeutic window exists. TDM is not considered necessary by default for most SSRIs and SNRIs, due to large interindividual differences in drug concentrations in the blood and the consequent lack of a reliable therapeutic window [25]. Exceptions are cases where adherence to therapy is suspected [25].

Evidence from the Literature: Summary

It can be concluded that:

1. There is some evidence from seven prospective studies that pharmacogenetics-guided treatment with antidepressants leads to a greater likelihood of remission of depressive symptoms and better treatment response than standard care.

2. No studies were found comparing the effect of pharmacogenetics-based treatment on the occurrence of adverse events with standard care in psychiatric patients taking or about to take antidepressants.

3. No studies were found comparing the effect of treatment based on pharmacogenetics with standard care with or without TDM in psychiatric patients who are or will be taking antipsychotics.

Dosing Guidelines

Since the share of drug metabolism catalyzed by CYP2C19, CYP2D6, and other enzymes is not uniform across psychiatric drugs, when it comes to meaningful guidelines, each drug needs to be considered separately. In 2005, the Dutch Pharmacogenetic Working Group (DPWG) formulated dosing advice based on pharmacogene metabolizer status (www.Kennisbank.knmp.nl); updated guidelines from DPWG and/or the Clinical Pharmacogenetics Implementation Consortium (CPIC) are provided (see www.Pharmgkb.org). Although such advice has been accepted worldwide with subtle differences, it is nonetheless still rarely used in clinical settings [6].

Recently a Dutch guideline, "Pharmacogenetics in Daily Psychiatric Clinical Practice," was drafted as assigned by the Dutch Psychiatric Association (NVvP) with funding from the Dutch Royal Medical Association (KNMG) [18]. The main goal of this guideline was to provide guidance on how genotyping could be used to contribute to the best clinical psychiatric practice. The purpose was to address basic questions such as when to genotype, how to request genotyping, which genes to investigate, and how to interpret the genotype results. Patients can also order genotyping via commercial companies, but this usually results in the outcome of more genes, for which not always sufficient evidence is present to be used in clinical practice. This guideline provides a description of dosing advice to be used in clinical psychiatric practice, based on current scientific evidence available. Because currently, insufficient data are available on the effects of genes involved in the pharmacodynamics of psychotropic drugs, these were excluded but will be included in the updates to this guideline when more knowledge about the clinical applicability becomes available [18]. In the Netherlands, there is a unique situation because of the fact that 16 hospital pharmacies offer non-commercial pharmacogenetic testing. These tests are reimbursed by Dutch health insurance companies. The DPWG and the infrastructure in this small country make for good working alliances and cooperation between professionals from different centers in different areas and with worldwide collaborations. With this to our knowledge first clinical psychiatric guideline drawn up by clinicians working together with other professionals, a start can be made by implementing pharmacogenetics in clinical psychiatry at a larger scale. Through alignment with other initiatives as for example the CPIC and the recently started pan-European PSY-PGx research consortium that was set up by van Westrhenen (www.PSY-PGx-org), an international effort could be undertaken to establish worldwide clinical guidelines for implementation of pharmacogenetics in psychiatry.

Pharmacogenetic Recommendations for Psychiatric Practice

The main recommendations for clinical use for pharmacogenetics in psychiatric practice from the Dutch guideline are summarized in Box 24.1.

Box 24.2 contains specific recommendations for antidepressants.

Patient Example: Implementing Pharmacogenetics in Patient Care

Box 24.3 highlights a persona based on a real patient who visited a non-commercial outpatient pharmacogenetics clinic that the author instituted in 2017 and where she has seen over 200 patients. This persona approach is often used in user-driven information and communication technology (ICT) research and development projects. The persona highlighted here received personalized medication advice based on their pharmacogenetic profile, medication history, diagnosis, and comedication. They consented in presenting their anonymized case.

Conclusions

Pharmacogenetics is rarely used in clinical settings other than in oncology, because it is difficult to translate the results to complex real-life patient settings; people often suffer from multiple disorders and are therefore taking combinations of medications, which can influence the metabolism of the central nervous system (CNS) active drugs. This phenomenon is called phenoconversion: conversion of, for example, extensive metabolizers into phenotypic intermediate or even poor metabolizers owing to the effects of concomitant medications on enzyme inhibition and induction, thereby modifying clinical response to drugs. This has mostly not been taken into account in clinical studies and there is a real risk that genotype-focused studies

---

Box 24.1 General Recommendations for All Psychopharmaca

- When considering genotyping, inform the patient and involve the patient in order to achieve shared decision making with regard to genotype.
- When genotype information is already available at the time of the prescription, use this information to select the right drug and the right dose for the right patient.
- Consider genotyping, when there is an indication (side effects or inefficacy of CYP2D6 and CYP2C19). Preemptive genotyping is therefore not recommended yet for psychotropic drugs.
- For some psychotropic drugs determination of CYP1A2, CYP2C9, and/or CYP3A4 can be of added value, but only determine those after consultation of a clinical pharmacologist or PharmD with pharmacogenetic expertise.
- Ensure that available genotyping results are recorded in the (electronic) patient file and that this information is shared with medication prescribers (as the GP) as well as the pharmacy.
- Consult a clinical pharmacologist or PharmD with specific knowledge in pharmacogenetics when in doubt before adjusting the drug dosage
- For a psychotropic drug where no dose recommendation is provided (see Table 24.2): consider a switch to a different medicine form from a similar drug class, when there is a genetic variant in a CYP enzyme that is involved in the metabolization.

Table 24.2 Effect of genotyping on dosage, indicated as percentage of commonly prescribed dosage, as indicated by the Royal Dutch Pharmacist's Association (KNMP)

Medicine	CYP2D6			CYP2C19			Relevant enzymes[#]
	PM	IM	UM	PM	IM	UM	
Amitriptyline	50%	60%	125%	70%*	80%*	140%*	CYP2D6, CYP2C19
Aripiprazol	max 10 mg/day	100%	100%	70%*	90%*	140%*	CYP2D6, CYP3A4
Citalopram	100%	100%	100%	50%	75%	100%	CYP2D6, CYP2C19, CYP3A4
Clomipramine	50%	70%	150%	65%*	75%*	130%*	CYP2D6, CYP2C19 (CYP3A4, CYP1A2)
Doxepine	40%	80%	200%	50%	90%	120%	CYP2D6 (CYP1A2, CYP3A4, 2C19)
Escitalopram	100%	100%	100%	50%	75%	150%	CYP2C19 (CYP3A4, CYP2D6)
Fluoxetine	100%	100%	100%				CYP2D6 (CYP2C19)
Haloperidol	50%	100%	Not specified				CYP2D6, CYP3A4
Imipramine	30%	70%	170%	70%	100%	100%	CYP2D6, CYP2C19
Nortriptyline	40%	60%	160%				CYP2D6, CYP2C19
Mirtazapine	100%	100%	100%				CYP2D6, CYP1A2, CYP3A4
Paroxetine	100%	100%	Not specified				CYP2D6
Pimozide	25%	60%	100%				CYP2D6, CYP3A4, CYP1A2
Risperidon	100%	100%	100%				CYP2D6 (CYP3A4)
Sertraline	100%	100%	100%	max 50mg/day	Max 100 mg	100%	CYP2C19 (CYP2D6, CYP2C9, CYP2B6, CYP3A4)
Venlafaxine	Not specified	Not specified	150%	40%*	90%*	125%*	CYP2D6, CYP3A4
Zuclopentixol	50%	75%	Not specified				

Of note: these percentages do not take into account co-medication, age, diet, renal function, or comorbidity. Enzymes in parentheses only have a minor contribution in the metabolization.[#]

Also see www.kennisbank.knmp.nl for recent updates or consult a pharmacologist or PharmD.*

Abbreviations: IM: intermediate metabolizer, PM: poor metabolizer; UM: ultrarapid metabolizer;

Reference: van Westrhenen et al., *Frontiers in Pharmacology* 2021 [25]

may therefore have missed clinically strong pharmacogenetic associations [6].

Recently in the UK, Biobanks PGx allele and phenotype frequencies for 487,409 participants were analyzed, including CYP2C19 and CYP2D6. For 14 CPIC pharmacogenes known to influence human drug response, it was found that 99.5% of individuals may have an atypical response to at least 1 drug; on average they may have an atypical response to 10.3

drugs. Nearly 24% of participants had been prescribed a drug for which they were predicted to have an atypical response [19].

Although the scientific evidence for the *CYP2C19* and *CYP2D6* genes seems strong enough to recommend clinical application, larger international and non-industry-funded implementation studies demonstrating feasibility and cost-effectiveness in real-world settings are lacking [6]. Real-world settings include people who

Box 24.2 Specific Recommendations per Drug Class

Antidepressants

Consider genotyping:

- In patients experiencing side effects or lack of efficacy after treatment with an adequate dose of an SSRI or SNRI. (see Figure 24.1). Genotyping should be considered especially in patients who experienced side effects or inefficacy with multiple psychotropic drugs with a similar CYP metabolism.
- In patients experiencing side effects or unexplained high or low blood drug levels in patients using TCA (tricyclic antidepressants).
- When next to above, there are side effects and/or inefficacy with other (somatic) pharmaca with similar CYP metabolism.

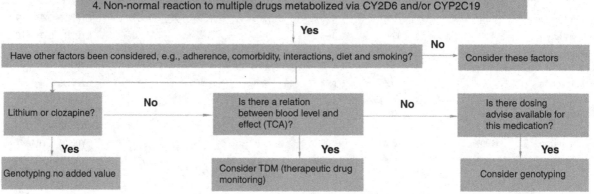

Figure 24.1 Flowchart of pharmacogenetics in psychiatry (courtesy R. van Westrhenen 2020 [6]).

Box 24.3 Angela Hoogakkers: Mood Disorder

Angela Hoogakkers, a 42-year-old woman from Bonaire, came to the PSY-PGx outpatient clinic because she suffered from a depressive disorder, moderate to severe, and had already tried three different antidepressants (SSRIs) that were not effective but caused nausea and fatigue with difficulties concentrating. Her family history was positive for depressive disorder (father) and she had a gastric bypass in 2014, iron deficiency anemia that was adequately corrected in 2016, and hypothyroidism that was also adequately treated.

When she was seen she had recently started imipramine 125 mg/day with low blood levels.

Genotyping showed: (1) CYP1A2: *1L/*1L (poor metabolizer), (2) CYP2C19: *1/*17 (1 hyperactive allele, but normal metabolizer), (3) CYP2D6: *3/*29 (1 less active allele, intermediate metabolizer = less enzyme activity) and (4) 3A4: *1G/*1G (2 less active alleles, intermediate metabolizer = less enzyme activity).

She was advised to use imipramine but in lower dosage than normal (70% of "standard dose").

After starting her new personalized medication, Angela felt more confident in using her medicine and was able to start working out again. After 2 months she was able to return to work. This relieved the workload on her colleagues and enabled the company to take on new commissions, strengthening their business. Angela concluded that she would recommend the pharmacogenetic-based individualized medication strategy to every patient and convinced her father to also attend the PSY-PGx outpatient clinic.

use more than one drug, for instance, which is something that the current guidelines do not yet cover. Possible obstacles in terms of feasibility include the availability of an efficient system to generate, deliver, and implement genotyping in the clinical prescription of psychiatric medication. At this time, despite gene-dosing advice for antidepressants (SSRIs, SNRIs, and TCAs) as well as for many antipsychotics, these are all prescribed to patients with almost no genotyping during treatment, not even when side effects occur or a psychopharmacotherapy is ineffective [6]. It is therefore recommended to consider genotyping, when there is an indication (side effects or inefficacy of *CYP2D6* and *CYP2C19*). Preemptive genotyping is therefore not recommended yet for psychotropic drugs [18].

References

1. Vieta E, Colom F. Therapeutic options in treatment resistant depression. *Ann Med* 2011;**43**:7, 512–30. doi: 10.3109/07853890.2011.583675.

2. Swedish Research Council on Health Technology Assessment (SBU). *Treatment of Depression: A Systematic Review.* 2004. ISBN 91-87890-87-9, 91-87890-887, 91–87890-94–12004.

3. Walker E, Kestler L, Bollini A, Hochman K. Schizophrenia: etiology and course. *Annu Rev Psychol.* 2004;**55**:410–30. doi.org/10.1146/annurev .psych.55.090902.141950.

4. Altar CA, Carhart J, Allen JD, et al. Clinical utility of combinatorial pharmacogenomics-guided antidepressant therapy: evidence from three clinical studies. *Mol Neuropsychiatry* 2015;**1**(3):145–55. doi: 10.1159/ 000430915.

5. Porcelli S, Drago A, Fabbri C, et al. Pharmacogenetics of antidepressant response. J *Psychiatry Neurosci* 2011.**36**(2):87–113.

6. van Westrhenen R, Aitchison KJ, Ingelman-Sundberg M, Jukic MM. Pharmacogenomics of antidepressants and antipsychotic treatment: how far have we got and where are we going? *Front Psych* 2020;**11**:94 https://doi.org/10.3389/ fpsyt.2020.00094

7. Zhou Y, Lauschke VM. The genetic landscape of major drug metabolizing cytochrome P450 genes – an updated analysis of population-scale sequencing data. *Pharmacogenomics J* 2022;**22**:284–93. https://doi.org/1 0.1038/s41397-022-00288-2

8. Ingelman-Sundberg M, Persson, Jukic MM. Polymorphic expression of CYP2C19 and 2D6 in the developing and adult human brain causing variables in cognition, risk for depression and suicide: the search for endogenous substrates. *Pharmacogenomics* 2014:**15** (15):1841–4.

9. Zackrinsson AL, Lindblom B, Ahler J. High frequency of occurrence of CYP2D6 gene duplication/ multiduplication in indicating ultrarapid metabolism among suicide cases. *Clin Pharmacol Ther* 2011;**3**:354-9.

10. Hall-Flavin DK, Winner JG, Allen JD, et al. Using a pharmacogenomic algorithm to guide the treatment of depression. *Transl Psychiatry* 2012;**2**:e172. doi:10.1038/tp.2012.99.

11. Hall-Flavin DK, Winner JG, Allen JD, et al. Utility of integrated pharmacogenomic testing to support the treatment of major depressive disorder in a psychiatric outpatient setting. *Pharmacogenet Genomics* 2013;**23**(10):535–48. doi: 10.1097/ FPC.0b013e3283649b9a. PubMed PMID: 24018772.

12. Winner JG, Carhart JM, Altar CA, et al. A prospective, randomized, double-blind study assessing the clinical impact of integrated pharmacogenomic testing for major depressive disorder. *Discov Med* 2013;**16**(89):219–27. PubMed PMID: 24229738

13. Singh AB. Improved antidepressant remission in major depression via a pharmacokinetic pathway polygene pharmacogenetic report. *Clin Psychopharmacol Neurosci* 2015;**13**(2):150–6. doi: 10.9758/cpn.2015.13.2.150.

14. Perez V, Salavert A, Espadaler J, et al. Efficacy of prospective pharmacogenetic testing in the treatment of major depressive disorder: results of a randomized, double-blind clinical trial. *BMC Psychiatry* 2017;**14**:**17**(1):250. doi: 10.1186/s12888-017-1412-1.

15. Bradley PJ, Shiekh M, Mehra V, et al. Improved efficacy with targeted pharmacogenetic-guided treatment of patients with depression and anxiety: randomized clinical trial demonstrating clinical utility. *J Psych Res* 2018;**96**:100–107. doi: 10.1016/.jpsychires.2017.09.024

16. Greden JF, Parikh SV, Rothschild AJ, et al. Impact of pharmacogenomics in major depressive disorder in the GUIDED trial: a large, patient- and rater-blinded, randomized, controlled study. *J Psychiatr Res* 2019;**111**:59–67 doi: 10.1038/tp.2012.99.

17. Han, C, Wing S-M, Bahk, W-M, et al. A pharmacogenomic-based antidepressant treatment for patients with major depressive disorder: results from an 8-week, randomized, single-blinded clinical trial. *Clin Psychopharmacol Neurosci* 2018;**16**:469–80.

18. Tiwari AK, Zai CC, Altar CA, et al. Clinical utility of combinatorial pharmacogenomic testing in depression: a Canadian patient- and rater-blinded, randomized, controlled trial. *Transl Psychiatry* 2022;**12**:101. https:// doi.org/10.1038/s41398-022-01847-8

19. Oslin D.W, Lynch KG, Shih MC, et al. Effect of pharmacogenomic testing for drug-gene interactions on medication selection and remission of symptoms in major depressive disorder: the PRIME Care

Randomized Clinical Trial. *JAMA* 2022;**328**(2):151–61. https://doi.org/10.1001/jama.2022.9805

20. Shan X, Zhao W, Qiu Y, et al. Preliminary clinical investigation of combinatorial pharmacogenomic testing for the optimized treatment of depression: a randomized single-blind study. *Front Neurosci* 2019;**13**:960. https://doi.org/10.3389/fnins.2019.00960

21. McCarthy MJ, Chen Y, Demodena A, et al. A prospective study to determine the clinical utility of pharmacogenetic testing of veterans with treatment-resistant depression. *J Psychopharmacol* 2021;**35**(8):992–1002. https://doi.org/10.1177/02698811211015224

22. Perlis RH, Dowd D, Fava M, Lencz T, Krause DS. Randomized, controlled, participant- and rater-blind trial of pharmacogenomic test-guided treatment versus treatment as usual for major depressive

disorder. *Depress Anxiety* 2020;**37**(9):834–41. https://doi.org/10.1002/da.23029

23. Vos CF, ter Hark SE, Schellekens AFA, et al. Effectiveness of genotype-specific tricyclic antidepressant dosing in patients with major depressive disorder: a randomized clinical trial. JAMA Netw Open 2023;**6**(5):e2312443. doi:10.1001/jamanetworkopen.2023.12443

24. Hiemke C, Bergemann N, Clement HW, et al. Consensus guidelines for therapeutic Drug monitoring in neuropsychopharmacology: update 2017. *Pharmacopsychiatry* 2018;**51**:9–62

25. van Westrhenen R, van Schaik RHN, van Gelder T, et al. Policy and practice review: a first guideline on the use of pharmacogenetics in clinical psychiatric practice. *Front Pharmacol* 2021;**12**:640032. doi.org/10.3389/fphar.2021.640032

Chapter 25

Mood Disorders: Therapeutic Challenges in the Medically Ill Patient

Peter A. Shapiro, Luis Pereira, Jon A. Levenson, and Chineze Worthington

Introduction

Mood disorders, especially depressive disorders, occur more commonly in persons with medical illness than in the general population. The lifetime prevalence of major depressive disorder is 5–10% in primary care, and up to 20–50% for patients with various serious and chronic medical conditions. Depression may occur as an independent comorbidity or an antecedent risk factor for or a complication of medical illness [1–5]. Bidirectional risk relationships are common, creating a psychosomatic vicious circle. These relationships may be mediated by biological factors (e.g., atherosclerosis, hypothalamic–pituitary–adrenal [HPA] axis dysfunction, inflammation, thyroid disease), behavioral factors (e.g., smoking, nonadherence to healthy lifestyle and medical treatment, risky behaviors), and psychosocial factors (e.g., social support, stigma, socioeconomic disadvantage and inequity, beliefs about illness).

Depression increases the risk acquiring and accumulating chronic medical conditions [6–8], and medical illness increases the likelihood of acquiring depression [9]. The high prevalence of bipolar disorder in people living with AIDS [10,11] can be explained at least in part by the association between manic symptoms and risky behaviors, a risk factor for HIV infection [12,13]. Mood disorders cause suffering and disability and are associated with reduced adherence to medical treatment and healthy lifestyle, and with increased morbidity and mortality of many illnesses [6,14–17], all reasons to think their treatment is important. However, diagnosis and treatment can be challenging.

Given the scope of the literature on psychiatric care of the medically ill, what follows is necessarily a selective and impressionistic review of challenges in treatment of mood disorders in this broad population.

Diagnosis

The Range of Moods

The differential diagnosis of mood disorders in patients with medical illness includes normal sadness and unhappiness, adjustment disorders, "primary" depressive and bipolar disorders, and "secondary" mood disorders. In the context of troubling circumstances such as medical illness, the boundaries between these categories can be hard to establish. Many patients are unhappy but not impaired in functioning (e.g., in managing their illness), and not so subjectively distressed by their unhappiness as to seek treatment. For these patients, no psychiatric diagnosis is justified.

DSM-5 Diagnoses

Adjustment disorders are characterized by subjective distress or impairment in functioning that arises following exposure to a stressor; symptoms may resemble those of a mood disorder but are insufficient in duration or number to warrant a mood disorder diagnosis. The DSM-5 notes that adjustment disorder is the most common diagnosis in psychiatric consultation in the general hospital setting, comprising nearly 50% of diagnoses [18].

"Primary" mood disorders include major depressive disorder, persistent depressive disorder, bipolar I and bipolar II disorders, and cyclothymic disorder. Diagnostic criteria for major depression and bipolar disorder include the important exclusion criterion that the illness is not best attributable to another mental disorder, or to the physiological effects of a substance, substance withdrawal, or another medical condition. (Among mood disorders, premenstrual dysphoric disorder is unique in that it is linked to a specific, normal physiological process that is not in itself a "medical condition"). Prototypical symptoms of depressive disorder include many "somatic" symptoms that might be attributable to medical illness or medications, such as abnormal sleep, low appetite, low energy, and fatigue, which makes distinguishing between primary mood disorders and secondary mood disorders challenging. But the distinction is important, since failure to address a reversible medical cause of mood symptoms may prevent successful treatment.

The Limited Value of Standard Rating Scales

Symptom rating scales such as the Hospital Anxiety and Depression Scale [19], PHQ-9 [20], and Beck Depression Inventory [21] are useful but imprecise for diagnosis, because symptoms may be present but better attributed to underlying medical illness or treatment than to a primary mood disorder. Diagnosis based on exclusion of potentially medically confounded symptoms, blanket inclusion of all symptoms without regard to potential "medical" confounding, and substitution of additional psychological symptoms in place of somatic symptoms have all been suggested as alternatives to attempts to attribute symptoms to primary mood disorder versus mood disorder secondary to a medical condition or substance, but none of these approaches has been proven best. An "inclusive approach" will have more sensitivity but less specificity in diagnosis of primary mood disorder. Nonprototypical symptoms such as nonadherence to medical therapy or somatization are sometimes used by clinicians as evidence of a depressive disorder, though without validation. Still, use of screening instruments is recommended as a standard of care in heart disease and cancer treatment [22,23].

Mood Disorders Secondary to Medical Condition

Secondary mood disorders are common. Illnesses whose physiological effects may lead directly to mood disorder include cerebrovascular disease, stroke, Parkinson's disease, multiple sclerosis, thyroid disease, and adrenal insufficiency, all of which may cause symptoms of depression [1,24]. Hyperthyroidism and hypercortisolemic conditions (Cushing's syndrome) may lead to mood elevation and symptoms of hypomania, mania, or mixed mood disorder. Neurosyphilis, lupus, and autoimmune encephalitis may present with manic, depressive, or psychotic symptoms. Anemia, heart failure, hypoxia, sleep apnea, renal failure, chronic liver disease, autoimmune and chronic inflammatory disorders, low serum testosterone (e.g., in hypogonadism associated

with HIV) [25], and some cancers may cause symptoms such as fatigue, low energy, sleep disturbance, and appetite disturbance, sometimes with sadness and depressed mood. Inadequate treatment of pain is a common cause of emotional distress that may manifest with withdrawal and apparent depressed mood. Other illnesses associated with secondary manic syndromes include brain tumors, seizure disorders, viral encephalitis, Wilson's disease, and frontotemporal dementia. In persons living with AIDS, opportunistic infections, antiretroviral treatment, and central nervous system inflammatory response to HIV can result in a secondary manic syndrome [26–29].

Inflammation

Inflammation blurs the boundary between primary and secondary mood disorder and points to the systemic nature of mood disorders. Patients with major depressive disorder and patients with elevated depression symptoms have elevated circulating C-reactive protein and circulating inflammatory cytokines including interleukin 6 (IL-6) and tumor necrosis factor-alpha, and several studies have found that anti-inflammatory treatment with NSAIDs, cytokine inhibitors, statins, minocycline, or steroids is effective in reducing symptoms of depression, both as monotherapy and as augmentation of other antidepressants [30]. Conversely, elevated inflammatory markers predict onset of depression symptoms, and exacerbations of somatic inflammatory diseases such as rheumatoid arthritis provoke depression symptoms. Depressive syndromes arise after infections and after hospitalizations for autoimmune disorders [31]. Exogenously administered inflammatory cytokines such as interferon alpha treatment for hepatitis or certain malignancies cause symptoms of lassitude, fatigue, depressed mood, an effect blocked by pretreatment with serotonin reuptake inhibitors [32,33].

Mood Disorders Secondary to Medications

Numerous commonly used medications have mood effects. Corticosteroids cause both mood elevation and depression. Biologic agents such as interferon alpha and antithymocyte globulin and novel monoclonal antibody agents such as basiliximab, alemtuzumab, and rituximab have a range of neuropsychiatric side effects, including fatigue and depressed mood [34]. Sympathomimetic bronchodilators may cause anxiety or mood elevation. Amiodarone, a potent antiarrhythmic agent, can cause hypothyroidism, with subsequent depressed mood. Beta-adrenergic blockers may be associated with fatigue and, less commonly, with clinical depression [35]. Antiretroviral medications, including integrase strand transfer inhibitors (INSTIs), which are currently used as first-line for treatment-naïve HIV patients, can cause or exacerbate depressive symptoms [36,37]. Other medications associated with depression include gonadotropin-releasing hormone agonists, mefloquine, and progestin in intrauterine devices and implanted contraceptives [38]. Depression symptoms occasionally occur as an adverse effect of other medications including trimethoprim-sulfamethoxazole, valacyclovir, valganciclovir, mycophenolate, and tacrolimus [15]. The association of isotretinoin with depression has been cast into doubt by recent studies (e.g., Chen et al. [39]).

Steroids

Corticosteroids are used for many medical conditions including autoimmune disorders, asthma, sepsis, pain, nausea, spinal cord compression, and cancer chemotherapy. They may cause mania, hypomania, anxiety, depression including psychotic depression, psychosis, delirium, agitation, and cognitive impairments, and are the most common cause of mania in cancer patients. The likelihood of mood effects increases with higher doses; the prevalence of new psychiatric symptoms approaches 20% in patients receiving over 80 mg of prednisone (or the equivalent) per day, but symptoms can occur during dose escalation, while at peak dosage, or during dose tapering [40]. Hypomanic-manic symptoms are the most common side effect [41].

Other Conditions That Might Be Mistaken for Depression

Oher conditions occurring in patients with medical illness are sometimes mistaken for depressive episodes, including hypoactive delirium, demoralization, and apathy [18,42–45]. Space does not allow for further review of these topics here.

Treatment

General Considerations

Engagement with treatment and appropriate goal setting are prerequisites to successful treatment of depression in the medically ill. Barriers to engagement include denial of distress or impairment, "normalization" of depressive symptoms in the context of illness, and the balance of perceived or actual burden versus benefit of depression treatment superimposed on the burdens posed by the patient's medical situation. Realistic goal setting improves the possibility of treatment success.

Treatment for mood disorders in the medically ill begins with diagnosis and appropriate intervention for causes of secondary mood disorders that can be mitigated, for example by treating thyroid disease or stopping drugs causing psychiatric side effects. Psychotherapy and psychopharmacological management are effective treatments for mood syndromes in the medically ill.

Psychotherapy

Support groups, brief counseling, supportive psychotherapy, cognitive behavioral therapy, problem-solving therapy, and interpersonal psychotherapy are the most frequently utilized nonpharmacological interventions. Effectiveness of psychotherapy to reduce depressive symptoms has been demonstrated for a variety of specific medical conditions including coronary heart disease and congestive heart failure [46–48], cancer [49,50], HIV [51–53], palliative care [54,55], and adolescents with chronic illnesses [56]. However, for many medical conditions no trials of psychotherapy for depression have been reported. Treatment may need to be especially focused on adjustment to illness, reframing illness-related cognitions, goal setting, and behavioral activation.

Psychopharmacology

Pharmacological treatment choices may be tailored to match target symptoms, for example, using mirtazapine, an antidepressant with antinausea effects, to treat depression in a patient with chemotherapy-associated nausea, or a relatively activating agent such as bupropion or a psychostimulant to address depression in a patient sedated by opioid pain medication. Pharmacological treatment must take into account physiological changes due to illness, altered drug metabolism, drug side effects, and drug interactions (Table 25.1). A detailed review is beyond the scope of this chapter, as entire volumes are devoted to this topic (e.g., Levenson and Ferrando [57]). Common practice is to begin medication trials at low doses and advance dosage cautiously. Even in nominally therapeutic doses and with nominally therapeutic blood levels, medication side effects may be particularly problematic in patients with medical illness. As a general rule, drugs that have a short half-life of elimination, that do not depend on phase 1 hepatic metabolism, and that have little effect on hepatic metabolism of other medications are to be preferred. Serotonin reuptake inhibitors and mirtazapine are first-line antidepressants with demonstrated benefit in treatment of depression in many medical conditions including heart disease, HIV, cancer, and stroke [58–63].

Altered End Organ Sensitivity

Ill and elderly patients may respond to medications at lower than typical doses. They may also be more sensitive to side effects. Some medical conditions are specifically associated with propensity to side effects. For example, AIDS patients and patients with Lewy body dementia are unusually prone to extrapyramidal side effects of antipsychotic medication.

Drug Metabolism

Drug metabolism may be affected by illness. Generally, oral and intramuscular (IM) absorption of psychotropic medications is unaffected by medical illness. However, conditions and procedures that affect gastric and small bowel function, such as pernicious anemia, Crohn's disease, and Roux-en-Y gastric bypass, may reduce drug absorption. Immediate release and liquid formulation of medications are preferable to extended-release forms. Conditions and treatments associated with decreased acid secretion accelerate dissolution of enteric coated medications and may increase drug absorption. P-glycoprotein efflux transporters in the gut wall limit absorption of many medications. For patients unable to take enteral medication, there may be no adequate IM or intravenous (IV) substitute. Chronic renal disease is associated with reduced intestinal CYP3A4 and P-glycoprotein, leading to reduced first-pass metabolism and increased bioavailability of CYP3A4 substrates [64]. Low cardiac output states may result in poor perfusion of peripheral tissues and reduced absorption of IM medications. Right-sided-heart failure causes hepatic congestion and cirrhosis and gut wall edema.

Drug distribution depends on lipid solubility, first-pass hepatic metabolism (for enteral medications), and protein binding. Distribution of drugs that are highly lipid-soluble is altered when fat stores are depleted by chronic illness. Ascite fluid and edema increase the volume of distribution of water-soluble drugs. When catabolic states, liver disease, or inadequate intake result in reduced plasma proteins, protein binding of psychotropic drugs in plasma is reduced and free drug relatively increased. Therapeutic drug level monitoring that does not take into account the effects of reduced protein binding may lead to underestimation of the level of biologically active free drug.

Most psychotropic drugs undergo hepatic metabolism into water-soluble metabolites that are then eliminated in urine. Exceptions include lithium, gabapentin, desvenlafaxine, paliperidone, pregabalin, levetiracetam, selegiline, and amphetamines, which are largely or entirely dependent on renal excretion. Hepatic metabolism usually involves cytochrome enzymes catalyzing reduction or oxidation reactions (phase 1 metabolism) followed by conjugation reactions utilizing uridine 5'-diphosphate glucuronosyl-transferase (UGT) (phase 2 metabolism). Chronic liver disease impairs phase 1 more than phase 2 metabolism. In heart failure, reduced hepatic artery blood flow may impair phase 1 metabolism. Chronic renal disease also reduces hepatic metabolism. For drugs highly dependent on renal excretion, acute or chronic renal failure may require significant dosage reduction. For renal failure patients on hemodialysis, lithium is typically given as a single dose following each dialysis session.

Side Effects and Drug Interactions

Typical side effects of antidepressants, mood stabilizers and antipsychotic drugs may be turned to advantage (e.g., improved appetite and sleep, antinausea effects) or limit or contraindicate treatment (e.g., cardiac arrhythmias, valproic acid–induced thrombocytopenia) (see Table 25.1).

Psychotropic and general medical drugs may have direct additive or offsetting effects ("pharmacodynamic" interaction) or interact via effects of one drug on the metabolism or bioavailability of the other ("pharmacokinetic" interaction) [64,65]. These interactions may be helpful or problematic, depending on the situation. Many psychotropic drugs prolong cardiac repolarization (indexed on the electrocardiogram QT interval), or inhibit the metabolism of other QT-interval prolonging medications, raising the risk of lethal polymorphic ventricular tachycardia (torsades de pointes). Some common medications with large QT prolongation effects are listed in Table 25.2 [66]. The sedating effect of opiates for cancer pain may be offset by the stimulating effect of methylphenidate used as an adjunctive antidepressant, a helpful pharmacodynamic interaction, but the effect of citalopram, an antidepressant known to

Table 25.1 Drugs commonly used for treatment of mood disorders: side effects, cytochrome, P-glycoprotein, and UGT effects – a selective list

Drugs	Common or especially serious side effects	Cytochrome effects	P-glycoprotein, UGT effects
Tricyclic antidepressants	Anticholinergic effects (e.g., blurry vision, delirium, dry mouth, constipation, urinary retention); orthostatic hypotension; tachycardia, heart block; exacerbation of narrow angle glaucoma; weight gain; sexual dysfunction; sedation	2D6 inhibitors: desipramine	P-gp inhibitors: amitriptyline, imipramine, desipramine
Serotonin reuptake inhibitors	Abdominal pain, weight loss or weight gain, diarrhea hepatotoxicity tremor sedation or insomnia bleeding, inhibition of platelet function sexual dysfunction prolonged QT interval (citalopram) SIADH serotonin syndrome	2D6 inhibitors: Paroxetine, fluvoxamine 3A4 inhibitors: fluoxetine, sertraline (at high dose) Pan-inhibitors: fluvoxamine, fluoxetine	P-gp inhibitors: sertraline, paroxetine
MAOIs	Orthostatic hypotension; sedation; weight gain; hypertensive crisis	Tranylcypromine: 1A2, 3A4 inhibitor; Phenelzine: 3A4 inhibitor	
Trazodone	Priapism, sedation		P-gp inducer
Nefazodone	hepatotoxicity sedation	Strong 3A4 inhibitor, and 3A4 substrate	
Mirtazapine	Increased appetite; sedation; antinausea; agranulocytosis (rare)	2D6, 3A4 substrate	
Bupropion	Decreased appetite; hypertension; reduced seizure threshold	2D6 inhibitor	
SNRIs	Abdominal pain, weight loss or weight gain, diarrhea; hepatotoxicity Tremor; sedation or insomnia; hypertension; sexual dysfunction	Duloxetine: 2D6 inhibitor	
Maprotiline			P-gp inhibitor
Milnacipran, levomilnacipran	Weight gain; sexual dysfunction; SIADH		
Vortioxetine	Nausea		
Vilazodone	Diarrhea, nausea; headache		
Lithium	Folliculitis, acne, exacerbation of psoriasis; Tremor; polyuria, nephrogenic diabetes insipidus, chronic renal failure; sinus node dysfunction; leukocytosis		

Table 25.1 (cont.)

Drugs	Common or especially serious side effects	Cytochrome effects	P-glycoprotein, UGT effects
Valproic acid	Thrombocytopenia; neutropenia; hepatotoxicity; pancreatitis, polycystic ovary syndrome; SIADH, sedation, weight gain	Substrate and inducer for CYP2A and CYP2C	UGT substrate and inhibitor
Carbamazepine	Neutropenia, thrombocytopenia; hepatotoxicity Sedation; weight gain	Induces all CYP450 enzymes; 3A4 substrate	UGT substrate and inducer. P-gp substrate
Lamotrigine	Stevens–Johnson syndrome	UGT inducers reduce lamotrigine blood level	UGT and P-gp substrate
Phenothiazines	QT interval prolongation Orthostatic hypotension Sedation Weight gain Extrapyramidal system effects: dystonic reactions, parkinsonism, akathisia, tardive dyskinesia Neuroleptic malignant syndrome		Chlorpromazine P-gp inhibitor, fluphenazine, trifluperazine
butyrophenones	QT interval prolongation Orthostatic hypotension Sedation Weight gain Extrapyramidal system effects: dystonic reactions, parkinsonism, akathisia, tardive dyskinesia	Haloperidol: 2D6 inhibitor	Haloperidol: P-gp inhibitor
Pimozide	QT interval prolongation Orthostatic hypotension Sedation Weight gain Extrapyramidal system effects: dystonic reactions, parkinsonism, akathisia, tardive dyskinesia		P-gp inhibitor
Second generation antipsychotics	Weight gain, impaired glycemic control, dyslipidemia (metabolic syndrome); QT prolongation; sedation orthostatic hypotension; hyperprolactinemia (especially risperidone); extrapyramidal system effects, tardive dyskinesia; neutropenia (especially, clozapine); Neuroleptic malignant syndrome sedation; Thrombocytopenia (quetiapine); Elevated prolactin, galactorrhea (especially risperidone) anti-emetic effect(olanzapine)	2D6 substrates; aripiprazole, brexpiprazole, cariprazine, chlorpromazine, clozapine, iloperidone, olanzapine, risperidone. 3A4 substrates: aripiprazole, brexpiprazole, cariprazine, clozapine, iloperidone, lurasidone, quetiapine, ziprasidone	Risperidone: P-gp inhibitor
Psychostimulants	Increased heart rate and blood pressure; appetite suppression; insomnia; psychosis; tics		

Abbreviation: P-gp: P-glycoprotein; SIADH: syndrome of inappropriate antidiuretic hormone secretion; UGT: uridine 5'-diphosphate glucuronosyltransferase.

Reference: Owen and Crouse, 2016 [64]; Flockhart et al., 2021 [68]

Table 25.2 Selected drugs that prolong QT interval

Antiretrovirals: indinavir, ritonavir

Cardiac medications: amiodarone, diltiazem, disopyramide, dofetilide, procainamide, quinidine, sotalol, verapamil,

Methadone

Ondansetron

Antibiotics: azithromycin, ciprofloxacin, clarithromycin, erythromycin, levofloxacin, moxifloxacin, trimethoprim-sulfamethoxazole

Antifungals: fluconazole, ketoconazole

Antimalarial: chloroquine

Psychotropics: thioridazine, citalopram, ziprasidone, phenothiazine antipsychotics (especially thioridazine), haloperidol

Tamoxifen

Source: Crediblemeds.org [125]; Beach et al., 2013 [66]

prolong the QT interval, combined with the effect of methadone, which also prolongs the QT interval, could result in a lethal cardiac arrhythmia – an undesirable pharmacodynamic interaction. Thiazide diuretics increase serum lithium level. The antiplatelet effects of selective serotonin reuptake inhibitors (SSRIs) combine with anticoagulant or antiplatelet treatment to increase bleeding risk. Many psychotropic drugs inhibit cytochrome P450 2D6 or 3A4, reducing the elimination and raising the blood level of the substrates of those enzymes, with subsequent potential exacerbation of the substrate's adverse effects. For example, bupropion and paroxetine are potent 2D6 inhibitors and reduce clearance of most beta-blockers, which could result in bradycardia, hypotension, and syncope. Inhibition of cytochrome enzymes by antidepressants may interfere with conversion of pro-drugs such as codeine, tramadol, and tamoxifen to their active metabolites.

Many websites provide lists of QT-interval prolonging medications, cytochrome, P-glycoprotein, and UGT system effects of medications, medication side effects, and drug–drug interactions, and when patients require treatment with both psychotropic and numerous other medications, reviewing the medication list for potential interactions is often revealing [67–69].

Psychedelics and Ketamine

In two widely noted trials, psilocybin was found to have beneficial effects on existential distress, mood and anxiety in patients with cancer and terminal illness [70,71]. Studies using lysergic acid diethylamide (LSD), 3,4-methylenedioxy-methamphetamine (MDMA), and psilocybin provide preliminary evidence of efficacy in

reduction of symptoms of depression and anxiety in chronically ill patients [72]. A recent systematic review of intravenous ketamine administration in the immediate postoperative period found statistically significant effects of ketamine on depressive symptoms on postoperative days 1 and 3 after surgery, but not at 7-day or 30-day follow-up. The beneficial effect was most pronounced in patients with preexisting high depression symptoms [73]. Trials of psilocybin and MDMA have excluded patients with uncontrolled hypertension and prolonged QT interval, severe cardiac disease, significant renal or hepatic dysfunction, brain metastases, primary brain disorders, personal or family history of psychotic disorders, and bipolar disorder. Adverse effects of acute administration of psilocybin and ketamine include increased heart rate and blood pressure, nausea, and headache, as well as adverse psychological responses. More research is needed to define the range of applicability and safety of psychedelics [74,75]. Psychedelic-assisted therapy is also illegal in most states in the United States, except in clinical trials, further limiting its availability and applicability [72,76].

ECT and TMS

Electroconvulsive therapy (ECT) is a safe and effective treatment for depression in the medically ill under most circumstances [77]. ECT causes an initial momentary bradycardia followed by sinus tachycardia and elevated blood pressure [78], which can be managed with appropriate monitoring and medication. Cardiac arrhythmias and acute coronary syndrome are the most frequent complications of ECT [77], but case reports and small case series describe safe ECT in patients with heart transplants, pacemakers, heart failure, and recent myocardial infarction [79–82], and even after prior ECT-induced Takotsubo cardiomyopathy [83]. However, cardiac conditions such as unstable angina and recurrent ventricular ectopy may contraindicate its use. In patients with Parkinson's disease, ECT improves both mood and motor symptoms [84]. ECT is safe in pregnancy and in treatment of post-stroke depression [85].

There are few studies of other brain-stimulation therapies for depression in the medically ill [86]. Several small studies indicate that transcranial magnetic stimulation (TMS) may be effective for post-stroke depression [87,88], with equivocal findings in Parkinson's disease [88]. Additional studies are needed to define the scope of potential application of these noninvasive therapies with low adverse effect burden.

Stepped-Care, Collaborative-Care Models

Team-based, collaborative-care, stepped-care models for treatment of depression in the medically ill have been of considerable interest since the report of the IMPACT trial for late-life depression treatment in primacy care [89,90]. These models depend on screening, review of case registries, and the central role of a behavioral care manager. The care manager engages patients with positive depression screens and delivers interventions such as brief counseling, behavioral activation, and problem-solving therapy; the primary care provider is responsible for prescribing antidepressants under the guidance of the behavioral care manager and consulting psychiatrist, and the consulting psychiatrist provides case registry review and case supervision with the care manager. Treatment intensity is "stepped up" when patients do not respond to initial low-intensity interventions. In addition to wide adoption in primary care clinics [91], collaborative care models have been tested and found helpful in treatment of depression in patients with recent acute coronary events [92,93], coronary bypass surgery [94], diabetes and cardiovascular disease in primary care [90,95,96], and cancer [97,98]. However, collaborative care models are demanding to implement and sustain. Barriers include resistance from primary care providers, inadequate training and overburdening of behavioral care managers, and high operating cost [96,99,100].

Exercise

Exercise is an effective treatment for depression symptoms in a number of medical conditions including coronary disease and heart failure [101,102], cancer [103,104], hemodialysis patients [105], and ankylosing spondylitis [106], but optimal dose, intensity, and duration of treatment are open questions.

Mood Disorders in the Terminally Ill and Patients Requesting Hastened Death

Depressive symptoms, demoralization, and major depression may emerge during the care of the terminally ill patient, and major depression is associated with hopelessness and desire for hastened death (DHD) [107,108]. Risk factors for depression in palliative care settings include poorly controlled pain, severe debility, dependency on others for basic needs, and inadequately managed physical symptoms (pain, dyspnea, fatigue, weakness, nausea/vomiting, pruritus, insomnia). Past psychiatric history of a mood disorder and low social or community support are also important factors in the assessment. Distinguishing DHD from acute suicidality is essential, as the suicidal terminally ill patient requires a higher level of acute care. A recent meta-analysis found a nearly twofold increased standardized mortality ratio (SMR) due to suicide in cancer patients compared to the general population. Clinical factors enhancing suicide risk included worse prognosis, more advanced stage, and time since diagnosis; suicide risk was highest within the first year after diagnosis, mostly accounted for by confounding with cancers with poor prognosis [109].

Requests for hastened death are sometimes resolved by better management of pain, nausea, shortness of breath, or other troubling somatic symptoms, particularly if that management improves comorbid depression [110,111]. Nevertheless, existential distress and greatly impaired quality of life with no hope for significant improvement may not be entirely remediable [42,112], contributing to requests for physician-assisted suicide and physician-assisted death (i.e., euthanasia). "Hopeless" cases create cognitive dissonance and emotional distress for healthcare providers when rescue fantasies, which are ubiquitous among physicians, cannot be realized [113]; this distress may result in either failure to shift to palliative and comfort-focused care or over-readiness to participate in hastening death. Patients with end-stage renal disease dependent on hemodialysis and heart failure patients maintained on left ventricular assist devices (LVADs) may hasten their own deaths by sabotaging treatment (intentionally missing dialysis or disconnecting or damaging the LVAD). A framework for achieving conceptual agreement in evaluating requests for hastened death via dialysis discontinuation has been proposed by Bostwick and Cohen [114], and increased awareness of desire for death via termination of LVAD therapy has led to the institution of extensive advance care planning prior to LVAD implantation at some institutions [115]. But when a patient who requests discontinuation of a life-extending treatment meets clinical criteria for diagnosis of a mood disorder, it may be difficult to arrive at consensus about how best to proceed. "Medical Assistance in Dying," that is, physician-assisted suicide and euthanasia, is now legal in many jurisdictions in Europe, the United States, and Canada, despite widespread concerns [116,117]. Further review on this topic is beyond the scope of this discussion.

Several psychotherapy interventions have been designed specifically for patients near the end of life, aiming to alleviate existential distress and reduce depression and anxiety [112]. Meaning-centered psychotherapy is a semistructured program focusing on identifying past meaningful life experience and creating meaningful experience in the time remaining in one's life; its effectiveness has been demonstrated in clinical trials [118,119]. However, it has not been tested as treatment for major depressive disorder.

Dignity-conserving psychotherapy (DCP) is an intervention designed for care of terminally ill patients in hospice settings who have active depressive symptoms including demoralization. DCP is a legacy-building approach that involves a semistructured interview reviewing the patient's life experience and seeking to articulate important life lessons that the patient can transmit as a legacy, thereby fostering generativity until the very end of life. The interview is transcribed and edited into a written "Dignity Document" that the patient can then share with loved ones. The intervention has been tested in clinical trials and shown to improve mood and quality of life in terminally ill patients, but it has not been tested as treatment for major depressive disorder [120,121].

Managing Cancer and Living Meaningfully (CALM) therapy is an individual supportive/expressive psychosocial intervention for treating and preventing depressive symptoms in advanced cancer patients. Components of CALM include enhanced communication with the oncology team to improve symptom management, an opportunity to reflect on the self and important relationships, and attending to spiritual well-being and concerns around mortality [122,123].

Pharmacotherapeutic approaches to treating depressive disorders in end- of-life care include standard antidepressants and stimulants. Response to standard antidepressant medications typically occurs over a period of weeks, while stimulant effects may be apparent within a few days, which may be especially valuable to alleviate suffering in terminally ill patients. Concerns about stimulant habituation and dependence are obviated by the patient's expected death. Stimulants have beneficial effects on mood, fatigue, well-being, and appetite and counteract opioid-induced sedation. No randomized trial has been conducted to evaluate the effectiveness of psychostimulants for this purpose. For newer interventional approaches for depression such as psychedelics, ketamine and esketamine, and transcranial magnetic stimulation (TMS), additional studies are needed.

The Emotional Burden on Care Providers

Treating mood disorders in medically ill patients may challenge treaters to acknowledge and manage their own discomfort about disability, sickness, disfigurement, and death, and the limitations of their ability to cure and to rescue, while providing a safe space for patients to express grief, fear, sadness, and anger. Psychotherapy with dying patients includes maintaining hope for the future that remains and helping the patient to address "unfinished business", as well as nonabandonment, presence, and bearing witness to the patient's suffering [124]. Existential despair, feelings of meaninglessness, depression, and exhaustion can affect the depression care provider as well as the ill and dying patient, but having a clear sense of one's role, doing what can be done, and accepting the inevitability of loss and grief as part of life help to maintain the treater's sense of vitality and the meaningfulness of the work.

Concluding Remarks

Much is known about the treatment of mood disorders in the medically ill, but much remains to be learned. Improvements in diagnosis, perhaps with the aid of new biomarkers, and better and more available therapies, with fewer complications due to adverse effects and drug interactions, are much to be desired. While the often-profound suffering that attends serious illness and the approach of death may be an existential reality that cannot be entirely resolved, treatment of mood disorders in the medically ill can improve patients' wellbeing and be rewarding for the clinician.

References

1. Rosenblat JD, Kurdyak P, Cosci F, et al. Depression in the medically ill. *Aust N Z J Psychiatry*. 2020;**54**(4):346–66.

2. Bobo WV, Yawn BP, St. Sauver JL, et al. Prevalence of combined somatic and mental health multimorbidity: patterns by age, sex, and race/ethnicity. *J Gerontol A Biol Sci Med Sci*. 2016;**71**(11):1483–91.

3. Thom R, Silbersweig DA, Boland RJ. Major depressive disorder in medical illness: a review of assessment, prevalence, and treatment options. *Psychosom Med*. 2019;**81**(3):246–55.

4. Mitchell AJ, Chan M, Bhatti H, et al. Prevalence of depression, anxiety, and adjustment disorder in oncological, haematological, and palliative-care settings: a meta-analysis of 94 interview-based studies. *Lancet Oncol*. 2011;**12**(2):160–74.

5. Rezaei S, Ahmadi S, Rahmati J, et al. Global prevalence of depression in HIV/AIDS: a systematic review and meta-analysis. *BMJ Support Palliat Care*. 2019;**9**(4):404–12.

6. Bobo WV, Grossardt BR, Virani S, et al. Association of depression and anxiety with the accumulation of chronic conditions. *JAMA Netw Open*. 2022;**5**(5): e229817.

7. Poole L, Steptoe A. Depressive symptoms predict incident chronic disease burden 10 years later: findings from the English Longitudinal Study of Ageing (ELSA). *J Psychosom Res*. 2018;**113**:30–6.

8. Xu X, Mishra GD, Jones M. Depressive symptoms and the development and progression of physical multimorbidity in a national cohort of Australian women. *Health Psychol*. 2019;**38**(9):812–21.

9. Carroll S, Moon Z, Hudson J, et al. An evidence-based theory of psychological adjustment to long-term physical health conditions: applications in clinical practice. *Psychosom Med*. 2022.

10. de Sousa Gurgel W, da Silva Carneiro AH, Barreto Rebouças D, et al. Prevalence of bipolar disorder in a HIV-infected outpatient population. *AIDS Care*. 2013;**25**(12):1499–503.

11. Lopes M, Olfson M, Rabkin J, et al. Gender, HIV status, and psychiatric disorders: results from the National Epidemiologic Survey on Alcohol and Related Conditions. *J Clin Psychiatry*. 2012;**73**(3):384–91.

12. Meade CS, Bevilacqua LA, Key MD. Bipolar disorder is associated with HIV transmission risk behavior among patients in treatment for HIV. *AIDS Behav*. 2012;**16**(8):2267–71.

13. Hunt GE, Malhi GS, Cleary M, Lai HM, Sitharthan T. Prevalence of comorbid bipolar and substance use disorders in clinical settings, 1990–2015: systematic review and meta-analysis. *J Affect Disord*. 2016;**206**:331–49.

14. Gehi A, Haas D, Pipkin S, Whooley MA. Depression and medication adherence in outpatients with coronary heart disease: findings from the Heart and Soul Study. *Arch Intern Med*. 2005;**165**:2508–13.

15. Nakamura ZM, Nash RP, Quillen LJ, et al. Psychiatric care in hematopoietic stem cell transplantation. *Psychosomatics*. 2019;**60**(3):227–37.

16. Gonzalez JS, Batchelder AW, Psaros C, Safren SA. Depression and HIV/AIDS treatment nonadherence: a review and meta-analysis. *J Acquir Immune Defic Syndr*. 2011;**58**(2):181–7.

17. Uthman OA, Magidson JF, Safren SA, Nachega JB. Depression and adherence to antiretroviral therapy in low-, middle- and high-income countries: a systematic review and meta-analysis. *Curr HIV/AIDS Rep*. 2014;**11**(3):291–307.

18. American Psychiatric Association. *Diagnostic and Statistical Manual of Mental Disorders: DSM-5*. 5th ed. Washington, DC: American Psychiatric Association, 2013.

19. Zigmond AS, Snaith RP. The Hospital Anxiety and Depression Scale. *Acta Psychiatr Scand*. 1983;**67**:3610370.

20. Kroenke K, Spitzer RL, Williams JB. The PHQ-9. Validity of a brief depression severity measure. *J Gen Intern Med*. 2001;**16**:606–13.

21. Beck AT, Steer RA. *Manual for the Beck Depression Inventory*. San Antonio, TX: Psychological Corporation, 1993.

22. Lichtman JH, Froelicher ES, Blumenthal JA, et al. Depression as a risk factor for poor prognosis among patients with acute coronary syndrome: systematic review and recommendations: a scientific statement from the American Heart Association. *Circulation*. 2014;**129**:1350–69.

23. Andersen BL, DeRubeis RJ, Berman BS, et al. Screening, assessment, and care of anxiety and depressive symptoms in adults with cancer: an American Society of Clinical Oncology guideline adaptation. *J Clin Oncol.* 2014;**32**(15):1605–19.

24. Empana JP, Boutouyrie P, Lemogne C, Jouven X, van Sloten TT. Microvascular contribution to late-onset depression: mechanisms, current evidence, association with other brain diseases, and therapeutic perspectives. *Biol Psychiatry.* 2021;**90**(4):214–25.

25. Wong N, Levy M, Stephenson I. Hypogonadism in the HIV-infected man. *Curr Treat Options Infect Dis.* 2017;**9**(1):104–16.

26. Johannessen DJ, Wilson LG. Mania with cryptococcal meningitis in two AIDS patients. *J Clin Psychiatry.* 1988;**49**(5):200–1.

27. Aslam SP, Carroll KA, Naz B, Alao AO. Valacyclovir-induced psychosis and manic symptoms in an adolescent young woman with genital herpes simplex. *Psychosomatics.* 2009;**50**(3):293–6.

28. Wright JM, Sachdev PS, Perkins RJ, Rodriguez P. Zidovudine-related mania. *Med J Aust.* 1989;**150** (6):339–41.

29. Shah MD, Balderson K. A manic episode associated with efavirenz therapy for HIV infection. *AIDS.* 2003;**17**(11):1713–14.

30. Köhler-Forsberg O, Lyndholm CN, Hjorthøj C, et al. Efficacy of anti-inflammatory treatment on major depressive disorder or depressive symptoms: meta-analysis of clinical trials. *Acta Psychiatr Scand.* 2019;**139**(5):404–19.

31. Kohler O, Krogh J, Mors O, Benros ME. Inflammation in depression and the potential for anti-inflammatory treatment. *Curr Neuropharmacol.* 2016;**14**(7):732–42.

32. Musselman DL, Lawson DH, Gumnick JF, et al. Paroxetine for the prevention of depression induced by high-dose interferon alpha. *N Engl J Med.* 2001;**344**:961–6.

33. Sarkar S, Schaefer M. Antidepressant pretreatment for the prevention of interferon alfa-associated depression: a systematic review and meta-analysis. *Psychosomatics.* 2014;**55**(3):221–34.

34. Sotelo JL, Musselman D, Nemeroff C. The biology of depression in cancer and the relationship between depression and cancer progression. *Int Rev Psychiatry.* 2014;**26**(1):16–30.

35. Ko DT, Hebert PR, Coffey CS, et al. Beta-blocker therapy and symptoms of depression, fatigue, and sexual dysfunction. *JAMA.* 2002;**288**:351–7.

36. Harris M, Larsen G, Montaner JS. Exacerbation of depression associated with starting raltegravir: a report of four cases. *AIDS.* 2008;**22**(14):1890–2.

37. Hoffmann C, Llibre JM. Neuropsychiatric adverse events with dolutegravir and other integrase strand transfer inhibitors. *AIDS Rev.* 2019;**21**(1):4–10.

38. Patten SB, Barbui C. Drug-induced depression: a systematic review to inform clinical practice. *Psychother Psychosom.* 2004;**73**(4):207–15.

39. Chen YH, Wang WM, Chung CH, et al. Risk of psychiatric disorders in patients taking isotretinoin: a nationwide, population-based, cohort study in Taiwan. *J Affect Disord.* 2022;**296**:277–82.

40. Kenna HA, Poon AW, de los Angeles CP, Koran LM. Psychiatric complications of treatment with corticosteroids: review with case report. *Psychiatry Clin Neurosci.* 2011;**65**(6):549–60.

41. Ismail MF, Lavelle C, Cassidy EM. Steroid-induced mental disorders in cancer patients: a systematic review. *Future Oncol.* 2017;**13**(29):2719–31.

42. Kissane DW. Demoralization: a life-preserving diagnosis to make for the severely medically ill. *J Palliat Care.* 2014;**30**(4):255–8.

43. Robinson S, Kissane DW, Brooker J, Burney S. A review of the construct of demoralization: history, definitions, and future directions for palliative care. *Am J Hosp Palliat Care.* 2016;**33**(1):93–101.

44. Oba H, Kobayashi R, Kawakatsu S, et al. Non-pharmacological approaches to apathy and depression: a scoping review of mild cognitive impairment and dementia. *Front Psychol.* 2022;**13**:815913.

45. Gracia-García P, Modrego P, Lobo A. Apathy and neurocognitive correlates: review from the perspective of "precision psychiatry." *Curr Opin Psychiatry.* 2021;**34**(2):193–8.

46. Freedland KE, Skala JA, Carney RM, et al. Treatment of depression after coronary artery bypass surgery: a randomized controlled trial. *Arch Gen Psychiatry.* 2009;**66**(4):387–96.

47. Freedland KE, Carney RM, Rich MW, Steinmeyer BC, Rubin EH. Cognitive behavior therapy for depression and self-care in heart failure patients: a randomized clinical trial. *JAMA Intern Med.* 2015;**175**(11):1773–82.

48. Berkman LF, Jaffe AS, editors. Results of the ENRICHD (Enhancing Recovery in Coronary Heart Disease) trial. Scientific Sessions of the American Heart Association, November 2001, Anaheim, California.

49. Jassim GA, Whitford DL, Hickey A, Carter B. Psychological interventions for women with non-metastatic breast cancer. *Cochrane Database Syst Rev.* 2015;(**5**):CD008729.

50. Li M, Fitzgerald P, Rodin G. Evidence-based treatment of depression in patients with cancer. *J Clin Oncol.* 2012;**30**(11):1187–96.

51. Safren SA, Bedoya CA, O'Cleirigh C, et al. Cognitive behavioural therapy for adherence and depression in patients with HIV: a three-arm randomised controlled trial. *Lancet HIV*. 2016;3(11):e529-e38.

52. Heckman TG, Markowitz JC, Heckman BD, et al. A randomized clinical trial showing persisting reductions in depressive symptoms in HIV-infected rural adults following brief telephone-administered interpersonal psychotherapy. *Ann Behav Med*. 2018;52(4):299–308.

53. Markowitz JC, Kocsis JH, Fishman B, et al. Treatment of depressive symptoms in human immunodeficiency virus-positive patients. *Arch Gen Psychiatry*. 1998;55(5):452–7.

54. Raue PJ, McGovern AR, Kiosses DN, Sirey JA. Advances in psychotherapy for depressed older adults. *Curr Psychiatry Rep*. 2017;19(9):57.

55. Fulton JJ, Newins AR, Porter LS, Ramos K. Psychotherapy targeting depression and anxiety for use in palliative care: a meta-analysis. *J Palliat Med*. 2018;21(7):1024–37.

56. Morey A, Loades ME. Review: how has cognitive behaviour therapy been adapted for adolescents with comorbid depression and chronic illness? A scoping review. *Child Adolesc Ment Health*. 2021;26(3):252–64.

57. Levenson JL, Ferrando SJ, editors. *Clinical Manual of Psychopharmacology in the Medically Ill*. 2nd ed. Arlington, VA: APA Publishing, 2016.

58. Shapiro PA. management of depression after myocardial infarction. *Curr Cardiol Rep*. 2015;17(10):1–9.

59. Jones M, Corcoran A, Jorge RE. The psychopharmacology of brain vascular disease/poststroke depression. *Handb Clin Neurol*. 2019;165:229–41.

60. Sherr L, Clucas C, Harding R, Sibley E, Catalan J. HIV and depression–a systematic review of interventions. *Psychol Health Med*. 2011;16(5):493–527.

61. Eshun-Wilson I, Siegfried N, Akena DH, et al. Antidepressants for depression in adults with HIV infection. *Cochrane Database Syst Rev*. 2018;1(1): CD008525.

62. Panjwani AA, Li M. Recent trends in the management of depression in persons with cancer. *Curr Opin Psychiatry*. 2021;34(5):448–59.

63. Rabin EE, Kim M, Mozny A, et al. A systematic review of pharmacologic treatment efficacy for depression in older patients with cancer. *Brain Behav Immun Health*. 2022;21:100449.

64. Owen JA, Crouse EL. Pharmacokinetics, pharmacodynamics, and principles of drug-drug interactions. In JL Levenson, SJ Ferrando, editors. *Clinical Manual of Psychopharmacology in the Medically Ill*. 2nd ed. Arlington, VA: APA Publishing; 2016; 3–45.

65. Smith CM, Hicks PB, Lindefjeld JK, et al. Antiretrovirals and psychotropics: drug interactions and complications. In J Bourgeois, M Adler Cohen, G Makurumidze, editors. *HIV Psychiatry: A Practical Guide for Clinicians*: Springer, 2022; 415–76.

66. Beach SR, Celano CM, Noseworthy PA, Januzzi JL, Huffman JC. QTc prolongation, Torsades de Pointes, and psychotropic medications. *Psychosomatics*. 2013;54(1):1–13.

67. CredibleMeds.org. www.crediblemeds.org

68. Flockhart DA, Thacker D, McDonald C, Desta Z. The Flockhart Cytochrome P450 Drug-Drug Interaction Table: Division of Clinical Pharmacology, Indiana University School of Medicine [updated 2021]. Available from: https://drug-interactions.medicine.iu.edu.

69. Liverpool Uo. HIV Drug Interactions 2022. Available from: HIV-druginteractions.org.

70. Ross S, Bossis A, Guss J, et al. Rapid and sustained symptom reduction following psilocybin treatment for anxiety and depression in patients with life-threatening cancer: a randomized controlled trial. *J Psychopharmacol*. 2016;30(12):1165–80.

71. Griffiths RR, Johnson MW, Carducci MA, et al. Psilocybin produces substantial and sustained decreases in depression and anxiety in patients with life-threatening cancer: a randomized double-blind trial. *J Psychopharmacol*. 2016;30(12):1181–97.

72. Rosa WE, Sager Z, Miller M, et al. Top ten tips palliative care clinicians should know about psychedelic-assisted therapy in the context of serious illness. *J Palliat Med*. 2022;25(8):1273–81.

73. Wang J, Sun Y, Ai P, et al. The effect of intravenous ketamine on depressive symptoms after surgery: a systematic review. *J Clin Anesth*. 2022;77:110631.

74. Schimmel N, Breeksema JJ, Smith-Apeldoorn SY, et al. Psychedelics for the treatment of depression, anxiety, and existential distress in patients with a terminal illness: a systematic review. *Psychopharmacology (Berl)*. 2022;239(1):15–33.

75. Reiche S, Hermle L, Gutwinski S, et al. Serotonergic hallucinogens in the treatment of anxiety and depression in patients suffering from a life-threatening disease: a systematic review. *Prog Neuropsychopharmacol Biol Psychiatry*. 2018;81:1–10.

76. Yaden DB, Nayak SM, Gukasyan N, Anderson BT, Griffiths RR. The potential of psychedelics for end of life and palliative care. *Curr Top Behav Neurosci*. 2022;56:169–84.

77. Espinoza RT, Kellner CH. Electroconvulsive therapy. *N Engl J Med*. 2022;386(7):667–72.

78. Wells DG, Davies GG. Hemodynamic changes associated with electroconvulsive therapy. *Anesthesia Analgesia*. 1987;**66**:1193–5.

79. Dolenc TJ, Barnes RD, Hayes DL, Rasmussen KG. Electroconvulsive therapy in patients with cardiac pacemakers and implantable cardioverter defibrillators. *Pacing Clin Electrophysiol*. 2004;**27**(9):1257–63.

80. Lee HB, Jayaram G, Teitelbaum ML. Electroconvulsive therapy for depression in a cardiac transplant patient. *Psychosomatics*. 2001;**42**(4):362–4.

81. Magid M, Lapid MI, Sampson SM, Mueller PS. Use of electroconvulsive therapy in a patient 10 days after myocardial infarction. *J ECT*. 2005;**21**(3):182–5.

82. Rayburn BK. Electroconvulsive therapy in patients with heart failure or valvular heart disease. *Convuls Ther*. 1997;**13**(3):145–56.

83. Kent LK, Weston CA, Heyer EJ, Sherman W, Prudic J. Successful retrial of ECT two months after ECT-induced takotsubo cardiomyopathy. *Am J Psychiatry*. 2009;**166**(8):857–62.

84. Takamiya A, Seki M, Kudo S, et al. Electroconvulsive therapy for Parkinson's disease: a systematic review and meta-analysis. *Mov Disord*. 2021;**36**(1):50–8.

85. Hermida AP, Glass OM, Shafi H, McDonald WM. Electroconvulsive therapy in depression: current practice and future direction. *Psychiatr Clin North Am*. 2018;**41**(3):341–53.

86. Valiengo LC, Benseñor IM, Lotufo PA, Fraguas R Jr., Brunoni AR. Transcranial direct current stimulation and repetitive transcranial magnetic stimulation in consultation-liaison psychiatry. *Braz J Med Biol Res*. 2013;**46**(10):815–23.

87. Shen Y, Cai Z, Liu F, Zhang Z, Ni G. Repetitive transcranial magnetic stimulation and transcranial direct current stimulation as treatment of poststroke depression: a systematic review and meta-analysis. *Neurologist*. 2022.

88. Hordacre B, Comacchio K, Williams L, Hillier S. Repetitive transcranial magnetic stimulation for post-stroke depression: a randomised trial with neurophysiological insight. *J Neurol*. 2021;**268**(4):1474–84.

89. Unutzer J, Katon W, Callahan CM, et al. Collaborative care management of late-life depression in the primary care setting: a randomized controlled trial. *JAMA*. 2002;**288**(22):2836–45.

90. Katon WJ, Lin EHB, Von Korff M, et al. Collaborative care for patients with depression and chronic illnesses. *N Engl J Med*. 2010;**363**(27):2611–20.

91. Coleman KJ, Magnan S, Neely C, et al. The COMPASS initiative: description of a nationwide collaborative approach to the care of patients with depression and diabetes and/or cardiovascular disease. *Gen Hosp Psychiatry*. 2017;**44**:69–76.

92. Davidson KW, Rieckmann N, Clemow L, et al. Enhanced depression care for patients with acute coronary syndrome and persistent depressive symptoms: coronary psychosocial evaluation studies randomized controlled trial. *Arch Intern Med*. 2010;**170**(7):600–8.

93. Davidson KW, Bigger JT, Burg MM, et al. Centralized, stepped, patient preference–based treatment for patients with post–acute coronary syndrome depression: Codiacs vanguard randomized controlled trial. *JAMA Intern Med*. 2013;**173**(11):997–1004.

94. Rollman BL, Belnap BH, LeMenager MS, et al. telephone-delivered collaborative care for treating post-CABG depression: a randomized controlled trial. *JAMA*. 2009;**302**:2095–103.

95. Katon WJ, Von Korff M, Lin EHB, et al. The Pathways Study: a randomized trial of collaborative care in patients with diabetes and depression. *Arch Gen Psychiatry*. 2004;**61**(10):1042–9.

96. Rossom R, Solberg L, Magnan S, et al. Impact of a national collaborative care initiative for patients with depression and diabetes or cardiovascular disease. *Gen Hosp Psychiatry*. 2017;**44**:77–85.

97. Sharpe M, Walker J, Holm Hansen C, et al. Integrated collaborative care for comorbid major depression in patients with cancer (SMaRT Oncology-2): a multicentre randomised controlled effectiveness trial. *Lancet*. 2014;**384**(9948):1099–108.

98. Walker J, Hansen CH, Martin P, et al. Integrated collaborative care for major depression comorbid with a poor prognosis cancer (SMaRT Oncology-3): a multicentre randomised controlled trial in patients with lung cancer. *Lancet Oncol*. 2014;**15**(10):1168–76.

99. Whitebird RR, Solberg LI, Jaeckels NA, et al. Effective implementation of collaborative care for depression: what is needed? *Am J Manag Care*. 2014;**20**(9):699–707.

100. Coleman KJ, Hemmila T, Valenti MD, et al. Understanding the experience of care managers and relationship with patient outcomes: the COMPASS initiative. *Gen Hosp Psychiatry*. 2017;**44**:86–90.

101. Blumenthal J, Babyak MA, O'Connor C, et al. Effects of exercise training on depressive symptoms in patients with chronic heart failure: The HF-ACTION randomized trial. *JAMA*. 2012;**308**(5):465–74.

102. Blumenthal JA, Sherwood A, Babyak MA, et al. Exercise and pharmacological treatment of depressive symptoms in patients with coronary heart disease: results from the UPBEAT (Understanding the Prognostic Benefits of Exercise and Antidepressant Therapy) study. *J Am Coll Cardiol*. 2012;**60**(12):1053–63.

103. Marconcin P, Marques A, Ferrari G, et al. Impact of exercise training on depressive symptoms in cancer patients: a critical analysis. *Biology (Basel)*. 2022;**11**(4).

104. Salam A, Woodman A, Chu A, et al. Effect of post-diagnosis exercise on depression symptoms, physical functioning and mortality in breast cancer survivors: a systematic review and meta-analysis of randomized control trials. *Cancer Epidemiol*. 2022;**77**:102111.

105. Bernier-Jean A, Beruni NA, Bondonno NP, et al. Exercise training for adults undergoing maintenance dialysis. *Cochrane Database Syst Rev*. 2022;**1**(1): CD014653.

106. Lane B, McCullagh R, Cardoso JR, McVeigh JG. The effectiveness of group and home-based exercise on psychological status in people with ankylosing spondylitis: a systematic review and meta-analysis. *Musculoskeletal Care*. 2022.

107. Breitbart W, Rosenfeld B, Pessin H, et al. Depression, hopelessness, and desire for hastened death in terminally ill patients with cancer. *JAMA*. 2000;**284**(22):2907–11.

108. Parpa E, Tsilika E, Galanos A, Nikoloudi M, Mystakidou K. Depression as mediator and or moderator on the relationship between hopelessness and patients' desire for hastened death. *Support Care Cancer*. 2019;**27**(11):4353–8.

109. Heinrich M, Hofmann L, Baurecht H, et al. Suicide risk and mortality among patients with cancer. *Nat Med*. 2022;**28**(4):852–9.

110. O'Mahony S, Goulet J, Kornblith A, et al. Desire for hastened death, cancer pain and depression: report of a longitudinal observational study. *J Pain Symptom Manage*. 2005;**29**(5):446–57.

111. Breitbart W, Rosenfeld B, Gibson C, et al. Impact of treatment for depression on desire for hastened death in patients with advanced AIDS. *Psychosomatics*. 2010;**51**(2):98–105.

112. Rosa WE, Chochinov HM, Coyle N, Hadler RA, Breitbart WS. Attending to the existential experience in oncology: dignity and meaning amid awareness of death. *JCO Glob Oncol*. 2022;**8**: e2200038.

113. Hetzler PT 3rd, Dugdale LS. How do medicalization and rescue fantasy prevent healthy dying? *AMA J Ethics*. 2018;**20**(8):E766–73.

114. Bostwick JM, Cohen LM. Differentiating suicide from life-ending acts and end-of-life decisions: a model based on chronic kidney disease and dialysis. *Psychosomatics*. 2009;**50**(1):1–7.

115. Nakagawa S, Yuzefpolskaya M, Colombo PC, Naka Y, Blinderman CD. Palliative care interventions before left ventricular assist device implantation in both bridge to transplant and destination therapy. *J Palliative Med*. 2017.doi: 10.1089/jpm.2016.0568.

116. Li M, Watt S, Escaf M, et al. Medical assistance in dying – implementing a hospital-based program in Canada. *N Engl J Med*. 2017;**376**(21):2082–8.

117. Mathews JJ, Hausner D, Avery J, et al. Impact of medical assistance in dying on palliative care: a qualitative study. *Palliat Med*. 2021;**35**(2):447–54.

118. Breitbart W, Rosenfeld B, Gibson C, et al. Meaning-centered group psychotherapy for patients with advanced cancer: a pilot randomized controlled trial. Psychooncology. 2010;**19**(1):21–8.

119. Breitbart W, Poppito S, Rosenfeld B, et al. Pilot randomized controlled trial of individual meaning-centered psychotherapy for patients with advanced cancer. *J Clin Oncol*. 2012;**30**(12):1304–9.

120. Chochinov HM, Hack T, Hassard T, et al. Dignity therapy: a novel psychotherapeutic intervention for patients near the end of life. *J Clin Oncol*. 2005;**23**(24):5520–5.

121. Chochinov HM, Kristjanson LJ, Breitbart W, et al. Effect of dignity therapy on distress and end-of-life experience in terminally ill patients: a randomised controlled trial. *Lancet Oncol*. 2011;**12**(8):753–62.

122. Hales S, Lo C, Rodin G. *Managing Cancer and Living Meaningfully (CALM) Treatment Manual: An Individual Psychotherapy for Patients with Advanced Cancer*. Toronto, Canada: Princess Margaret Cancer Centre, University Health Network; 2015.

123. Rodin G, Lo C, Rydall A, et al. Managing Cancer and Living Meaningfully (CALM): a randomized controlled trial of a psychological intervention for patients with advanced cancer. *J Clin Oncol*. 2018;**36**(23):2422–32.

124. Eissler K. *The Psychiatrist and the Dying Patient*. New York: Int Univ Press; 1955.

125. CredibleMeds.org. Risk Categories for Drugs that Prolong QT & induce Torsades de Pointes (TdP). Available from: crediblemeds.org.

The Treatment of Mood Disorders in Children and Adolescents

Ioanna Douka and Argyris Stringaris

Unipolar Depression

Significance of Depression in Children and Adolescents

Depressive disorders are a leading cause of disability in adolescents [1], and it has its origins early in life with a cumulative estimated prevalence of 10% by age 16 [2]. Whilst depression is less common in children, its incidence starts peaking during adolescence, the time at which the female preponderance (2:1) of the disease manifests itself [3,4]. Adolescents are up to 30 times more likely to die of suicide [5], and suicide is the second leading cause of the death among ages 15–19 years in the United States [6].

Establishing a Treatment Plan

Following an in-depth diagnostic assessment, the first step in the therapeutic approach is establishing a treatment plan. Current guidelines recommend collaboration with patients and their families for a successful treatment plan [7]. Psychoeducation of both patients and their family members about depression contributes to decrease of nonadherence and stigmatization [8]. In addition, education of the school personnel plays a significant role as accommodations of the schedule and the workload may be necessary. Furthermore, schoolperformance reflects the disease's progression and should be part of the patient's evaluation [8].

Collaborative care between primary care clinicians or pediatricians and a mental health specialist is also essential, especially with patients with treatment-resistant depression (TRD) or when the primary care clinician lacks experience in the treatment of major depressive disorder (MDD) [9].

Evaluation of Treatment Response

Definitions of treatment response are presented in Table 26.1. Measurement of treatment response has

recently been increasingly debated in child psychiatry. It is important to try to integrate information from multiple informants [11]. Depending on clinician time and preference, standardized instruments can be used.

The K-SADS [12], for example, is a semi-structured interview, whilst the DAWBA [13] is a structured interview schedule that is also available in electronic form; however, these are typically used for diagnostic purposes and rarely as follow-up measures.

The patient's perspective is increasingly recognized and measures such as the Mood and Feelings Questionnaire or the QIDS can be used to ascertain a number of symptoms and severity of depression. Such measures can also be collected from the parents.

The Children's Depression Rating Scale (CDRS) [14] is a clinician-rated instrument that captures depression severity and is used in anti-depressant trials. Standardized clinical instruments such as the clinician-administered CDRS [14] and the patient-completed Mood and Feelings Questionnaire (MFQ) include both child/adolescent forms and parent forms [15]. Although the CDRS has been the gold standard instrument in pediatric MDD trials, the short version of the

Table 26.1 Definitions of treatment response

Remission	No or minimal symptoms of depression after treatment
Response	>50% Improvement in depression symptoms
Partial response	25–49% Improvement in depression symptoms
No response	<25% Improvement in depression symptoms
Relapse	Worsening of depressive symptoms during remission
Recurrence	The emergence of a new episode after recovery

Source: Dwyer et al., 2020 [10]

MFQ is a brief, easy-to-complete, standardized scale filled in by the patients and their parents. Evidence in adults suggest that the use of standardized scales may improve treatment outcome; however, there is no available evidence for the pediatric population.

Functional outcomes are also important indexes of treatment response. Psychosocial and academic functioning, like teachers' reports on school performance and environmental conditions, should be reviewed frequently [8,14].

First-Line Treatment: Depression

Cognitive Behavioral Therapy (CBT)

Both the National Institute for Health and Care Excellence (NICE) and the American Academy of Child and Adolescent Psychiatry (AACAP) recommend that psychotherapy be offered as a component of treatment for childhood and adolescent depression and should be the first line for mild depression [8,16]. Note that currently there are no available randomized controlled trials (RCTs) supporting the superiority of psychotherapy as first line over pharmacotherapy. There are several forms of psychotherapies, but evidence from meta-analyses suggests that cognitive behavioral therapy (CBT) as well as interpersonal therapy (IPT) appeared to be more effective in comparison with other psychological interventions [17,18]. For moderate to severe cases, a combination of CBT with pharmacotherapy is the method of choice. Even though CBT has an established role in treatment of pediatric depression, a recent RCT found no additional benefit of CBT added to medication (selective serotonin reuptake inhibitors [SSRIs]) and active clinical care [19]. Moreover, meta-analytic evidence suggests that the overall effect size of psychotherapy for depression is poor and estimated to be around $p = 0.3$ [20]. Given the emerging evidence regarding the significance of combination treatment, the NICE Surveillance Group comments that combining CBT and antidepressant medication may not be as beneficial as previously thought [16].

Pharmacotherapy

Overall, pharmacotherapy for depression in adolescents is an issue of ongoing debate despite the many RCTs that have been conducted. Many antidepressant trials have failed to demonstrate a separation from placebo or shown a relatively small one. This state of affairs has been attributed to various factors including an inherently lower response propensity of youth to antidepressants. Overall, there is a high placebo response rate in youth (around 50% in many trials), which itself has been interpreted as the result of various factors, including the recruitment of not-so-ill and therefore spontaneously remitting patients, the problems associated with multisite studies [21], and the differences between National Institutes of Health–funded and industry-sponsored studies [22].

It should also be noted that particularly in youth, there are high rates of spontaneous remission [23], and that, according to some studies, up to 50% of those experiencing one depressive episode may not experience another one.

Table 26.2 presents the recommended SSRI doses in pediatric populations.

Table 26.2 Recommended SSRI doses in pediatric populations

	Starting dose (mg/day)	Typical dose range (mg/day)	Level of evidence in MDD	US Food and Drug Administration indications
Citalopram	10–20	20–40	C	–
Escitalopram	5–10	10–40	A	MDD
Fluoxetine	10–20	20–80	A	MDD, OCD
Fluvoxamine	25–50	50–300	C	OCD
Paroxetine	10–20	20–60	C	–
Sertraline	25–50	100–200	A	OCD

Abbreviations: MDD: major depressive disorder; OCD: obsessive-compulsive disorder.

Fluoxetine

Fluoxetine is the only medication approved by the US Food and Drug Administration (FDA) for treatment of depression in children of 8 years old and above. Fluoxetine is the most studied drug [24] and the one that in trials shows a higher drug response than placebo [8,24]. But is this a true pharmacological difference? One possible explanation may lie in the fact that fluoxetine has a longer half-life than other SSRIs. Specifically, the half-life of fluoxetine is estimated to be 1–4 days and 7–15 days for its metabolite, which makes it also favorable regarding withdrawal [10] concerns [25,26]. Also, someone should take into consideration the design and the higher standards of the fluoxetine studies.

Contra-indications: fluoxetine should not be used in patients with long-QT syndrome.

Other SSRIs

Escitalopram is approved by the FDA for children older than 12 years. Two large RCTs demonstrated the efficacy of escitalopram in treatment of depression in adolescents but not in children [27]. A meta-analysis of the two studies didn't emerge as significant, but showed there was a trend for greater response or remission with escitalopram than placebo [28].

Sertraline or citalopram may be used as an alternative SSRI when there is no response to fluoxetine [16]. Pooled analysis of two RCTs demonstrated that sertraline was superior to placebo in depressed children and adolescents [29]. Because citalopram is associated with long-QT syndrome in children, which is dose dependent, the FDA recommends that the maximum dose should not exceed 40 mg per day. Also, it should be used with caution in patients with hepatic impairment. Paroxetine is not effective in the treatment of depression in children and adolescents with a meta-analysis of four RCTs showing no difference between medication and placebo [30].

Alternative Pharmacological Agents

Venlafaxine

Few RCTs have examined the efficacy of serotonin and norepinephrine reuptake inhibitors (SNRIs) in depressed children and adolescents but have shown no differences between medication and placebo. Venlafaxine trials have demonstrated an age effect being superior to placebo in adolescents but not in children [31]. However, venlafaxine is associated with cardiovascular side effects. Also, a meta-analysis found an increased risk of suicidality in pediatric patients treated with venlafaxine [24].

Tricyclic Antidepressants (TCAs)

Tricyclic antidepressants (TCAs) are not recommended for treatment in children and adolescents [16] and have an unfavorable side effect profile [32]. In addition, different meta-analyses demonstrated that the effect of TCAs for treatment of depression in children and adolescents is marginal and limited in adolescents [32,33].

Is Medication Treatment Effective?

The average SSRI response rate in children and adolescents is 59% and the average placebo response rate is 46%. The number needed to treat (NNT) ranges from 3 to 10, which means that you have to treat 3 to 10 people with the drug in order to prevent one additional bad outcome and the number needed to harm (NNH) from 112 to 200, which means that for every 112 to 200 patients given antidepressant medication, one experienced adverse effects. It is now generally accepted the overall risk:benefit profile favors the use of antidepressants for the treatment of MDD in the pediatric population [34]. Also, children and adolescents with MDD appear with higher placebo response rates than other mental disorders, like anxiety disorders [35]. Several factors may contribute to this phenomenon. First, we must take into consideration that the placebo response includes the placebo effect, the effect of the standard of care (depressed patients may be more susceptible) and the ratio of the patients who are experiencing spontaneous remission in the placebo arm [36]. Secondly, most of the industrial pediatric antidepressant trials have excluded severely ill patients, which might have resulted in greater drug–placebo difference [37], and their increased number of sites have been associated with higher placebo response rates. In contrast, studies funded by the National Institute of Mental Health (NIMH) are characterized by methodological strengths and present with lower placebo rates and greater antidepressant efficacy [22].

Adverse Effects of SSRIs in Children and Adolescents

Acute

True estimation of the rate of side effects remains challenging. Usually most of the SSRI side effects present early in treatment or worsen with dose increase [38] and tend to subside over 1 to 2 weeks or with dose reduction [8]. Most common side effects include nausea, headaches, gastrointestinal (GI) distress, sleep disturbances (insomnia, sedation, nightmares, and vivid dreams), akathisia, diaphoresis, and sexual side effects.

In children and adolescents, a behavioral activation syndrome has been observed that presents with hyperactivity, impulsivity, insomnia, and disinhibition. It is more common in younger children, usually manifests early in treatment (first 2–3 weeks) [39], and it should be differentiated from manic symptoms.

Serotonin Syndrome

Very rarely, SSRIs have been associated with serotonin syndrome; however, the risk is very low when they are used as a monotherapy and increases when they are combined with other serotoninergic agents, for example, migraine treatment (triptans), other antidepressants, cough suppressant (dextromethorphan) and pain medication (tramadol) [40]. Also, serotonin syndrome has been observed in adolescents using 3,4-methylenedioxy methamphetamine (MDMA), or "Ecstasy" [41].

Long-Term Side Effects

Additionally, another possible side effect of SSRIs in children and adolescents is reduction in projected growth [42]. However, there is limited evidence to further support this association.

Suicidality in SSRIs

Suicidality in adolescents treated with SSRIs is the subject of a long debate. The FDA has a "black box" warning for young people treated with SSRIs regarding increased suicidality. This decision was strongly based on a meta-analytic report of industry-sponsored antidepressant pediatric trials [43]. A debate ensued in the aftermath of the report [44] with some authorities arguing that the black box warning may pose a greater risk for suicidal behavior in adolescents. Since the warning, a decline in SSRI prescriptions has been linked with an increase in suicides in adolescents [45]. Note also that no suicides have been reported during any antidepressant trial [37] and a meta-analysis found no statistically significant risk difference in reported suicide ideation between treatment and placebo arm [34]. Furthermore, an epidemiological study supports an inverse relationship between rates of SSRI prescriptions and rates of suicide in the adolescent population [46].

Risk of Bipolar Disorder

As already discussed, behavioral activation and agitation that may present after prescription of SSRIs should be differentiated from symptoms of hypomania or mania. In fact, manifestation of mania after initiation of SSRIs is now thought to be a relatively rare event [47].

Significance of Early Treatment

In order to complete an adequate trial, treatment of 8 weeks at a therapeutic dose or above is recommended. No signs of response by the end of this interval indicate the need of an alternative treatment. It's worth mentioning that recent data suggest that most of the patients respond to treatment the first 2 weeks, with some patients showing significant improvement even from the first week [48,49]. Moreover, this early response may be predictive of overall response [50] and reflect changes in cognitive processing observed in experimental studies described by Harmer's group in Oxford [51]. It is reasonable, though, for patients with severe depression symptoms or persistent suicidality who have no signs of response by 6 weeks to switch to another agent sooner [52]. For children with no adequate symptom relief after 4 weeks, current guidelines suggest increasing the dose to the maximum tolerated recommended dose [8]. There is no evidence in children of efficacy of SSRIs at a subtherapeutic level, neither for acute nor maintenance treatment. Therefore, we cannot consider an adequate trial unless a therapeutic dose is achieved [53].

Treatment-Resistant Depression

Definitions of treatment-resistant and treatment-refractory depression are presented in Table 26.3. It is estimated that one-third of pediatric MDD patients won't respond to treatment. Predictors of poor response include severe or prolonged depression episode, greater functional impairment, substance abuse, hopelessness, increased suicidal ideation, family conflict, and anhedonia [54,55]. Also, evidence from the TORDIA study suggests that the presence of subsyndromal manic symptoms may negatively predict treatment response [56].

Table 26.3 Definitions of treatment-resistant and treatment-refractory depression

Treatment-resistant depression	Clinically impairing depression symptoms despite an adequate trial of an evidence-based psychotherapy and an antidepressant with Grade A evidence for treating depression in pediatric population (fluoxetine, escitalopram, sertraline)
Treatment-refractory depression	Clinically impairing depression symptoms despite an adequate trial of an evidence-based psychotherapy and at least 2 antidepressants with Grade A evidence for treating depression in pediatric population (fluoxetine, escitalopram, sertraline)

Source: Dwyer et al., 2020 [10]

TORDIA

Evidence from the TORDIA study suggest that adolescents with SSRI-resistant MDD improve when they switch to another SSRI or venlafaxine.

The response rate is equally higher in both cases when it is combined with CBT. However, venlafaxine carries a greater side effect burden in contrast with SSRIs. Besides the TORDIA study there is limited evidence of children and adolescents' treatment-refractory management and decisions are based largely in adult literature. To create an evidence-based clinical strategy, Dwyer et al. have recommended a 10-stage treatment-resistant definition table with its respective management (see Table 26.4). This table has been extracted from the combination of the limited pediatric and adult literature and can serve as a clinical guidance for pediatric treatment-resistant depression [10].

Ketamine

There is now one available published RCT of small sample size conducted in a cross-over design that examines the efficacy and safety of ketamine in children and adolescents and it shows ketamine to be superior to the benzodiazepine that was used as a control with an effect size of 0.75 [57]. In adults, multiple RCTs signified efficacy of ketamine. Currently only esketamine is FDA approved for treatment-refractory depression in adults [58,59].

Electroconvulsive Therapy (ECT)

Currently there are no RCTs of electroconvulsive therapy (ECT) in the pediatric population and conclusions about safety and efficacy can be extracted only from adult studies. Thus, ECT is considered for treatment only in children above 12 years and when they meet certain criteria. These criteria include the following:

- There is failure to respond to at least two adequate trials of appropriate psychopharmacological agents accompanied by at least one psychotherapy trial.

- The symptomatology is severe, persistent, significantly disabling, or life threatening.
- ECT can be considered earlier when the patient is unable to tolerate pharmacological treatment or for patients who are severely incapacitated and cannot take medication [8,60].

Treatment of Comorbidities

Addressing comorbid disorders is essential, as they may negatively influence the progression of depression, increase the risk of suicide and the functional impairment of the patient [8]. The disorder that causes the greatest distress or impairment should be treated initially. Also, some comorbidities, such as anxiety disorders, respond to the same pharmacological treatment as depression and CBT.

Additionally, depression increases the risk for substance abuse disorder (SUD), and the existence of comorbid SUD negatively affects the prognosis of depression [61]. The same applies to eating disorders and is important that clinicians screen for these disorders [62].

Treatment Duration

In order to avoid depression relapse, treatment should be continued for at least 6–12 months [8]. After an asymptomatic period of 6–12 months, it should be decided whether the patient should be under maintenance treatment or discontinue treatment [8]. Generally, duration of maintenance phase may last 1 year or longer and is recommended for patients with history of recurrent, severe, or prolonged depressive episodes, suicidal behavior, and other negative environmental factors (e.g., family disruption or psychopathology, lack of community support) [8]. When cessation of pharmacological treatment is decided in order to minimize the possibility of discontinuation syndrome, antidepressants should be tapered. A gradual decrease of 25–50% per week is recommended.

Table 26.4 10 stages of treatment resistance in pediatric depression

Stage	Definition (substantial residual symptoms of depression despite . . .)	Treatment modalities				
		Therapy	SSRI	Alternative antidepressants	Augmentation	Interventional techniques
0	No previous treatment for depression					
1	Previous counseling for depression of unclear modality or efficacy	?				
2	Previous evidence-based therapy for depression	Y				
3	A single pharmacological trial of FDA-approved antidepressant for depression (fluoxetine, escitalopram, sertraline) of adequate duration and at the **minimally** recommended dose	Y*	?			
4	A single pharmacological trial of FDA-approved antidepressant for depression (fluoxetine, escitalopram, sertraline) of adequate duration and at the **maximally** tolerated dose	Y*	1			
5	Two trials of adequate dose and duration with SSRI medications	Y*	2–2+			
6	At least two trials of adequate dose and duration with SSRI medications + at least one trial with an alternative antidepressant (SNRI, bupropion or mirtazapine) or evidence-based	Y*	2–2+	1		

Table 26.4 (cont.)

Stage	Definition (substantial residual symptoms of depression despite . . .)	Treatment modalities				
		Therapy	SSRI	Alternative antidepressants	Augmentation	Interventional techniques
	augmentation strategy in adults (antipsychotics, lithium, bupropion, mirtazapine, stimulant medications)					
7	At least two trials of adequate dose and duration with SSRI medications + at least two trials with an alternative antidepressant agents or augmentation strategies with evidence of efficacy in adults	Y*	2–2+	2		
8	At least two trials of adequate dose and duration with SSRI medications + at least one trial with an alternative antidepressant agent (SNRI, bupropion or mirtazapine) AND at least two augmentation strategies with evidence of efficacy in adults	Y*	2–2+	1	2	
9	At least two trials of adequate dose and duration with SSRI medications + at least two trials with an alternative antidepressant agent or augmentation strategies with evidence of efficacy in adults + a somatic treatment (repetitive transcranial magnetic stimulation [rTMS] or ketamine)	Y*	2–2+	1	2	Repetitive transcranial magnetic stimulation (rTMS) or ketamine**

Table 26.4 (cont.)

Stage	Definition (substantial residual symptoms of depression despite . . .)	Treatment modalities				
		Therapy	SSRI	Alternative antidepressants	Augmentation	Interventional techniques
10	At least two trials of adequate dose and duration with SSRI medications + at least two trials with an alternative antidepressant agents or augmentation strategies with evidence of efficacy in adults + electroconvulsive therapy (ECT)	Y*	2–2 +	1	2	ECT**

Y*= Multiple different types of evidence-based psychotherapy should be trialed in parallel with pharmacological treatments and should be specified along with stage of pharmacological treatment resistance.

**= As per current treatment guidelines, interventional techniques may be considered starting around stage 7 of treatment resistance or potentially in exceptional cases such as ECT in psychotic depression not responsive to antipsychotic augmentation or ECT/ketamine in severely suicidal patients who have past stage 4 or 5 of treatment resistance [10].

References

1. Murray CJL. Disability-adjusted life years (DALYs) for 291 diseases and injuries in 21 regions, 1990-2010: a systematic analysis for the Global Burden of Disease Study 2010. *Lancet.* 2012 December;**380**(9859):2197–223.

2. Costello EJ. Prevalence and development of psychiatric disorders in childhood and adolescence. *Arch Gen Psychiatry.* 2003;**60**(8):837–44.

3. Thapar A. Depression in adolescence. *Lancet.* 2012 March;**379**(9820):1056–67.

4. Maughan B, Collishaw S, Stringaris A. Depression in childhood and adolescence. *J Can Acad Child Adolesc Psychiatry.* 2013 February;**22**(1):35–40.

5. Brent DA. Major depressive disorder. *New Dir Ment Health Serv.* 1992 Summer;(54):39–44.

6. CDC WONDER. About underlying cause of death, 1999–2020. [cited 2021 May 19]. Available from: http://wonder.cdc.gov/ucd-icd10.html.

7. Goodyer IM, Wilkinson PO. Therapeutics of unipolar major depressions in adolescents. *J Child Psychol Psychiatry.* 2019;**60**(3):232–43.

8. Birmaher B, Brent D; AACAP Work Group on Quality Issues, et al. Practice parameter for the assessment and treatment of children and adolescents with depressive disorders. *J Am Acad Child Adolesc Psychiatry.* 2007;**46**(11):1503–26.

9. Cheung AH, Zuckerbrot RA, Jensen PS, et al.; GLAD-PC STEERING GROUP. Guidelines for Adolescent Depression in Primary Care (GLAD-PC): part II. Treatment and ongoing management. *Pediatrics.* 2018;**141**(3):e20174082

10. Dwyer JB, Stringaris A, Brent DA, Bloch MH. Annual research review: defining and treating pediatric treatment-resistant depression. *J Child Psychol Psychiatry.* 2020 March;**61**(3):312–32.

11. Reyes ADL, Augenstein TM, Wang M, et al. The validity of the multi-informant approach to assessing child and adolescent mental health. *Psychol Bull.* 2015 July;**141**(4):858–900.

12. Kaufman J, Birmaher B, Brent D, et al. Schedule for Affective Disorders and Schizophrenia for School-Age Children-Present and Lifetime Version (K-SADS-PL): initial reliability and validity data. *J Am Acad Child Adolesc Psychiatry.* 1997 July;**36**(7):980–8.

13. Goodman R, Ford T, Richards H, Gatward R, Meltzer H. The Development and Well-Being Assessment: description and initial validation of an integrated assessment of child and adolescent

psychopathology. *J Child Psychol Psychiatry*. 2000 July;**41**(5):645–55.

14. Poznanski EO, Grossman JA, Buchsbaum Y, et al. Preliminary studies of the reliability and validity of the Children's Depression Rating Scale. *J Am Acad Child Psychiatry*. 1984;**23**(2):191–7.

15. Daviss WB, Birmaher B, Melham NA, et al. Criterion validity of the Mood and Feelings Questionnaire for depressive episodes in clinic and non-clinic subjects. *J Child Psychol Psychiatry*. 2006;**47**(9):927–34.

16. National Institute for Health and Clinical Excellence (NICE). Depression in children and young people: NICE guideline. London, 2005. [Cited 2007 August 14.]

17. Eckshtain D, Kuppens S, Ugueto A, et al. Meta-analysis: 13-year follow-up of psychotherapy effects on youth depression. *J Am Acad Child Adolesc Psychiatry*. 2020;**59**(1):45–63.

18. Zhou X, Hetrick SE, Cuijpers P, et al. Comparative efficacy and acceptability of psychotherapies for depression in children and adolescents: a systematic review and network meta-analysis. *World Psychiatry*. 2015;**14**(2):207–22.

19. Goodyer IM, Dubicka B, Wilkinson P, et al. A randomised controlled trial of cognitive behaviour therapy in adolescents with major depression treated by selective serotonin reuptake inhibitors. The ADAPT trial. *Health Technol Assess*. 2008;**12**(14):iii–iv; ix–60.

20. Weisz J, Southern-Gerow MA, Gordis EB, et al. Cognitive-behavioral therapy versus usual clinical care for youth depression: an initial test of transportability to community clinics and clinicians. *J Consult Clin Psychol*. 2009;**77**(3):383–96.

21. Bridge JA, Birmaher B, Iyengar S, et al. Placebo response in randomized controlled trials of antidepressants for pediatric major depressive disorder. *Am J Psychiatry*. 2009 January;**166**(1):42–9.

22. Walkup JT. Antidepressant efficacy for depression in children and adolescents: industry- and NIMH-funded studies. *Am J Psychiatry*. 2017;**174**: 430–7.

23. Whiteford HA, Harris MG, McKeon G, et al. Estimating remission from untreated major depression: a systematic review and meta-analysis. *Psychol Med*. 2010 August;**43**(8):1569–85.

24. Cipriani A, Zhou X, Del Giovana C, et al. Comparative efficacy and tolerability of antidepressants for major depressive disorder in children and adolescents: a network meta-analysis. *Lancet*. 2016;**388**(10047):881–90.

25. Wilens TE, Cohen L, Biederman J, et al. Fluoxetine pharmacokinetics in pediatric patients. *J Clin Psychopharmacol*. 2002;**22**(6):568–75.

26. Findling RL, McNamara NK, Stansbrey RJ, et al. The relevance of pharmacokinetic studies in designing efficacy trials in juvenile major depression. *J Child Adolesc Psychopharmacol*. 2006;**16**:131–45.

27. Emslie GJ, Ventura D, Korotzer A, Turkodimitris S. Escitalopram in the treatment of adolescent depression: a randomized placebo-controlled multisite trial. *J Am Acad Child Adolesc Psychiatry*. 2009;**48**(7):721–9.

28. Hetrick SE, McKenzie JE, Cox GR, et al. Newer generation antidepressants for depressive disorders in children and adolescents. *Cochrane Database Syst Rev*. 2012 Nov 14;**11**(11):CD004851.

29. Wagner KD, Ambrosini P, Rynn M, et al. Efficacy of sertraline in the treatment of children and adolescents with major depressive disorder: two randomized controlled trials. *JAMA*. 2003;**290**(8):1033–41.

30. Hetrick SE, McKenzie JE, Bailey AP, et al. Newer generation antidepressants for depressive disorders in children and adolescents: a network meta-analysis. *Cochrane Database Syst Rev*. 2021;**2021**(5): CD013674.

31. Emslie GJ. Venlafaxine ER for the treatment of pediatric subjects with depression: results of two placebo-controlled trials. *J Am Acad Child Adolesc Psychiatry*. 2007;**46**:479–88.

32. Hazell P, Mirzaie, M. Tricyclic drugs for depression in children and adolescents. *Cochrane Database Syst Rev*. 2013; June18;**2013**(6):CD002317.

33. Tsapakis EM, Soldani F, Tondo L, Baldessanni RJ. Efficacy of antidepressants in juvenile depression: meta-analysis. *Br J Psychiatry*. 2008 July;**193**(1): 10–17.

34. Bridge JA, Iyengar S, Salary CB, et al. Clinical response and risk for reported suicidal ideation and suicide attempts in pediatric antidepressant treatment: a meta-analysis of randomized controlled trials. *JAMA*. 2007;**297**:1683–96.

35. Cohen D, Deniau E, Maturana A, et al. Are child and adolescent responses to placebo higher in major depression than in anxiety disorders? A systematic review of placebo-controlled trials. *PLoS One*. 2008; 3(7):e2632.

36. Cohen D, Consoli A, Bodeau N, et al. Predictors of placebo response in randomized controlled trials of psychotropic drugs for children and adolescents with internalizing disorders. *J Child Adolesc Psychopharmacol*. 2010;**20**:39–47.

37. Wilkinson P, Kelvin R, Roberts C, et al. Clinical and psychosocial predictors of suicide attempts and nonsuicidal self-injury in the Adolescent Depression Antidepressants and Psychotherapy Trial (ADAPT). *Am J Psychiatry*. 2011 May;**168**(5):495–501.

38. Walkup J, Labellarte M. Complications of SSRI treatment. *J Child Adolesc Psychopharmacol*. 2001; **11**: 1–4.

39. Safer DJ, Magno Zito J. Treatment-emergent adverse events from selective serotonin reuptake inhibitors by age group: children versus adolescents. *J Child Adolesc Psychopharmacol*. 2006;**16**:159–69.

40. Dwyer JB, Bloch MH. Antidepressants for pediatric patients. *Curr Psychiatr*. 2019;**18**:26–42 F.

41. Dobry Y, Rice T, Sher L. Ecstasy use and serotonin syndrome: a neglected danger to adolescents and young adults prescribed selective serotonin reuptake inhibitors. *Int J Adolesc Med Health*. 2013;**25**:193–9.

42. Nilsson M, Joliat MJ, Miner CM, et al. Safety of subchronic treatment with fluoxetine for major depressive disorder in children and adolescents. *J Child Adolesc Psychopharmacol*. 2004;**14**:412–17.

43. Hammad TA, Laughren T, Racoosin J. Suicidality in pediatric patients treated with antidepressant drugs. *Arch Gen Psychiatry*. 2006;**63**:332–9.

44. Fornaro M, Anastasia A, Valchera A, et al. The FDA "black box" warning on antidepressant suicide risk in young adults: more harm than benefits? *Front Psychiatry*. 2019;**10**:294.

45. Garland EJ, Kutcher S, Virani A, et al. Update on the use of SSRIs and SNRIs with children and adolescents in clinical practice. *J Can Acad Child Adolesc Psychiatry*. 2016;**25**:4–10.

46. Olfson M, Shafer D, Marcus SC, Greenbergt T. Relationship between antidepressant medication treatment and suicide in adolescents. *Arch Gen Psychiatry*. 2003;**60**:978–82.

47. Baldessarini RJ, Faedda GL, Offidani E, et al. Antidepressant-associated mood-switching and transition from unipolar major depression to bipolar disorder: a review. *J Affect Disord*. 2013;**148**:129–35.

48. Nierenberg AA, Farabaugh AH, Alpert JE, et al. Timing of onset of antidepressant response with fluoxetine treatment. *Am J Psychiatry*. 2000 September;**157**(9):1423–8.

49. Taylor MJ, Freemantle N, Geddes JR, Bhagwagar Z. Early onset of selective serotonin reuptake inhibitor antidepressant action: systematic review and meta-analysis. *Arch Gen Psychiatry*. 2006 November; **63** (11):1217–23.

50. Varigonda AL, Jakobovski E, Taylor MJ, et al. Systematic review and meta-analysis: early treatment responses of selective serotonin reuptake inhibitors in pediatric major depressive disorder. *J Am Acad Child Adolesc Psychiatry*. 2015;**54**:557–64.

51. Murphy SE, Capitão LP, Giles SLC, et al. The knowns and unknowns of SSRI treatment in young people with depression and anxiety: efficacy, predictors, and mechanisms of action. *Lancet Psychiatry*. 2021 September;**8**(9):824–35.

52. Dwyer JB, Stringaris A, Brent DA, Bloch MH. Annual research review: defining and treating pediatric treatment-resistant depression. *J Child Psychol Psychiatry*. 2020 Mar;**61**(3):312–32.

53. Jakubovski E, Varigonda Al, Freemantle N, et al. Systematic review and meta-analysis: dose-response relationship of selective serotonin reuptake inhibitors in major depressive disorder. *Am J Psychiatry*. 2016; **173**:174–83.

54. McMakin DL, Olino TM, Porta G., et al. Anhedonia predicts poorer recovery among youth with selective serotonin reuptake inhibitor treatment-resistant depression. *J Am Acad Child Adolesc Psychiatry*. 2012; **51**:404–11.

55. Vitiello B, Emslie G, Clarke G, et al. Long-term outcome of adolescent depression initially resistant to selective serotonin reuptake inhibitor treatment: a follow-up study of the TORDIA sample. *J Clin Psychiatry*. 2011;**72**(3):388–96.

56. Maalouf FT, Porta G, Vitiello B, et al. Do sub-syndromal manic symptoms influence outcome in treatment resistant depression in adolescents? A latent class analysis from the TORDIA study. *J Affect Disord*. 2012;**138**:86–95.

57. Dwyer JB, Landeros-Weisenberger A, Johnson JA, et al. Efficacy of intravenous ketamine in adolescent treatment-resistant depression: a randomized midazolam-controlled trial. *Am J Psychiatry*. 2021 April 1;**178**(4):x.

58. Sanacora G, Frye MA, McDonald W, et al. A consensus statement on the use of ketamine in the treatment of mood disorders. *JAMA Psychiatry*. 2017 April;**74**(4):399–405.

59. Daly EJ, Singh JB, Fedgchin M, et al. Efficacy and safety of intranasal esketamine adjunctive to oral antidepressant therapy in treatment-resistant depression: a randomized clinical trial. *JAMA Psychiatry*. 2018 February;**75**(2):139–48.

60. Ghaziuddin N, Kutcher SP, Knapp P, et al. Practice parameter for use of electroconvulsive therapy with adolescents. *J Am Acad Child Adolesc Psychiatry*. 2004;**43**:1521–39.

61. Carton L, Pignon B, Baguet A, et al. Influence of comorbid alcohol use disorders on the clinical patterns of major depressive disorder: a general population-based study. *Drug Alcohol Depend*. 2018 June;**187**:40–7.

62. Puccio F, Fuller-Tyszkiewicz M, Ong D, Krug I. A systematic review and meta-analysis on the longitudinal relationship between eating pathology and depression. *Int J Eat Disord*. 2016 February;**49**(5): 439–54.

Chapter 27

Considerations about the Treatment of Mood Disorders in Elderly Patients

Lokesh Shahani and Louis A. Faillace

Depressive symptoms affect 8% to 16% of community-dwelling elders and higher numbers in long-term care settings [1]. The Epidemiologic Catchment Area Study, a community-based structured survey, detected major depression in 1.4% to 3.7% of its 5,723 elderly respondents [2]. Depression in older adults can represent chronic, recurrent, or new-onset symptomatology. In many cases, the onset of depression occurs after age 60.

The timing of this chapter cannot be more appropriate. According to the U.S. Census Bureau's 2017 National Population Projections, the year 2030 marks an important demographic turning point in the United States. By 2030, all baby boomers will be older than age 65, which will expand the size of the older population so that 1 in every 5 residents will be retirement age [3]. Considering the growing geriatric population, the appropriate management of geriatric mood disorder is very important.

Assessment

The assessment of a patient includes detailed history from both patient and informant covering aspects such as recent change in mood, medical illness, drug and alcohol use, adverse life events, and available support systems. An examination with special importance on suicidal ideation and plans, delusions, and cognitive impairment is an essential component of the assessment. An issue of particular importance is the assessment of suicidal risk. Any deliberate self-harm in an older person should be taken very seriously, especially in patients with a depressive disorder.

To rule out medical conditions that may simulate or exacerbate depression, the laboratory assessment can include a chemistry profile with liver function tests, blood urea nitrogen, creatinine, thyroid function tests, vitamin B12 and folate levels, complete blood count, clean-catch urinalysis, chest x-ray, electrocardiogram, and neuroimaging study. Because many older adults are on prescribed medications for their medical comorbidities, it is imperative to rule out

depression that is secondary to the use of pharmacological agents. Antihypertensive agents such as reserpine, methyldopa, beta blockers, clonidine, calcium channel blockers, and angiotensin-converting enzyme inhibitors have been associated with inducing depressive symptoms [4]. Systemic corticosteroids such as prednisone have also been associated with depression as well as with mania [4]. Lipid-lowering agents, selective estrogen receptor modulators, nonsteroidal anti-inflammatory drugs, interferon, histamine-2 receptor antagonists, sedative-hypnotics such as benzodiazepines or barbiturates, and opioids have also been associated with mood symptoms [4]. If medication-induced depression is suspected, elimination of these medications from the patient's treatment regimen or their replacement with medications less likely to affect the central nervous system is recommended.

Depression in later life can present with symptoms that differ from those of depression in younger adults. Elderly depressed patients are more likely to report poor appetite and are less likely to endorse crying spells, sadness, feeling fearful, being bothered, or feeling that life is a failure, compared with younger adults. Screening for depressive disorder in older people can be achieved with the Geriatric Depression Scale [5], which has been validated and widely used in elderly subjects. It is quick to administer and exists in several versions (ranging from 4 to 30 items). The severity of a diagnosed case of depression can be assessed with the Montgomery–Asberg Depression Rating Scale (MADRS) [6] or the Hamilton Rating Scale for Depression (HRSD) [7]. Both have been validated in elderly depressed subjects [8] and are useful in assessing response to treatment.

Treatment

The first effective step in successfully treating depression is to break down the barriers that prevent treatment from being provided in the first place. Education about depressive disorder and its treatments is vital in building a trusting and therapeutic relationship with the patient. It may include the following:

- Counseling the patient that depression is a treatable disorder
- Explaining that antidepressants are nonaddictive
- Discussing the importance of compliance
- Explaining that acute treatment in older people may typically last for 6–8 weeks at the minimum, and that medications should be stopped only after discussing with the treatment provider

Pharmacotherapy

The response or remission rates in older adults are similar to those of younger adults. In a large meta-analysis that included 51 randomized clinical trials involving patients 55 years or older, 48% patients achieved a response, very similar to response rates of the 53.8% [9] and 50.1% found in younger adult patients [10]. Antidepressants are beneficial for older patients with depression, but the effects are modest. A meta-regression including 3,690 patients 60 years or older found that with increasing age, antidepressant efficacy decreased [11]. Antidepressants may be less effective in older patients because they have a greater burden of somatic disorders such as cardiovascular diseases and ischemic brain changes (manifested as white matter hyperintensities in magnetic resonance imaging [MRI]) and because their physicians have a tendency to prescribe suboptimal doses of antidepressants.

Pharmacological interventions are safe and effective in treating older adults, especially when the depression is severe and the patient is experiencing more debilitating neurovegetative symptoms such as anhedonia, insomnia, poor concentration, appetite disturbances, or psychomotor retardation or agitation; guilt or delusions; or suicidal ideation. The choice of antidepressant should be guided by clinical factors such as the patient's symptoms, concurrent medical problems, medications currently taken, and antidepressant side effect profile and by the practical issues of medication cost and insurance coverage. Special considerations should be placed on adverse effect profile or drug interactions' and hepatic and renal metabolism of the drug.

Published geriatric guidelines provide guidance to clinicians not only on which antidepressant to use but also on initial dosages, titration, and how long to wait before switching antidepressants [12,13]. Both the 2001 US Expert Consensus Guidelines [12] and the 2006 guidelines from the Canadian Coalition for Seniors' Mental Health [13] recommend the use of selective serotonin reuptake inhibitors (SSRIs) as first-line antidepressant, favoring citalopram and sertraline. However, since the publications of these guidelines, citalopram has been associated with dose-dependent increases in the QTc interval. Based on these findings, the US Food and Drug Administration (FDA) has issued a warning about the potential of citalopram to induce an increase in QTc, with a recommendation to avoid dosages above 20 mg/day in older patients [14]. The FDA did not deem the smaller increase in QTc observed with escitalopram to be clinically significant and did not issue recommendations for escitalopram. While geriatric guidelines recommend low initial dosages and titrations slower than those recommended in younger patients, target doses are similar.

More recently, a section on "special populations" in the updated 2016 guidelines from the Canadian Network for Mood and Anxiety Treatments (CANMAT) include specific recommendations for elderly patient with late-life depression [15]. In this context, the recommended first-line antidepressants comprise duloxetine, mirtazapine, nortriptyline (with "level 1 evidence") and bupropion, citalopram, escitalopram, desvenlafaxine, sertraline, venlafaxine, and vortioxetine (with "level 2 evidence")

The treatment of depression is divided into acute, continuation, and maintenance phases. In general, the dose of antidepressant for an elderly patient is preferably half of that recommended for a younger adult patient because of the pharmacodynamic effects of antidepressants and on pharmacokinetic parameters including drug distribution, metabolism, and elimination. Although an initial partial response may be seen within 1 to 3 weeks, older patients may take up to 6 to 8 weeks to respond to a therapeutic antidepressant dose. Geriatric guidelines recommend switching to another antidepressant after about 4 weeks at a therapeutic or maximum tolerated dose in the absence of meaningful response (i.e., at least 6–8 weeks of treatment).

Current guidelines suggest that in cases of nonresponse, clinicians should switch to another antidepressant within the same class or another class [15]. Augmentation is favored over switching when a partial response is observed with first-line treatment, as there is a risk of worsening (or discontinuation symptoms) upon stopping this first-line antidepressant. In cases of partial response, these guidelines suggest combining the initial SSRI or serotonin-norepinephrine reuptake inhibitor (SNRI) with bupropion or nortriptyline or augmenting it with lithium after up to 8 weeks (i.e., 12 weeks of treatment). This recommendation is supported based on results of several small trials [16]. Recent studies emphasize the use of atypical antipsychotic (aripiprazole and quetiapine) as an augmentation agent in the treatment of nonpsychotic major depressive disorder (MDD) in adults [17].

After the acute response or remission of depression, a continuation treatment phase begins. Monitoring for ongoing effectiveness, side effects, and treatment adherence is recommended for 6 to 12 months, with the objectives of consolidating gains and preventing relapse. Expert guidelines recommend that patients continue the dose of antidepressant that achieved the acute response or remission [12]. After the continuation phase, many patients are advised to enter a maintenance phase of treatment to prevent illness recurrence. Factors such as the number and severity of depressive episodes, response to treatment, concomitant anxiety symptoms, and delayed response to treatment during the first episode may be important considerations when planning maintenance treatment duration. Expert consensus guidelines recommend that treatment extend for 1 or more years after a severe first episode and for 3 or more years after a third or subsequent episode [12].

Psychotherapy

Depression-specific psychotherapy is recommended as an initial treatment choice for patients with mild to moderate depression [18]. Psychotherapy is considered comparable with the effectiveness of antidepressants. Cognitive behavioral therapy is the best-studied psychotherapeutic intervention. A meta-analysis of randomized controlled psychotherapy trials for late-life depression demonstrated that psychotherapy was effective, but the magnitude of the effect varies widely with the type of control group [19]. The influence of physical diseases, frailty, and cognitive impairment on the efficacy or feasibility of psychotherapy has not been assessed. However, especially for these patients, tolerance of antidepressants may be poor, so psychotherapy may be an effective alternative.

Electroconvulsive Therapy

Electroconvulsive therapy (ECT) remains an important treatment of geriatric patients with severe depressive illness and a limited number of other severe psychiatric conditions. Since its introduction, ECT has been one of the most effective treatments for psychiatric illness. Studies have demonstrated that ECT may be more effective in the elderly than in other age groups [20,21]. ECT must be a treatment consideration in the elderly, particularly in instances of medication resistance or intolerance. Despite concerns regarding medical comorbidities in the geriatric population, ECT remains a fairly safe treatment option with few medical contraindications [22]. The evidence base supports ECT's use as an effective treatment in a variety of neuropsychiatric conditions in the elderly, including depression, mania, psychosis, and catatonia.

Despite ECT's efficacy, concerns regarding its side effect burden may reduce its appeal. Many clinicians remain concerned about the cognitive effects of ECT, particularly retrograde amnesia, especially in the geriatric population where neurocognitive dysfunction is common at baseline. Recent studies have examined the relationship of ECT to preexisting memory impairment and demonstrated that ECT may not significantly worsen these difficulties [20].

Studies of ECT in the elderly indicate response rates greater than 63%. Spaans et al. demonstrated geriatric depressed patients receiving ECT achieved remission faster and had a significantly higher remission rate: 63.8%, compared with 33.3% for medication [21]. The Prolonging Remission in Depressed Elderly (PRIDE) study demonstrated similar results, where 62% of patients remitted and 70% responded. Older age positively predicted speed and response to ECT. The PRIDE study confirmed this finding, noting that patients more than 70 years old were 1.89 times more likely to respond than those 60 to 69 years old, and a larger portion of those greater than 70 years old remitted (69.7%) compared with those who were 60 to 69 years old (55.0%) [20].

Geriatric Bipolar Disorder

Bipolar disorder in geriatric patients includes illness of new onset (late-onset bipolar disorder), as well as bipolar disorder that first manifested in earlier life and has persisted. The Epidemiologic Catchment Area Survey reported a 12-month prevalence rate of 0.1% of bipolar disorder among those aged 65 years or older [2]. Similarly, the US National Comorbidity Survey Replication (NCS-R) reported lifetime prevalence rate of 1% among those aged 60 years or older [23]. In contrast to relatively low numbers in the community studies, data from clinical settings suggest that geriatric bipolar disorder is relatively common. Prevalence rates ranging from 4% to 8% in geriatric psychiatry inpatient units [24] and 17% of elders presenting to psychiatric emergency rooms [25] are reported.

Bipolar disorder has been associated with significant morbidity, high rates of mortality, and considerable use of mental health services [26]. Late-onset mania is described as a syndrome with multiple causes, including drugs (steroids) and metabolic, infectious, and structural cerebrovascular diseases such as stroke and tumor [27]. Late-onset mania warrants complete investigation for underlying cerebral pathology.

Treatment

Given the complex nature of geriatric bipolar disorder, comorbidity, and behavioral disturbances, inpatient intervention may be required for stabilization, safety, and medical and psychiatric diagnostic workup. As with all patients with bipolar disorder, treatment may differ depending on illness polarity, symptom severity, and phase (acute vs. stabilization vs. maintenance treatment).

Treatment of Acute Mania

The GERI-BD randomized controlled trial of lithium versus valproate for acute treatment of bipolar mania/hypomania in adults aged 60 years and older demonstrated that both lithium and divalproex were adequately tolerated and efficacious; however, lithium was associated with a greater reduction in mania scores over 9 weeks [28]. Lithium is less prescribed in the elderly because of concerns regarding tolerability and multiple medical comorbidities. However, lithium may be the preferred choice for older adults with classic mania and minimal neurological impairment [29]. It is suggested that geriatric bipolar disorder patients may respond to lower lithium levels compared with younger adults [28]. In the elderly, side effects of lithium include cognitive impairment, ataxia or gait abnormalities, tremor, urinary frequency or renal deterioration, hypothyroidism, weight gain, rash or cutaneous abnormalities, worsening of arthritis, and peripheral edema. Older adults are more prone to acute lithium toxicity because of reduced renal clearance, vulnerability to medical comorbidity (especially cardiovascular abnormalities), and drug–drug interactions with angiotensin-converting enzyme inhibitors, calcium antagonists,

thiazide and loop diuretics, and non-steroidal anti-inflammatory drugs [30].

Valproate has been suggested to be effective in geriatric bipolar disorder. Valproate may also be associated with more risk in the elderly than in younger patients. The free serum valproate level should be checked in addition to total levels in geriatric patients, especially in patients being co-administered aspirin, warfarin, digoxin, and phenytoin, wherein protein displacement can occur. Pancreatitis and fatal hepatotoxicity are rare side effects associated with valproate [30].

All the second-generation antipsychotics except for clozapine are FDA approved for acute bipolar mania. In a secondary data analysis of patients aged 50 years or older, patients treated with olanzapine demonstrated an improvement in manic symptoms when compared with patients treated with divalproex [31]. Quetiapine is a potentially useful treatment option among older adults with bipolar I mania, compared with younger adults, as suggested by a recent post hoc analysis of two quetiapine monotherapy clinical trials comparing those aged 55 years or greater with younger adults [32]. This study demonstrated that both older and younger patients treated with quetiapine had significant improvement from baseline on mania scores compared with placebo-treated patients. Side effects of particular concern with antipsychotic treatment in the elderly include weight gain, metabolic abnormalities, sedation, extrapyramidal symptoms, fall risk, and neuroleptic malignant syndrome.

A particular concern in geriatric patients is the potentially increased mortality associated with antipsychotic medications. The FDA has placed a black box warning on all atypical and typical agents warning of the significant increased risk of death in elderly patients with dementia [33]. The FDA has reported a warning of a 1.6- to 1.7-fold increase in mortality from all causes for older adult patients with dementia-related psychosis [33]. The warning was based on the FDA's review of 17 placebo-controlled trials of olanzapine, aripiprazole, risperidone, or quetiapine to treat dementia-related behavioral problems. Among these patients, specific causes of death included cardiac disorders (25%), cerebrovascular disease (8%), pulmonary disease (8%), cancer (7%), and diabetes (3%) [34]. Although the atypical antipsychotic drugs are an extremely useful and important part of treatment in younger patients with bipolar disorder, and are considered the first-line treatment, their role in treatment for elders with bipolar disorder needs further study.

Treatment of Bipolar Depression

Lithium, the anticonvulsant lamotrigine, and selected atypical antipsychotics, including quetiapine and olanzapine/fluoxetine combination, have demonstrated efficacy in treatment of bipolar depression.

An open-label trial of add-on lamotrigine to current maintenance mood-stabilizing medication in elderly adults with bipolar depression demonstrated significant improvement in depression symptoms and improvement in functional status [35]. A recent meta-analysis of placebo-controlled trials in bipolar depression suggested that quetiapine and olanzapine are effective and rapidly acting as both adjunct therapies and monotherapy in bipolar depression [36]. Among patients treated with atypical antipsychotics, older age is significantly associated with metabolic syndrome and patients with metabolic syndrome have a doubled 10-year coronary heart disease risk [37].

A post hoc analysis combined results from two double-blind, randomized, placebo-controlled studies of quetiapine in bipolar depression. The analysis demonstrated improvement in depression scores as compared to placebo, with effect size and discontinuation rates similar in older adults as compared to younger adults [38]. The most common reasons for discontinuation were adverse events in groups treated with quetiapine (most frequently sedation, somnolence, and dizziness) and lack of efficacy in groups treated with placebo, with no age-related differences.

The role of antidepressant drugs as part of the bipolar treatment is controversial. However, the overall risk may be relatively low in geriatric bipolar disorder patients. Schaffer and colleagues conducted a population-based retrospective cohort design study that used the administrative databases for all individuals aged 66 years and older in a Canadian healthcare network. Bipolar disorder patients who received a prescription for an antidepressant medication were compared with a control group of randomly selected subjects from the eligible bipolar disorder population who did not receive a prescription for an antidepressant medication during the same surveillance period. During total 5,135 person-years of follow-up, antidepressant use among elderly bipolar disorder patients was associated with decreased rates of hospitalization for manic/mixed episodes [39].

Maintenance Drug Treatment of Bipolar Disorder

Data from the National Institute of Mental Health-funded Systematic Treatment Enhancement Program for Bipolar Disorder (STEP-BD) study on prescription patterns and recovery status, in younger subjects aged 20 to 59 years and older subjects aged 60 years and older, showed that 78.5% of older patients versus 66.8% of younger patients achieved a recovered status. Those who achieved a recovered status took an average of 2.05 medications, with no difference between the age groups. The older group had 29.5% of patients on lithium versus 37.8% of younger patients. Lithium dosing was lower among individuals aged 50 years and older, but 42.1% of recovered bipolar disorder elders achieved recovery with lithium alone compared with only 21.3% of the younger group [40].

Lamotrigine received FDA approval for the maintenance treatment of bipolar disorder based on results of placebo-controlled 18-month trial [41,42]. A secondary analysis of bipolar disorder in adults aged 55 years and older suggested that overall, lamotrigine was more effective in delaying bipolar depressive relapse and lithium was more effective in delaying mania [43]. In a recent retrospective analysis of older adults with unipolar depression and bipolar disorder, which compared each patient to their own clinical course before and after lithium treatment, the probability of relapse and recurrence, suicidal behavior, and severity of mood disturbance was significantly decreased by lithium maintenance [44].

Various atypical antipsychotics have received FDA approval for the maintenance treatment of bipolar disease. However, their efficacy and tolerability in older adults has not been established. A large randomized open-label study compared lithium and valproate monotherapies and combination treatment (BALANCE trial) for maintenance of bipolar disorder [45]. Combination treatment or lithium monotherapy seemed superior to treatment with valproate alone in prevention of relapse over a 2-year study period. Older and younger subgroups did not seem to differ with respect to treatment response to monotherapy versus combination therapy.

Conclusion

Mood disorders in the elderly are a growing source of morbidity and mortality. Unfortunately, mood disorders in later life are often not appropriately diagnosed and treated. Appropriate, prompt diagnosis and treatment of late life mood disorders can significantly improve the quality of life of patients and families and may prove life changing. Current treatments can help older adults with mood disorders.

References

1. Kyomen HH, Gottlieb GL. Financial issues in the delivery of geriatric psychiatric care. In BJ Sadock, VA Sadock, P Ruiz, editors. *Comprehensive Textbook of Psychiatry IX*. Philadelphia: Lippincott Williams and Wilkins, 2009; 4185–93.

2. Weissman MM, Bruce ML, Leaf PJ, et al. Affective disorders. In LN Robins, DA Regier, editors. *Psychiatric Disorders in America: The Epidemiologic Catchment Study*. New York: Free Press, 1991; 53–80.

3. U.S. Census Bureau. Older people projected to outnumber children for first time in U.S. history. Press release number CB18-41. March 13, 2018. Available at www.census.gov/newsroom/press-releases/2018/cb18-41-population-projections.html

4. Kotlyar M, Dysken M, Adson DE. Update on drug-induced depression in the elderly. *Am J Geriatr Pharmacother* 2005;3(4):288–300.

5. Yasavage JA, Brink TL, Rose TL et al. Development and validation of a geriatric depression screening scale: a preliminary report. *J Psychiatr Res* 1983;17: 37–49.

6. Montgomery SA, Asberg M. A new depression scale intended to be sensitive to change. *Br J Psychiatry* 1979;134:382–9.

7. Hamilton M. A rating scale for depression. *J Neurol Neurosurg Psychiatry* 1960;2356–62.

8. Mottram P, Wilson K, Copeland J. Validation of the Hamilton Depression Scale and Montgomery and Asberg rating scales in terms of AGECAT depression cases. *Int J Geriatr Psychiatry* 2000;15:111 3–19.

9. Kok RM, Nolen WA, Heeren TJ. Efficacy of treatment in older depressed patients: a systematic review and meta-analysis of double-blind randomized controlled trials with antidepressants. *J Affect Disord* 2012;141 (2–3):103–15.

10. Papakostas GI, Fava M. Does the probability of receiving placebo influence clinical trial outcome? A meta-regression of double-blind, randomized clinical trials in MDD. *Eur Neuropsychopharmacol* 2009;19 (1):34–40.

11. Calati R, Salvina Signorelli M, Balestri M, et al. Antidepressants in elderly: metaregression of double-blind, randomized clinical trials. *J Affect Disord* 2013;147(1–3):1–8.

12. Alexopoulos GS, Katz IR, Reynolds CF 3rd, et al. The expert consensus guideline series. Pharmacotherapy of depressive disorders in older patients. *Postgrad Med* 2001; Spec No Pharmacotherapy:1–86.

13. Canadian Coalition for Seniors' Mental Health. National guidelines for seniors' mental health – the assessment and treatment of depression. 2006. Available at: http://ccsmh.ca/ccsmh-nationalguidelines-for-seniors-mental-health

14. Food and Drug Administration. FDA drug safety communication: revised recommendations for Celexa (citalopram hydrobromide) related to a potential risk of abnormal heart rhythms with high doses. 2012. Available at: www.fda.gov/Drugs/DrugSafety/ucm297391.htm

15. MacQueen GM, Frey BN, Ismail Z, et al.; CANMAT Depression Work Group. Canadian Network for Mood and Anxiety Treatments (CANMAT) 2016 clinical guidelines for the management of adults with major depressive disorder section 6. Special populations: youth, women, and the elderly. *Can J Psychiatry* 2016;61(9):588–603.

16. Cooper C, Katona C, Lyketsos K, et al. A systematic review of treatments for refractory depression in older people. *Am J Psychiatry*. 2011;168(7):681–8.

17. Zhou X, Ravindran AV, Qin B, et al. Comparative efficacy, acceptability, and tolerability of augmentation agents in treatment-resistant depression: systematic review and network meta-analysis. *J Clin Psychiatry* 2015;76(4):487–98.

18. American Psychiatric Association. *Practice Guideline for the Treatment of Patients with Major Depressive Disorder*. 3rd ed. Arlington, VA: American Psychiatric Association, 2010.

19. Huang AX, Delucchi K, Dunn LB, Nelson JC. A systematic review and meta-analysis of psychotherapy for late-life depression. *Am J Geriatr Psychiatry* 2015 Mar;23(3):261–73.

20. Kellner CH, Husain MM, Knapp RG, et al. Right unilateral ultrabrief pulse ECT in geriatric depression: phase 1 of the PRIDE study. *Am J Psychiatry* 2016;173 (11): 1101–9.

21. Spaans HP, Sienaert P, Bouckaert F, et al. Speed of remission in elderly patients with depression: electroconvulsive therapy v. medication. *Br J Psychiatry* 2015;206(1):67–71.

22. Tørring N, Sanghani SN, Petrides G, et al. The mortality rate of electroconvulsive therapy: a systematic review and pooled analysis. *Acta Psychiatr Scand* 2017;135(5):388–97.

23. Kessler RC, Berglund P, Demler O, et al. Lifetime prevalence and age-of-onset distributions of DSM-IV

disorders in the National Comorbidity Survey Replication. *Arch Gen Psychiatry* 2005;**62**(6):593–602.

24. Yassa R, Nair V, Nastase C, et al. Prevalence of bipolar disorder in a psychogeriatric population. *J Affect Disord* 1988;**14**(3):197–201.

25. Depp CA, Lindamer LA, Folsom DP, et al. Differences in clinical features and mental health service use in bipolar disorder across the lifespan. *Am J Geriatr Psychiatry* 2005;**13**(4):290–8.

26. Bartels SJ, Forester B, Miles KM, et al. Mental health service use by elderly patients with bipolar disorder and unipolar depression. *Am J Geriatr Psychiatry* 2000;**8**:160–6.

27. Evans DL, Byerly MJ, Greer RA. Secondary mania: diagnosis and treatment. *J Clin Psychiatry* 1995;**56** (Suppl 3):31–7.

28. Young RC, Mulsant BH, Sajatovic M, et al. GERI-BD: a randomized double-blind controlled trial of lithium and divalproex in the treatment of mania in older patients with bipolar disorder. *Am J Psychiatry* 2017 Nov 1;**174**(11):1086–93.

29. Shulman KI, Rochon P, Sykora K, et al. Changing prescription patterns for lithium and valproic acid in old age: shifting practice without evidence. *BMJ* 2003;**326**(7396):960–1.

30. Sajatovic M. Treatment of bipolar disorder in older adults. *Int J Geriatr Psychiatry* 2002;**17**(9):865–73.

31. Bayer JL, Siegal A, Kennedy JS. Olanzapine, divalproex and placebo treatment, non-head to head comparisons of older adults acute mania. 10th Congress of the International Psychogeriatric Association. Nice, France, September 9–14, 2001.

32. Sajatovic M, Calabrese JR, Mullen J. Quetiapine for the treatment of bipolar mania in older adults. *Bipolar Disord* 2008;**10**(6):662–71.

33. Food and Drug Administration. FDA Public Health Advisory: deaths with antipsychotics in elderly patients with behavioral disturbances. April 11, 2005. Available at https://psychrights.org/drugs/FDAatypicalswarning4elderly.pdf

34. Kales HC, Valenstein M, Kim HM, et al. Mortality risk in patients with dementia treated with antipsychotics versus other psychiatric medications. *Am J Psychiatry* 2007;**164**:1568.

35. Sajatovic M, Gildengers A, Al Jurdi R, et al. *Multi-Site, Open-Label, Prospective Trial of Lamotrigine for Geriatric Bipolar Depression.* Hollywood, FL: American College of Neuropsychopharmacology (ACNP), 2009.

36. Cruz N, Sanchez-Moreno J, Torres F, et al. Efficacy of modern antipsychotics in placebo-controlled trials in bipolar depression: a meta-analysis. *Int J Neuropsychopharmacol* 2010;**13**(1):5–14.

37. Correll CU, Frederickson AM, Kane JM, et al. Metabolic syndrome and the risk of coronary heart disease in 367 patients treated with second-generation antipsychotic drugs. *J Clin Psychiatry* 2006;**67**(4):575–83.

38. Sajatovic M. *Quetiapine for the Treatment of Depressive Episodes in Adults Aged 55 to 65 Years with Bipolar Disorder.* New Orleans, LA: American Association of Geriatric Psychiatry (AAGP), 2007.

39. Schaffer A, Mamdani M, Levitt A, et al. Effect of antidepressant use on admissions to hospital among elderly bipolar patients. *Int J Geriatr Psychiatry* 2006;**21**(3):275–80.

40. Al Jurdi RK, Marangell LB, Petersen NJ, et al. Prescription patterns of psychotropic medications in elderly compared with younger participants who achieved a "recovered" status in the systematic treatment enhancement program for bipolar disorder. *Am J Geriatr Psychiatry* 2008;**16** (11):922–33.

41. Calabrese JR, Bowden CL, Sachs G, et al. A placebo-controlled 18-month trial of lamotrigine and lithium maintenance treatment in recently depressed patients with bipolar I disorder. *J Clin Psychiatry* 2003;**64**(9):1013–24.

42. Bowden CL, Calabrese JR, Sachs G, et al. A placebo-controlled 18-month trial of lamotrigine and lithium maintenance treatment in recently manic or hypomanic patients with bipolar I disorder. *Arch Gen Psychiatry* 2003;**60**(4):392–400.

43. Sajatovic M, Gyulai L, Calabrese JR, et al. Maintenance treatment outcomes in older patients with bipolar I disorder. *Am J Geriatr Psychiatry* 2005;**13**(4):305–11.

44. Lepkifker E, Iancu I, Horesh N, et al. Lithium therapy for unipolar and bipolar depression among the middle-aged and older adult patient subpopulation. *Depress Anxiety* 2007;**24**(8):571–6.

45. BALANCE Investigators and Collaborators, Geddes JR, Goodwin GM, et al. Lithium plus valproate combination therapy versus monotherapy for relapse prevention in bipolar I disorder (BALANCE): a randomised open-label trial. *Lancet* 2010;**375**(9712):385–95.

Evidence-Based Psychological Interventions for Bipolar Disorders

Thomas D. Meyer and Jan Scott

Introduction

Over the past 30 years there have been many studies of psychosocial aspects of bipolar disorders (BD) and increasing arguments for psychological as well as pharmacological treatments for individuals with BD [1]. While this represents a significant leap forward from the situation in the 1960s, the clinical reality is that systematic research into the effectiveness of psychosocial treatments for BD is still in its infancy. This is especially true when work on BD is compared with the amount of empirical evidence accumulated over decades for talking therapies in other areas, especially major depression or anxiety disorders.

Until relatively recently, the mainstay of BD treatment was pharmacotherapy alone. The reliance on medication arose for several reasons. First, aetiologic models highlighted the key role of genetic and biological factors in BD. However, the preeminent position of these topics in the research agenda was misconstrued as indicating that medication was not just the primary treatment, but the only appropriate and necessary intervention. Second, there was a misconception that individuals with BD made a full inter-episode recovery and returned to their premorbid level of functioning (which was often erroneously reported as above average). Third, there was only a limited acknowledgement of the extent of medication non-adherence and that such problems could be addressed with psychotherapy.

The very early stages of psychotherapy research for BD were characterized by only a few, uncontrolled studies that investigated the efficacy of psychological treatments, even including psychodynamic approaches [2–5], and the first randomized controlled trial (RCT) was published by Cochran in 1984 [6], which focused on a very brief interpretation. It was not before the 1990s when the development of evidence-based adjunctive psychological treatments were intensified; and these efforts were largely driven by the increased acknowledgement that a significant proportion of

individuals with BD reported subsyndromal symptoms, functional impairments in everyday life, and recurrent mood episodes, despite a wide range of available pharmacological treatment options [7,8].

As demonstrated in other chapters, evidence has clarified the importance of stress-vulnerability models that highlight the interplay between psychological, social and biological factors in BD, demonstrated the significant morbidity and impairment of functioning experienced by individuals with the disorder and highlighted that non-adherence is a significant barrier to good outcomes with mood stabilizer prophylaxis. As such, it has become clear that additional psychological and social support may benefit individuals with BD. Furthermore, evidence indicated that adjunctive psychotherapies improved outcomes for severe and chronic depressive and psychotic disorders [9,10].

While the above reduced resistance to introducing some psychosocial interventions for individuals with BD and their significant others, there were still some barriers to overcome. For example, few psychodynamic or psychoanalytic therapists regarded individuals with BD as appropriate candidates for traditional therapy interventions, and many private practitioners were concerned about liability and safety issues related to manic episodes [1]. While manualized psychotherapies were being developed, few researchers had developed BD-specific models. Furthermore, RCTs were focused on existing and new medications, and there was a lack of funding and/or empirical support for therapy RCTs. Last but not least, even as demand for therapies began to rise, there were few clear indicators regarding when or how to incorporate such approaches into day-to-day practice.

Since 2000, the landscape has changed dramatically. Systematic research has explored cognitive, behavioural, emotional and interpersonal problems in BD and how to implement constructive interventions that target these issues; it also highlighted the critical role of both critical life events and affective style, expressed emotion as well as interpersonal support in those families where one or more person is diagnosed with BD; research also demonstrated that psychoeducation about the disorder, especially delivered in group format and allied to self-monitoring and self-management, can enhance clinical outcomes. The development of specific psychological therapies for BD has been a necessary advance in the field of therapeutics. Indeed, not only individuals with BD and their significant others, but also many psychopharmacologists have welcomed the introduction of psychosocial interventions. However, concerns have been raised that the value of adjunctive therapies (compared with general supportive interventions) may have been over-stated. For instance, one expert supported the role of psychosocial approaches in general but commented that 'psycho-education is bound to be better than psycho-ignorance', and that more evidence was required regarding active ingredients of therapies. So at present, there is a debate regarding the clinical significance of the gains reported with some specific therapies and whether current clinical practice guidelines have made recommendations regarding adjunctive therapies that exceed the available evidence [11,12].

Give all of the above, this chapter briefly outlines the rationale for using psychological therapies in combination with medication in the treatment of adult clients with BD. Concerns regarding the evidence for efficacy is examined by specifically highlighting a recent network meta-analysis that explored not only which therapies may be beneficial to individuals with BD, but also which therapy components (often shared across models) are most likely to enhance outcomes in general and/or by episode polarity. The latter is detailed because it may offer new directions for the developments of psychological interventions in BD. Finally, we highlight some of the likely developments in research in the field and how these might translate to clinical practice in the next decade.

The Rationale for Psychological Treatments

Several psychobiosocial models have been developed that guided treatment development. One of the most influential theories about depression, initially focused on unipolar depression [13,14] was expanded to BD. The basic idea is that latent negative beliefs, so-called schemata (e.g., 'nobody loves me'), are activated by current life events (e.g., criticism from a loved one, failure in an exam), which then leads to negative thoughts, emotions and behaviours, manifesting itself as clinical depression if the symptoms last and are sufficiently severe. This basic idea was expanded to bipolar depression but also hypomania and mania, that is, underlying positive beliefs can lead to changes in behaviour, thinking and emotions that spiral into mania [15–18] (see Figure 28.1). Several studies demonstrated similarities between unipolar and bipolar depression in dysfunctional attitudes and selectivity for negative stimuli [19–22]. While there is also some evidence for positivity biases in cognition related to vulnerability to mania [23–26], hypomania and mania are characterized by coexistence of both negative and positive cognitions [19,22,27]. The latter makes sense given the prevalence of mixed states.

The cognitive model does not negate the relevance of genetic and biological factors, but it focuses more on psychological processes that can be targeted with psychotherapeutic strategies. The model highlights the role of stress which has shown to affect onset and course [28,29] with individuals with BD being especially sensitive to certain classes of life events: the first group of stressors are those affecting circadian / sleep–wake rhythms, such as flights across time zones, birth of a baby, change in work hours [30–33]. While the exact mechanisms of how the disruption in circadian rhythms translates into clinically relevant mood episodes are not fully understood, within a cognitive model attribution and appraisal processes following changes in internal states (e.g., activation level, energy, fatigue) can help conceptualize the emergence of mania or depression under these circumstances. Adopting the theoretical perspective from an interpersonal or family focus [34,35], it is easy to see how interpersonal conflicts at home or at work or a breakup of a relationship will interfere with the sleep–wake rhythm and set of the process; the other group of stressors highly relevant for BD are those that affect the 'behaviour activation system' (BAS), a neurobiological system that regulates goal-directed activation and motivation [36,37]. Examples for events that dysregulate this system would be passing/failing an exam, a promotion at work, assignment of a highly valued project, or participation in a sports tournament. The assumption is that BD is associated with a hypersensitive BAS with regards to any external or internal cues for reward or reinforcement or its loss [38–41].

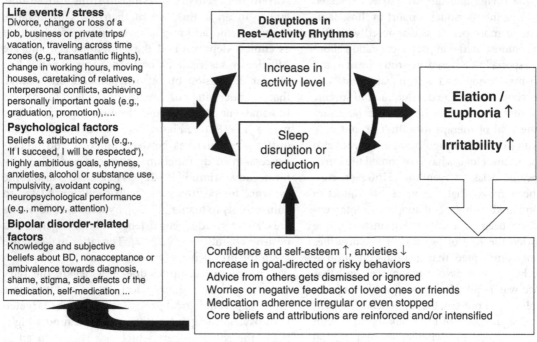

Figure 28.1 CBT conceptualization of (hypo)mania (adapted from Meyer [16,17]).

Table 28.1 Shared elements of evidence-based psychosocial treatments for BD

1. Psychoeducation is seen as a core element to allow the individual to become an expert for their own condition and help with motivation to actively engage in treatment.
2. A theory-driven individualized case formulation for each patient (and family) is developed.
3. Transparency about the therapy model is shared with the patient and (where applicable) the family.
4. The individualized case formulation provides the jointly agreed basis for any therapeutic techniques used (e.g., self-monitoring, medication adherence).
5. The active role of the patient and their engagement in the process of change are emphasized (e.g., tailored exercises or homework assignment between sessions).
6. The development of self-management strategies and other skills that can be applied outside of therapy is the focus of treatment.

(Adapted from Miklowitz and Scott [44])

While the different psychotherapeutic modalities differ in what processes they focus on during treatments, they all agree on the core elements of therapy to achieve the overarching goal of psychological treatments in BD of relapse prevention, alleviating symptoms and restoring psychosocial functioning and quality of life (see Table 28.1).

Synthesizing Evidence about Psychological Therapies

When considering the whole range of adjunctive psychological treatments for BD, most systematic reviews and meta-analyses conclude that they reduce recurrence of mood episodes and improve symptoms and/or psychosocial impairment [42–45]. Given that the research in this area is still in its early stages, it is not surprising that some reviews claim that the evidence base is only low to moderate [46–48]. However, all these meta-analyses have never compared the relative efficacy of those psychosocial treatments with each other and only considered the active treatment relative to its control condition. This gap in the literature was addressed by a network meta-analysis published by Miklowitz and colleagues in 2021 [49].

Since the 1990s, Miklowitz et al. [49] identified that there have been > 300 published RCTs of adjunctive psychological interventions for individuals with BD. These show considerable heterogeneity, with sample sizes ranging from < 20 to > 300 participants, trial durations of 1 to > 20 months and widely varying quality of methodology, including reliability and validity of outcome measures and statistical analyses employed. Further, it should be acknowledged that these therapy RCTs often have additional limitations that are not encountered in pharmacological studies (e.g., greater problems with double-blinding; difficulties with reproducibility of the therapy in different centres and delivery of consistent optimal exposure to the intervention). One way to try to compensate for some of these problems is to synthesize the available evidence from RCTs that meet minimum quality assurance criteria. There have been many attempts to do this, and since the mid-1990s, there have been > 100 articles reviewing findings from studies of psychological interventions for BD, of which about 40% purportedly offered systematic evaluations of the literature. Further, as of December 2020, we identified 24 published meta-analyses of pooled outcome data from RCTs (usually regarded as the highest quality of evidence).

As already indicated above, all the systematic reviews and meta-analyses indicate that individuals who are offered one of the four key therapies – Cognitive Behavioural Therapy (CBT), Family-Focused Treatment (FFT), Interpersonal and Social Rhythm Therapy (IPSRT) and Group Psychoeducation (PED) – are likely to show significantly greater benefit than those offered treatment as usual (TAU), and most also demonstrate some advantage when compared with supportive therapies (plus TAU). However, these publications again highlight the modest quality of many trials, the pooled meta-analyses rarely include the same RCTs and they report inconsistent findings, and there are few indicators of whether some specific therapies are more useful than others or should be targeted at selected clinical subpopulations. This is frustrating, as patients and clinicians need to be able to decide between the alternative interventions available and balance the relative risks and benefits of each modality. One way to try to explore this issue is to undertake a network meta-analysis (NMA). This technique has been widely employed in pharmacology research, as it combines direct estimates of outcomes (comparison of treatments within the same study) and indirect estimates of outcomes (comparisons

of treatments across studies using a common comparator condition such as TAU) in a single analysis. Importantly, the combination of direct and indirect evidence increases the precision of the effect estimate between two interventions [50].

Although a well-conducted NMA can potentially provide insights into the comparative effectiveness of available interventions, it is noteworthy that the analysis is more complex than the classic (pair-wise comparison) meta-analytic model, and relatively minor errors in data management (e.g., method of imputing missing data) can significantly impact the treatment hierarchies generated and/or undermine the interpretation of findings. As such, NMA is best undertaken by an expert in this approach, and it is unsurprising that only two research groups have taken up the challenge to date. The most recent NMA had access to a larger number of RCTs that met specific quality assurance criteria than the earlier NMA and also explored different components of the most widely used therapies. The latter allowed investigators to determine which shared components of the therapies (e.g., sleep–wake regulation) were most strongly associated with good clinical outcomes. Given these additional methodological advantages, and the involvement of one of the chapter authors in the second publication, we focus on the key findings of the NMA reported by Miklowitz and colleagues [49]. (Please note that full details of the NMA methods and statistical analyses are beyond the scope of this chapter; here we focus only on key outputs and their clinical relevance).

The publication utilized data from 3,888 participants included in 40 RCTs (37 concerning adults and 3 concerning adolescents) published from 1984 onwards; 38 trials compared two treatment arms (e.g., therapy plus TAU versus TAU), while one compared 3 and the other compared 4 arms. Examination of the eligible publications identified that seven separate categories of intervention had been employed in the trials, namely: CBT, IPSRT, Family/Conjoint therapy (including family-focused therapy, multifamily groups or caregiver-only groups), psychoeducation (group or individual), brief psychoeducation (i.e., 6 sessions or fewer in an individual, family or group format), supportive therapy or TAU (defined as medication management with a physician, including regular sessions in which symptoms and side effects were evaluated). Before undertaking the NMA, the investigators then examined the therapy manuals and, as shown in Table 28.2, they identified 14 separate therapy elements that were employed in one or more of the interventions.

The NMA then examined which therapy was most useful for preventing relapse (return of acute mood symptoms following a period of remission), which was for acute stabilization of depressive and manic symptoms and which was most likely to be associated with therapy dropout. Then the investigators examined which therapy components were most strongly associated with relapse prevention and/or acute symptom stabilization.

We produced an adapted diagram representing the NMA output in Figure 28.2. The straight lines identify the connections between the seven intervention categories (termed nodes). In any network plot, the thickness of the connections corresponds to the number of studies performing each treatment comparison, while the size of the nodes corresponds to the number of studies comparing each treatment. If there is no line directly connecting two nodes, then the NMA will not report direct estimates (although it is possible to report indirect estimates).

As shown in Figure 28.2, the most robust comparisons regarding relapse prevention are for CBT, Family/Conjoint Therapy, and psychoeducation and TAU. As in previous meta-analyses, the NMA confirmed that several of the specific therapies such as Family/Conjoint Therapy (odds ratio [OR] for reduction in relapse rate = 0.30; 95% confidence

Table 28.2 Therapy components

Component	Definition
Therapeutic technique	
Psychoeducation: information only	Information-giving (without skill development/practice)
Psychoeducation: information plus active skill practice	Information-giving with skills development and practice
Self-monitoring assignments	Patient tracks moods, sleep, thoughts and/or medication adherence between sessions
Self-management assignments	Patient learns to recognize early signs of illness episodes and to implement preventative strategies in a timely manner
Cognitive restructuring	Patient learns to challenge self-defeating thoughts and beliefs and to develop and rehearse adaptive thinking
Keeping regular social rhythms	Patient learns to recognize and regulate daily activities (e.g., eating and exercise patterns) and sleep–wake schedules (with the aim of influencing mood states)
Behavioural activation assignments	Patient plans activities to increase engagement with environment or to modulate stimulation
Behavioural problem solving	Coaching on how to identify and define problems, generate and evaluate solutions and implement chosen solutions
Interpersonal problem solving	Patient is encouraged to identify interpersonal habits and patterns and to consider alternative ways of managing social problems
Communication training	Coaching, typically of families or groups, on effective speaking and listening skills with in-session rehearsal
Mode of delivery	
Individual format	Sessions are limited to the individual patient
Group format	Sessions primarily occur with other patients or families
Family format	Sessions primarily occur in a family or couples format
Caregiver-only format	Caregivers participate (e.g., in group psychoeducation or a support program), but individuals with BD do not

(adapted from Miklowitz et al., 2021 [49])

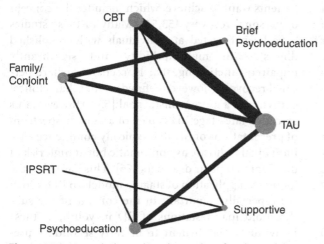

Figure 28.2 Network plot to show the number of studies and the types of comparisons made between therapies aimed at reducing relapse in BD (adapted and modified from Miklowitz et al., 2021 [49]).

In this network plot, the straight lines identify the connections between the seven different interventions examined (which are termed nodes). Here, the thickness of the connections corresponds to the number of studies performing each treatment comparison, while the size of the nodes corresponds to the number of studies comparing each treatment. If there is no line directly connecting two nodes, then the NMA will not report direct estimates (although it is possible to report indirect estimates). To give two examples: there is a large number of studies comparing CBT with TAU (larger circles and thick connecting line). In contrast, overall there are fewer studies of IPSRT that were eligible for this network meta-analysis, but IPSRT is one of the few therapies to be compared with another psychological intervention (i.e., supportive therapy). The thickness of the line demonstrates there were few such studies, but nevertheless, it is important to compare psychological treatments as well as comparing psychological treatments to TAU.

Abbreviations: CBT: Cognitive Behavioural Therapy; IPSRT: Interpersonal and Social Rhythm Therapy; TAU: treatment as usual.

intervals [CI]: 0.17, 0.53) and CBT (OR = 0.52, 95% CI: 0.34, 0.79) were more effective at preventing relapse than TAU. However, the novel findings from the NMA of therapy components was that relapse prevention was best achieved with a psychoeducation technique that incorporated active skills learning and practice and self-monitoring of symptoms and daily rhythms. This means also that psychoeducation modules in any therapy that used an 'information only' approach, such as didactic lecture models and/or modules composed of brief psychoeducation, were insufficient. Regarding the format, delivering these two components (i.e., psychoeducation with active skill practice and self-monitoring) in a family or group format was more effective for reducing relapse rates than the same strategies delivered in an individual format (OR = 0.12; 95% CI: 0.02, 0.94).

Many individuals with BD commence therapy when they have acute symptoms, so the NMA also examined which therapies and then which shared therapy components were most efficient at stabilizing depressive or manic symptoms. For depression, evidence favoured CBT compared to TAU (standardized mean difference [SMD] = −0.32; 95% CI: −0.64, −0.01). Further, when therapy components were examined, the elements found to be most effective for acute stabilization were cognitive restructuring (SMD = -1.26; 95% CI: –2.10, –0.35) and regulating daily rhythms (SMD = −0.78; 95% CI: −1.28, −0.24). When these components were combined, they were clearly more effective than TAU (SMD = −2.07; 95% CI: −3.23 to −0.85). The most efficacious treatment components for stabilizing baseline mania symptoms were cognitive restructuring (SMD = −1.0, 95% CI: −2.15 to 0.16), regulating daily rhythms (SMD = −0.42; 95% CI: −1.08 to 0.28) and communication training (SMD = -0.80; 95% CI: −2.23 to 0.63). Fewer individuals with manic symptoms were included in the RCTs, so although findings for mania were similar to those for depression, they are weaker and less reliable. For example, there was a trend for CBT to be the most useful approach for stabilization of manic symptoms (SMD = −0.32; 95% CI: −0.65, +0.01). Likewise, the component analysis (again with trends towards significance) indicated that the most efficacious techniques for stabilizing manic symptoms were regulating daily rhythms, basic cognitive restructuring and communication training, especially when this combination of components was offered in a group or family format rather than an individual format.

Overall, we suggest the NMA does offer important insights that can be used by researchers in the field of adjunctive psychological therapies for BD. For instance, the NMA indicates that evidence for efficacy is stronger for some therapies (PED, FFT, CBT) than others (e.g., brief PED, IPSRT), but that these findings should be balanced against evidence that the likelihood of dropping out of CBT was higher than for FFT or IPSRT. The NMA also highlighted the need for more information about when and whether to employ specific therapies for individuals experiencing manic symptoms. Most importantly, the component analysis demonstrated that the techniques that were most useful for stabilization of depressive symptoms (e.g., cognitive restructuring, regulating daily rhythms) differed from those that are most effective in relapse prevention (e.g., family or group psychoeducation with active skills training). These findings should allow therapists who practice different models of intervention to collaborate in devising new therapy manuals that incorporate the shared active ingredients and to design modules that can be used during different phases of BD. Also, evidence that the use of group or family formats is as effective or more effective than individual formats could help re-think how therapy programmes are delivered in day-to-day clinical settings, which may be especially useful given the need to increase access to trained therapists.

Future Directions

There are many gaps and limitations in our understanding of the optimal application of psychological interventions for individuals with BD, and we still have many questions to resolve regarding the 'who, what, why and when'. For example, even though we have increasing evidence regarding efficacy across a range of clinical settings and subpopulations, this needs to be complemented by more comparative effectiveness research, including pragmatic trials and observational studies of real-world clinical cohorts [51]. These studies often have limited resources for monitoring outcomes, but as noted by the Institute of Medicine in the United States, they can focus on patient-related outcomes and use of self-ratings in broader clinical samples than recruited to RCTs [52].

More recently, studies of psychotherapy in BD have shifted from focusing primarily on reducing symptoms and preventing recurrence (which perhaps represents a traditional medical approach) to incorporating more assessments of what individual patients want to achieve, which includes the concept of personal recovery [53,54]. Many of these studies have been targeted at individuals with established illness, with multimorbidity and significantly impaired functioning, that is, scenarios where personal recovery (however defined) rather than clinical euthymia is a more realistic goal [55]. However, this so-called late-stage BD is part of an entire spectrum of presentations of BD that typically commence with individuals who are asymptomatic but at high risk of developing bipolar disorders [56]. This has led to the increased application of staging models to BD, which are especially important in the context of the subthreshold manifestations of BD in youth, as these individuals may benefit from early secondary preventative psychological interventions [57]. While few studies have sufficient statistical power to reliably demonstrate that they prevent progression to full-threshold BD, psychological interventions do appear to have a favourable benefit-to-risk ratio, can be used without medication in the very early stages of BD and so appear to be acceptable to individuals with high risk of or recent onset of BD [58–60]. What is not yet known is how early interventions should be attempted, that is, is it appropriate to offer interventions to the offspring of parents with BD, even if the children and adolescents are asymptomatic, or should they be targeted at a range of high-risk individuals [61]?

As well as extending knowledge about the range of individuals with BD who might benefit from psychological interventions, we still need to address major gaps in our understanding of the mechanisms, mediators and moderators of outcome. For example, there is evidence that the patients' memory for the content of previous therapy sessions might not be as solid as needed to learn and implement changes [62], and there is preliminary evidence that verbal learning and memory might affect the course of treatment differently depending on the intervention prescribed [63]. Furthermore, given the high level of comorbidity in BD, it is essential to state that only very studies specifically target comorbidities, such as substance use disorders [64,65]. Currently, it is not known how to best address co-existing mental health problems in BD, that is, is it better to address them sequentially or simultaneously as part of an integrative case formulation? Also, these complex presentations have increased the use of multi-model interventions that draw active ingredients from a range of interventions and develop optimal combinations that best match to the identified individual needs of the patient and, on many occasions, those of their family as well [65].

Conclusions

While the existing research shows that efficacious psychosocial treatments exist to improve the lives of individuals with BD and their families, there are few effectiveness studies and gaps that hinder reliable translation and generalizability of interventions to the spectrum of individuals who present with this complex and multifaceted disorder. As such, there needs to be more effort and funding invested in implementational science for existing therapies and further work on the role of additional self-guided, digital or virtual approaches. This is critically important as, despite recommendations for the use of psychological treatments in most clinical practice guidelines, most individuals with BD still do not have access to psychosocial treatments [66–68].

References

1. Scott J. Psychotherapy for bipolar disorder. *Br J Psychiatry*. 1995;**167**(5):581–8.

2. Benson R. The forgotten treatment modality in bipolar illness: psychotherapy. *Dis Nerv Syst*. 1975;**36**(11):634–9.

3. Davenport YB, Ebert MH, Adland ML, Goodwin FK. Couples group therapy as an adjunct to lithium maintenance of the manic patient. *Am J Orthopsychiatry*. 1977;**47**(3):495.

4. Mayo JA. Marital therapy with manic-depressive patients treated with lithium. *Comp Psychiatry*. 1979;**20**(5):419–26.

5. Shakir SA, Volkmar FR, Bacon S, Pfefferbaum A. Group psychotherapy as an adjunct to lithium maintenance. *Am J Psychiatry*. 1979;**136**(4A):455–6.

6. Cochran SD. Preventing medical noncompliance in the outpatient treatment of bipolar affective disorders. *J Consult Clin Psychol*. 1984;**52**(5):873.

7. Goldberg JF, Harrow M. A 15-year prospective follow-up of bipolar affective disorders: comparisons with unipolar nonpsychotic depression. *Bipolar Disord*. 2011;**13**(2):155–63.

8. Treuer T, Tohen M. Predicting the course and outcome of bipolar disorder: a review. *Eur Psychiatry*. 2010;**25**(6):328–33.

9. Paykel ES, Scott J, Teasdale JD, et al. Prevention of relapse in residual depression by cognitive therapy: a controlled trial. *Arch Gen Psychiatry*. 1999;**56**(9):829–35.

10. Sensky T, Turkington D, Kingdon D, et al. A randomized controlled trial of cognitive-behavioral therapy for persistent symptoms in schizophrenia resistant to medication. *Arch Gen Psychiatry*. 2000;**57**(2):165–72.

11. Scott J, Colom F. Gaps and limitations of psychological interventions for bipolar disorders. *Psychother Psychosom*. 2008;**77**(1):4–11.

12. Fountoulakis KN, Tohen M. Interpreting the findings of a meta-analysis of psychosocial interventions in bipolar disorder. *JAMA Psychiatry*. 2021;**78**(4):447–8.

13. Beck A. *Depression: Clinical, Experimental and Theoretical Aspects*. New York: Harper and Row, 1967.

14. Beck AT. *Cognitive Therapy of Depression*: New York: Guilford Press, 1979.

15. Meyer T, Hautzinger M. Psychotherapie bei bipolaren affektiven Störungen – Ein Überblick über den Stand der Forschung. *Verhaltenstherapie*. 2000;**10**(3):177–86.

16. Meyer TD. Hypomanie und Manie (chapter 18). In B Röhrle, F Caspar, PF Schlottke, editors. *Lehrbuch der klinisch-psychologischen Diagnostik*. Stuttgart: Kohlhammer, 2008; 433–74.

17. Meyer TD. Manie (chapter 6). In W Rief, E Schramm, B Strauss, editors. *Psychologische Psychotherapie: Ein Kompetenzorientiertes Lehrbuch München*. Elsevier Urban & Fischer, 2021; 99–108.

18. Newman CF, Leahy RL, Beck AT, Reilly-Harrington NA, Gyulai L. *Bipolar Disorder: A Cognitive Therapy Approach*. Washington, DC: American Psychological Association, 2002.

19. Lyon HM, Startup M, Bentall RP. Social cognition and the manic defense: attributions, selective attention, and self-schema in bipolar affective disorder. *J Abnorm Psychol*. 1999;**108**(2):273.

20. Pavlickova H, Varese F, Turnbull O, et al. Symptom-specific self-referential cognitive processes in bipolar disorder: a longitudinal analysis. *Psychol Med*. 2013;**43**(9):1895–907.

21. Reilly-Harrington NA, Alloy LB, Fresco DM, Whitehouse WG. Cognitive styles and life events interact to predict bipolar and unipolar symptomatology. *J Abnorm Psychol*. 1999;**108**(4):567.

22. Scott J, Pope M. Cognitive styles in individuals with bipolar disorders. *Psychol Med*. 2003;**33**(6):1081.

23. Lex C, Hautzinger M, Meyer TD. Cognitive styles in hypomanic episodes of bipolar I disorder. *Bipolar Disord*. 2011;**13**(4):355–64.

24. Meyer TD, Hautzinger M, Bauer IE. A mania-related memory bias is associated with risk for relapse in bipolar disorder. *J Affect Disord*. 2018;**235**:557–64.

25. Schönfelder S, Langer J, Schneider EE, Wessa M. Mania risk is characterized by an aberrant optimistic update bias for positive life events. *J Affect Disord.* 2017;**218**:313–21.

26. Lam D, Wright K, Smith N. Dysfunctional assumptions in bipolar disorder. *J Affect Disord.* 2004;**79**(1–3):193–9.

27. Fletcher K, Parker G, Manicavasagar V. Behavioral Activation System (BAS) differences in bipolar I and II disorder. *J Affect Disord.* 2013;**151**(1):121–128.

28. Lex C, Bazner E, Meyer TD. Does stress play a significant role in bipolar disorder? A meta-analysis. *J Affect Disord.* 2017;**208**:298–308.

29. Aldinger F, Schulze TG. Environmental factors, life events, and trauma in the course of bipolar disorder. *Psychiatry Clin Neurosci.* 2017;**71**(1):6–17.

30. Inder ML, Crowe MT, Porter R. Effect of transmeridian travel and jetlag on mood disorders: evidence and implications. *Aus N Z J Psychiatry.* 2016;**50**(3):220–7.

31. Malkoff-Schwartz S, Frank E, Anderson B, et al. Stressful life events and social rhythm disruption in the onset of manic and depressive bipolar episodes: a preliminary investigation. *Arch Gen Psychiatry.* 1998;**55**(8):702–7.

32. Murray G, Harvey A. Circadian rhythms and sleep in bipolar disorder. *Bipolar Disord.* 2010;**12**(5):459–72.

33. Shen GH, Alloy LB, Abramson LY, Sylvia LG. Social rhythm regularity and the onset of affective episodes in bipolar spectrum individuals. *Bipolar Disord.* 2008;**10**(4):520–9.

34. Frank E. *Treating Bipolar Disorder: A Clinician's Guide to Interpersonal and Social Rhythm Therapy.* New York: Guilford Press, 2005.

35. Miklowitz DJ. *Bipolar Disorder: A Family-Focused Treatment Approach.* 2nd ed. New York: Guilford Press; 2010.

36. Depue RA, Iacono WG. Neurobehavioral aspects of affective disorders. *Annu Rev Psychol.* 1989;**40**(1):457–92.

37. Johnson SL. Mania and dysregulation in goal pursuit: a review. *Clin Psychol Rev.* 2005;**25**(2):241–62.

38. Alloy LB, Abramson LY. The role of the behavioral approach system (BAS) in bipolar spectrum disorders. *Cur Dir Psychol Sci.* 2010;**19**(3):189–94.

39. Alloy LB, Nusslock R, Boland EM. The development and course of bipolar spectrum disorders: an integrated reward and circadian rhythm dysregulation model. *Annur Rev Clin Psychol.* 2015;**11**:213–50.

40. Johnson SL, Edge MD, Holmes MK, Carver CS. The behavioral activation system and mania. *Annu Rev Clin Psychol.* 2012;**8**:243–67.

41. Kwan JW, Bauer IE, Hautzinger M, Meyer TD. Reward sensitivity and the course of bipolar disorder: a survival analysis in a treatment seeking sample. *J Affect Disord.* 2020;**261**:126–30.

42. Chatterton ML, Stockings E, Berk M, Barendregt JJ, Carter R, Mihalopoulos C. Psychosocial therapies for the adjunctive treatment of bipolar disorder in adults: network meta-analysis. *Br J Psychiatry.* 2017;**210**(5):333–41.

43. Macheiner T, Skavantzos A, Pilz R, Reininghaus EZ. A meta-analysis of adjuvant group-interventions in psychiatric care for patients with bipolar disorders. *J Affect Disord.* 2017;**222**:28–31.

44. Miklowitz DJ, Scott J. Psychosocial treatments for bipolar disorder: cost-effectiveness, mediating mechanisms, and future directions. *Bipolar Disord.* 2009;**11**:110–22.

45. Schöttle D, Huber CG, Bock T, Meyer TD. Psychotherapy for bipolar disorder: a review of the most recent studies. *Curr Opin Psychiatry.* 2011;**24**(6):549–55.

46. Lynch D, Laws K, McKenna P. Cognitive behavioural therapy for major psychiatric disorder: does it really work? A meta-analytical review of well-controlled trials. *Psychol Med.* 2010;**40**(1):9–24.

47. Oud M, Mayo-Wilson E, Braidwood R, et al. Psychological interventions for adults with bipolar disorder: systematic review and meta-analysis. *Br J Psychiatry.* 2016;**208**(3):213–22.

48. Szentagotai-Tatar A, David D. Evidence-based psychological interventions for bipolar disorder. In D David, SJ Lynn, GH Montgomery, editors. *Evidence-Based Psychotherapy: The State of the Science and Practice.* Wiley Blackwell, 2018; 37–61.

49. Miklowitz DJ, Efthimiou O, Furukawa TA, et al. Adjunctive psychotherapy for bipolar disorder: a systematic review and component network meta-analysis. *JAMA Psychiatry.* 2021;**78**(2):141–50.

50. Cipriani A, Higgins JP, Geddes JR, Salanti G. Conceptual and technical challenges in network meta-analysis. *Ann Inter Med.* 2013;**159**(2):130–7.

51. Etain B, Scott J, Cochet B, et al. A study of the real-world effectiveness of group psychoeducation for bipolar disorders: is change in illness perception a key mediator of benefit? *J Affect Disord.* 2018;**227**:713–20.

52. Jonas DE, Mansfield AJ, Curtis P, et al. Identifying priorities for patient-centered outcomes research for serious mental illness. *Psychiatr Serv.* 2012;**63**(11):1125–30.

53. Jones SH, Smith G, Mulligan LD, et al. Recovery-focused cognitive–behavioural therapy for recent-onset bipolar disorder: randomised controlled pilot trial. *Br J Psychiatry.* 2015;**206**(1):58–66.

54. Murray G, Leitan ND, Thomas N, et al. Towards recovery-oriented psychosocial interventions for bipolar disorder: quality of life outcomes, stage-sensitive treatments, and mindfulness mechanisms. *Clin Psychol Rev*. 2017;**52**:148–63.

55. Tremain H, Fletcher K, Scott J, et al. The influence of stage of illness on functional outcomes after psychological treatment in bipolar disorder: a systematic review. *Bipolar Disord*. 2020;**22** (7):666–92.

56. Berk M, Conus P, Lucas N, et al. Setting the stage: from prodrome to treatment resistance in bipolar disorder. *Bipolar Disord*. 2007;**9**(7):671–8.

57. Vallarino M, Henry C, Etain B, et al. An evidence map of psychosocial interventions for the earliest stages of bipolar disorder. *Lancet Psychiatry*. 2015;**2**(6):548–63.

58. Leopold K, Bauer M, Bechdolf A, et al. Efficacy of cognitive-behavioral group therapy in patients at risk for serious mental illness presenting with subthreshold bipolar symptoms: results from a prespecified interim analysis of a multicenter, randomized, controlled study. *Bipolar Disord*. 2020;**22**(5):517–29.

59. Miklowitz DJ, Schneck CD, Singh MK, et al. Early intervention for symptomatic youth at risk for bipolar disorder: a randomized trial of family-focused therapy. *J Am Acad Child Adolesc Psychiatry*. 2013;**52** (2):121–31.

60. Scott J, Meyer TD. Brief research report: a pilot study of Cognitive Behavioral Regulation Therapy (CBT-REG) for young people at high risk of early transition to bipolar disorders. *Front Psychiatry*. 2020;**11**:616829.

61. Davison J, Scott J. Should we intervene at stage 0? A qualitative study of attitudes of asymptomatic youth at increased risk of developing bipolar disorders and parents with established disease. *Early Interv Psychiatry*. 2018;**12**(6):1112–19.

62. Lee JY, Harvey AG. Memory for therapy in bipolar disorder and comorbid insomnia. *J Consult Clin Psychol*. 2015;**83**(1):92.

63. Bauer IE, Hautzinger M, Meyer TD. Memory performance predicts recurrence of mania in bipolar disorder following psychotherapy: a preliminary study. *J Psychiatr Res*. 2017;**84**:207–13.

64. Crowe M, Eggleston K, Douglas K, Porter RJ. Effects of psychotherapy on comorbid bipolar disorder and substance use disorder: a systematic review. *Bipolar Disord*. 2021;**23**(2):141–51.

65. Biseul I, Icick R, Seguin P, Bellivier F, Scott J. Feasibility and acceptability of the 'HABIT' group programme for comorbid bipolar and alcohol and substance use disorders. *Clin Psychol Psychother*. 2017;**24**(4):887–98.

66. Barbato A, Vallarino M, Rapisarda F, et al. Do people with bipolar disorders have access to psychosocial treatments? A survey in Italy. *Int J Soc Psychiatry*. 2016;**62**(4):334–44.

67. Crusey A, Schuller K, Trace J. Access to care barriers for patients with bipolar disorder in the United States. *J Healthc Qual Res*. 2020;**35**(3):167–72.

68. Rummel-Kluge C, Kluge M, Kissling W. Frequency and relevance of psychoeducation in psychiatric diagnoses: results of two surveys five years apart in German-speaking European countries. *BMC Psychiatry*. 2013;**13**(1):1–5.

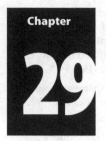

Chapter 29

Evidence-Based Psychotherapeutic Approaches for Depressive Disorders

Robin B. Jarrett and Jeffrey R. Vittengl

Worldwide, major depressive disorder (MDD) affects over 300 million people or 4.4% of the population and increases the risk of: impairment in social roles, nonpsychiatric illnesses, disability, and death through its link to suicide [1]. Accessing prompt and effective treatment can reduce these risks, as well as the associated suffering and burdens, when patients learn to recognize their symptoms and participate in evidence-based treatments that improve the lifetime trajectory of illness that is too often chronic and/or recurrent. Depressed adults tend to prefer psychotherapy over the modal prescription for antidepressant medication [2,3], which is equally (but not more) effective than the psychotherapy described herein [4]. For these reasons, it is incumbent on our field to improve understanding of and access to evidence-based psychotherapy for people with depressive disorders.

The purpose of this chapter is to identify contemporary evidence-based psychotherapeutic approaches for adults with depression. We use "depression" broadly to refer to unipolar, nonpsychotic, negative affective (and related) syndromes with functional impairment (e.g., as referenced by the American Psychiatric Association's *Diagnostic and Statistical Manual* as major depressive disorder [5] and by the *International Classification of Diseases* [6] as depressive disorders). We focus on the most recognized, contemporary evidence-based psychotherapies for depression, including traditional and newer forms of cognitive behavioral therapy, interpersonal psychotherapy, brief dynamic psychotherapy, and supportive psychotherapy. We offer a basic understanding of the potential for these depression-specific psychotherapies to promote response, remission, relapse prevention, and recovery in adults with major depressive disorder. We summarize the findings that permit these psychotherapies to be termed "evidence based," defined as clinical practices that are based on research findings. To connect these summaries with

research findings, the reader can compare the following psychotherapies in light of existing treatment metrics (e.g., effect sizes). Effect sizes for antidepressant medications are also included for comparison. For simplicity we focus on evidence-based psychotherapy as a solitary therapy but direct the reader to the literature on their efficacious use in combination with [7] or after [8] antidepressant medication.

Evidence-Based and Emerging Evidence-Based Psychotherapies for Adults with Major Depressive Disorder

Several evidence-based psychotherapies for depression are described below and summarized in Table 29.1. To differentiate these treatments, we emphasize unique aspects of their conceptualizations of depression and therapeutic processes. However, we appreciate that the treatments' average effects on depression appear similar in the current research literature [9]. We note the hypothesis that a moderate to large portion of the treatments' effects may be achieved through "common factors," although the evidence of such factors is largely indirect at this time [10]. We also note that emerging transdiagnostic therapy shows promised with effect sizes ranging from 0.65 to 0.80 (standardized mean differences in symptom scores; depending on type of comparator) even when remote, internet delivery is used [11]. We assert that these trends away from disorder-specific psychotherapy offer a potentially efficient approach not only to facilitating dissemination but also to understanding and treating the core symptoms shared among mood, anxiety, and related or comorbid disorders. We also note parallel trends in transdiagnostic neuroscience models that have identified commonalities in brain structure or function among psychiatric disorders [12].

Table 29.1 Summary of selected evidence-based psychotherapies and antidepressant medications for depression: theory and treatment metrics

1. Cognitive behavioral therapies (CBT)

1a. Cognitive therapy (CT)

Conceptualization of depression: Negatively biased information processing structures are activated by perceived stress or loss to produce depressed mood and maladaptive behavior, such as avoidance and withdrawal.

Therapeutic processes and activities: The therapist and patient collaborate to increase the patient's engagement with sources of reinforcement and adaptive functioning (behavioral activation) and then to identify and change negatively biased cognition including automatic thoughts and schema (cognitive restructuring).

Example treatment manuals or descriptions: Beck et al. (1979) [13]; Jarrett and Kraft (1997) [14]

Acute effect size estimate: SMD = 0.95 (CI 0.77–1.14)[a]; U3 = 83%[†]; U3 R = 45%[††]

Continuation/maintenance effect size estimate: RD = 0.20 (CI 0.11–0.28)[b]; NNT = 5.0[†††]

1b. Behavioral activation (BA)

Conceptualization of depression: Similar to CT but emphasizing reducing behavioral withdrawal and avoidance and increasing behavioral engagement as treatment targets.

Therapeutic processes and activities: The therapist and patient collaborate to increase the patient's engagement with sources of reinforcement and adaptive functioning. BA is a component of CT.

Example treatment manuals or descriptions: Jacobson et al. (2001) [15]; Martell et al. (2010) [16]

Acute effect size estimate: SMD = 1.05 (CI 0.80–1.30)[a]; U3 = 85%[†]; U3 R = 49%[††]

Continuation/maintenance effect size estimate: not established

1c. Mindfulness-based cognitive therapy (MBCT)

Conceptualization of depression: Dysphoria activates depressogenic cognition (e.g., rumination) and behavior (e.g., avoidance) that then escalate into a major depressive episode.

Therapeutic processes and activities: Patients learn to monitor thoughts and moods nonjudgmentally and with self-compassion, rather than assuming that negative thoughts and mood accurately match reality. Patients engage in mindfulness mediation exercises to decenter and disengage from depressogenic cognition to prevent or reduce effects of depressive cognitive content on mood and behavior.

Example treatment manuals or descriptions: Segal et al. (2013) [17]; Baer and Walsh (2016) [18]

Acute effect size estimate: SMD = 0.71 (CI 0.41–1.01)[a]; U3 = 76%[†]; U3 R = 36%[††]

Continuation/maintenance effect size estimate: RD = 0.21 (CI 0.09–0.32)[b]; NNT = 4.8[†††]

1d. Acceptance and commitment therapy (ACT)

Conceptualization of depression: Individuals' attempts to resist or control their negative thoughts and emotions are often counterproductive and lead to an increase in depressive mood and behavior.

Therapeutic processes and activities: Patients learn to accept, rather than resist or attempt to control, their negative thoughts and emotions while committing to and working toward personal goals grounded in values and adaptive functioning.

Example treatment manuals or descriptions: Hayes et al. (1999) [19]; Zettle (2007) [20]

Acute effect size estimate: SMD = 0.74 (CI 0.61–0.87)[a]; U3 = 77%[†]; U3 R = 37%[††]

Continuation/maintenance effect size estimate: not established

1e. Cognitive behavioral analysis system of psychotherapy (CBASP)

Conceptualization of depression: Depression results from immature (pre-logical, pre-causal) patterns of thinking and feeling, particularly those related to interpersonal behavior and social relationships, in which depressed persons fail to understand the consequences of their behaviors.

Therapeutic processes and activities: Patients learn to think more rationally and logically about their emotions and behaviors, including learning connections between their behaviors and outcomes of social situations, and they rehearse improved social–interpersonal skills to reach desired outcomes.

Example treatment manuals or descriptions: McCullough (2000) [21]; McCullough (2003) [22]

Acute effect size estimate: SMD = 0.42 (CI 0.08–0.76)[c]; U3 = 66%[†]; U3 R = 26%[††]

Continuation/maintenance effect size estimate: RD = 0.18[d]; NNT = 5.6[†††]

2. Interpersonal psychotherapy (IPT)

Conceptualization of depression: Depression is a medical illness (not the patient's fault) that occurs in an interpersonal context and relates to difficulty fulfilling and adjusting to social roles and resolving interpersonal losses.

Table 29.1 (cont.)

Therapeutic processes and activities: Treatment focuses on an identified area of interpersonal stress (e.g., role transition or dispute, complicated grief). The therapist facilitates the patient's expression of negative emotion, assertion of needs and wishes, and development of new skills applied in the interpersonal context.

Example treatment manuals or descriptions: Markowitz and Weissman (2004) [23]; Weissman et al. (2000) [24]

Acute effect size estimate: SMD = 0.60 (CI 0.34–0.86)[a]; U3 = 73%[†]; U3 R = 32%[††]

Continuation/maintenance effect size estimate: RD = 0.16 (CI 0.04–0.37)[b]; NNT = 6.3[†††]

3. Brief psychodynamic therapy (BPT)

Conceptualization of depression: Depression results from childhood adversity that produces inaccurate perceptions of the self and the world manifest in stress-generating thoughts and behaviors.

Therapeutic processes and activities: A supportive therapist interprets patient–therapist interactions as a means to assess and reduce discrepancies between the patient's actual and desired self and relations with the external world.

Example treatment manuals or descriptions: De Jonghe et al. (2013) [25]; Davanloo (2005) [26]; Malan (1963/2001) [27]

Acute effect size estimate: SMD = 0.39 (CI 0.16–0.62)[a]; U3 = 65%[†]; U3 R = 25%[††]

Continuation/maintenance effect size estimate: not established

4. Nondirective supportive therapy (NDST)

Conceptualization of depression: Arguably less specifically articulated but also less relevant, given the therapeutic process, than for other treatments in this table. Depression may result from adverse or unsupportive environments.

Therapeutic processes and activities: A caring, warm, and open therapist helps the patient feel listened to and understood, conveys empathy and therapeutic optimism, facilitates the patient's expression of emotion, and encourages the patient's problem solving, but does not teach a specific set of skills to regulate thought, behavior, or emotion.

Example treatment manuals or descriptions: Rogers (1961) [28]; Novalis et al. (2019) [29]

Acute effect size estimate: SMD = 0.58 (CI 0.42–0.75)[a]; U3 = 72%[†]; U3 R = 31%[††]

Continuation/maintenance effect size estimate: not established

5. Antidepressant medication plus clinical management

Conceptualization of depression: Depression is a medical illness resulting from underlying abnormal pathophysiology, typically in brain functioning.

Therapeutic process and activities: Review of signs, symptoms, and treatment effects, including side effects in the context of a supportive relationship.

Example of treatment manual: Fawcett et al. (1987) [30]

Acute effect size estimate: SMD = 0.30 (CI 0.26–0.34)[e]; U3 = 62%[†]; U3 R = 22%[††]

Continuation/maintenance effect sizes estimate: RD = 0.19 (CI 0.16–0.22)[f], NNT = 5.3[†††]

Abbreviations: SMD = standardized mean difference in symptom severity between target treatment and control groups. CI = 95% confidence interval. RD = risk difference; the absolute reduction in relapse/recurrence proportions in treatment versus control groups.

a. Cuijpers et al. (2020) [9] meta-analysis; psychotherapy versus mixed control groups (waitlist, treatment as usual [TAU], or other)

b. Biesheuvel-Leliefeld et al. (2015) [31] meta-analysis; psychotherapy versus TAU

c. Van Bronswijk et al. (2019) [32] meta-analysis; psychotherapy plus TAU versus TAU alone

d. Klein et al. (2004) [33] randomized controlled trial; CBASP versus assessment-only

e. Cipriani et al. (2018) [34] meta-analysis; medication versus pill placebo

f. Kato et al. (2021) [35] meta-analysis; medication versus pill placebo

[†] U3 is the estimated proportion of treated patients who are nominally better (lower symptom scores) than the average control patient (Cohen, 1988) [36]. U3 is derived from the preceding SMD: $U3 = \Phi(SMD)$, where Φ is the cumulative distribution function of the standard normal distribution.

[††] U3 R is the estimated proportion of treated patients who are *reliably* better (statistically significantly lower symptom scores) than the average control patient (Vittengl and Jarrett, 2014)[37]. UR3 is derived from the preceding SMD: $U3\ R = \Phi(SMD-1.07)$, where Φ is the cumulative distribution function of the standard normal distribution, and 1.07 is the reliable change index (Jacobson and Truax, 1991) [38], expressed in standard deviation units and assuming symptom measure reliability = 0.85 and two-tailed alpha = 0.05.

[†††] NNT is the number needed to treat; how many patients would need to receive the target treatment versus control to prevent one additional relapse or recurrence (Kraemer and Kupfer, 2006) [39]. NNT is derived from the preceding RD: $NNT = 1/RD$.

To quantify evidence for the efficacy of the treatments, we report effect sizes from recent meta-analyses when available. Acute-phase treatment focuses on depression symptom reduction. Accordingly, for acute-phase efficacy, we report the standardized mean difference (SMD) effect size, computed as the difference between the average symptom level of target treatment and control (e.g., treatment as usual, waitlist), divided by the standard deviation of the symptom measure. Values of 0.2, 0.5, and 0.8 are often interpreted as "small," "moderate," and "large," respectively [36]. As shown in Table 29.1, acute-phase effect sizes are mostly moderate-large for the psychotherapies reviewed here. These effect sizes are generally comparable to those observed for acute-phase antidepressant medication and resulted in both modalities being classified as first line treatment choices for patients and clinicians [40].

We report additional statistics derived from SMD that may have more intuitive interpretations. In particular, U3 is the estimated proportion of patients in the target treatment who have at least nominally lower symptoms (e.g., ≥ 1 point on the Beck Depression Inventory [BDI] [41] or Hamilton Rating for Depression [HRSD] [42]) than the average patient in the control group [36]. Similarly, UR3 is the proportion of patients in the target treatment who have *reliably* lower symptoms (e.g., $\geq 8-9$ points on the BDI or HRSD) than the average control group patient [37,43]. The U3 and U3R estimates in Table 29.1 are often roughly 70–80% and 30–40%, respectively, suggesting that most patients are helped, although fewer are helped *substantively*, by these psychotherapies. These estimates highlight the need for innovation and improvement in treatment strategies.

Continuation phase treatment aims to produce remission within and prevent relapse of the index episode, while maintenance phase treatment seeks to promote full recovery without the emergence of a new episode or a recurrence. To quantify continuation/maintenance treatment effects, we report the absolute risk difference (RD) effect size, computed as the difference between proportions of patients relapsing/recurring in target treatment versus control groups [39]. Values of 0.1, 0.3, and 0.5 might be interpreted as "small," "moderate," and "large," respectively. Available RD estimates are all small-moderate (see Table 29.1), and we note the opportunity for several reviewed treatments to be systemically tested in continuation or maintenance phases and thus fill the

existing gaps in Table 29.1. Computed from RD, we also reported the "number needed to treat" (NNT), an estimate of how many patients would need to be treated with the target treatment instead of control (e.g., no additional treatment, treatment as usual, clinical management) to prevent an additional relapse/recurrence. Most NNT values are 5–6, suggesting that prevention is substantive but far from assured. These effect sizes reflect outcomes comparable to or better than continuation/maintenance antidepressant medication [31,40].

Cognitive behavioral therapies (CBTs) for depression share efforts to mitigate relations among depressive cognitive content, mood, and functional behavior but vary in conceptual and therapeutic emphases. A frequently researched and prototypical CBT is Beck's cognitive therapy (CT) [13]. This time-limited acute-phase treatment (e.g., 16–20 one-hour sessions over 3–4 months) includes both behavioral activation and cognitive restructuring in the context of a collaborative relationship between the patient and therapist. In particular, CT aims first to increase patients' adaptive behavior and engagement with sources of reinforcement (e.g., at work, leisure, social relationships), while also identifying and changing depressive cognition, such as negative automatic thoughts (e.g., "I'm no good, I always lose.") and schema (broader views about the self, world, and future; e.g., "To be truly happy, I must be loved by all").

As shown in Table 29.1, acute-phase CT lowers mean depressive symptom levels to a large extent compared to control groups (SMD = 0.95). Roughly 8 in 10 CT patients are nominally better (U3 = 83%), and nearly half are reliably better (U3 R = 45%), than the average control group patient. Cognitive therapy modifications or extensions have also been developed to prevent relapse [44]. For example, Jarrett and colleagues first reported that an 8-month, 10-session continuation-phase treatment [45] produced preventive effects superior to assessment-only [46,47] or pill placebo [48] and comparable to continuation antidepressant medication [48]. Absolute reduction in proportions of patients relapsing with continuation CT versus control average roughly 20% (RD = 0.20), equivalent to NNT = 5.

Behavioral activation (BA), a component of CT, has been tested as a stand-alone treatment for depression (see Table 29.1). Acute-phase effect sizes for BA and CT appear comparable [9]. Some suggest that this is indirect evidence for nonspecific factors common to both BA and CT plus specific BA processes may account for CT's acute-phase benefits [10,15]. It is also recognized that since overt and covert behaviors are correlated, it is difficult to influence one without affecting the other. The research base is not as well developed for acute-phase BA, and BA has not yet been tested rigorously as a continuation or maintenance treatment for depression.

Newer forms of CBT have also shown to be helpful as acute and/or continuation/maintenance treatments for depression (see Table 29.1). These so-called third-wave CBTs include mindfulness-based cognitive behavioral therapy (MBCT) and acceptance and commitment therapy (ACT).

Different from traditional CT that focuses on identifying and modifying negatively biased cognition and behavior with undesired consequences, MBCT teaches patients to experience or observe their mood and thoughts, and possibly to simply note depression-related cognitive content (e.g., negative automatic thoughts, rumination) without reaction outside of mindfulness meditation. By changing patients' reactions to negative thoughts, depressive mood and other symptoms are hypothesized to decrease in MBCT. This treatment can be provided in a group format, including 8 weekly sessions lasting 2–2.5 hours each, sometimes followed by less frequent booster sessions. (mindful meditations, with similarities to MBCT, can also be accessed through adjunctive online resources in vivo and on demand, which may increase its potential if shown to be "generically" effective and without substantial risk for selected patients). Initially developed as a continuation/maintenance treatment [49], MBCT has been tested as an acute-phase treatment as well [50,51]. Acute and continuation/maintenance effects of MBCT appear comparable to those for CT (see Table 29.1).

Broadly similar to MBCT, ACT aims to teach patients to accept negative emotions and distance themselves from the experience of cognitive content, rather than attempting to change these experiences, while also working toward personally valued goals for committed and adaptive functioning. For example, ACT patients may practice "cognitive diffusion" to become nonjudgmentally mindful of themselves and their external circumstances, while also being committed to behavior that reflects their stated values. Although components of ACT and MBCT potentially overlap, delivery of ACT appears to have been tested in more formats (e.g., individual, group, self-help)

and variable durations (e.g., 1–30 sessions) [52–54]. While the number of studies is smaller, the emerging efficacy of acute-phase ACT suggests similarity to CT. Although ACT has yet to be rigorously evaluated as a continuation or maintenance treatment, ACT may reduce residual symptoms of MDD [55].

Cognitive behavioral analysis system of psychotherapy (CBASP) was developed specifically for adults with chronic depression (e.g., major depressive disorder lasting 2 or more years, dysthymia, or persistent mood disorder) [21]. This treatment is based in developmental and psychodynamic theories, conceptualizing depression as a consequence of immature (childlike) thinking and social behavior. Patients receiving CBASP learn to make their thinking more rational and to improve their social–interpersonal functioning based on the consequences they experience in implementing actions planned during therapy. Specifically, CBASP teaches patients to differentiate between actual versus desired outcomes in interpersonal situations, understand the consequences of their behavior, improve the accuracy of their views of the therapist by differentiating patients' historical reactions to influential persons (e.g., parents), and practice new skills to reach desired social–interpersonal outcomes. This treatment has been time limited in clinical trials (e.g., 20–32 sessions over 4–12 months) [33,56], although CBASP was developed to be provided through remission without imposing time limits [22]. The focus of CBASP on chronic and treatment-resistant depression may help explain the somewhat smaller acute-phase effect size (SMD = 0.42) compared to other CBTs (see Table 29.1). The continuation/maintenance effect size estimate (RD = 0.18) is based on a single randomized clinical trial [33]; thus, additional research is needed to clarify the benefit of CBASP for patients who have responded or remitted.

Interpersonal psychotherapy (IPT) was developed as part of an early randomized clinical trial of depression treatments [57] and has conceptual roots in psychodynamic and developmental theories relevant to depression (e.g., concerning attachment, grief, early relationships) [58]. From IPT's perspective, depression is medical illness, avoiding blame and stigma for symptoms, while also emphasizing the bidirectional influences within the social–interpersonal environment. During IPT, interpersonal assessment first identifies a current problem area (e.g., bereavement, conflict with others about a new or ongoing social role as a spouse, parent, child, worker) that becomes the focus of treatment. The IPT therapist offers guidance and reinforcement for developing, rehearsing, and troubleshooting application of new skills to solve the interpersonal problem. This treatment is typically time limited (e.g., 16–20 sessions over 3–4 months) and can be applied as an acute or continuation/maintenance treatment with effect sizes comparable to CT (see Table 29.1).

Brief psychodynamic therapy (BPT) includes a number of related treatments [25–27] that are not distinguished here. These BPTs view depression as the product of early adversity (e.g., physical and/or emotional, particularly from caregivers), perhaps in combination with biological vulnerabilities. Early adverse experiences are hypothesized to lead to depressogenic misperceptions of the self and the external world, which are reinforced by current behaviors that generate further stress and dissatisfaction [59]. Treatment with BPT is time limited (e.g., 10–30 sessions over 10–26 weeks) [60] and supportive, rather than attempting fundamental personality change, as in traditional long-term psychoanalysis. The active BPT therapist focuses on improving the patient's relations to the self and world, using interpretation of the therapeutic relationship and in-session behaviors to address problematic styles of thinking, emoting, and behaving. Perhaps in part because the treatment aims to be curative [25], BPT has been tested primarily as an acute-phase rather than as continuation/maintenance treatment for depression. Although BPD's acute-phase SMD (0.39) appears somewhat lower than those for CBTs, differences were not statistically significant in a recent meta-analysis [9].

Nondirective supportive psychotherapy (NDSP) has several potentially distinguishable variants [61] that we collapse here to simplify. Historically, NDSP was sometimes provided to patients deemed unlikely to benefit from psychoanalysis, although Rogers developed NDSP as a first-choice treatment [28]. Current conceptualizations of NDSP emphasize "common factors," such as an open, warm, affirming therapist who conveys therapeutic optimism, understanding, and empathy, facilitates the patient's expression of affect, and encourages the patient's problem solving [56,62]. The therapist may provide basic education about depression (e.g., defining symptoms and related psychosocial issues) but does not actively educate the patient in a specific set of skills or techniques. In randomized clinical trials, NDSP produced acute-phase outcomes superior to control groups

and not significantly different from CBTs, IPT, or BPT [9]. However, NDSP has not been tested rigorously as a continuation- or maintenance-phase treatment for depression.

Conclusion

Evidence-based psychotherapies offer patients and clinicians opportunities to treat the symptoms and functioning impairment of depression with and without adjunctive antidepressant medication, in person or remotely with individuals or groups of adults. Using a collaborative, shared decision-making partnership [63] that emphasizes the evidence-based options for the acute, continuation, and maintenance phases of treatment of depression allows the clinician and patient to make informed choices based on data, preference, and practicalities.

The findings herein are based on existing studies. As the databases and sample sizes increase in number and diversity, it may be possible to better understand any potential differences in efficacy among psychotherapies (along with delivery platforms), which patients have the best outcomes with a given psychotherapy, which psychotherapies are easiest for patients and providers to learn, and what critical components of each therapy are best disseminated through which methods. As findings increase, it will also become apparent where transdiagnostic psychotherapies fit in the available array of evidence-based choices. Such an understanding (informed by progress in neuroscience and public health) will not only advance a mechanistic understanding of how evidence-based psychotherapy for depression and related disorders work, but also will allow the most important elements of these treatment strategies to be disseminated and made accessible both within health systems and in communities worldwide.

Acknowledgement

We appreciate the editorial assistance of Karen Meltzer and Ofelia Chapa in formatting the citations for this chapter.

References

1. World Health Organization. Depression and other common mental disorders: global health estimates. 2017. Available at: www.who.int/publications-detail-redirect/depression-global-health-estimates (Accessed May 14, 2021)

2. M. Olfson, S.C. Marcus. National trends in outpatient psychotherapy. *Am J Psychiatry* 2010; **167**(12):1456–63.

3. R.K. McHugh, S.W. Whitton, A.D. Peckham, J.A. Welge, M.W. Otto. Patient preference for psychological vs pharmacologic treatment of psychiatric disorders: a meta-analytic review. *J Clin Psychiatry* 2013; **74**(6):595–602.

4. G. Gartlehner, B.N. Gaynes, H.R. Amick, et al. Comparative benefits and harms of antidepressant, psychological, complementary, and exercise treatments for major depression: an evidence report for a clinical practice guideline from the American college of physicians. *Ann Intern Med* 2016; **164** (5):331–41.

5. American Psychiatric Association. *Diagnostic and Statistical Manual of Mental Disorders: DSM-5*. 5th ed. Washington, DC: American Psychiatric Association, 2013.

6. World Health Organization. ICD 11: classifying disease to map the way we live and die. 2018. Available at: www.who.int/news-room/spotlight/int ernational-classification-of-diseases (Accessed May 14, 2021).

7. P. Cuijpers, L. de Wit, E. Weitz, G. Andersson, M.J.H. Huibers. The combination of psychotherapy and pharmacotherapy in the treatment of adult depression: a comprehensive meta-analysis. *J Evid-Based Psychother* 2015; **15**(2):147–68.

8. B.W. Dunlop, D. LoParo, B. Kinkead, et al. Benefits of sequentially adding cognitive-behavioral therapy or antidepressant medication for adults with nonremitting depression. *Am J Psychiatry* 2019; **176** (4):275–86.

9. P. Cuijpers, E. Karyotaki, L. de Wit, D.D. Ebert. The effects of fifteen evidence-supported therapies for adult depression: a meta-analytic review. *J Soc Psychother Res* 2020; **30**(3):279–93.

10. P. Cuijpers, M. Reijnders, M.J. H. Huibers. The role of common factors in psychotherapy outcomes. *Annu Rev Clin Psychol* 2019; **15**(1):207–31.

11. J.M. Newby, A. McKinnon, W. Kuyken, S. Gilbody, T. Dalgleish. Systematic review and meta-analysis of transdiagnostic psychological treatments for anxiety and depressive disorders in adulthood. *Clin Psychol Rev* 2015; **40**:91–110.

12. M. Goodkind, S.B. Eickhoff, D.J. Oathes, et al. Identification of a common neurobiological substrate for mental illness. *JAMA Psychiatry* 2015; **72**(4):305–15.

13. A.T. Beck, A.J. Rush, B.F. Shaw, G. Emery. *Cognitive Therapy of Depression*. New York: Guilford Press, 1979.

14. R.B. Jarrett, D. Kraft. Prophylactic cognitive therapy for major depressive disorder. *Sess Psychother Pract* 1997; **3**(3):65–79.

15. N.S. Jacobson, C.R. Martell, S. Dimidjian. Behavioral activation treatment for depression: returning to contextual roots. *Clin Psychol Sci Pract* 2001; **8**(3):255.

16. C.R. Martell, S. Dimidjian, R. Herman-Dunn. *Behavioral Activation for Depression: A Clinician's Guide*. New York: Guilford Press, 2010.

17. Z.V. Segal, J.M.G. Williams, J.D. Teasdale. *Mindfulness-Based Cognitive Therapy for Depression: A New Approach to Preventing Relapse*. 2nd ed. New York : Guilford Press, 2013.

18. R. Baer, E. Walsh. Treating acute depression with mindfulness-based cognitive therapy – treating depression. In A. Wells, P. Fisher, editors. *Treating Depression: MCT, CBT and Third Wave Therapies*. West Sussex: Wiley-Blackwell, 2016; 344–68. Available at: https://onlinelibrary-wiley-com.foyer.s wmed.edu/doi/abs/10.1002/9781119114482.ch14 (Accessed May 12, 2021).

19. S.C. Hayes, K.D. Strosahl, K.G. Wilson. *Acceptance and Commitment Therapy: An Experiential Approach to Behavior Change*. New York: Guilford Press, 1999.

20. R.D. Zettle. *ACT for Depression: A Clinician's Guide to Using Acceptance & Commitment Therapy in Treating Depression*. Oakland: New Harbinger, 2007.

21. J.P. McCullough. *Treatment for Chronic Depression: Cognitive behavioral Analysis System of Psychotherapy*. New York: Guilford Press, 2000.

22. J.P. McCullough. Treatment for chronic depression using cognitive behavioral analysis system of psychotherapy (CBASP). *J Clin Psychol* 2003; **59** (8):833–46.

23. J.C. Markowitz, M.M. Weissman. Interpersonal psychotherapy: principles and applications. *World Psychiatry* 2004; **3**(3):136–9.

24. M.M. Weissman, J.C. Markowitz, G.L. Klerman. *Comprehensive Guide to Interpersonal Psychotherapy*. New York: Basic Books, 2000.

25. F. de Jonghe, S. de Maat, R. Van, et al. Short-term psychoanalytic supportive psychotherapy for depressed patients. *Psychoanal Inq* 2013; **33**(6): 614–25.

26. H. Davanloo. *Intensive Short-Term Dynamic Psychotherapy*. Philadelphia: Lippincott Williams & Wilkins, 2005.

27. D. Malan. *A Study of Brief Psychotherapy*. New York: Routledge, 1963/2001.

28. C.R. Rogers. *On Becoming a Person: A Therapist's View of Psychotherapy*. Boston: Houghton Mifflin, 1961.

29. P.M. Novalis, V. Singer, R. Peele. *Clinical Manual of Supportive Psychotherapy*. 2nd ed. Washington, DC: American Psychiatric Association; 2019.

30. J. Fawcett, P. Epstein, S.J. Fiester, I. Elkin, J.H. Autry. Clinical management–imipramine/placebo administration manual. NIMH treatment of depression collaborative research program. *Psychopharmacol Bull* 1987; **23**(2):309–24.

31. K.E.M. Biesheuvel-Leliefeld, G.D. Kok, C.L.H. Bockting, et al. Effectiveness of psychological interventions in preventing recurrence of depressive disorder: meta-analysis and meta-regression. *J Affect Disord* 2015; **174**:400–10.

32. S. van Bronswijk, D. Moopen, L. Beijers, H.G. Ruhe, F. Peeters. Effectiveness of psychotherapy for treatment-resistant depression: a meta-analysis and meta-regression. *Psychol Med* 2019; **49**(3):366–79.

33. D.N. Klein, N.J. Santiago, D. Vivian, et al. Cognitive behavioral analysis system of psychotherapy as a maintenance treatment for chronic depression. *J Consult Clin Psychol* 2004; **72**(4):681–8.

34. A. Cipriani, T.A. Furukawa, G. Salanti, et al. Comparative efficacy and acceptability of 21 antidepressant drugs for the acute treatment of adults with major depressive disorder: a systematic review and network meta-analysis. *Lancet* 2018; **391** (10128):1357–66.

35. M. Kato, H. Hori, T. Inoue, et al. Discontinuation of antidepressants after remission with antidepressant medication in major depressive disorder: a systematic review and meta-analysis. *Mol Psychiatry* 2021; **26** (1):118–33.

36. J. Cohen. *Statistical Power Analysis for the Behavioral Sciences*. 2nd ed. Hillsdale, NJ: Erlbaum; 1988.

37. J.R. Vittengl, R.B. Jarrett. Major depressive disorder. In S.G. Hoffman, W. Rief, editors. *The Wiley Handbook of Cognitive Behavioral Therapy*. New York: Wiley-Blackwell, 2014; 1131–60. Available at: https://onlinelibrary.wiley.com/doi/ab s/10.1002/9781118528563.wbcbt48 (Accessed May 17, 2021).

38. N.S. Jacobson, P. Truax. Clinical significance: a statistical approach to defining meaningful change in psychotherapy research. *J Consult Clin Psychol* 1991; **59**(1):12.

39. H.C. Kraemer, D.J. Kupfer. Size of treatment effects and their importance to clinical research and practice. *Biol Psychiatry* 2006; **59**(11):990–6.

40. American Psychological Association. APA clinical practice guideline for the treatment of depression across three age cohorts. Available at www.apa.org/d epression-guideline (Accessed May 12, 2021).

41. A.T. Beck, C.H. Ward, M. Mendelson, J. Mock. Erbaugh. An inventory for measuring depression. *Arch Gen Psychiatry* 1961; **4**:561–71.

42. M. Hamilton. A rating scale for depression. *J Neurol Neurosurg Psychiatry* 1960; **23**(1):56–62.

43. R.B. Jarrett, J.R. Vittengl. Efficacy of cognitive-behavioral therapy for depression. In P.L. Fisher, A. Wells, editors. *Treating Depression: Principles and Practice of MCT, CBT, and Third Wave Therapies*. New York: Wiley, 2016; 52–80.

44. C.L. Bockting, S.D. Hollon, R.B. Jarrett, W. Kuyken, D. Dobson. A lifetime approach to major depressive disorder: the contributions of psychological interventions in preventing relapse and recurrence. *Clin Psychol Rev* 2015; **41**:16–26.

45. R.B. Jarrett, J.R. Vittengl, L.A. Clark. Preventing recurrent depression. In M.A. Whisman, editor. *Adapting Cognitive Therapy for Depression: Managing Complexity and Comorbidity*. New York: Guilford Press, 2008; 132–56.

46. R.B. Jarrett, M.R. Basco, R. Risser, et al. Is there a role for continuation phase cognitive therapy for depressed outpatients? *J Consult Clin Psychol* 1998; **66** (6):1036–40.

47. R.B. Jarrett, D. Kraft, J. Doyle, et al. Preventing recurrent depression using cognitive therapy with and without a continuation phase: a randomized clinical trial. *Arch Gen Psychiatry* 2001; **58**(4):381.

48. R.B. Jarrett, A. Minhajuddin, H. Gershenfeld, E.S. Friedman, M.E. Thase. Preventing depressive relapse and recurrence in higher-risk cognitive therapy responders: a randomized trial of continuation phase cognitive therapy, fluoxetine, or matched pill placebo. *JAMA Psychiatry* 2013; **70**(11):1152.

49. J.D. Teasdale, Z.V. Segal, J.M.G. Williams, et al. Prevention of relapse/recurrence in major depression by mindfulness-based cognitive therapy. *J Consult Clin Psychol* 2000; **68**(4):615–23.

50. J.R. van Aalderen, A.R.T. Donders, F. Giommi, et al. The efficacy of mindfulness-based cognitive therapy in recurrent depressed patients with and without a current depressive episode: a randomized controlled trial. *Psychol Med* 2012; **42**(5):989–1001.

51. M. de Jong, F. Peeters, T. Gard, et al. A randomized controlled pilot study on mindfulness-based cognitive therapy for unipolar depression in patients with chronic pain. *J Clin Psychiatry* 2018; **79**(1):26–34.

52. E.M. Forman, J.D. Herbert, E. Moitra, P.D. Yeomans, P.A. Geller. A randomized controlled effectiveness trial of acceptance and commitment therapy and cognitive therapy for anxiety and depression. *Behav Modif* 2007; **31**(6):72–99.

53. E.B. Kroska, A.I. Roche, M.W. O'Hara. How much is enough in brief acceptance and commitment therapy? A randomized trial. *J Context Behav Sci* 2020; **15**:235–44.

54. M. Fledderus, E.T. Bohlmeijer, M.E. Pieterse, K.M.G. Schreurs. Acceptance and commitment therapy as guided self-help for psychological distress and positive mental health: a randomized controlled trial. *Psychol Med* 2012; **42**(3):485–95.

55. T. Østergaard, T. Lundgren, I. Rosendahl, et al. Acceptance and commitment therapy preceded by attention bias modification on residual symptoms in depression: a 12-month follow-up. *Front Psychol* 2019; **10**.

56. E. Schramm, L. Kriston, I. Zobel, et al. Effect of disorder-specific vs nonspecific psychotherapy for chronic depression: a randomized clinical trial. *JAMA Psychiatry* 2017; **74**(3):233–42.

57. G.L. Klerman, A. Dimascio, M. Weissman, B. Prusoff, E.S. Paykel. Treatment of depression by drugs and psychotherapy. *Am J Psychiatry* 1974; **131**(2):186–91.

58. J.C. Markowitz, M.M. Weissman. Interpersonal psychotherapy: past, present and future. *Clin Psychol Psychother* 2012; **19**(2):99–105.

59. P. Luyten, S.J. Blatt. Psychodynamic treatment of depression. *Psychiatr Clin North Am* 2012; **35** (1):111–29.

60. E. Driessen, J.J.M. Dekker, J. Peen, et al. The efficacy of adding short-term psychodynamic psychotherapy to antidepressants in the treatment of depression: a systematic review and meta-analysis of individual participant data. *Clin Psychol Rev* 2020; **80**:1–10.

61. J.C. Markowitz. What is supportive psychotherapy? *Focus* 2014; **12**(3):285–9.

62. J.H. Kocsis, A.J. Gelenberg, B.O. Rothbaum, et al. Cognitive behavioral analysis system of psychotherapy and brief supportive psychotherapy for augmentation of antidepressant nonresponse in chronic depression: the REVAMP trial. *Arch Gen Psychiatry* 2009; **66**(11):1178–88.

63. E. Duncan, C. Best, S. Hagen. Shared decision making interventions for people with mental health conditions. *Cochrane Database Syst Rev* 2010;**2010**(1): CD007297.

Chapter 30

Rating Instruments for Mood Disorders in Clinical Practice

Danielle Hett and Steven Marwaha

Introduction

"Mood disorders" is a broad term used to refer to several types of mental disorders that primarily affect a person's mood and associated functioning. In the *Diagnostic and Statistical Manual of Mental Disorders* (DSM-5) [1], mood disorders are now grouped separately into depressive and bipolar disorders, with the main disorders being Major Depressive Disorder (MDD), Bipolar I Disorder, Bipolar II Disorder and other conditions such as cyclothymic disorder. In brief, individuals with MDD (often referred to as clinical depression) experience periods of intense sadness and feelings of hopelessness, alongside deficits in their physical and cognitive functioning, such as trouble sleeping or having a poor appetite and concentration. In bipolar disorders, individuals experience intense mood swings, fluctuating from extreme lows (i.e., depression) to extreme highs – often referred to as mania. Mania can be defined as a "persistently elevated, expansive, or irritable mood" lasting for at least one week and be present most of the day, nearly every day [1]. However, some individuals may experience a milder form of mania, known as hypomania, whereby the symptoms only need to last for four consecutive days. To be diagnosed with bipolar I disorder, individuals must have experienced at least one episode of mania, whereas those considered to have bipolar II disorder must have had at least one episode of current or past hypomania and at least one episode of current or past major depression. Both depressive and bipolar disorders are among some of the leading causes of disability worldwide [2], and unfortunately both are often under-recognised and misdiagnosed.

One way to support the timely and accurate assessment of these mood disorders is via the use of valid, reliable, sensitive to change, effective and user-friendly ratings tools. Further, evaluation of the effectiveness of treatments tends to rely heavily on changes in symptoms, thus the use of reliable ratings tools is imperative, whether for research studies or at the clinical interface.

Several rating scales exist for both depressive and bipolar disorders and can typically be divided into either clinician-rated (i.e., completed by the clinician only), self-rated (i.e., completed by the patient) or in some cases, a mixture of both [3].

This chapter will discuss some of the most widely used rating tools for both depressive and bipolar disorders and outline the evidence supporting their psychometric properties (e.g., validity, reliability, sensitivity) and practicality (e.g., user-friendly) for use in research and clinical practice. Following this, the chapter will highlight additional rating tools that are playing an emerging role in mood disorders research and clinical practice, such as those assessing for affective instability, a core trait-like feature known to underpin the development and emergence of mood disorder symptoms, and the use of digital mood-monitoring tools. Lastly, this chapter will conclude with a summary of the current ratings tools and their future role in clinical practice.

Rating Instruments for Major Depressive Disorder (MDD)

Clinician-Rated Instruments

Hamilton Depression Rating Scale (HDRS/HAM-D)

One of the most widely used clinician-administered rating tools for depression is the Hamilton Depression Rating Scale (HDRS), also known as the HAM-D [4]. The HDRS is designed to be administered during a clinical interview with a patient, and clinicians rate the intensity or frequency of depressive symptoms based on their observations of the patient during the interview. Two versions of the HDRS exist, one composed of 17 items (original version) and the other of 21 items, with the 17-item version most typically used in practice. Items assess depressive symptoms and are defined by anchor point descriptions that increase in severity on a scale of 0 (e.g., "*absent*") to 4 (e.g., "*patient reports virtually only these feeling states in his/her spontaneous verbal and non-verbal communication*"). A score ≤ 7 is considered to be within the normal range or indicate clinical remission, whereas scores of > 20 are deemed indicative of moderate to severe depression. In research studies, two HDRS outcomes are deemed important to mark a clinically significant change in scores. The first is response to treatment, marked by a 50% reduction in HDRS total scores from baseline to trial end and the other is remission, which is typically characterised by a score of 7 or less on the HDRS total score [5]. Authors report good internal consistency (0.76–0.92) and inter-rater reliability (0.87–0.95). However, it is not without its limitations, namely, it has been argued that the HDRS represents a multidimensional measure of depression, as opposed to a measure of the core symptoms of depression [6], and because of this, its sensitivity to change has been challenged [7,8].

The Montgomery–Asberg Depression Rating Scale (MADRS)

The Montgomery–Asberg Depression Rating Scale (MADRS) consists of 10 items aimed at evaluating depression symptoms (e.g., "*apparent sadness*"; "*reduced appetite*"; "*concentration difficulties*") [9]. Each item is rated using an associated severity scale from 0 ("*no abnormality*") to 6 ("*severe*"), with higher scores indicating greater severity. Nine of these items are based on patient report, with the final item based on the rater's observation during the interview. Research shows that the MADRS has high inter-rater reliability (0.89–0.97), which is maintained even when being tested among raters from different disciplines (e.g., nurse vs. psychiatrist) [10]. It also has the added benefit of being easy to administer, taking approximately 15–20 minutes to complete. The MADRS is considered to be superior to the HDRS [11] as unlike the HDRS, it does not focus largely on somatic symptoms of depression, but rather on more core mood symptoms such as sadness, pessimistic thoughts and tension. Consequently, the MADRS has been designed to be particularly sensitive to changes in treatment effects and is frequently used within randomised controlled trials (RCTs) and clinical practice.

Self-Rated Instruments

Beck Depression Inventory (BDI)

Currently one of the most widely used self-report depression scales is the Beck Depression Inventory (BDI) [12]. This 21-item scale examines key symptoms of depression including mood, pessimism, sense of failure, self-dissatisfaction, guilt, punishment, self-dislike and suicidality, among many others. Each item is rated on a 4-point scale, ranging from 0 (*least*) to 3 (*most*), with total summed scores ranging from 0–63 and higher scores indicating greater depressive symptoms and total scores of 14–19, 20–28 and 29–63 are regarded as mild, moderate and severe depression, respectively [12]. Two subscales can be calculated from the BDI, including a cognitive-affective subscale and a somatic-performance subscale. Research has consistently shown the BDI to have good internal consistency (0.9) and test-retest reliability (0.73–0.96) [13], including across a range of populations such as adult inpatients, adult outpatients and adolescents [14–16]. It is also found to demonstrate acceptable sensitivity and specificity in detecting depression, further supporting its use as a diagnostic tool in clinical practice [17], although further research on its sensitivity and specificity properties is needed. Overall, the BDI is considered a reliable, user-friendly and cost-effective tool to assess symptoms of depression.

Patient Health Questionnaire (PHQ-9)

The Patient Health Questionnaire (PHQ-9) is a rapid and widely used tool to detect and monitor the severity of depression symptoms [18]. The PHQ-9 consists of nine items, and each one assesses for a symptom of depression (e.g., "*little interest or pleasure in doing things?*") and patients answer each item by rating how often they have felt this way over the past two weeks, using a scale of 0 (not at all) to 3 (nearly every day). The agreed standard cut-off for depression is a total score of ≥ 10 [18–20]. Although originally developed to be used in primary care settings, it has been well used within community-based settings [21] and has been translated into several languages and used worldwide. It has good internal consistency (Cronbach's alphas 0.70–0.93) [22–24], sensitivity and specificity [25].

Quick Inventory of Depressive Symptomology (QIDS)

The Quick Inventory of Depressive Symptomology (QIDS) [26] is a brief 16-item scale developed from the 30-item Inventory of Depressive Symptomology [27] to assess for nine depression symptom domains outlined in the DSM (i.e., sadness, concentration, self-criticism, suicidal ideation, interest, energy/fatigue, sleep disturbance, appetite, agitation). Symptoms are assessed in relation to the past seven days, and total scores range from 0 to 27, with higher scores indicating a more severe depression. A meta-analysis ($N = 37$ studies; $N = 17,118$ participants) assessing the psychometric properties of the QIDS concluded that the QIDS is a unidimensional tool with acceptable consistency; however, it highlighted that more studies outside of the United States are needed to justify the increased use of QIDS in clinical practice [28]. Additionally, the QIDS is found to correlate highly ($r = 0.86$) with and have comparable sensitivity to that of the HDRS [26].

Rating Instruments for Bipolar Disorder

Clinician-Rated Instruments for Bipolar Mania

The Young Mania Rating Scale (YMRS)

The most commonly used mania scale is the Young Mania Rating Scale (YMRS) [29]. This 11-item scale is based on a patient's subjective report of their condition over the previous 48 hours, with additional information being included based on the clinician's observation of the patient during the clinical interview. Each of the 11 items (e.g., *"elevated mood"*; *"sleep"*; *"irritability"*) uses a 5-point severity scale, each with definitions. For instance, with the elevated mood item, a rating of 0 relates to *"absent"*, whereas a rating of 4 relates to *"euphoric, inappropriate laughter, singing"*. Four of the 11 items are graded on a scale of 0 to 8 (i.e., *"irritability"*, *"speech"*, *"thought content"* and *"disruptive/aggressive behaviour"*) and are given twice the weight of the other items. Scores of 20 are considered mild mania, and this is the usually the threshold score used for inclusion in clinical trials [30], whereas scores of 26 and 38 are considered moderate and severe mania, respectively. However, other cut-offs for clinically relevant manic symptoms are also recommended in sub-populations research, such as scores of ≥ 9 [31,32]. Authors report good inter-rater reliability (0.93) and good internal reliability (Cronbach's alpha coefficients 0.80–0.91) [29], and further research has found the YMRS to have high sensitivity (0.93) [33]. There are several benefits to the YMRS as it is widely adopted (allowing for comparison of study results), brief (approximately 15–30 minutes) and easy to use.

The Clinical Global Impression-Bipolar (CGI-BP)

The Clinical Global Impression-Bipolar (CGI-BP) tool [34] was adapted from the Clinical Global Impression scale to assess global illness severity and changes in patients with bipolar disorder. It includes three core bipolar symptom scales: mania, depression and an overall scale. Each of these scales is rated separately on global severity, change from baseline and changes from the worst self-nominated phase of a patient's current episode. The CGI-BD has many advantages as a rating tool as it is quick to administer (< 5 minutes) and allows for a global consideration of all aspects of a patient's mental health condition and behaviour. To ensure that clinicians administer and complete the CGI-BD in a comparable way (i.e., improved inter-rater agreement), authors have developed user guides. Interclass correlations for mania, depression and overall severity are found to be good (> 0.93).

Longitudinal Interval Follow-up Evaluation (LIFE)

The Longitudinal Interval Follow-up Evaluation (LIFE) [35] is a gold standard tool used to assess the longitudinal course and morbidity of psychiatric disorders. The LIFE consists of a semi-structured interview to assess for key psychosocial, psychopathological and treatment information over a given follow-up period. At the start of the interview, participants are reminded of the beginning and end-point dates for which the assessment period is referring, and similar to its use for other psychiatric disorders, when the LIFE is used to assess depressive and bipolar disorders, participants are prompted for their retrospective recollections of DSM-IV symptoms they had during the nominated time period (e.g., 16 weeks [36]). At this point, the interviewer rates the weekly level of psychopathology that occurred during the time period and assigns a weekly score for each mood syndrome using a 7-point scale from 0 (*"no symptoms at all"*) to 6 (*"full criteria met; very severe"*). The LIFE has sound psychometric properties, including good internal consistency [37], high intraclass correlation coefficients for rating changes in symptoms [35] and test-retest reliability [38].

Clinician-Rated Instruments for Bipolar Depression

Compared to the rating tools developed to assess symptoms of bipolar mania, there is a paucity of research and tools designed to specifically assess bipolar depressive symptoms. This is concerning, given that patients with bipolar frequently experience depressive episodes compared to manic [39,40]. Typically, bipolar depression is rated using either the HDRS [41] or the MADRS [9], both of which were developed for assessing unipolar depressive symptoms, and they fail to assess the full spectrum of depression symptoms that may be more commonly observed in bipolar depression, such as hypersomnia. Further, these tools fail to distinguish bipolar depression that may occur with mixed and atypical symptoms [42]. To address the lack of specificity found in the HDRS and MADRS for bipolar depression, new rating tools have been developed, namely, the Bipolar Depression Rating Scale (BDRS) [43].

Bipolar Depression Rating Scale (BDRS)

The Bipolar Depression Rating Scale (BDRS) [43] consists of brief (i.e., 15 minutes) 20-item scale designed to specifically assess for bipolar depressive symptoms. Symptom severity for each item (e.g., "*reduced energy and activity*"; "*reduced social engagement*"; "*anhedonia*") is assessed using a 4-item scale of 0 (*no symptoms present*) to 3 (*severe symptoms*), and the authors have developed a semi-structured scoring manual for clinicians, providing operationalised anchor points to help aid inter-rater reliability. Authors report that the BDRS appears to have good internal consistency (Cronbach's alpha of 0.92) and strong correlations with other well-known reliable tools such as the MADRS ($r = 0.91$) and the HAM-D ($r = -0.74$). It has also been found to be sensitive to change in the context of clinical trials [44], as well as being sensitive to the examination of depressive symptoms present in both depressive and mixed episode states [45].

Self-Rated Instruments

Internal State Scale (ISS)

The Internal State Scale (ISS) [3] is a 15-item self-report measure that captures individuals' subjective mood experiences using a Likert-type scale, and unlike other measures, it does not focus on the typical symptoms of (hypo)mania as outlined in the DSM-5 (e.g., decreased sleep). To complete the ISS, respondents are asked to read each of the 15 statements relating to their mood (e.g., "*today my mood is changeable*", "*today I feel irritable*", "*today I feel impulsive*") and rate on an 11-point scale (0 = *not at all/ rarely*, to 100 = *very much so/ much of the time*) the extent to which that statement aligns with their mood over the past 24 hours. The final statement refers to a global mood item, whereby respondents are asked to

rate how they feel using an 11-point scale (0 = *depressed* to 100 = *manic*), with a mid-point marker of "*normal*". It is composed of four principal components yielding four subscales: Activation, Wellbeing, Perceived Conflict, Depression Index. Both the Activation and Wellbeing subscales can be used to determine mood state in BD (i.e., euthymia/(hypo)manic, mixed state, depression) and the Activation, Depression Index and Perceived Conflict subscales can be used to capture symptom severity. The ISS is deemed to be a reliable and promising self-rating tool for (hypo)mania [46] and is found to correlate highly with clinician ratings of mania and depression (Cronbach's alpha 0.81–0.92) [3]. Meyer et al.'s [46] review paper found 13 independent studies offering evidence for the validity and reliability of the ISS, including evidence for its test-retest reliability [47,48] and its internal consistency [3,49,50].

An important marker of validity for clinical practice is sensitivity to change and the ISS yields promising results in this domain also. For instance, Bauer and colleagues [3] reported that in both healthy controls and patients, mood state was associated with ISS scores over time. That is, when individuals remained in the same mood state, no significant changes were found in the ISS scores; however, when manic patients become euthymic/depressed, ISS scores decreased, a finding that has since been replicated [51].

Altman Self-Rating Mania Scale (ASRM)

The Altman Self-Rating Mania Scale (ASRM) [52] is a brief (i.e., 5 minutes) self-rating scale designed to assess for the presence and/or severity of manic symptoms and is often used in clinical practice as a screening tool to facilitate diagnostic assessment or used in research. The ASRM is composed of five statement groups (i.e., cheerfulness, self-confidence, sleep, talkativeness, activity levels), whereby respondents are asked to reach each statement within the group and select the statement that best describes how they have been feeling *over the past week*. For example, the first group of questions relates to how cheerful/happy the respondent has been feeling, and here they are asked to rate the statement that best describes how they have been feeling in each group on a 5-point scale from 0 (= "*I do not feel happier or more cheerful than usual*) to 4 (= "*I feel happier or more cheerful than usual all of the time*"). Scores from each of the five groups are added together to give a total score (ranging from 0 to 20), with greater scores indicated higher likelihood of (hypo)mania. This is also found to be a reliable tool [46] with evidence of good internal consistency (Cronbach's alpha scores ranging from 0.57 to 0.84) [52–55], good test-re-test reliability ($r = 0.86$–0.89) and evidence of convergent validity when compared against the YMRS [29,52,53]. It has also been found to successfully differentiate healthy controls versus manic patients [56]. Following principal components analysis, the original ASRM publication found three factors, mania, psychotic symptoms and irritability, and a sensitivity score of 85.5%.

Self-Report Manic Inventory (SRMI)

The Self-Report Manic Inventory (SRMI) [57] is composed of 47 statements related to (hypo)mania symptoms, whereby respondents are asked to read each statement and state whether it is a "true" or "false" reflection of their mood state and behaviour in the month prior to admission / current date. Factor analysis has found evidence of two symptom clusters linked to energised dysphoria (e.g., racing thoughts) and hedonistic euphoria (e.g., elation) [57,58]. It has been found to have high internal (Cronbach's alpha = 0.94) and test-retest reliability (0.79–0.86) [57,58] as well as moderate convergent validity when compared to the ASRM [51], the ISS and the YMRS [59]. It has also been found to be sensitive to detect mood changes over time [51]. For instance, one study found that the SRMI was able to detect significant decreases in manic symptoms compared to baseline, and that these changes were comparable to the changes detected in the YMRS (a clinician-rated tool), which was administered alongside the SRMI [58].

Affective Instability

Affective instability (AI) can be defined as *"rapid oscillations of intense affect, with a difficulty in regulating these oscillations or their behavioural consequences"* [60] and is a transdiagnostic symptom [61] featured in several psychiatric conditions, including mood disorders such as depression [60] and bipolar disorders [62]. The literature makes little differentiation between the terms "affective" and "mood" instability. There is a growing body of literature outlining the central role of AI in the development of mood disorders. For instance, individuals with MDD have greater AI compared to those without MDD [63], and baseline AI scores have been found to positively predict the likelihood of having lifetime major depression [64]. Similarly, AI is present within bipolar disorders, with research showing that compared to healthy controls, individuals with BD report higher rates of AI [65,66] and that AI within BD is associated with a worsened clinical trajectory (e.g., suicide attempts, earlier age of onset) [66].

Thus, AI appears to be a clinically relevant characteristic that influences the course of mood disorders and may be worthwhile measuring within clinical practice to aid clinical decision making. Some core elements of AI are oscillation, intensity, control and subjective ability to regulate affect and its behavioural consequences, [60] and some measures that tap into these elements have been developed. Some of the most well-known and commonly used self-report measures are the Affective Lability Scale (ALS) [67], the Affective Intensity Measure (AIM) [68] and the Affective Control Scale (ACS) [69], all which will be discussed in turn below.

Affective Lability Scale (ALS)

The ALS [67] is the most commonly used scale to assess rapid oscillations of affect and has been used across a range of diagnostic groups. The ALS measures individual proneness to rapid shifts from different emotional states (e.g., anxiety, depression, hypomania). The full version consists of 54 questions split into six subscales assessing variations between normal mood and elevated mood states such as elation, anger, depression and anxiety. There is also a shorter version, made up of 18 items, which is based on a three-factor model of AI (anxiety/depression, depression/elation and anger) and is highly correlated with the original version ($r = 0.94$) [70]. Both versions demonstrate good psychometric properties such as high internal consistency (Cronbach's alpha coefficients ranging from 0.77–0.92).

Affective Intensity Measure (AIM)

The AIM [68] assesses intensity by examining emotional reactions to typical life events. In its full version it is made up of 40 items, although a shorter 20-item version is also available. Each item (e.g., *"when I feel happiness, it is a quiet type of contentment"*) is rated on a 6-point scale from 0 (*never*) to 5 (*almost always*). Authors report high internal consistency (Cronbach's alpha > 0.90), test-retest reliability and criterion-related validity.

Affective Control Scale (ACS)

The ACS [69] was developed to measure fear of strong emotions, namely, fear of losing control of one's emotional experience and/or reaction to the experience

[71] and is composed of 42 items related to fear of emotions (e.g., "*depression could really take over me, so it is important to fight off sad feelings*"). Participants are asked to rate the extent to which they agree with each item using a scale of 1 (*very strongly disagree*) to 7 (*very strongly agree*). Williams and colleagues [69] highlighted the detrimental role that fear of emotion can play in the development of several clinical disorders such as depression and mania, and consequently the ACS assesses fear of four specific emotional states (subscales): anxiety, anger, depressed mood and positive mood.

Research shows that lower perceived emotional control is found among clinical populations (i.e., BD, borderline personality disorder, psychosis and depression), compared to healthy controls [72], further supporting the need to assess for components of AI within routine clinical practice. Evidence suggests that the ACS has sound psychometric properties, with authors reporting good internal consistency (0.94), test-retest reliability (0.66–0.77) and construct validity. More recent work offers support for the specificity and predictive validity of the ACS [73], and it has been found to correlate well with sensitivity to emotions [71,74] and an inability to effectively regulate one's emotions [75–77].

Electronic Mood Monitoring

Whether it be self-report or clinician-rated, the accurate assessment of mood and/or AI is a fundamental component to both the diagnosis and prognosis of mood disorders such as depression and BD. Unlike the classical description of depression and bipolar disorder, which have been episodic in nature, we know that mood instability is frequently superimposed on this picture. Thus, effective, sensitive and accurate mood-monitoring tools are needed to capture mood fluctuations and aid clinical decision making.

Traditionally, daily mood assessments have relied heavily on one-time paper-based assessment tools. Yet, given that mood fluctuations are often experienced on a daily basis, it is thought that these one-time assessment tools are more likely capturing "mood state" (which refers to a more prolonged state or disposition), and not all the mood fluctuations that are commonly experienced within a day-to-day period. Further, there are key barriers to the adherence of these paper-based tools, such as low compliance and retrospective recall bias [78].

One approach to better assess for mood and the temporal pattern of AI is by using the experience sampling method (ESM) [79,80], which prompts people to rate the intensity of different emotions at several timepoints in the day, over several days/weeks, as they occur in real time in their natural environment. Due to the frequency of these mood ratings, researchers have employed digital technologies (e.g., smartphone apps, text messaging) as a way to facilitate participant completion of these ratings. Over the past decade there has been a shift towards employing these digital technologies to monitor mood within mood disorder patients, and this is evidenced by several review papers that seek to evaluate the effectiveness of electronic mood-monitoring methods [78,81–84].

There are several benefits to the use of electronic mood monitoring, namely, that it offers ecological momentary assessments [85], providing real-time data on mood within naturalistic settings and thus increasing the ecological validity of the data. Second, it eliminates the need for costly and error-prone data entry associated with paper-based one-time assessment methods and, although not cost-free, telemonitoring is found to be more cost-effective than traditional interviews [84]. Third, it is found to be a reliable assessment method, with studies showing that compared to clinical ratings of depression, electronic mood monitoring is found to be a valid and reliable tool [78]. Lastly, electronic mood-monitoring methods have been found to improve access to professional care for patients [86,87].

Self-management is a core clinical component to the treatment of depressive and bipolar disorders [88,89] and part of this includes self-monitoring one's mood. Research has found that self-monitoring is associated with improved illness insight/self-awareness and longer symptom-free intervals among those with recurrent depression [90,91], as well as promoting help-seeking behaviour [92], better communication with clinicians [93,94] and feelings of empowerment among patients [95]. Consequently, self-monitoring via ESM is being increasingly used as a tool within mental healthcare [96,97] and recent work examining patient (BD) and clinician experiences of ESM in clinical practice outlines that ESM is perceived as helpful in aiding patients to cope better and improve their awareness of symptoms and that both patients and clinicians advocate for increased personalisation and embedding of ESM in clinical care [98].

Conclusion

In sum, based on the current literature, it appears that the assessment of mood disorders is more advanced for some areas compared to others. Several clinician-rated and self-rated tools appear to be more commonly used in both research and clinical practice, contributing to the evidence surrounding their psychometric properties. The majority of them have the added benefit of being brief and user-friendly, further supporting their utility in clinical practice. However, there appears to be only one validated measure for bipolar depression that is commonly used; thus, future research may benefit from exploring the development of new bipolar depressive measures, as well as measures for other, more difficult-to-treat forms of depression (i.e., treatment-resistant depression, TRD). Finally, with the growing evidence surrounding the use of digital technologies / ESM to monitor mood, it appears that clinical practice would greatly benefit from embedding these methods into routine clinical care. For instance, mood-disorder patients could self-monitor their mood digitally, and these results could be automatically shared with their practitioner to help aid clinical monitoring and the early identification of any potential relapse episodes. This would allow clinicians to promote treatment approaches (e.g., early intervention / relapse-prevention plans) to help prevent a full relapse and prevent the patient from further mood deterioration.

References

1. American Psychiatric Association. *Diagnostic and Statistical Manual of Mental Disorders: DSM-5*. 5th ed. Washington, DC: American Psychiatric Association, 2013.

2. World Health Organisation (WHO). Depressive disorder (depression). 2023. Available from: www.who.int/news-room/fact-sheets/detail/depression.

3. Bauer MS, Crits-Christoph P, Ball WA, et al. Independent assessment of manic and depressive symptoms by self-rating: scale characteristics and implications for the study of mania. *Arch Gen Psychiatry*. 1991;48(9):807–12.

4. Hamilton M. Development of a rating scale for primary depressive illness. *Br J Soc Clin Psychol*. 1967;6(4):278–96.

5. Zimmerman M, Posternak MA, Chelminski I. Is the cutoff to define remission on the Hamilton Rating Scale for Depression too high? *J Nerv Ment Dis*. 2005;193(3):170–5.

6. Bagby RM, Ryder AG, Schuller DR, Marshall MB. The Hamilton Depression Rating Scale: has the gold standard become a lead weight? *Am J Psychiatry*. 2004;161(12):2163–77.

7. Bech P. The responsiveness of the different versions of the Hamilton Depression Scale. *World Psychiatry*. 2015;14(3):309.

8. Hieronymus F, Emilsson JF, Nilsson S, Eriksson E. Consistent superiority of selective serotonin reuptake inhibitors over placebo in reducing depressed mood in patients with major depression. *Mol Psychiatry*. 2016;21(4):523–30.

9. Montgomery SA, Åsberg M. A new depression scale designed to be sensitive to change. *Br J Psychiatry*. 1979;134(4):382–9.

10. Davidson J, Turnbull CD, Strickland R, Miller R, Graves K. The Montgomery-Åsberg Depression Scale: reliability and validity. *Acta Psychiatr Scand*. 1986;73(5):544–8.

11. Carmody TJ, Rush AJ, Bernstein I, et al. The Montgomery Äsberg and the Hamilton ratings of depression: a comparison of measures. *Eur Neuropsychopharmacol*. 2006;16(8):601–11.

12. Beck AT, Ward C, Mendelson M, Mock J, Erbaugh J. Beck Depression Inventory (BDI). *Arch Gen Psychiatry*. 1961;4(6):561–71.

13. Wang Y-P, Gorenstein C. Psychometric properties of the Beck Depression Inventory-II: a comprehensive review. *Braz J Psychiatry*. 2013;35(4):416–31.

14. Gomes-Oliveira MH, Gorenstein C, Neto FL, Andrade LH, Wang YP. Validation of the Brazilian Portuguese version of the Beck Depression Inventory-II in a community sample. *Braz J Psychiatry*. 2012;34(4):389–94.

15. Kojima M, Furukawa TA, Takahashi H, et al. Cross-cultural validation of the Beck Depression Inventory-II in Japan. *Psychiatry Res*. 2002;110(3):291–9.

16. Segal DL, Coolidge FL, Cahill BS, O'Riley AA. Psychometric properties of the Beck Depression Inventory-II (BDI-II) among community-dwelling older adults. *Behav Modif*. 2008;32(1):3–20.

17. Homaifar BY, Brenner LA, Gutierrez PM, et al. Sensitivity and specificity of the Beck Depression Inventory-II in persons with traumatic brain injury. *Arch Phys Med Rehabil*. 2009;90(4):652–6.

18. Kroenke K, Spitzer RL, Williams JB. The PHQ-9: validity of a brief depression severity measure. *J Gen Intern Med*. 2001;16(9):606–13.

19. Spitzer R, Kroenke K, Williams J. Validation and utility of a self-report version of PRIME-MD: the PHQ primary care study. Primary Care Evaluation of Mental Disorders. Patient Health Questionnaire. *JAMA*. 1999;282(18):1737–44.

20. Gilbody S, Richards D, Brealey S, Hewitt C. Screening for depression in medical settings with the Patient Health Questionnaire (PHQ): a diagnostic meta-analysis. *J Gen Intern Med*. 2007;**22**(11):1596–602.

21. van der Zwaan GL, van Dijk SE, Adriaanse MC, et al. Diagnostic accuracy of the Patient Health Questionnaire-9 for assessment of depression in type II diabetes mellitus and/or coronary heart disease in primary care. *J Affect Disord*. 2016;**190**:68–74.

22. McGuire L, Kiecolt-Glaser JK, Glaser R. Depressive symptoms and lymphocyte proliferation in older adults. *J Abnorm Psychol*. 2002;**111**(1):192.

23. Beard C, Hsu K, Rifkin L, Busch A, Björgvinsson T. Validation of the PHQ-9 in a psychiatric sample. *J Affect Disord*. 2016;**193**:267–73.

24. Kocalevent R-D, Hinz A, Brähler E. Standardization of the depression screener patient health questionnaire (PHQ-9) in the general population. *Gen Hosp Psychiatry*. 2013;**35**(5):551–5.

25. Levis B, Benedetti A, Thombs BD. Accuracy of Patient Health Questionnaire-9 (PHQ-9) for screening to detect major depression: individual participant data meta-analysis. *BMJ*. 2019;**365**:1476.

26. Rush AJ, Trivedi MH, Ibrahim HM, et al. The 16-Item Quick Inventory of Depressive Symptomatology (QIDS), clinician rating (QIDS-C), and self-report (QIDS-SR): a psychometric evaluation in patients with chronic major depression. *Biol Psychiatry*. 2003;**54**(5):573–83.

27. Trivedi MH, Rush A, Ibrahim H, et al. The Inventory of Depressive Symptomatology, Clinician Rating (IDS-C) and Self-Report (IDS-SR), and the Quick Inventory of Depressive Symptomatology, Clinician Rating (QIDS-C) and Self-Report (QIDS-SR) in public sector patients with mood disorders: a psychometric evaluation; Psychometrics of the QIDS in public sector patients; MH Trivedi and others. *Psychol Med*. 2004;**34**(1):73.

28. Reilly TJ, MacGillivray SA, Reid IC, Cameron IM. Psychometric properties of the 16-item Quick Inventory of Depressive Symptomatology: a systematic review and meta-analysis. *J Psychiatr Res*. 2015;**60**:132–40.

29. Young RC, Biggs JT, Ziegler VE, Meyer DA. A rating scale for mania: reliability, validity and sensitivity. *Br J Psychiatry*. 1978;**133**(5):429–35.

30. Tohen M, Jacobs TG, Grundy SL, et al. Efficacy of olanzapine in acute bipolar mania: a double-blind, placebo-controlled study. *Arch Gen Psychiatry*. 2000;**57**(9):841–9.

31. Strejilevich S, Martino DJ, Murru A, et al. Mood instability and functional recovery in bipolar disorders. *Acta Psychiatr Scand*. 2013;**128** (3):194–202.

32. Marwaha S, Hett D, Johnson S, et al. The impact of manic symptoms in first-episode psychosis: findings from the UK National EDEN study. *Acta Psychiatr Scand*. 2021;**144**(4):358–67.

33. Mohammadi Z, Pourshahbaz A, Poshtmashhadi M, et al. Psychometric properties of the Young Mania Rating Scale as a mania severity measure in patients with bipolar I disorder. *Pract Clin Psychol*. 2018;**6**(3):175–82.

34. Spearing MK, Post RM, Leverich GS, Brandt D, Nolen W. Modification of the Clinical Global Impressions (CGI) Scale for use in bipolar illness (BP): the CGI-BP. *Psychiatry Res*. 1997;**73**(3):159–71.

35. Keller MB, Lavori PW, Friedman B, et al. The Longitudinal Interval Follow-Up Evaluation: a comprehensive method for assessing outcome in prospective longitudinal studies. *Arch Gen Psychiatry*. 1987;**44**(6):540–8.

36. Morriss R, Lobban F, Riste L, et al. Clinical effectiveness and acceptability of structured group psychoeducation versus optimised unstructured peer support for patients with remitted bipolar disorder (PARADES): a pragmatic, multicentre, observer-blind, randomised controlled superiority trial. *Lancet Psychiatry*. 2016;**3**(11):1029–38.

37. Leon AC, Solomon DA, Mueller TI, et al. A brief assessment of psychosocial functioning of subjects with bipolar I disorder: the LIFE-RIFT. *J Nerv Ment Dis*. 2000;**188**(12):805–12.

38. Warshaw MG, Keller MB, Stout RL. Reliability and validity of the longitudinal interval follow-up evaluation for assessing outcome of anxiety disorders. *J Psychiatr Res*. 1994;**28**(6):531–45.

39. Tondo L, H Vazquez G, J Baldessarini R. Depression and mania in bipolar disorder. *Curr Neuropharmacol*. 2017;**15**(3):353–8.

40. Judd LL, Akiskal HS, Schettler PJ, et al. The long-term natural history of the weekly symptomatic status of bipolar I disorder. *Arch Gen Psychiatry*. 2002;**59** (6):530–7.

41. Hamilton M. A rating scale for depression. *J Neurol Neurosurg Psychiatry*. 1960;**23**(1):56.

42. Serretti A, Olgiati P. Profiles of "manic" symptoms in bipolar I, bipolar II and major depressive disorders. *J Affect Disord*. 2005;**84**(2–3):159–66.

43. Berk M, Malhi G, Mitchell P, et al. Scale matters: the need for a Bipolar Depression Rating Scale (BDRS). *Acta Psychiatr Scand*. 2004;**110**:39–45.

44. Berk M, Dodd S, Dean OM, et al. The validity and internal structure of the Bipolar Depression Rating Scale: data from a clinical trial of N-acetylcysteine as adjunctive therapy in bipolar disorder. *Acta Neuropsychiatr*. 2010;**22**(5):237–42.

45. Bruschi A, Mazza M, Camardese G, et al. Psychopathological features of bipolar depression: Italian validation of the Bipolar Depression Rating Scale (I-BDRS). *Front Psychol*. 2018;**9**:1047.

46. Meyer TD, Crist N, La Rosa N, et al. Are existing self-ratings of acute manic symptoms in adults reliable and valid? – A systematic review. *Bipolar Disord*. 2020;**22**(6):558–68.

47. Dodd AL, Mansell W, Morrison AP, Tai S. Extreme appraisals of internal states and bipolar symptoms: the Hypomanic Attitudes and Positive Predictions Inventory. *Psychol Assess*. 2011;**23**(3):635.

48. Huang C-L, Yang Y-K, Chen M, et al. Patient- and family-rated scale for bipolar disorder symptoms: internal state scale. *Kaohsiung J Med Sci*. 2003;**19**(4):170–5.

49. Mansell W, Jones SH. The Brief-HAPPI: a questionnaire to assess cognitions that distinguish between individuals with a diagnosis of bipolar disorder and non-clinical controls. *J Affect Disord*. 2006;**93**(1–3):29–34.

50. Mackali Z, Akkaya C, Aydemir Ö. The Turkish adaptation, validity, and reliability of the internal states scale. *Arch Neuropsychiatry*. 2016;**53**(3):222.

51. Altman E, Hedeker D, Peterson JL, Davis JM. A comparative evaluation of three self-rating scales for acute mania. *Biol Psychiatry*. 2001;**50**(6):468–71.

52. Altman EG, Hedeker D, Peterson JL, Davis JM. The Altman Self-Rating Mania Scale. *Biol Psychiatry*. 1997;**42**(10):948–55.

53. Ng TH, Johnson SL. Rejection sensitivity is associated with quality of life, psychosocial outcome, and the course of depression in euthymic patients with bipolar I disorder. *Cogn Ther Res*. 2013;**37**(6):1169–78.

54. Weinstock LM, Broughton MK, Tezanos KM, et al. Adjunctive yoga versus bibliotherapy for bipolar depression: a pilot randomized controlled trial. *Ment Health Phys Activity*. 2016;**11**:67–73.

55. Stange JP, Molz AR, Black CL, et al. Positive overgeneralization and Behavioral Approach System (BAS) sensitivity interact to predict prospective increases in hypomanic symptoms: a behavioral high-risk design. *Behav Res Ther*. 2012;**50**(4):231–9.

56. Alvarez M. [Translation and adaptation in the Spanish environment of the Altman Self-Rating Mania Scale]. *Actas Esp Psiquiatr*. 2005;**33**(3):180–7.

57. Shugar G, Schertzer S, Toner BB, Di Gasbarro I. Development, use, and factor analysis of a self-report inventory for mania. *Compr Psychiatry*. 1992;**33**(5):325–31.

58. Bräunig P, Shugar G, Krüger S. An investigation of the Self-Report Manic Inventory as a diagnostic and severity scale for mania. *Compr Psychiatry*. 1996;**37**(1):52–5.

59. Cooke RG, Krüger S, Shugar G. Comparative evaluation of two self-report mania rating scales. *Biol Psychiatry*. 1996;**40**(4):279–83.

60. Marwaha S, Balbuena L, Winsper C, Bowen R. Mood instability as a precursor to depressive illness: a prospective and mediational analysis. *Aust N Z J Psychiatry*. 2015;**49**(6):557–65.

61. Broome M, Saunders K, Harrison P, Marwaha S. Mood instability: significance, definition and measurement. *Br J Psychiatry*. 2015;**207**(4):283–5.

62. Stange JP, Sylvia LG, da Silva Magalhaes PV, et al. Affective instability and the course of bipolar depression: results from the STEP-BD randomised controlled trial of psychosocial treatment. *Br J Psychiatry*. 2016;**208**(4):352–8.

63. Houben M, Van Den Noortgate W, Kuppens P. The relation between short-term emotion dynamics and psychological well-being: a meta-analysis. *Psychol Bull*. 2015;**141**(4):901.

64. Eldesouky L, Thompson RJ, Oltmanns TF, English T. Affective instability predicts the course of depression in late middle-age and older adulthood. *J Affect Disord*. 2018;**239**:72–8.

65. Aminoff SR, Jensen J, Lagerberg TV, et al. An association between affective lability and executive functioning in bipolar disorder. *Psychiatry Res*. 2012;**198**(1):58–61.

66. Henry C, Van den Bulke D, Bellivier F, et al. Affective lability and affect intensity as core dimensions of bipolar disorders during euthymic period. *Psychiatry Res*. 2008;**159**(1–2):1–6.

67. Harvey PD, Greenberg BR, Serper MR. The Affective Lability Scales: development, reliability, and validity. *J Clin Psychol*. 1989;**45**(5):786–93.

68. Larsen RJ, Diener E, Emmons RA. Affect intensity and reactions to daily life events. *J Pers Soc Psychol*. 1986;**51**(4):803.

69. Williams KE, Chambless DL, Ahrens A. Are emotions frightening? An extension of the fear of fear construct. *Behav Res Ther*. 1997;**35**(3):239–48.

70. Look AE, Flory JD, Harvey PD, Siever LJ. Psychometric properties of a short form of the Affective Lability Scale (ALS-18). *Pers Individ Dif*. 2010;**49**(3):187–91.

71. Berg CZ, Shapiro N, Chambless DL, Ahrens AH. Are emotions frightening? II: an analogue study of fear of emotion, interpersonal conflict, and panic onset. *Behav Res Ther*. 1998;**36**(1):3–15.

72. Marwaha S, Price C, Scott J, et al. Affective instability in those with and without mental disorders: a case control study. *J Affect Disord*. 2018;**241**:492–8.

73. Hughes CD, Gunthert K, Wenze S, German R. The subscale specificity of the Affective Control Scale: ecological validity and predictive validity of feared emotions. *Motivation Emotion*. 2015;**39**(6):984–92.

74. Salters-Pedneault K, Gentes E, Roemer L. The role of fear of emotion in distress, arousal, and cognitive interference following an emotional stimulus. *Cogn Behav Ther*. 2007;**36**(1):12–22.

75. Robins CJ, Keng SL, Ekblad AG, Brantley JG. Effects of mindfulness-based stress reduction on emotional experience and expression: a randomized controlled trial. *J Clin Psychol*. 2012;**68**(1):117–31.

76. Beck JG, Davila J. Development of an interview for anxiety-relevant interpersonal styles: preliminary support for convergent and discriminant validity. *J Psychopathol Behav Assess*. 2003;**25**(1):1–9.

77. Riskind JH, Kleiman EM. Looming cognitive style, emotion schemas, and fears of loss of emotional control: two studies. *Intl J Cogn Ther*. 2012;**5**(4):392–405.

78. Faurholt-Jepsen M, Munkholm K, Frost M, Bardram JE, Kessing LV. Electronic self-monitoring of mood using IT platforms in adult patients with bipolar disorder: a systematic review of the validity and evidence. *BMC Psychiatry*. 2016;**16**(1):1–14.

79. Larson R, Csikszentmihalyi M. The experience sampling method. In M Csikszentmihalyi. *Flow and the Foundations of Positive Psychology*. Springer, 2014; 21–34.

80. Csikszentmihalyi M, Larson R. Validity and reliability of the experience-sampling method. In M Csikszentmihalyi. *Flow and the Foundations of Positive Psychology*. Springer, 2014; 35–54.

81. van der Watt A, Odendaal W, Louw K, Seedat S. Distant mood monitoring for depressive and bipolar disorders: a systematic review. *BMC Psychiatry*. 2020;**20**(1):1–14.

82. Dubad M, Winsper C, Meyer C, Livanou M, Marwaha S. A systematic review of the psychometric properties, usability and clinical impacts of mobile mood-monitoring applications in young people. *Psychol Med*. 2018;**48**(2):208–28.

83. Bopp JM, Miklowitz DJ, Goodwin GM, et al. The longitudinal course of bipolar disorder as revealed through weekly text messaging: a feasibility study. *Bipolar Disord*. 2010;**12**(3):327–34.

84. Miklowitz DJ, Price J, Holmes EA, et al. Facilitated integrated mood management for adults with bipolar disorder. *Bipolar Disord*. 2012;**14**(2):185–97.

85. Shiffman S, Stone AA, Hufford MR. Ecological momentary assessment. *Annu Rev Clin Psychol*. 2008;**4**:1–32.

86. Wenze SJ, Armey MF, Miller IW. Feasibility and acceptability of a mobile intervention to improve treatment adherence in bipolar disorder: a pilot study. *Behav Modif*. 2014;**38**(4):497–515.

87. Depp CA, Ceglowski J, Wang VC, et al. Augmenting psychoeducation with a mobile intervention for bipolar disorder: a randomized controlled trial. *J Affect Disord*. 2015;**174**:23–30.

88. Jones S, Deville M, Mayes D, Lobban F. Self-management in bipolar disorder: the story so far. *J Ment Health*. 2011;**20**(6):583–92.

89. Houle J, Gascon-Depatie M, Bélanger-Dumontier G, Cardinal C. Depression self-management support: a systematic review. *Patient Educ Couns*. 2013;**91** (3):271–9.

90. Kordy H, Wolf M, Aulich K, et al. Internet-delivered disease management for recurrent depression: a multicenter randomized controlled trial. *Psychother Psychosom*. 2016;**85**(2):91–8.

91. Kauer SD, Reid SC, Crooke AHD, et al. Self-monitoring using mobile phones in the early stages of adolescent depression: randomized controlled trial. *J Med Internet Res*. 2012;**14**(3):e1858.

92. BinDhim NF, Alanazi EM, Aljadhey H, et al. Does a mobile phone depression-screening app motivate mobile phone users with high depressive symptoms to seek a health care professional's help? *J Med Internet Res*. 2016;**18**(6):e5726.

93. Murnane EL, Cosley D, Chang P, et al. Self-monitoring practices, attitudes, and needs of individuals with bipolar disorder: implications for the design of technologies to manage mental health. *J Am Med Inform Assoc*. 2016;**23**(3):477–84.

94. Bilderbeck AC, Saunders KE, Price J, Goodwin GM. Psychiatric assessment of mood instability: qualitative study of patient experience. *Br J Psychiatry*. 2014;**204** (3):234–9.

95. Simons C, Hartmann J, Kramer I, et al. Effects of momentary self-monitoring on empowerment in a randomized controlled trial in patients with depression. *Eur Psychiatry*. 2015;**30**(8):900–6.

96. van Os J, Verhagen S, Marsman A, et al. The experience sampling method as an mHealth tool to support self-monitoring, self-insight, and personalized health care in clinical practice. *Depress Anxiety*. 2017;**34**(6):481–93.

97. Bos FM, Snippe E, Bruggeman R, Wichers M, van der Krieke L. Insights of patients and clinicians on the promise of the experience sampling method for psychiatric care. *Psychiatr Serv*. 2019;**70**(11):983–91.

98. Bos FM, Snippe E, Bruggeman R, et al. Recommendations for the use of long-term experience sampling in bipolar disorder care: a qualitative study of patient and clinician experiences. *Int J Bipolar Disord*. 2020;**8**(1):1–14.

Chapter 31

Service Delivery for Mood Disorders

Karine Macritchie

Introduction

Mood disorders are common, debilitating conditions that carry a high risk of suicide. Clear guidelines exist on effective, evidence-based treatments, and several promising new therapies are emerging. Despite this, for many healthcare providers, the goal of an effective, comprehensive service for mood disorders remains elusive. In consequence, mood disorders are often under-recognised and undertreated.

Following their review of the epidemiology of mood disorders and suicide 20 years ago, Nierenberg et al. (2001) concluded that 'the widespread underdiagnosis and undertreatment of major depression and bipolar disorder contribute to an unacceptable risk of suicide, a preventable tragedy'. A more recent World Health Organisation community household survey of 21 countries concluded that 'only a minority of participants with major depressive disorder received minimally adequate treatment' (Thornicroft et al., 2017). The authors called for substantial improvements in care for major depressive disorder, with 'fundamental transformations in community education and outreach, supply of treatment and the quality of services'. Initial reports from the Bipolar Commission in the United Kingdom (Bipolar UK, 2022) called for wide-ranging service improvements. These included earlier diagnosis, better specialist services and in-patient care and continuity of care across the phases of illness. A need to provide pragmatic early warning symptom response plans and education on more general bipolar self-management strategies was identified. The need to address suicide rates was emphasised.

Healthcare providers certainly face considerable challenges in establishing and maintaining services for mood disorders. Services must offer evidence-based treatments from a variety of disciplines. They must span primary healthcare / family practice, from increasingly specialist mental health services to expert programmes. They must offer care across the age range from childhood and adolescence through working life to older age. Service provision should address each phase of mood disorders, every degree of severity and every level of complexity. Physical and mental health comorbidities should be addressed. The means to assess and manage high rates of suicide and other forms of risk should be incorporated. In addition to major depressive disorder, persistent depressive disorder and bipolar disorder, programmes should be available to diagnose and manage disruptive mood dysregulation disorder and premenstrual dysphoric disorder.

In this chapter, the components of services for mood disorders are outlined, and several problematic issues are discussed. Recent examples of service development are described. The general elements of a business case for service development are outlined. Finally, the key issues of staff recruitment, retention and training are considered.

The Components of a Comprehensive Mood Disorders Service

The components of services for mood disorders services are summarised in Table 31.1. The nature of mood disorders and their treatment has been discussed in detail elsewhere in this volume; issues particularly relevant to service provision are considered in this section. These are diagnosis, the efficient and timely referral to appropriate services, continuity of care, and the management of risk.

Diagnosis

Clearly, the diagnosis of a mood disorder is fundamental to successful clinical management and recovery. However, diagnosis presents a considerable difficulty in clinical practice, especially in primary care where major depression is significantly unrecognised. Many

Table 31.1 The components of a comprehensive mood disorders service

Timely diagnosis and formulation, including recognition of physical and mental health comorbidities.
Risk assessment and management.
Efficient and timely referral to appropriate services, addressing clinical need and risk.
Treatment planning and implementation, potentially involving several clinical disciplines.
Medication initiation and monitoring.
Access to neurostimulation treatments.
Evidence-based psychotherapy and psychoeducation.
Physical health monitoring.
Ongoing review for acute episodes.
Regular reviews of maintenance treatment.
Occupational therapy and vocational support to promote functional recovery.
Access to social and financial support and advice.
Support/education for family and friends.
Optimal continuity of care across the phases of illness.

people with bipolar disorder wait long periods for a correct diagnosis. This lack of recognition may lead to prolonged periods of suffering and inadequate or inappropriate treatments (Scott and Leboyer, 2011).

Delayed diagnosis is also financially costly. In 2008, the King's Fund estimated the total annual service cost for patients with bipolar disorder in England to be £1.6 billion. Potential healthcare savings from early detection in 75% of new cases were estimated to be £16.4 million (McCrone et al., 2008). A retrospective study from the California Medicaid Programme over a 6-year period found that while the cost of care for patients with recognised bipolar disorder rose by 82%, the cost of care for those with a delayed diagnosis rose by 171% (McCombs et al., 2006).

Screening for depressive symptoms can be done quickly and effectively, for instance using the Patient Health Questionnaire-2, which contains two questions relating to low mood, hopelessness and anhedonia (Kroenke et al., 2003) or the longer Patient Health Questionnaire-9 (Spitzer et al., 1999). Screening for bipolar disorder can be performed through the further investigation of suspected current or past episodes of hypomania or mania identified using the Mood Disorder Questionnaire (Hirschfeld, 2002).

Efficient and Timely Referral to Appropriate Services, Given Clinical Need and Risk

When an acute depressive episode is identified in primary care, the context and form of treatment will depend on its severity and the presence of risks. Should the patient be managed in primary care, or is a specialist home-treatment team or in-patient care required? Patients with depression may be treated in primary care / family practice initially but should be referred to specialist services speedily if they fail to respond or only respond partially to two treatments – either two short trials of antidepressants or one antidepressant and a course of psychotherapy. During this period, there should be robust risk monitoring.

Patients with suspected bipolar disorder should be referred to specialist mental health services for diagnostic confirmation and management. An acute episode should be managed in mental health services because of the need for specialist treatment and risk management. An established case of bipolar disorder may be managed in primary care during the maintenance phase, with careful attention to ongoing monitoring for medication efficacy, side effects and physical health. However, the maintenance phase of treatment is often an opportunity for psychoeducation and psychotherapy. Questions about the effectiveness and the acceptability of maintenance pharmacological treatment should lead to early re-referral to specialist services.

For all mood disorders, treatment failure may be evident in recurrent episodes and frequent admissions, or the presence of chronic, treatment-resistant symptoms. These factors indicate the need for specialist review: they may require an expert opinion in a tertiary service.

Risk Assessment and Management

The long-term risk of suicide in mood disorders is at least 10% (Angst et al., 2005). The period of suicide risk extends beyond admission: the time immediately following discharge is a period of particular suicide risk (Appleby et al., 2013). Other risks include those of self-harm, violence to others, self-neglect, risk of exploitation, reputational risk and any risk to children and vulnerable adults. Again, these risks may necessitate referral specialist services. Their management may require in-patient rather than community care.

The anti-suicidal effect of long-term treatment with lithium in depression and bipolar disorder is supported by an increasing body of evidence (Smith and Cipriani, 2017). Lithium treatment requires attention to safe prescribing, the careful monitoring of adverse effects and blood results and attention to potential medication interactions. The safety and effectiveness of lithium treatment can be improved by a formal lithium clinic pathway (National Institute for Health and Care Excellence, 2015). Similarly, a digital app that meets safety and governance standards may support lithium prescribing, monitoring and education.

Continuity of Care and Links with Other Services

Continuity of care across the phases of illness is important, but in some countries, there is increasing disconnection between in-patient and community specialist services, and between mental health services and primary care / family practice. Discontinuity between adolescent and adult services can be particularly problematic (Royal College of Psychiatrists, 2017): with bipolar disorder, this transition may occur at the time of the first early episodes. Clinical services should be linked with others to address comorbidities, including anxiety disorders and addictions services. It is essential that patients can be referred to partner organisations to address psychosocial issues, such as financial pressures, accommodation needs and employment problems. It can be seen that patients with mood disorders services may require access to programmes offered by several agencies that are funded by a variety of sources.

Service Development for Mood Disorders

Service development should improve adherence to existing guidelines. Over time, service providers may also be required to respond to the recommendations of newly revised treatment guidelines and, in some cases, to the development of new treatments.

Large-scale service development rarely takes place 'de novo'. Long-term initiatives leading to full-service transformation are infrequent. In the United Kingdom, the ambitious NHS Long Term Plan is a central government-funded initiative that will provide an opportunity to develop mental health services further (NHS Long Term Plan, 2019). One approach to this challenge is the development of diagnosis-defined pathways of care, including pathways for mood disorders. The success of large programmes of this kind requires long-term commitment that persists, despite changes in annual financial settlements, organisational managerial structural changes and changes in clinical and managerial personnel.

In most cases, service development occurs through the addition of new programmes: several examples are discussed below. Some programmes are national initiatives. The needs of individual local services may be identified by systematically conducting a 'gap analysis' that compares current service provision with guideline recommendations. In this section, examples of national and local initiatives are described.

Improving Access to Psychological Therapies

The 'Improving Access to Psychological Therapies' (IAPT) is a national programme that provides therapies for depression and anxiety, established some 10 years ago in England. Although the programme made welcome steps to increase the availability of psychological therapies in primary care (family practice) (Wakefield et al., 2021), the programme's capacity to address the needs of more complex cases was subsequently questioned (Martin et al., 2022).

A more specialised demonstration site psychotherapy programme for bipolar disorder, 'Improving Access to Psychological Therapies – Severe Mental Illness Bipolar Disorder' (IAPT-SMI BD) (Jones et al., 2018), reported improvement in personal recovery, quality of life, work and social functioning and mood and anxiety symptoms.

The Bipolar Education Programme Cymru

Group psychoeducation is thought to reduce recurrences and reduce admissions and duration of hospital admissions, to lead to better treatment adherence and to reduce stigma (Soo et al., 2018). The Bipolar Education Programme Cymru (Wales) was funded by the United Kingdom National Lottery. It was developed by the National Centre for Mental Health at Cardiff University and the Mental Health Cardiff and Vale University Health Board Service and is now available in several locations in Wales.

Specialist Out-Patient Clinics for Bipolar Disorder

In a Danish study, Kessing et al. (2013) conducted a randomised controlled trial of a specialised out-patient treatment for those in the early course of bipolar disorder and recently discharged from hospital. The trial design was a pragmatic one, with few exclusion criteria. The trial offered two interventions: a programme of psychoeducation and the prescribing of evidence-based pharmacotherapy, based on British Association for Psychopharmacology guidelines (Goodwin and Consensus Group, 2009 – subsequently updated). This was compared to standard treatment comprising access to standard out-patient mental health services and treatment with a general practitioner and a psychiatrist. Over a mean follow-up period of two and a half years, there was a 40% reduction in the risk of re-admission compared to those on standard treatment. The authors demonstrated that the additional costs for the specialist clinic were more than compensated by savings in the cost of admissions.

The OPTIMA Mood Disorders Service is another specialist service for bipolar disorder, which was established by the South London and Maudsley NHS Foundation Trust in 2015 (Macritchie et al., 2019). Based on the Kessing (2013) study, the service focused on the management of those experiencing the most frequent admissions to hospital in the Trust. Using a combination of individually tailored medication and psychoeducation, the service aims to consolidate recovery from bipolar episodes and to optimise maintenance treatment, while working towards functional recovery. The financial case for this programme was partly based on the premise that by improving the management of bipolar disorder in this group, there would be cost savings in a reduction in admissions and other demands on services. The service did significantly reduce intra-individual admission rates. It also reduced home-treatment team spells of care, but not to a statistically significant degree. This may have been because OPTIMA was well placed to support people in engaging with home-treatment care during a window of opportunity that exists before the need for in-patient care becomes inevitable (Macritchie et al., 2019).

The Incorporation of New Therapies into Existing Services

For emerging treatments, decisions about their incorporation into existing services will require evaluation of the evidence base and sensitivity to existing regulatory frameworks. Careful attention to clinical governance and operational protocols will be required. One example of this is the establishment of programmes offering ketamine and related compounds as therapeutic agents in the treatment of treatment-resistant depression (Bayes et al., 2021). In the future, services may be required to address new treatment targets, for instance, therapies for the cognitive dysfunction associated with bipolar disorder (Strawbridge et al., 2021).

Building a Business Case for Local Service Development

In presenting a business case for a new service, a funding body is often invited to invest money in order to benefit from clinical improvements and financial savings in the future. In creating a case for local service development, the first step is to identify an area of unmet clinical need. Unmet clinical need may become apparent through clinical experience or through service user and carer consultation. It can be confirmed and quantified through clinical audit or in a gap analysis.

Having identified the absence of a recommended treatment or service, the case for service development is constructed. First, the costs of the absence of a service are estimated. In addition to the personal cost to the service user and those who care for them, the clinical and financial costs to the service provider are summarised. For instance, as demonstrated above, failure to optimise maintenance treatment in bipolar disorder can lead to episode recurrence. In addition to the damaging personal consequences for the individual patient, an admission to hospital can be highly financially costly. The cost savings from saved admissions may contribute to the cost of the new service.

A proposal for the new service is constructed in consultation with service users and stakeholder clinicians. Co-production with those who will use the service is an increasingly important feature of service development. A document demonstrating this consultation and co-production will strengthen the business case.

Information on the clinical effectiveness of the proposed intervention and its potential benefits may already be available in accounts of similar services in the literature. Financial estimations can be made when considering the size of the service and the proposed number of patients and clinicians. How much will this proposal cost? Can this proposal reduce costs elsewhere? Costs may include accommodation, staff costs and staff recruitment and training, but there may also be wider costs that may not be immediately obvious to a clinician. Partnership with local operational service managers and local health service accountants will ensure that the proposal will be both practicable and affordable.

The business case should include a statement of the primary outcome measure of the innovation, the duration of a pilot period and the timing of this assessment.

The completed business plan will be presented to the service provider's executive committee for adoption, and it can be used in consultation and negotiation processes with commissioning bodies and other stakeholder organisations.

Staff Recruitment, Retention and Training

The quality of any services is dependent on the skill, experience and motivation of its clinicians. The treatment of people with mood disorders requires trained clinicians from a range of disciplines, including psychiatrists, community psychiatric nurses, psychotherapists, in-patient and specialist service nurses and occupational therapists.

Staff recruitment, retention and training are the foundation of service provision, and should be addressed in financial planning. Training should include knowledge of the nature of mood disorders and their associated risk and management. The training will vary in content, duration and intensity, depending on the context of the clinician's work; refresher courses should be offered regularly.

For specialist mental health services, there should be opportunities for professional development and career planning. For some clinicians, their retention in the field of mood disorders will require pathways of career progression leading to senior clinical roles. For instance, in the United Kingdom, this could take the form of an Advanced Clinical Practitioner, credentialed by their professional body (NHS, People Plan, 2020). Local and national conferences and networks and the provision of mentors may support continuing professional development. In turn, these clinicians may advocate for and support further service improvements.

Conclusion

Mood disorders are common, debilitating illnesses with high suicide rates. There is strong evidence that mood disorders services do not meet the needs of the patients they serve, such that mood disorders are often under-recognised and undertreated. This diagnostic delay and undertreatment results in prolonged personal suffering. It also imposes substantial direct financial costs of care and broader indirect costs to society. A strong case can be made that these personal and financial costs can be reduced by service improvements that address the recognition and treatment of mood disorders.

There is a need to expand and maintain services for mood disorders across the tiers of healthcare systems. Opportunities for long-term, large-scale, transformative funded initiatives are much needed, but they are rare. Focused national and local service developments are more common. Staff recruitment, retention and training form the cornerstone of service provision. The first task for those wishing to build satisfactory services for mood disorders in the future is to interest, recruit and encourage clinicians to work in them, and to build career pathways in which they can flourish in this essential area of practice.

References

Angst J, Angst F, Gerber-Werder R, et al. Suicide in 406 mood disorder patients with and without medication. A forty to forty-four years follow-up. *Arch Suicide Res*. 2005;**9** 279–300.

Appleby L, Kapur N, Shaw J et al, The National Confidential Inquiry into Suicide and Homicide by People with Mental Illness. Annual Report: England, Northern Ireland, Scotland and Wales. The University of Manchester, July 2013. Available at https://documents.manchester.ac.uk/display.aspx?DocID=37595

Bayes A, Dong V, Martin D, et al. Ketamine treatment for depression: a model of care. *Aus N Z J Psychiatry*. 2021;**55**:1134–43.

Bipolar UK Commission. Hidden in Plain Sight: A Lived Experience Report by Bipolar UK. March 2022.

Goodwin GM, Consensus Group of the British Association of Psychopharmacology. Evidence-based guidelines for treating bipolar disorder: revised second edition – recommendations from the British Association for Psychopharmacology. *J Psychopharmacol*. 2009;**23**:346–88. (N.B. further updated guidelines were published in 2016).

Hirschfeld R. The Mood Disorder Questionnaire: a simple, patient-rated screening instrument for bipolar disorder. *Prim Care Companion J Clin Psychiatry*. 2002;**4**:9–11.

Jones SH, Akers N, Eaton J, et al. Improving Access to Psychological Therapies (IAPT) for people with bipolar disorder: summary of outcomes from the IAPT demonstration site. *Behav Res Ther*. 2018;**111**:27–35.

Kessing LV, Hansen HV, Hvenegaard A, et al. Treatment in a specialised out-patient mood disorder clinic v. standard out-patient treatment in the early course of bipolar disorder: randomised clinical trial. *Br J Psychiatry*. 2013;**202**:212–19.

Kroenke K, Spitzer RL, Williams JBW. The Patient Health Questionnaire-2: validity of a two-item depression screener. *Med Care*. 2003;**41**:1284–92.

Macritchie K, Mantingh T, Hidalgo-Mazzei D, et al. A new inner-city specialist programme reduces readmission rates in frequently admitted patients with bipolar disorder *Br J Psychiatry Bull*. 2019;**43**:58–60.

Martin C, Iqbal Z, Airey N D, Marks L. Improving Access to Psychological Therapies (IAPT) has potential, but is not sufficient. How can it better meet the range of primary mental health needs? *Br J Clin Psychol*. 2022;**61**:157–74.

McCombs JS, Ahn J, Tencer T, et al. The impact of unrecognised bipolar disorders among patients treated with depression with antidepressants in the fee-for services California Medicaid (Medi-Cal) program: a 6-year retrospective analysis. *J Affect Disord*. 2006;**97**:171–9.

McCrone P, Shanasiri S, Patel, A, et al. *Paying the Price: The Cost of Mental Health Care in England to 2026*. London: King's Fund, 2008. ISBN 978 1 87175714.

National Institute for Health and Care Excellence. The Impact of Introducing a Lithium Care Pathway. 2015. Available at: www.nice.org.uk/sharedlearning/the-impact-of-introducing-a-lithium-care-pathway

NHS. The NHS Long Term Plan. July 2019. Available at: www.longtermplan.nhs.uk/publication/nhs-long-term-plan/

NHS. We Are the NHS: People Plan 2020/21 – Action for Us All. July 2020. Available at: www.england.nhs.uk/wp-con tent/uploads/2020/07/we-are-the-nhs-action-for-all-of-us-f inal-march-21.pdf

Nierenberg AA, Gray SM, Grandin LD. Mood disorders and suicide. *J Clin Psychiatry*. 2001;**62**:27–30.

Royal College of Psychiatrists. Faculty of Child and Adolescent Psychiatry and Faculty of General Adult Psychiatry. Good Mental Health Services for Young People. Faculty Report CAP/GAP/01. 2017. Available at: www.rcps ych.ac.uk/docs/default-source/members/faculties/child-an d-adolescent-psychiatry/fr-cap-gap-01-good-mh-services-f or-young-peop.pdf?sfvrsn=606ce0ae_2

Scott J. Leboyer M. Conséquences du retard diagnostique dans la dépression bipolaire [Consequences of delayed diagnosis of bipolar disorders]. *L'Encéphale*. 2011;**37**:S173–S175.

Smith KA, Cipriani A. Lithium and suicide in mood disorders: updated meta-review of the scientific literature. *Bipolar Disord*. 2017;**19**:575–86.

Soo SA, Zhang ZW, Khong SJ, et al. Randomized controlled trials of psychoeducation modalities in the management of bipolar disorder: a systematic review. *J Clin Psychiatry*. 2018;**79**:17r11750.

Spitzer RL, Kroenke K, Williams JBW. Validation and utility of a self-report version of PRE-MD: the PHQ primary care study. Primary Care Evaluation of Mental Disorders. Patient Health Questionnaire. *JAMA*. 1999;**282**:1737–44.

Strawbridge R, Tsapekos D, Hodsoll J, et al. Cognitive remediation therapy for patients with bipolar disorder: a randomised proof-of-concept trial. *Bipolar Disord*. 2021;**23**:196–208.

Thornicroft G, Chatterji S, Evans-Lacko S, et al. Undertreatment of people with major depressive disorder in 21 countries. *Br J Psychiatry*. 2017;**210**:119–24.

Wakefield S, Kellett S, Simmonds-Buckley M, et al. Improving Access to Psychological Therapies (IAPT) in the United Kingdom. A systematic review and meta-analysis of 10 years of practice-based evidence. *Br J Clin Psychol*. 2021;**60**:1–37.

Index

Printed in the United States
by Baker & Taylor Publisher Services